Cerebrospinal Fluid in Clinical Neurology

Florian Deisenhammer • Finn Sellebjerg
Charlotte E. Teunissen • Hayrettin Tumani
Editors

Cerebrospinal Fluid
in Clinical Neurology

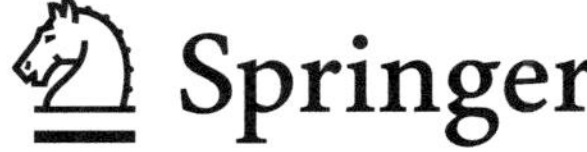

Editors
Florian Deisenhammer
Department of Neurology
Innsbruck Medical University
Innsbruck
Austria

Finn Sellebjerg
Danish Multiple Sclerosis Center
Department of Neurology
Rigshospitalet, University of Copenhagen
Copenhagen
Denmark

Charlotte E. Teunissen
Neurochemistry Laboratory and Biobank
Department of Clinical Chemistry
VU University Medical Center Amsterdam
Amsterdam
The Netherlands

Hayrettin Tumani
Department of Neurology
University of Ulm
Ulm
Germany

ISBN 978-3-319-34368-6   ISBN 978-3-319-01225-4   (eBook)
DOI 10.1007/978-3-319-01225-4
Springer Cham Heidelberg New York Dordrecht London

Foreword

It is a pleasure to see that CSF analysis continues to march ahead. Professor Florian Deisenhammer is to be congratulated for assembling a strong team, with diverse expertise, to give us a coherent picture of the current state of the art. His spectrum of people extends all the way from the bedside to the bench. They each give an in-depth analysis as well as useful tips about how to get the most information from this important liquid-biopsy of brain fluid.

From the bedside, among other experts, we have Prof. Kaj Blennow who has been a pioneer of CSF analysis in dementia whose work has withstood the test of time and continues to be fundamental for further progress on this ever increasing disease, as we all live longer. There is also useful information from several experts on less common diseases involved in molecular mimicry, or auto-immune syndromes, where again it is found that CSF can provide more useful information rather than only blood tests for the same antibodies, by using the ratio of specific antibody titers which can be normalized to the total antibody ratio. In addition to the traditional acute inflammatory diseases, there are also detailed chapters on chronic noninfectious inflammatory CNS diseases as well as chronic inflammatory diseases of the PNS. On a personal note, I am pleased to see my trusted colleague of many years, Geoff Keir, is still carrying on the basic work for CSF leakage syndromes.

From the bench, the very important pre-analytical role of CSF analysis is given a detailed account which should be heeded by all who are responsible for triage of CSF, since they can have a profound effect on the final results, depending on how samples are to be correctly handled. In addition, the crucial role for the technique of lumbar puncture is addressed.

Although much has been written about diagnostic criteria (not least in MS), nevertheless in terms of basic pathophysiology, CSF offers much more direct evidence than a number of other investigations for the role of immunology in the disease processes under differential consideration. One day we may even understand the exact molecular mechanisms.

This book is to be read by both practicing clinicians as well as those who are entrusted with the most careful analysis of such precious fluid with future promise.

London, UK   Emeritus Prof. Edward J. Thompson,
                                                         DSc, MD, PhD, FRCPath, FRCP

Preface

The analysis of cerebrospinal fluid (CSF) is an invaluable diagnostic aid in clinical neurology and can be obtained with relative ease by lumbar puncture. CSF analysis is amenable to various technologies applied in haematology, cytochemistry, clinical chemistry, microbiology and virology. There are not many constituents that are measured during routine diagnostic work-up, nevertheless the combination of these variables gives a wide range of patterns that are often typical for certain neurological diseases. Therefore, it takes a profound knowledge of the particularities of the CSF for analyses and also for reporting. The relative paucity of constituents in the CSF and their low concentration pose a certain methodological challenge; on the other hand it has the advantage of low background activity which makes it better accessible for exploration of new biomarkers. This development has led to discovery of a variety of diagnostic markers expanding the use of CSF in everyday clinical decision making.

In this book we try to give an up-to-date overview as to how the CSF can be applied in clinical neurology. The intention was to create a book of reference for which we invited numerous experts in the field to contribute. The chapters not only focus on technical aspects of CSF analyses but discuss CSF findings in a broader clinical context too.

We do hope you will enjoy reading and find the book helpful not only in your clinical work but also in increasing your knowledge in a wide range of CSF-related topics.

Innsbruck, Austria
Copenhagen, Denmark
Amsterdam, The Netherlands
Ulm, Germany

Florian Deisenhammer
Finn Sellebjerg
Charlotte E. Teunissen
Hayrettin Tumani

Acknowledgment
by Florian Deisenhammer

I want to thank my co-editors who not only contributed by writing chapters but also helped with the overall work by reviewing the single chapters by our authors and providing extremely valuable input. Further, I want to thank my long standing chief lab technician, Ingrid Gstrein, whose invaluable work made the Innsbruck CSF laboratory what it is today.

Contents

Part I

Basic Aspects of the Cerebrospinal Fluid

The History of Cerebrospinal Fluid

Florian Deisenhammer

Contents

Abstract

There is a long history of the CSF and its anatomical spaces dating back to ancient Egypt when it occurred first in human literature between 3000 and 2500 BC. The development of knowledge of this fluid goes hand in hand with the history of neuroanatomy. Many famous names in medical history turn up in context with the history of CSF such as Hippocrates, Galen of Pergamon, Leonardo da Vinci and François Magendie. Most authors feel that the first full account of the CSF was given by Domenico Cotugno in 1764, and for some time the fluid was referred to as "liquor cotugnii". There is also wide consensus that Heinrich

F. Deisenhammer
Department of Neurology,
Innsbruck Medical University, Innsbruck, Austria
e-mail: florian.deisenhammer@uki.at

© Springer International Publishing Switzerland 2015
F. Deisenhammer et al. (eds.), *Cerebrospinal Fluid in Clinical Neurology*,
DOI 10.1007/978-3-319-01225-4_1

Quincke performed the first diagnostic lumbar puncture in 1891 which paved the way for modern CSF diagnostic procedures.

This chapter provides milestones of the history of CSF, the associated neuroanatomy and the diagnostic use.

1.1 Introduction

The history of cerebrospinal fluid (CSF) is not restricted to the fluid itself but must be seen in context with the history of neuroanatomy, neurophysiology and neuropathology. Although a fluid within the skull and vertebral column has been described dating back as early as 2500 BC, the CSF as such has not been discovered before the sixteenth century. Several thoughts on the origin and function have been brought forward, e.g. the CSF replaced or corresponds the ocean as it surrounded all creatures in prehistoric times (Schaltenbrand 1953). For a long time, it was thought that the ventricles contain spirits rather than a fluidic substance, and after the discovery of the fluid, it took roughly two centuries to accept the CSF as a normal constituent in the eighteenth century.

1.2 The Edwin Smith Surgical Papyrus

In 1862 an antique dealer named Edwin Smith bought a papyrus scroll from a local dealer in Luxor, Egypt. This scroll is almost 5 m long and it turned out that it contains one of the most fascinating medical texts from ancient Egypt. It is the oldest known manuscript on traumatic injuries, mostly in the field of neurotrauma. The very scientific approach, omitting magic and spells, makes it outstanding compared to other documents from this age. It dates back to 1500 BC, the time of dynasties 16–17 in ancient Egypt, and it is believed to be a copy of a text written during the period of the old kingdom between 3000 and 2500 BC. Some authors speculated that the author of the original manuscript was Imhotep (Breasted 1930).

The Edwin Smith Papyrus is composed of 48 case reports describing various traumas beginning with the head followed by spinal cord and peripheral nerve injuries. Each case is neatly structured into examination, diagnosis, prognosis and treatment, followed by a gloss, which has been added as an explanation of the original text using terms that were unfamiliar at the time when the Smith Papyrus was written. The document is now displayed at the New York Academy of Medicine (Fig. 1.1).

Case number six is of utmost interest with respect to CSF. The patient had "a gaping wound in the head with compound comminuted fracture of the skull and rupture of the meningeal membrane" (Breasted 1930). In this case the meninges were described, but moreover, the word brain (marrow of the skull) occurs the first time in any kind of literature. Apart from the anatomical details, the fluid surrounding the brain, by which the author most likely refers to the cerebrospinal fluid, is

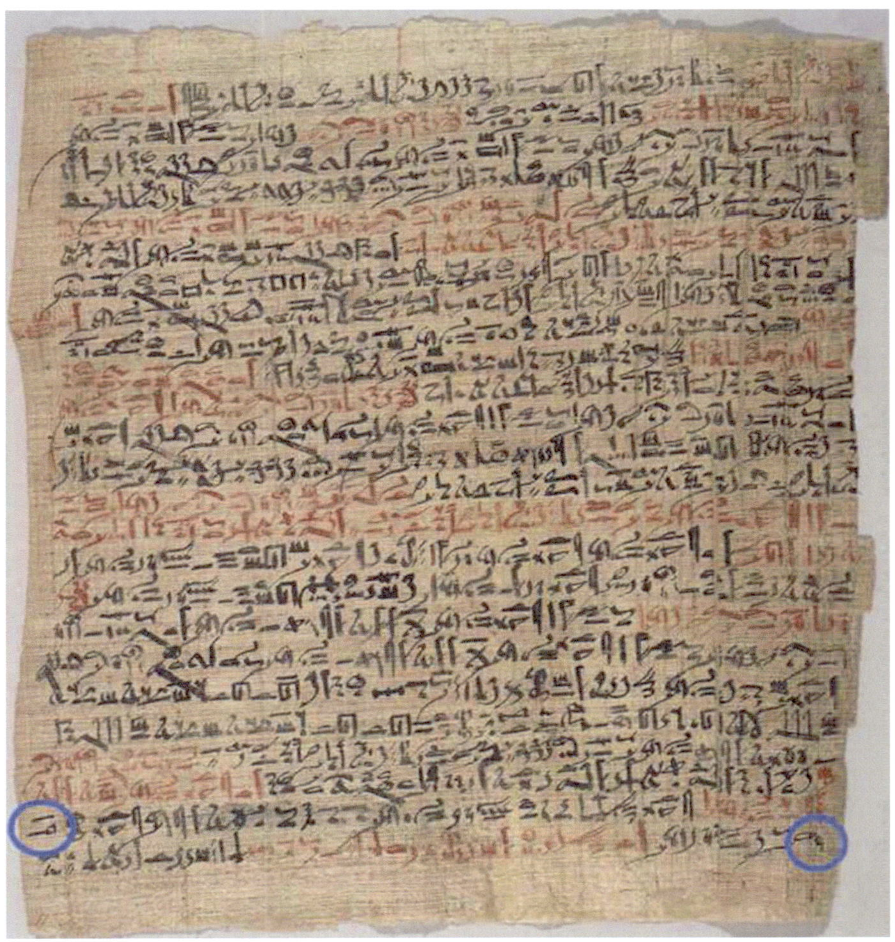

Fig. 1.1 *Bottom* of the second column of the Edwin Smith Papyrus. The hieroglyphs in *blue circles* refer to watery fluid in context with the surface of the brain (Courtesy of The New York Academy of Medicine Library)

also described in this case of brain injury. A number of authors therefore refer to the Smith Papyrus as the first occurrence of the CSF in the medical literature (Clarke and O'Malley 1996; Wilkins 1964) (Fig. 1.2a, b).

1.3 The Greek Physicians and Philosophers

After a long period of lack of documents regarding CSF, it was not before the times of the famous philosophers when further milestones in CSF discovery were achieved by physicians and scientists of ancient Greece (Woollam 1957).

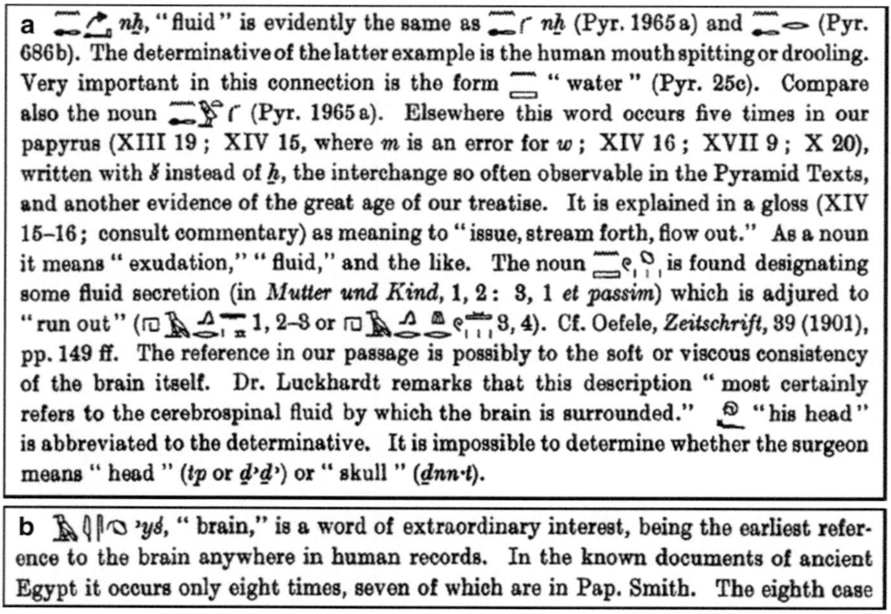

> **a** ___ *nḥ*, "fluid" is evidently the same as ___ *r nḥ* (Pyr. 1965 a) and ___ (Pyr. 686b). The determinative of the latter example is the human mouth spitting or drooling. Very important in this connection is the form ___ "water" (Pyr. 25c). Compare also the noun ___ *r* (Pyr. 1965 a). Elsewhere this word occurs five times in our papyrus (XIII 19 ; XIV 15, where *m* is an error for *w* ; XIV 16 ; XVII 9 ; X 20), written with *š* instead of *ḥ*, the interchange so often observable in the Pyramid Texts, and another evidence of the great age of our treatise. It is explained in a gloss (XIV 15–16 ; consult commentary) as meaning to "issue, stream forth, flow out." As a noun it means "exudation," "fluid," and the like. The noun ___ is found designating some fluid secretion (in *Mutter und Kind*, 1, 2 : 3, 1 *et passim*) which is adjured to "run out" (___ 1, 2–3 or ___ 3, 4). Cf. Oefele, *Zeitschrift*, 39 (1901), pp. 149 ff. The reference in our passage is possibly to the soft or viscous consistency of the brain itself. Dr. Luckhardt remarks that this description "most certainly refers to the cerebrospinal fluid by which the brain is surrounded." ___ "his head" is abbreviated to the determinative. It is impossible to determine whether the surgeon means "head" (*tp* or *ḏ'ḏ'*) or "skull" (*ḏnn·t*).

> **b** ___ *'yš*, "brain," is a word of extraordinary interest, being the earliest reference to the brain anywhere in human records. In the known documents of ancient Egypt it occurs only eight times, seven of which are in Pap. Smith. The eighth case

Fig. 1.2 (**a**) Self-explaining text from page 172 in Breasted's translation of the Edwin Smith Papyrus (Breasted 1930). (**b**) Text from page 166 in Breasted's translation of the Edwin Smith Papyrus (case six), mentioning the word brain for the first time in medical literature (Breasted 1930) (Public domain)

With Hippocrates CSF-related topics reappeared in the literature. The Corpus Hippocraticum dating back to the fifth century BC, a work of many different authors, describes the brain as an organ attracting water from the rest of the body as a pathological process.

In contrast to Hippocrates, Aristotle thought that the heart was the centre of intelligence and the task of the brain was to alleviate the temperature that came from the heart (Clarke and O'Malley 1996). In *Historia Animalium* he wrote of the membranes around the brain as well as the ventricles which can be found in the "great majority of animals" (Thompson 1910).

Herophilus was specifically interested in the anatomy of the nervous system. As a member of the Hippocratic School, he found the brain to be the centre of thoughts and soul, and the latter he placed to the ventricles. He described the fourth ventricle, the most important one to his mind, as well as the meninges, and his name is still associated with the confluence of sinuses, the torcula Herophili. Also, the choroid plexus appears in his scripts for the first time.

Of note however, there is no direct mentioning of the CSF itself in the ancient Greek literature.

1.4 Claudius Galenus (Galen of Pergamon)

Galen (AD 129–216), a physician and philosopher, was an extremely influential figure in that his work was standard knowledge until the sixteenth century when postmedieval medicine developed and got generally accepted.

Galen developed the famous pneuma (spirits) theory. There were three pneumas, the pneuma zoticon (vital spirit), pneuma physicon (natural spirit) and pneuma psychicon (animal spirit).

The pneuma in general enters the body via respiration into the lungs and through the pulmonary veins as well as the portal veins and reaches the blood where it mingles with the pneuma physicon of the body. The exchange between left and right ventricle of the heart transforms it to the pneuma zoticon, and finally it becomes the pneuma psychicon in the rete mirabile – a vascular network of tiny arteries – at the base of the brain. From there on it enters the anterior horns of the cerebral ventricles and spreads to the rest of the ventricular system. The interesting part is that the pneuma moves along the nerves and by that it operates the muscles (Woollam 1957). The rete mirabile tells us that the anatomical studies were done in oxen, because it does not occur in the human cerebral circulation. Dissection of human bodies was an absolute no-go at that time and in fact for a very long period thereafter. This and the compatibility with Christian trinity were reasons why the pneuma theory held up for more than a millennium.

Before the time of a more fact-based approach, the cerebral ventricles were given various functions; mostly the lateral ventricles were assigned to imagination, the third ventricle to cognition and the fourth ventricle to memory (Sudhoff 1914).

Apart from the flow of pneumas, Galen was ascribed to have discovered a "vaporous humor in the ventricles that provided energy to the entire body" (Conly and Ronald 1983), and also Torack referred to Galen discovering the CSF (Torack 1982). Moreover, he thought that the CSF was produced in the choroid plexus of lateral ventricles and from there passed on to the third and fourth ventricles, an idea that was picked up again only much later in history. Apart from a fluidlike substance in the ventricles, he suggested a fluid between the pia and dura mater. The arachnoid was not mentioned in his books.

This status of knowledge held up through the dark medieval times and was only further developed by the next generation of researchers during the renaissance.

1.5 Leonardo Da Vinci, Andreas Vesalius, Costanzo Varolio (Varolius) and Colleagues

Further advance in the discovery of ventricular and CSF functions started in the renaissance when dissection – particularly human dissection – was reintroduced in medical science. This allowed a more fact-based approach to medical research and started a new epoch in science in general. One milestone was a wax cast of the ventricular system by da Vinci which came, however, probably from an ox's brain as there were signs of the rete mirabile. Da Vinci used these casts for anatomical drawings of the human brain. His findings came to public knowledge only in the nineteenth century (Clark 1935). The first sketches of the ventricles showed a very vague picture of their topographical order which improved clearly after the wax casts were constructed (Fig. 1.3).

Andreas Vesalius became professor of surgery and anatomy in Padova and later taught at Bologna where he performed public dissections at the specifically designed anatomy theatre. He was strongly opposed to Galen's work and put much effort in rewriting human anatomy which ended in his most famous book *De humani corporis fabrica libri septem* (Vesalius 1543). Vesalius initiated a paradigm shift from philosophical approaches to anatomy towards fact-based description of the human body. In order to achieve this goal, he relied on dissection and apparently had access to skilled draughtspersons which led to an unprecedented accurate illustration not only of the ventricles but also of the whole central nervous system. He failed, however, to describe the inter-ventricular foramina explicitly but at least gave credit to a "watery humour" which often was found to fill the ventricles. In his illustration the arachnoid granulations as well as the choroid plexus were depicted in great detail (Singer 1952). Varolius, like Vesalius teaching at the University of Padova, further developed the idea of fluid filling the ventricles rather than spirits, and since then, the pneuma theory was finally left for good (Varolius 1573).

An anatomical fact that was not well covered by the above-mentioned anatomists is the existence of the arachnoid as an important border of the CSF space. The name of the membrane was created by Gerardus Blasius one century later (Blaes 1666). Raymond Vieussens and Frederik Ruysch completed the knowledge by describing its entirety shortly thereafter (Ruysch 1737; Vieussens 1685). Around that time, Antonio Pacchioni precisely described the arachnoid granulations, and he still stands for these structures eponymously (Pacchionus 1705).

1.6 The Next Generation of Neuroanatomists: Monro, Sylvius, Von Luschka and Magendie

It was now time to discover the relationship between the ventricles and the CSF itself. Interestingly, it was Galen who found a physical communication between the lateral and third ventricle which got forgotten for a long time. The first to describe the inter-ventricular foramen in a distinct and accurate way was Alexander Monro secundus, and he also made it clear that there were no other routes of communication between both laterals as well as between the lateral and third ventricles (Monro 1783). Since then these structures are eponymously known as foramina Monro. Monro was a Scottish anatomist at the University of Edinburgh where he succeeded his father Alexander Monro primus. There were of course others who hinted to or gave partial descriptions before mainly referring to the openings, sometimes as anus or vulva (Casserio 1627; Marchetti 1665). A similar precise account of the foramina was provided by Vicq d'Azyr previous to Monro but not published before 1805.

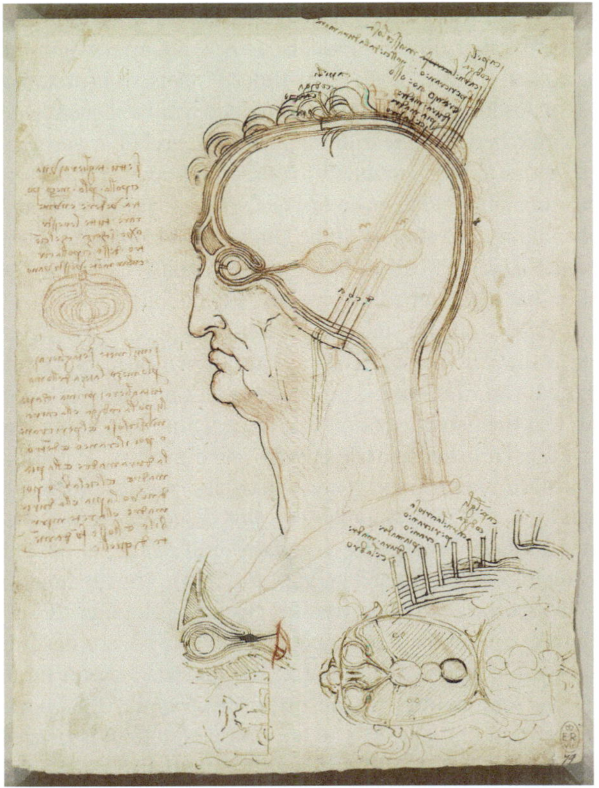

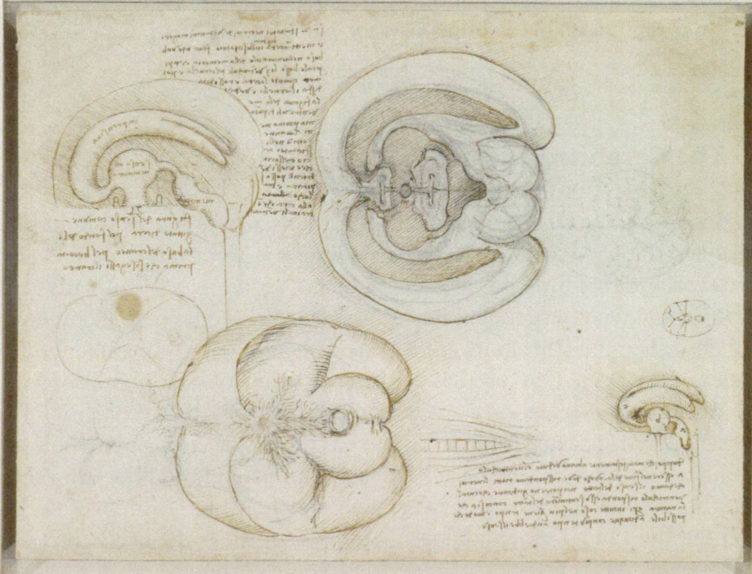

Fig. 1.3 View of the ventricles by Leonardo da Vinci before (*upper panel*) and after (*lower panel*) performing wax casts illustrating how facts influence knowledge. This fact-based approach was reintroduced during the Renaissance (Royal Collection Trust/© Her Majesty Queen Elizabeth II 2014)

The connection between the third and fourth ventricle, the aqueduct, has been described in full detail for the first time by Franciscus Sylvius after whom also the lateral cerebral sulcus is named (Baker 1909). Sometimes Franciscus is mixed up with Jacobus Sylvius, teacher of Andreas Vesalius, who provided a rather accurate description but misplaced it as a tube between the midbrain and the cerebellar vermis. Galen already placed a channel close to the aqueduct; it is thought however that this corresponded a portion of the subarachnoidal space of the midbrain. Julius Caesar Aranzi (Arantius), professor of anatomy and surgery at the University of Bologna, came closest to the description of the aqueduct before Sylvius. He actually named it aqueduct but still stuck to the belief that it contained the pneuma psychicon.

Finally, the efflux of CSF from the inner to the outer space – the lateral and median apertures – had to be discovered. There is no known description of these orifices in ancient and medieval literature. Maybe there was no momentum to look into this further as there was the general notion that the pneuma was not to leave the fourth ventricle. It is well established that Magendie gave the first account of the median aperture presenting a wax model of the ventricles including the foramen Magendie. As a profound novelty in brain anatomy, this discovery was a matter of debate for quite a while, not least because he was a difficult character described as vain, stubborn and rash by his contemporaries (Enersen 2014). The median foramen got finally accepted by the work of Key and Retzius (Key and Retzius 1876).

The history of the lateral apertures is less spectacular. They were described by von Luschka (foramina Luschka) (von Luschka 1855) and also by an interesting person named Swedenborg (see below) whose manuscript went unpublished and contained a detailed description of the CSF. The notion that the CSF is produced by the choroid plexus was introduced by Willis and finally established by von Luschka (Willis 1664), whereas its absorption by the arachnoid granulations was acknowledged by the landmark publication of Key and Retzius (Key and Retzius 1876) (Fig. 1.4).

1.7 The Cerebrospinal Fluid

It took a long time to full acceptance of the CSF as a physiological fluid filling the ventricles and the subarachnoidal space. Although it went rather unnoticed by the scientific world at that time because the publication was not specifically dedicated to CSF, it is now widely accepted that Domenico Felice Antonio Cotugno discovered and described the CSF in its entirety as a physiological constituent of the nervous system. In fact the CSF used to be referred to as liquor cotugnii for some time (Di and Yasargil 2008). He gave a quite precise account of the location of CSF in the subarachnoidal space of the brain as well as the spinal cord and in the ventricles, the circulation through the inter-ventricular foramina and the flow from the fourth ventricle through the foramina of Magendie and Luschka. Moreover, he made it clear that the fluid in all these compartments was of the same origin and of water-like appearance. Also, an approximate total volume was stated (Cotugno 1764). Interestingly, Cotugno believed that Albrecht von Haller had to be given credit for

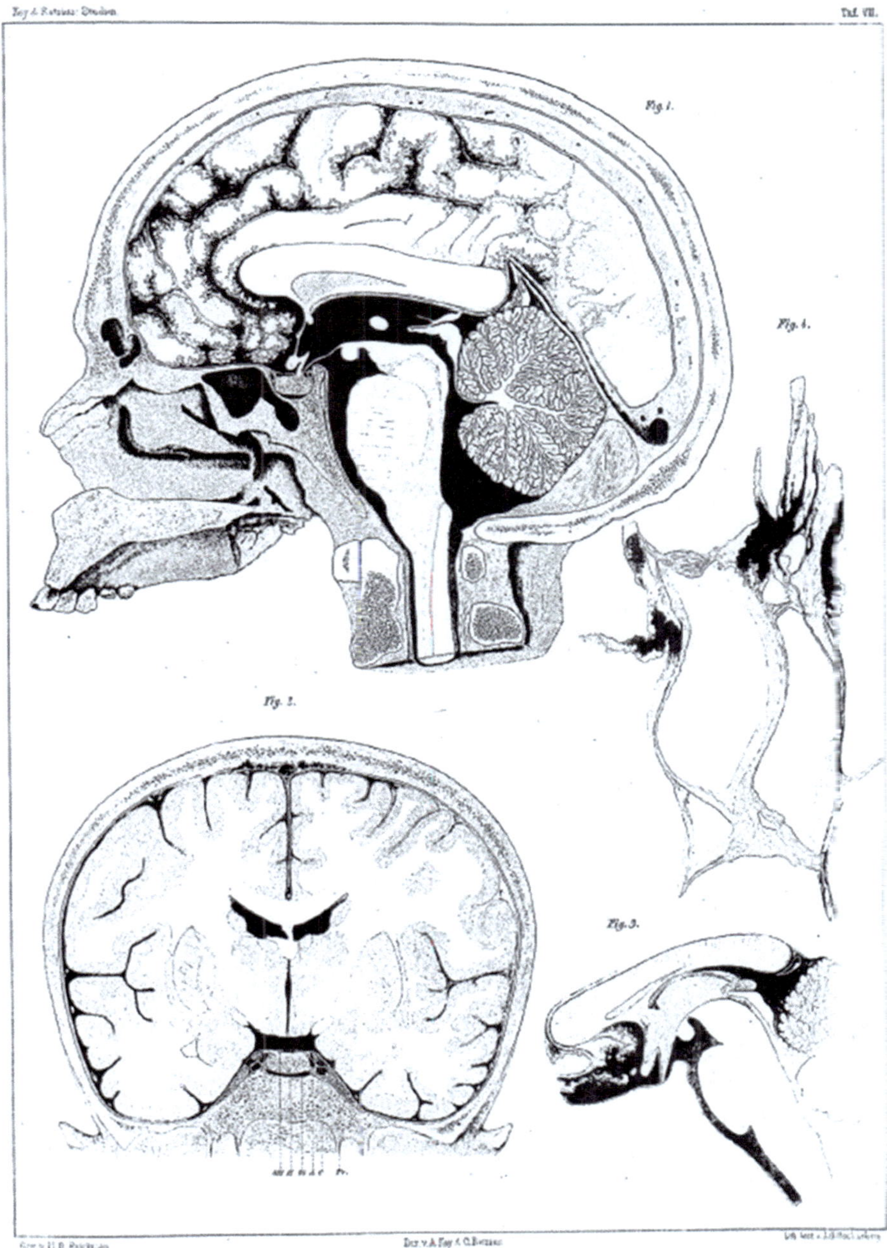

Fig. 1.4 Various sections of the brain demonstrating the subarachnoidal and ventricular spaces based on post-mortem injections with Berlin blue staining. Table VII, page 248 in Key and Retzius (1876) (With permission from the Bayerische Staatsbibliothek München, document signature urn:nbn:de:bvb: 12-bsb00002349-4)

discovery of CSF. Indeed von Haller was mostly right in his CSF work, he felt, however, that this "viscid" fluid evaporates after death and becomes gelatinous (von Haller 1762).

There were a few others who came close to be recognised as the discoverers of CSF but not quite. The first to be mentioned is Emanuel Swedenborg from Sweden, who was not a physician but was interested in science in general as well as in theology. One could say he was a multi-talent and so he performed also studies of anatomy and physiology. Many of his manuscripts were not immediately published, among them a paper which was published only in 1887 including a detailed description of the CSF very similar to Cotugno's discoveries (Gordh et al. 2007). However, the manuscripts must have been available before that time because in textbook (von Haller's 1803), there is a reference to Swedenborg's work (Herbowski 2013).

Much earlier in 1536, Niccolò Massa, Venetian physician and anatomist, discovered several anatomical novelties among which he described the existence of fluid in the ventricles of the human brain using post-mortem autopsies (Massa 1536). Mario Valsalva is generally given credit for discovering the spinal fluid which he obtained during a dissection of a dog's spinal cord (Woollam 1957).

The final breakthrough came with Francois Magendie who eventually established the place of CSF in neuroanatomy and physiology mainly by republishing Cotugno's previous work. He also stressed that the CSF is a normal rather than a pathological constituent of the human body, and most importantly he gave the name "liquide cerebrospinal" (Magendie 1842) which has been used since then.

1.7.1   Getting Access to the CSF for Diagnostic Testing

After getting familiar with the CSF as a physiological body fluid, it was about time to use it for diagnostic purposes. Again several physicians and scientists were involved, and although in close temporal relationship with others who performed punctures of the subarachnoidal space, it was Heinrich Irenaeus Quincke (Quincke 1891a, b) to whom the first diagnostic lumbar puncture has been ascribed by most authors (Hajdu 2003; Woollam 1957), although it must be said that the diagnostic part was secondary (Fig. 1.5).

Quincke's report at the conference in Wiesbaden included lumbar puncture (LP) in children with increased CSF pressure, one of whom had tubercular meningitis. The procedures dated back to 1888 and 1890 (Pearce 1994). The primary goal in Quincke's report in the Berliner Klinische Wochenschrift was to relieve intracranial pressure in five patients with cerebral tumours, subarachnoidal haemorrhage and hydrocephalus due to chronic meningitis. The outcome was recovery in two and death in three patients. The diagnostic part included measurement of opening and closing pressure as well as determination of protein concentrations.

Almost at the same time, Walter Essex Wynter described LP in order to decrease intracranial pressure in four children with tubercular meningitis with fatal outcome (Wynter 1891). In contrast to Quincke who used a fine cannula, he performed the LP with a Southey tube following incision in the lumbar region demonstrating the dura

Die Berliner Klinische Wochenschrift erscheint jeden Montag in der Stärke von 2 bis 3 Bogen gr. 4. — Preis vierteljährlich 6 Mark. Bestellungen nehmen alle Buchhandlungen und Postanstalten an.

BERLINER
KLINISCHE WOCHENSCHRIFT.

Organ für practische Aerzte.

Mit Berücksichtigung der preussischen Medicinalverwaltung und Medicinalgesetzgebung
nach amtlichen Mittheilungen.

Einsendungen wolle man portofrei an die Redaction (W. Steglitzerstrasse No. 68) oder an die Verlagsbuchhandlung von August Hirschwald in Berlin N.W. Unter den Linden No. 68 adressiren.

Redaction:
Prof. Dr. C. A. Ewald und Priv.-Docent Dr. C. Posner.

Expedition:
August Hirschwald, Verlagsbuchhandlung in Berlin.

Montag, den 21. September 1891.   № 38.   Achtundzwanzigster Jahrgang.

I. Die Lumbalpunction des Hydrocephalus.

Von
H. Quincke in Kiel.

Auf dem letzten Congress für innere Medicin[1]) beschrieb ich ein Verfahren zur Herabsetzung abnormen Druckes in den Hirnventrikeln durch Punction des Subarachnoidalraumes in der Lendengegend. Nachstehend berichte ich über weitere damit gemachte Erfahrungen.

Neigung nach unten annehmen und dadurch den Zwischenbogenraum mehr oder weniger decken. Die gewöhnlich querovale Gestalt kann — in der Projection auf die Hinterfläche des Körpers — dadurch erheblich verändert werden. Zuweilen springt die Crista an der Wurzel des Dornfortsatzes von unten her in die Lichtung des Interarcualraumes vor. So bestehen bedeutende individuelle Variationen, ohne dass sich constante Beziehungen zu Alter, Geschlecht oder Stärke der Knochen überhaupt finden

No.	Name	Alter	Krankheit	Ausgang der Krankheit	Dauer der Krankheit z. Zeit der Punction	Punction					Druck				Flüssigkeit		
						Zahl	Narkose?	Ort		Tiefe cm	in mm Wasser		in mm Hg		Menge ccm	Specifisch. Gewicht	Eiweissgehalt
											i. Aufg.	a. Ende	i. Aufg.	a. Ende			
6	Claus R.	25 J.	Tumor cerebri Hydrocephalus	†	16 Mon.	1. (5. April)	+	III.	I.-A.-R.	6	500	—	37	—	100	1018	6,2 p. M.
						2. (6. Mai)	+	III.	„	6,5 (4,7)	680	—	50	—	63	1011	7,4 p. M.
						3. (9. Mai) in morte	—	III.	„	—	—	—	—	—	35	1010	etwa gleich
7	Heinr. R.	39 J.	Hydroceph. chron. Mening. serosa	†	8 Tage	29. Juli	0	III.	„	5	150	35-50	11	2,5-3,5	20	1008	Spur
8	Peter P.	33 J.	Tumor cerebri (vorn links?)	genesen	5 Mon.	1. Juli	0	III.	„	—	180-210	—	13-15	—	32 in 20 Minut.	—	Spur
9	Auguste G.	20 J.	Hydroceph. chronicus? Meningitis serosa	genesen	5 Wochen	5. Juni	0	III.	„	?	150 160	90	11	8,5	32 in 15 Minut.	—	Spur
10	Johanne H.	22 J.	Haemorrhagia cerebri et ventriculorum cerebri	†	5 Tage	14. August	0	IV.	„	5,2	320	40	23,5	8	26	1011	7,8 p. M

Fig. 1.5 (**a**) Heading of Quincke's publication on LP in hydrocephalus (From Quincke (1891a), with kind permission of Springer Science + Business Media). (**b**) Results in Quincke's report on LP in five cases including clinical outcomes, location of LP, opening and closing pressure as well as volume, specific weight and protein contents of CSF (From Quincke (1891a), with kind permission of Springer Science + Business Media)

which probably served the purpose of constant CSF drainage better. Some chemical analyses of the obtained CSF were done such as albumen, glucose and chloride measurements as well as Fehling's reaction. The results of these measurements were rather qualitative than quantitative and therefore somewhat inconclusive in both Quincke's and Wynter's cases.

In the context of first LPs, it is worthwhile mentioning that spinal anaesthesia was introduced before. James Leonard Corning in 1885 described two experiments one in a dog and one in a man; in the latter he applied cocaine – possibly unintentionally – to the lumbar subarachnoidal space because the person complained of typical post-LP headache the next day (Corning 1885). Originally, he planned to apply the substance subcutaneously.

1.7.2 The Advance of Diagnostic Methods

Perhaps one should refer to Ludwig Lichtheim who first performed quantitative CSF analyses by determining protein and glucose in patients with tubercular meningitis (Lichtheim 1893) and found them elevated compared to a reference group of tumour patients. Quite remarkably, he clearly stated that the LP can be done easily and is a safe procedure and anaesthesia is not needed.

In his thesis William Mestrezat in 1911 gave a comprehensive account of normal values in the CSF for protein and glucose concentrations as well as pressure and cell constitutions (Mestrezat 1911). This is really the cradle of CSF diagnostics as these variables still constitute the basic CSF analysis, and by combining them, one gets relatively specific patterns for various infectious and haemorrhagic diseases (Deisenhammer et al. 2009). Subsequently, several authors published normal values of a great variety of CSF components. An extensive summary of these efforts can be found in Houston Merritt's and Frank Fremont-Smith's book *The Cerebrospinal Fluid* published in 1937 (Meritt and Fremont-Smith 1937).

The laboratory methods developed and with that came progress in CSF analyses. Microbiological staining and bacterial cultivation were used to provide direct evidence of bacterial meningitis, and differentiation of bacteria was made possible by the method developed by Hans Christian Gram in 1884 which is still in use today. Another staining method by Ziehl-Neelsen, also used nowadays, has enriched microbiological diagnostics for tubercle bacillus (Bulloch 1938). Wasserman developed the eponymic serologic reaction as a test for syphilis (von Wassermann and Plaut 1906), which, however, has been replaced by newer methods today.

The colloidal gold test, a precipitation method which specifically detects globulins excluding albumin, was introduced by Carl Friedrich Lange (Lange 1912). Further progress in CSF analytical progress was provided by Elvin Kabat who introduced electrophoresis in clinical neurology. Kabat and colleagues were able to demonstrate an increase of intrathecal immunoglobulin independent of serum concentrations, particularly in multiple sclerosis and neurosyphilis (Kabat et al. 1942). The refinement of electrophoretic methods towards higher resolution of immunoglobulins came about in 1959 by Ewald Frick who published an immunoelectrophoretic method which was further developed by Hans Link and finally turned into isoelectric focusing demonstrating CSF-restricted oligoclonal bands by Delmotte (Delmotte 1972; Frick 1959; Link 1967). This method is still widely used in diagnostic workup of CSF with some methodological adjustments until today. Although oligoclonal bands are not specific for multiple sclerosis (McLean et al. 1990), their diagnostic sensitivity and specificity for this disease is very high (beyond 90 % for each), which makes it difficult to understand why this test has been deleted from the diagnostic criteria in the latest version (Polman et al. 2011).

In recent decades the CSF has been investigated in a great number of diseases. A PubMed search for CSF and biomarkers shows roughly 50 hits at the end of the 1980s, around 100 hits at the end of the 1990s and more than 500 hits in the last couple of years.

References

Baker F (1909) The two Sylviuses. A historical study. Bull Johns Hopkins Hosp 20:329–339

Blaes G (1666) Anatomiae medullae spinalis et nervorum inde provenientium. Cammelinum, Amsterdam

Breasted JH (1930) The Edwin Smith surgical papyrus. Kessinger Legacy Reprints, Chicago

Bulloch W (1938) The history of bacteriology. Oxford University Press, London

Casserio G (1627) Tabulae Anatomicae LXXIIX. Bucretius, Venice

Clark K (1935) A catalogue of the drawings of Leonardo da Vinci in the collection of His Majesty the King at Windsor Castle

Clarke E, O'Malley CD (1996) The human brain and spinal cord. A historical study illustrated by writings from antiquity to the twentieth century. Norman Publishing, San Francisco

Conly JM, Ronald AR (1983) Cerebrospinal fluid as a diagnostic body fluid. Am J Med 75:102–108

Corning JL (1885) Spinal anaesthesia and local medication of the cord. N Y Med J 42:483–485

Cotugno D (1764) De Ischiade Nervosa Commentarius. Fratrem Simonios, Neapolis

Deisenhammer F, Egg R, Giovannon G, Hemmer B, Petzold A, Sellebjerg F, Teunissen C, Tumani H (2009) EFNS guidelines on disease specific CSF investigations. Eur J Neuro 16:760–770

Delmotte P (1972) Comparative results of agar electrophoresis and electrofocalization examination of gamma globulins of the cerebrospinal fluid. Acta Neurol Belg 72:226–234

Di IA, Yasargil MG (2008) Liquor cotunnii: the history of cerebrospinal fluid in Domenico Cotugno's work. Neurosurgery 63:352–358

Enersen OD (2014) Francois Magendie. www.whonamedit.com/doctor.cfm/2104.html.

Frick E (1959) Immunophoretic studies on cerebrospinal fluid. Klin Wochenschr 37:645–651

Gordh TE, Mair WG, Sourander P (2007) Swedenborg, Linnaeus and brain research–and the roles of Gustaf Retzius and Alfred Stroh in the rediscovery of Swedenborg's manuscripts. Ups J Med Sci 112:143–164

Hajdu SI (2003) A note from history: discovery of the cerebrospinal fluid. Ann Clin Lab Sci 33:334–336

Herbowski L (2013) The maze of the cerebrospinal fluid discovery. Anat Res Int 2013:1–8

Kabat EA, Moore DH, Landow H (1942) An electrophoretic study of the protein components in cerebrospinal fluid and their relationship to the serum proteins. J Clin Invest 21:571–577

Key A, Retzius G (1876) Studien in der Anatomie des Nervensystems und des Bindgewebes P.A. Norstedt & Söner, Stockholm

Lange C (1912) Die Ausflockung kolloidalen Goldes durch Zerebrospinalflüssigheit bei luetischer Affektionen des Zentralnervensystems. Z Chemother 1:44–78

Lichtheim L (1893) Re: the proposal of Quincke to withdraw cerebrospinal fluid by lumbar puncture in cases of brain disease. Dtsch Med Wochenschr 19:1234

Link H (1967) Immunoglobulin G and low molecular weight proteins in human cerebrospinal fluid. Chemical and immunological characterisation with special reference to multiple sclerosis. Acta Neurol Scand 43(Suppl 28):1–136

Magendie F (1842) Recherches physiologiques et cliniques sur le liquide céphalo-rachidien ou cérébro-spinal. Méquignon-Marvis fils, Paris

Marchetti P (1665) Observationum medico-chirurgicarum Sylloge. Wappler, Astelodamum

Massa N (1536) Nicolai Massa… Liber introductorius anatomiae siue dissectionis corporis humani. in [a]edibus Fra[n]cisci Bindoni, ac Maphei Pasini, socios, Venice

McLean BN, Luxton RW, Thompson EJ (1990) A study of immunoglobulin G in the cerebrospinal fluid of 1007 patients with suspected neurological disease using isoelectric focusing and the log IgG-Index. Brain 113:1269–1289

Meritt HH, Fremont-Smith F (1937) The cerebrospinal fluid. W. B. Saunders Company, Philadelphia

Mestrezat W (1911) Le liquide céphalo-rachidien normal et pathologique. Valeur clinique de l'examen chimique. Université de Montpellier, Montpellier

Monro A (1783) Observations on the structure and functions of the nervous system. Creech, Edinburgh

Pacchionus A (1705) De Glandulis Conglobatis Durae Meningis Humanae indeque Ortis Lymphaticis ad Piam Meningem productis. Cesarius Leopodinus University, Rome

Pearce JM (1994) Walter Essex Wynter, Quincke, and lumbar puncture. J Neurol Neurosurg Psychiatry 57:179

Polman CH, Reingold SC, Banwell B, Clanet M, Cohen JA, Filippi M, Fujihara K, Havrdova E, Hutchinson M, Kappos L, Lublin FD, Montalban X, O'Connor P, Sandberg-Wollheim M, Thompson AJ, Waubant E, Weinshenker B, Wolinsky JS (2011) Diagnostic criteria for multiple sclerosis: 2010 revisions to the McDonald criteria. Ann Neurol 69:292–302

Quincke HI (1891a) Die Lumbalpunction des Hydrocephalus. Berl Klin Wochenschr 28:929–933

Quincke HI (1891b) Über Hydrocephalus. Verh Congress Innere Med X:321–329

Ruysch F (1737) Opera omnia anatomico-medico-chirurgica. Apud Janssonio-Waesbergios, Amsterdam

Schaltenbrand G (1953) Normal and pathological physiology of the cerebrospinal fluid circulation. Lancet 1:805–808

Singer C (1952) Vesalius on the human brain. Oxford University Press, London

Sudhoff W (1914) Die Lehre von den Hirnventrikeln in textlicher und graphischer Tradition des Altertums und Mittelalters, 7:149–205. Arch Gesch Med 149

Thompson DW (1910) The works of Aristotle. In: Smith JA, Ross WD (eds) Historia Animalium. Clarendon Press, Oxford

Torack RM (1982) Historical aspects of normal and abnormal brain fluids. I. Cerebrospinal fluid. Arch Neurol 39:197–201

Varolius C (1573) De Nervis Opticis nonnulisque aliis praeter communem opinionem in Humano capite observatis. Meietti Fratres, Padova

Vesalius A (1543) De humani corporis fabrica libri septem. Basle Colophon, Basle

Vieussens R (1685) Neurographia universalis. Joannem Certe, Lyon

von Haller A (1762) Elementa Physiologiae corporis humani. Francisci Grasset, Lausanne

von Haller A (1803) First lines of physiology: translated from the third Latin edition. Obadiah Penniman & Co, Albany

von Luschka H (1855) Die Adergeflechte des menschlichen Gehirns. Georg Reimer, Berlin

von Wassermann A, Plaut F (1906) Über das Vorhandensein Syphilitischer Antistoffe in der cerebrospinalen Flüssigkeit von Paralytikern. Dtsch Med Wochenschr 32:1769–1772

Wilkins RH (1964) Neurosurgical classic XVII. J Neurosurg 21:240–244

Willis T (1664) Cerebri anatome: cui accessit nervorum descriptio et usus. Flesher, London

Woollam DH (1957) The historical significance of the cerebrospinal fluid. Med Hist 1:91–114

Wynter WE (1891) Four cases of tubercular meningitis in which paracentesis of the theca vertebralis was performed for the relief of fluid pressure. Lancet 1:981–982

Anatomy of CSF-Related Spaces and Barriers Between Blood, CSF, and Brain

2

Hayrettin Tumani

Contents

Abstract

Cerebrospinal fluid (CSF) circulates in cerebral ventricles and subarachnoid spaces which represent a compartment within the central nervous system (CNS) consisting of the components brain parenchyma, vascular system, and CSF space. The CSF space is separated from the vascular system by the blood-CSF barrier, whereas the blood-brain barrier responsible for maintaining the homeostasis of the brain is located between brain parenchyma and vascular system. Both barriers differ with regard to their morphological and functional properties, and they are permeable not only for small molecules but also for macromolecules and circulating cells. Aquaporin-4 is particularly prevalent in astrocytic membranes at the blood-brain and brain-CSF interfaces.

Alterations of lumbar CSF are influenced by processes of the CNS located adjacent to the ventricular and spinal CSF space but not by pathologies in cortical areas remote from the ventricles.

H. Tumani
Department of Neurology,
University of Ulm, Ulm, Germany
e-mail: hayrettin.tumani@uni-ulm.de

© Springer International Publishing Switzerland 2015
F. Deisenhammer et al. (eds.), *Cerebrospinal Fluid in Clinical Neurology*,
DOI 10.1007/978-3-319-01225-4_2

2.1 Anatomy of CSF Spaces

The anatomy of CSF spaces comprises all intracerebral ventricles, spinal and brain subarachnoid spaces, such as cisterns and sulci, and the central canal of the spinal cord (Fig. 2.1). The total volume of CSF space is between 90 and 150 mL in adults, and the spinal CSF space (subarachnoid space) makes up about 30 mL (Davson et al. 1970).

The CSF space is regarded as one of the four compartments within the central nervous system (CNS) consisting of the vascular system, the brain parenchyma with extracellular space (ECS) and intracellular space (ICS), and the CSF compartment (Felgenhauer 1995) (Fig. 2.2).

These compartments of the CNS are separated by a barrier system (blood-brain barrier (BBB) and blood-CSF barrier (BCB)) which is important for maintenance of the cerebral environment and protection of the brain from the systemic circulation. The barriers are not completely impermeable, as assumed in earlier times based on the trypan blue experiments by Ehrlich and Goldmann, but permeable even for macromolecules and circulating cells (Davson 1976; Felgenhauer 1995). Both barrier systems allow an exchange between compartments next to each other, while the blood-brain barrier and the blood-cerebrospinal barrier differ both morphologically and with regard to their transfer properties (Abbott et al. 2010). A barrier between the parenchyma of the brain and the CSF compartment has not yet been defined. It is also unclear whether the protein content of the extracellular space differs from that in the CSF compartment (Davson et al. 1970).

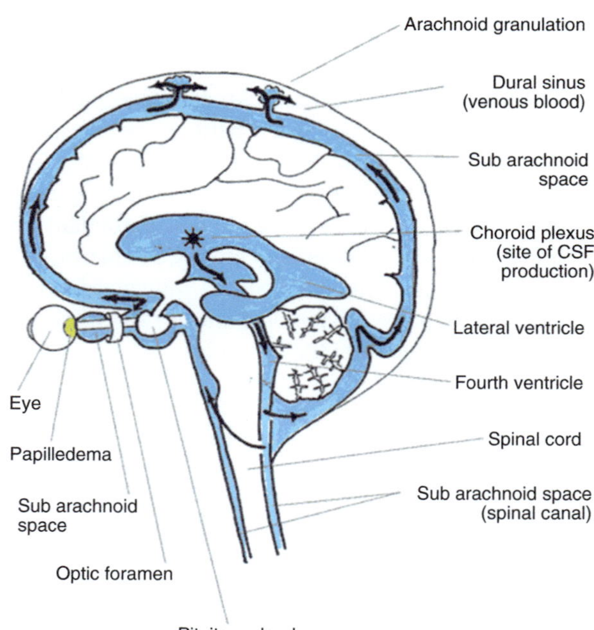

Fig. 2.1 CSF spaces and site of CSF production, circulation, and elimination (http://ihrfoundation.org/images/uploads/schematic_lg.gif)

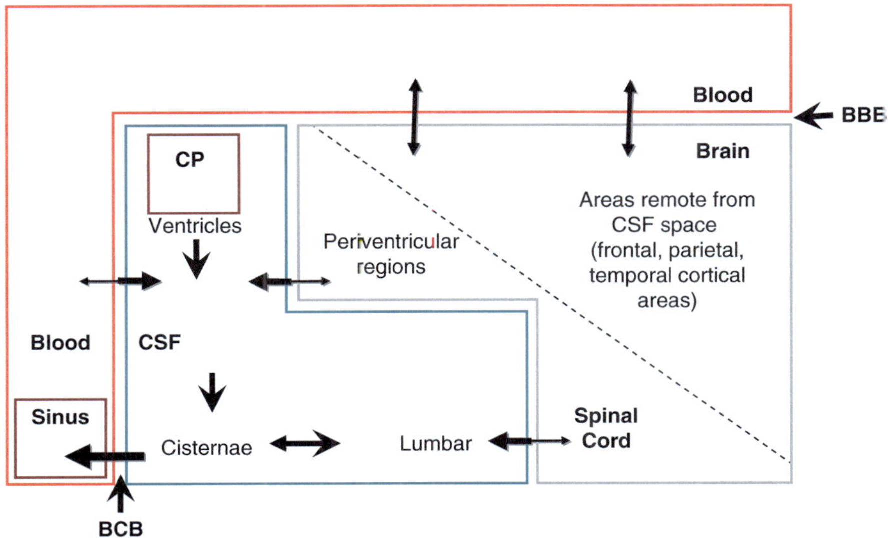

Fig. 2.2 The central nervous system (*CNS*) consists of compartments separated by blood-brain (━━━) and blood-CSF (━━━) barriers (*BBB, BCB*). Cerebrospinal fluid (*CSF*) is formed mostly at the choroid plexus and other sites along the BCB (80 %). Epithelia of the CSF space and the extracellular space of the CNS contribute a smaller fraction (20 %). *Arrows* indicate bulk flow within the CSF space and bilateral transfer processes across the barriers. *CP* choroid plexus

2.2 The Blood-Brain Barrier (BBB)

The concept of an anatomical barrier separating blood and CNS first emerged from the studies of Goldmann (1913) who injected trypan blue into the venous system and observed that staining occurred throughout the body, whereas only the brain and CSF remained unstained. When he injected the dye into the CSF, the CNS tissue including the leptomeninges was strongly stained (Goldmann 1913). The role of this barrier system is to protect the brain from the outside environment and to maintain homeostasis of the brain (Dunn and Wyburn 1972; Abbott et al. 2010).

The special components of the BBB include capillary walls of endothelial cells, the basal membrane, and the perivascular layer of astrocytic end-feet. The BBB structures comprise a large surface area of 12–18 m^2 in adult humans for exchange of humoral and cellular factors across this barrier (Abbott et al. 2010).

The capillary wall consists of a monolayer of non-fenestrated endothelial cells which form the functionally most important part of the BBB (Fig. 2.3) (Süssmuth et al. 2008). Where the endothelial cells overlap, their cell membranes are connected to each other by tight junction protein complexes known as zonulae occludentes. The tight junctions of the BBB consist of different integral membrane proteins including occludins, claudins, junctional adhesion molecules, and associated cytoplasmatic proteins (Koziara et al. 2006). The presence of tight junctions

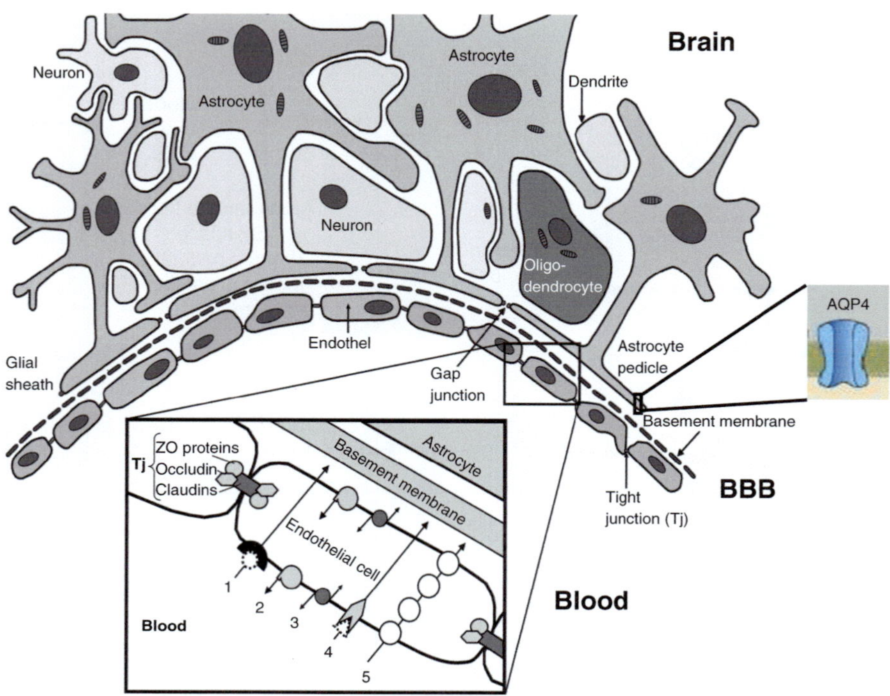

Fig. 2.3 Morphologic structure of the blood-brain barrier (*BBB*) and bidirectional transfer mechanisms (Modified according to Süssmuth et al. (2008)). *1* carrier-mediated transport, *2* efflux transport, *3* ion transport, *4* receptor-mediated transport, *5* transcytosis. *T* tight junction, *ZO* zonula occludens, *AQP4* aquaporin-4

and the lack of fenestrae severely restrict paracellular transport. Accordingly, any transport of molecules to the brain must occur via the transcellular route by passive diffusion or active transport, which may be adsorption mediated, carrier mediated, or receptor mediated (Koziara et al. 2006).

The endothelium basement membrane with a width of about 300–500 Å offers no barrier to the passage of hydrophilic molecules such as ferritin (Brightman 1965). The vascular system and the neuronal system are not in direct contact but are covered by a sheath made up from processes of neuroglial cells including astrocytes and oligodendrocytes. The astrocytes dominate the transport route from capillaries to the neuron as seen in electron microscopy (Dunn and Wyburn 1972). Their processes variously called pedicles, end plates, or foot plates form a sheath covering the neurons, dendrites, axons, and capillaries. Another part of the satellite cells closely located to the neurons is the oligodendrocytes. Besides forming the myelin sheaths in the CNS, oligodendrocytes also take part in the formation of the glial sheath covering neuronal and vascular cells. A further element of the BBB is the extracellular space with a width of about 200 Å that is labyrinthically ramifying between neurons, glial cells, and capillaries. It allows the unrestricted passage of ions and substances of colloidal size (Davson et al. 1970; Davson 1976).

Recent findings describe highly abundant AQP4 channels localized to perivascular and subpial end-foot membranes of astrocytes throughout the brain involved in regulation of extracellular space volume (Nagelhus and Ottersen 2013).

2.3   The Blood-CSF Barrier (BCB)

The BCB is formed by epithelial cells of the choroid plexus located in the four ventricles of the brain and the subarachnoid epithelial structures facing the CSF space in intracranial and spinal areas.

While the BBB is sealed by "tight junctions" and does not show any permanent fenestration, the BCB has several fenestrations ("gap junctions") and pinocytosis vesicles, which form a macrofilter for proteins (Goldstein and Betz 1986; Westergaard 1977) (Fig. 2.4).

The extent of passive transfer across the BCB depends on the hydrodynamic size of the proteins (Felgenhauer 1974; Felgenhauer et al. 1976; see also Chap. 4, Fig. 4.1. physiology of CSF). In addition, the respective blood concentration of a given protein and the permeability of the BCB influence the concentration of molecules in the CSF.

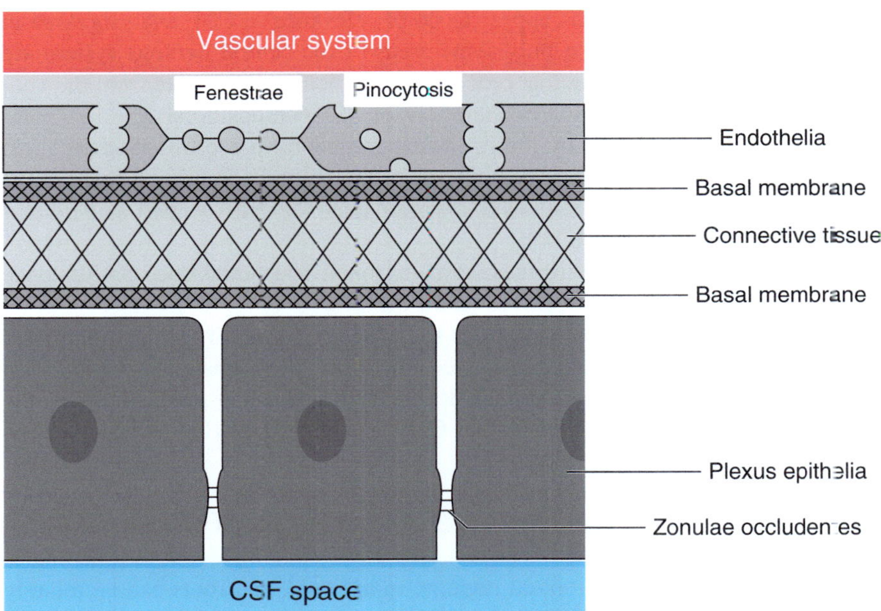

Fig. 2.4 Morphologic structure of the blood-CSF barrier (Modified according to Felgenhauer and Beuche (1999))

The CSF proteins are not only exposed to the structural properties of the barriers which have to be crossed on their way to the subarachnoid space (vessels, plexus choroideus, ventricle, cisterna, lumbar subarachnoid space) but also to physiological and biophysical processes along the craniocaudal neuraxis. Because the sum of multiple processes influences the empirical concentration of CSF proteins, the integrity of the BCB is referred to as BCB function rather than described by its morphological properties (Reiber 1994; Reiber and Felgenhauer 1987). According to Reiber, all factors contributing to increases of CSF protein concentration can be explained by a reduced CSF flow. A spinal block as well as polyradiculitis or purulent meningitis will lead to a reduced CSF flow which in turn will result in an increased CSF protein concentration.

The relationship between CSF flow and CSF protein concentration has been characterized by a flow rate formula by Reiber (1994) and can be explained mechanistically such that reduced CSF flow causes a holdup of proteins in the vascular system, which in turn leads to an increased gradient between blood and CSF compartments which finally will result in an increase of protein transfer across the BCB. According to this concept (Reiber 1994), any increase of CSF protein concentration can be ultimately attributed to reduced CSF flow rate independent of the underlying disease etiology.

2.4   Brain Areas Reflected by CSF Analysis

Only defined cerebral regions appear to be of relevance to CSF analysis done in lumbar CSF. This means that only some areas of the central nervous system are drained to the lumbar sac and that processes in cortical areas remote from the ventricles very often may not result in alterations of CSF composition.

This notion is supported by the following frequently made observation: focal cerebral lesions related to infectious or to autoimmune inflammation located in the frontal, temporal, or parietal regions of the brain may not be associated with inflammatory changes of the lumbar CSF.

For instance, CEA-producing metastasis in frontal brain areas does not influence CEA levels in the lumbar CSF (Jacobi et al. 1986).

As shown for the adhesion molecules sICAM-1 and sVCAM-1 in patients with MS, there is an inverse relationship between the distance of enhancing single lesion to the ventricular surface and the CSF levels of the adhesion molecules, i.e., the smaller the distance, the higher the CSF concentration (Felgenhauer 1995; Rieckmann et al. 1997) (Fig. 2.5).

Diseases localized in brain areas adjacent to CSF space are more easily accessible to CSF diagnostics. In this context, Felgenhauer introduced the term "CSF analytic brain" (Felgenhauer 1995). In contrast, CNS pathologies of the meninges, periventricular areas, temporobasal regions, spinal cord, and roots can be reliably detected by inflammatory changes of the CSF.

Therefore, analysis of the lumbar CSF allows only a topographically restricted assessment of inflammatory diseases of the CNS and may not rule out any inflammation of the CNS.

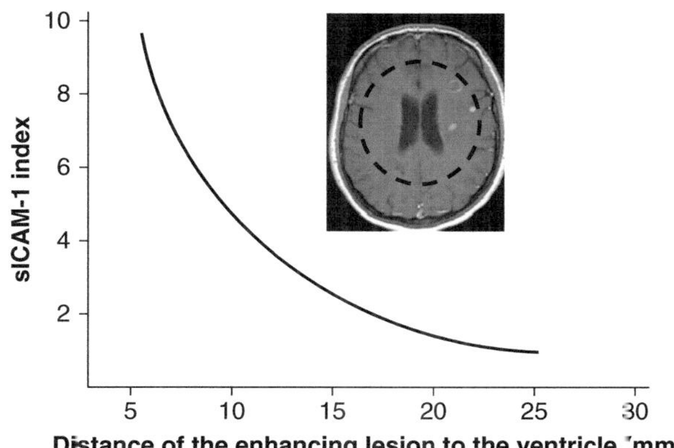

Fig. 2.5 Inverse relationship between the CSF index of the adhesion molecule sICAM-1 in patients with MS and the distance of enhancing single lesion to the ventricular surface (Modified according to Rieckmann et al. (1997))

References

Abbott NJ, Patabendige AA, Dolman DE, Yusof SR, Begley DJ et al (2010) Structure and function of the blood-brain barrier. Neurobiol Dis 37(1):13–25

Brightman MW (1965) The distribution within the brain of ferritin injected into cerebrospinal fluid compartments II. Parenchymal distribution. Am J Anat 117:193–220

Davson H (1976) The blood-brain barrier (review lecture). J Physiol 255:1–28

Davson H, Hollingsworth G, Segal MB (1970) The mechanism of drainage of the cerebrospinal fluid. Brain 93(4):665–678

Dunn JS, Wyburn GM (1972) The anatomy of the blood brain barrier: a review. Scott Med J 17(1):21–36

Felgenhauer K (1974) Protein size and cerebrospinal fluid composition. Klin Wochenschr 52:1158–1164

Felgenhauer K (1995) The filtration concept of the blood-CSF barrier as basis for the differentiation of CSF proteins. In: Greenwood J, Begley DJ, Segal MB (eds) New concepts of a blood-brain barrier. Plenum Press, New York, pp 209–217

Felgenhauer K, Beuche W (1999) Labordiagnostik neurologischer Erkrankungen. Verlag Stuttgart Thieme

Felgenhauer K, Schliep G, Rapic N (1976) Evaluation of the blood-CSF barrier by protein gradients and the humoral immune response within the central nervous system. J Neurol Sci 30:113–128

Goldmann EE (1913) Vitalfarbung am Zentralneirvensystem. Abh preuss Akad Wims Phys Math Kl I:1–60

Goldstein GW, Betz AL (1986) The blood-brain barrier. Sci Am 255(3):74–83

Jacobi C, Reiber H, Felgenhauer K (1986) The clinical relevance of locally produced carcinoembryonic antigen in cerebrospinal fluid. J Neurol 233(6):358–361

Koziara JM, Lockman PR, Allen DD, Mumper DJ (2006) The blood-brain barrier and brain drug delivery. J Nanosci Nanotechnol 6(9–10):2712–2735

Nagelhus EA, Ottersen OP (2013) Physiological roles of aquaporin-4 in brain. Physiol Rev 93:1543–1562

Reiber H (1994) Flow rate of cerebrospinal fluid (CSF)–a concept common to normal blood-CSF barrier function and to dysfunction in neurological diseases. J Neurol Sci 122:189–203

Reiber H, Felgenhauer K (1987) Protein transfer at the blood cerebrospinal fluid barrier and the quantitation of the humoral immune response within the central nervous system. Clin Chim Acta 163:319–328

Rieckmann P, Altenhofen B, Riegel A, Baudewig J, Felgenhauer K (1997) Soluble adhesion molecules (sVCAM-1 and sICAM-1) in cerebrospinal fluid and serum correlate with MRI activity in multiple sclerosis. Ann Neurol 41(3):326–333
Süssmuth SD, Landfester K, Tumani H, Ludolph AC, Brettschneider J (2008) Blood-brain barrier in neurodegenerative diseases: perspectives for nanomedicine. Eur J Nanomed 2:39–47
Westergaard E (1977) The blood-brain barrier to horseradish peroxidase under normal and experimental conditions. Acta Neuropathol 39(3):181–187

Physiology and Constituents of CSF

3

Hayrettin Tumani

Contents

Abstract

CSF protects the CNS in different ways involving metabolic homeostasis, supply of nutrients, functioning as lymphatic system, and regulation of intracranial pressure.

CSF is produced by the choroid plexus, brain interstitium, and the meninges, and it circulates in craniocaudal direction from ventricles to spinal subarachnoic space from where it is removed via craniocaudal lymphatic routes and venous system. The CSF is renewed 3–5 times daily, and its molecular constituents are mainly blood derived (80 %), while the remainder consists of brain-derived and intrathecally produced molecules (20 %).

The transfer of molecules between the blood–brain and blood–CSF barriers is selectively regulated by diffusion (e.g., passive or facilitated transport for proteins) or active transport (e.g., glucose). Aquaporin-4 channels, abundantly localized at the blood–brain interface, are involved in the regulation of extracellular space volume, potassium buffering, cerebrospinal fluid circulation, and interstitial fluid absorption.

H. Tumani
Department of Neurology,
University of Ulm, Ulm, Germany
e-mail: hayrettin.tumani@uni-ulm.de

© Springer International Publishing Switzerland 2015

25

F. Deisenhammer et al. (eds.), *Cerebrospinal Fluid in Clinical Neurology*,
DOI 10.1007/978-3-319-01225-4_3

The concentration of CSF constituents is influenced by multiple factors most significantly by blood concentration, protein size, blood–CSF barrier integrity, and intrathecal production.

3.1 Biological Function of CSF

The CSF is a clear colorless fluid with several protective functions within the nervous system involving structural, hydrodynamic, metabolic, and immunological aspects.

It is assumed that CSF and its spaces provide a mechanical protection system by acting as a cushion to protect the brain from hitting the own skull in case of fast and abrupt head movements and mild head traumas. In severe traumas such as traffic accidents or sports injuries, the protection system of the CSF may not suffice to avoid brain damage such as contusio cerebri. An animal model (miniature pig) has been developed as an appropriate model for studying CSF, spinal cord, and dura interactions during injury (Jones et al. 2012).

The CSF influences the metabolic homeostasis of the central nervous system (CNS) by maintaining the electrolytic environment and the systemic acid–base balance, serving as a medium for the supply of nutrients to neuronal and glial cells, functioning as a lymphatic system for the CNS by removing the degradation products of cellular metabolism, and transporting hormones, neurotransmitters, releasing factors, and other neuropeptides throughout the CNS.

According to a classical concept, CSF functions as a "sink" by which the various substances formed in the CNS tissue during its metabolic activity diffuse rapidly into the CSF, and from there, they are reabsorbed into the vascular system (Davson et al. 1970).

Enhanced removal of potentially neurotoxic waste products (e.g., β-amyloid clearance) that accumulate in the awake CNS occurs predominantly in natural sleep or anesthesia. This has been discussed as a consequence of an increase in convective exchange of cerebrospinal fluid with interstitial fluid (Xie et al. 2013; Iliff et al. 2012).

Moreover, CSF is directly involved in regulation of sleep–wake cycle via the prostaglandin D2 (PGD2) and prostaglandin-D-synthase (PGDS) system, both of which occur in a very high concentration in the CSF (Hayaishi 2000).

Immunoperoxidase staining and direct enzyme activity determination revealed that PGDS is mainly localized in the membrane systems surrounding the brain including the arachnoid membrane and choroid plexus (Blödorn et al. 1999). From there, PGDS is secreted into the CSF to become beta-trace, a major protein component of the CSF intrathecally produced (Tumani et al. 1998). PGD2 exerts its somnogenic activity by binding to PGD2 receptors exclusively localized at the ventrorostral surface of the basal forebrain suggesting that PGD2 may induce sleep via leptomeningeal PGD2 receptors localized on neurons in these areas (Hayaishi 2000).

Intrathecal application of anesthetics, steroids, or chemotherapies via puncture of lumbar CSF space is an established treatment option underscoring the importance of CSF as a route and medium for the supply of therapeutic compounds to neuronal and glial cells. In addition, pressure-related diseases such as intracranial hypotension and hypertension can be diagnosed, monitored, and treated by accessing the CSF space (spinal tap, lumbar catheter, lumbar blood patch, ventriculoperitoneal or lumboperitoneal shunt, etc.) (Torbey et al. 2004; Yadav et al. 2010).

Apart from being a transport medium, CSF serves as an important diagnostic tool in the evaluation of CNS diseases (Deisenhammer et al. 2009). It is the only tool besides brain biopsy to confirm or to rule out inflammatory processes within the CNS. Furthermore, it allows diagnostic evaluation of noninflammatory diseases such as intracranial bleeding and neoplastic and neurodegenerative processes as outlined in the following chapters of this book.

3.2 CSF Production, Circulation, and Absorption

CSF is mainly produced by the choroid plexus in the ventricles. The remainder of CSF is formed by the interstitium and the meninges. While the choroid plexus and brain parenchyma give rise to most of ventricular CSF, the meninges and dorsal roots contribute significantly to the formation of lumbar CSF (Stewart 1922; Davson et al. 1970; Cserr et al. 1992; Thompson and Zeman 1992). Recent findings suggest that aquaporin-4 channels abundantly localized at blood–brain interface contribute significantly to water flux in the pericapillary (Virchow–Robin) space and thereby to CSF production (Nagelhus and Ottersen 2013; Nakada 2014).

The amount of CSF produced at a rate of 0.3–0.4 mL min^{-1} is approximately 450–550 mL in 24 h. The overall CSF turnover ranges roughly between 3 and 5 times per day given a total volume of the CSF space in adults between 90 and 150 mL (Davson et al. 1970; Battal et al. 2011; Nakada 2014).

According to the classical concept, CSF circulates through the ventricles, the cisterns, and the subarachnoid space ultimately to be absorbed into the blood at the level of the arachnoid villi. Ten to fifteen percent of CSF is drained into the lymphatics that flow via the perineural spaces of the cranial and spinal nerves (Davson et al. 1970; Cserr et al. 1992).

The CSF circulation has been explained by two different concepts: (1) bulk flow (unidirectional circulation) and (2) pulsatile flow (back and forth motion). According to the bulk flow concept, a hydrostatic pressure causes a gradient between the site of its formation (choroid plexus in the ventricles with a slightly high pressure) and its site of absorption (arachnoid granulations with a slightly low pressure). In contrast recent insights into a new hydrodynamics of the CSF visualized by phase-contrast MR imaging provide evidence for the pulsatile flow concept, according to which circulation of the CSF results from pulsations related to cardiac cycle of the cerebral arteries (Battal et al. 2011; Bulat and Klarica 2011; Oreskovic and Klarica 2010; Greitz and Hannerz 1996).

A study on laboratory animals found that 77 % of the lumbar CSF pulse wave was caused by arterial and venous pulses in the spinal canal, and 23 % was caused by spinal transmission of the intracranial pressure pulse wave (Urayama 1994).

Based on the findings described above, CSF circulation appears much more complex and most likely is driven by a combination of directed bulk flow, pulsatile to-and-fro movement, and continuous bidirectional fluid exchange at the blood–brain barrier and the cell membranes at the borders between CSF and interstitial fluid spaces (Oreskovic and Klarica 2010; Brinker et al. 2014).

Traditional models of CSF physiology based on studies until the 1980s assumed that any absorption would require a CSF pressure higher than the intravascular pressure (McComb 1983). However, current concepts derived from studies on aquaporins and blood–brain interfaces postulate the involvement of osmotic forces in brain water homeostasis in addition to classical pressure gradient (Oreskovic and Klarica 2010; Brinker et al. 2014).

3.3 Transfer Mechanisms

All molecules stemming from the blood cross the blood–brain barrier or the blood–CSF barrier by diffusion (e.g., passive or facilitated transport for proteins) or via active transport (e.g. glucose).

The transfer properties of the blood–brain barrier are characterized by a characteristic identification line (Oldendorf curve) for the lipophilic transport of small molecules (Oldendorf et al. 1972). Substances of low solubility in olive oil (<1 %) have little chances to pass the blood–brain barrier. Substances insoluble in fat such as glucose and amino acids pass the barrier with the help of specific carrier molecules (Abbott et al. 2010). Lipid-soluble substances of a molecular weight of more than 500 Da also have problems passing the blood–brain barrier. However, larger molecules, even when insoluble in fat (hydrophilic), can pass the blood–CSF barrier more easily. This passage is governed by the Meyer–Overton rule (Nau et al. 1994; Honkanen et al. 1995). In "steady state," the ratio of CSF to serum concentrations of hydrophilic molecules correlates with the hydrodynamic radii of molecules (Felgenhauer 1974, 1995). The filtration line according to Felgenhauer (Fig. 3.1) shows these ratios in molecular level with a hydrodynamic radius of 1–100 Å.

The basic principles of secretion and transport at the blood–CSF barrier are identical to those of the blood–brain barrier. These are active transportation and facilitated diffusion, so that the inner lining of the plexus (epithelium) is either characterized by secretion or absorption of isotonic fluid (Davson et al. 1970). The most important transportation system at the blood–CSF barrier is the sodium$^+$/potassium$^+$ ATPase located at the apical ciliated ridge (microvilli) of the plexus choroideus (Keep et al. 1999). In addition, carboanhydrase for the exchange of HCO^{-3} and Cl^- plays a role. Blocking these transportation systems is used therapeutically (furosemide, acetazolamide) to reduce CSF formation (Carrion et al. 2001). Although the main route of transport is unidirectional from the blood to the subarachnoid space, there is also a bidirectional transport at the blood–CSF barrier (Oreskovic and Klarica 2010; Brinker et al. 2014). This way, certain substrates (inorganic ions, metabolites of neurotransmitters, antibiotics) can be removed from the brain and the CSF. According to a recent two-photon imaging study visualizing fluorescent tracers through a cranial window of living mice, a significant proportion

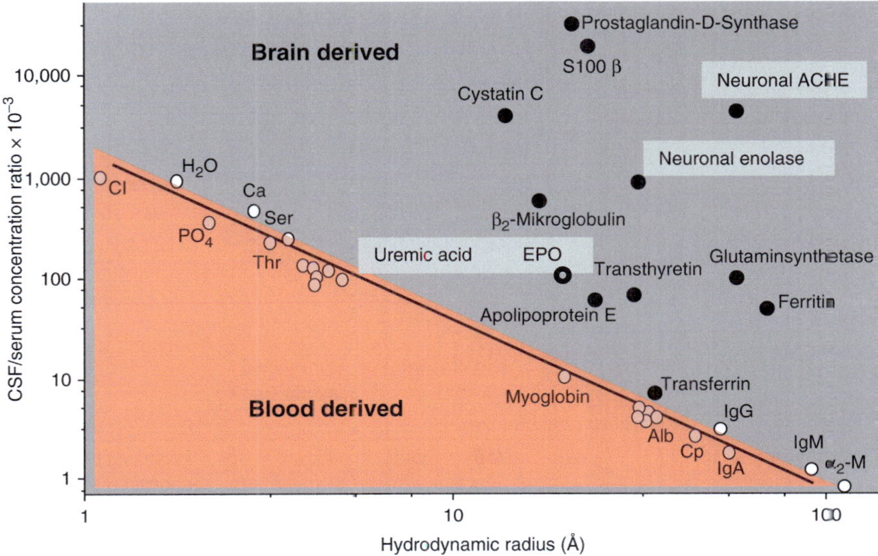

Fig. 3.1 Relationship between CSF–serum ratio of blood (*white circles*) and brain-derived (*black circles*) compounds and their hydrodynamic radius under "steady-state" conditions (Modified according to Felgenhauer (1995)). *Alb* albumin, *α2-M* α2-Makroglobulin, *Ca* calcium, *Cl* chloride *Cp* ceruloplasmin, *EPO* erythropoietin, *Ig* immunoglobulin, *PO₄* phosphate, *Ser* serine, *Thr* threonine)

of CSF recycles into the brain along paravascular pathways mediated by aquaporin-4 channels (Iliff et al. 2012). The authors conclude that AQP4-mediated water flow along vessels may be relevant for clearing brain interstitial water, interstitial waste, and soluble proteins.

3.4 CSF Proteins and Factors Influencing Their Concentration

The composition of the lumbar CSF has been intensively studied, since the introduction of the spinal tap more than a century ago (Quincke 1891; Wynter 1891). The CSF is a cell-free clear fluid and contains approximately 0.3 % plasma proteins, or approximately 150–450 mg/L, depending on age and sampling site (ventricular vs. lumbar).

The majority of the protein content of the lumbar CSF is blood derived (80 %), and the remainder consists of brain-derived or intrathecally produced proteins (20 %) (Fig. 3.1, Tables 3.1 and 3.2) (Felgenhauer 1974; Thompson and Zeman 1992).

Under physiological conditions, blood-derived proteins enter the CSF compartment via passive diffusion across the blood–CSF barrier. Depending on their molecular size and their blood concentration, CSF proteins of blood origin show a specific CSF-to-blood ratio The larger the protein size, the higher the concentration gradient between blood and CSF (e.g., IgM > IgA > IgG > albumin) (Fig. 3.1, Tables 3.1 and 3.2) (Felgenhauer 1974).

Table 3.1 Major blood-derived proteins in CSF (80 % of total CSF proteins)

Compound	CSF		Blood (serum or plasma)		CSF–serum ratio
	Reference range (mean)				
Total protein	200–500	mg/L	60–80	g/L	
Albumin	150–350	mg/L	35–55	g/L	$<8 \times 10^{-3}$
IgG	<40	mg/L	7–16	g/L	$<6 \times 10^{-3}$
IgA	<6	mg/L	0.7–4.0	g/L	$<4 \times 10^{-3}$
IgM	<1	mg/L	0.4–2.3	g/L	$<1.8 \times 10^{-3}$

Table 3.2 Mainly brain-derived proteins in CSF (20 % of total CSF proteins)

Compound	CSF		Blood (serum or plasma)		Intrathecal synthesis (%)	Noteworthiness
	Reference range (mean)					
Transthyretin	17	mg/L	250	mg/L	93	Produced by choroid plexus; thyroid transporter
Prostaglandin-D synthase (beta-trace)	15	mg/L	0.5	mg/L	>99	Marker for CSF fistula; enzyme and retinol transporter
Cystatin C (γ-Trace)	3	mg/L	0.5	mg/L	>99	Proteinase inhibitor
Apolipoprotein E	6	mg/L	93.5	mg/L	90	Lipid transporter
Neopterin	4.2	nmol/L	5.3	nmol/L	98	Marker for microglia and macrophage activity
Neuron-specific enolase (NSE)	5	mg/L	6	µg/L	>99	Marker for neuronal damage
Glial fibrillary acidic protein (GFAP)	0.12	mg/L	0		100	Marker for glial activity or damage
Ferritin	6	mg/L	120	µg/L	97	Marker for subarachnoid bleeding
S-100 protein	2.9	mg/L	0.12	µg/L	>99	Marker for glial activity or damage
Myelin basic protein (MBP)	0.5	mg/L	0		100	Marker for myelin damage
Tau protein	0.2	mg/L	0		100	Marker for neuronal and axonal damage
Neurofilaments	0.1	mg/L	0		100	Marker for axonal damage

When molecular size and serum levels are known, the CSF concentration of a given blood-derived protein can be calculated. A concentration in the CSF exceeding the calculated value indicates a local production of that given protein within the CNS, i.e., intrathecal synthesis (Felgenhauer 1995).

Erythropoietin (EPO) in CSF may serve as an example (Fig. 3.1): Based on the molecular weight (30 kd) and the corresponding hydrodynamic radius of 24 Å, the estimated CSF–serum ratio of EPO would be 0.01, if EPO found in CSF originated from the blood compartment via passive diffusion only. The CSF–serum concentration ratio of EPO in symptomatic controls (tension-type headache) appears however to be 0.126. Therefore, the approximate proportion of CSF EPO originating from intrathecal synthesis can be estimated being 92 % (Widl et al. 2007) Additional evidence for its intrathecal origin is that CSF EPO concentrations are independent of blood–CSF barrier function, i.e., there is no Q_{alb}.-related increase of EPO in the CSF.

Another way to determine the extent to which a given protein is produced within the CNS formula taking into account the serum concentration of the respective protein (e.g., IgG) and the albumin CSF-to-serum ratio can be used. Various formulae such as IgG index, IgG synthesis rate, and IgG(loc) have been developed to discriminate between blood- and brain-derived fractions of IgG (Link and Tibbling 1977; Tourtellotte et al. 1980; Reiber and Felgenhauer 1987).

Another important factor influencing the protein content is the permeability at the blood–CSF barrier (Felgenhauer et al. 1976). The function of the blood–CSF barrier is best characterized by the albumin CSF-to-serum ratio, since albumin is exclusively produced in the liver and not by the nervous system (Brettschneider et al. 2005).

In blood–CSF barrier dysfunctions (elevated albumin CSF–serum ratio), the concentration of proteins originating from blood (IgG, IgA, IgM) increases in accordance with a nonlinear hyperbolic function (Reiber 1994).

In contrast, CSF proteins which are predominantly synthesized in the CNS (>95 %) such as tau protein or NSE are not influenced by the respective blood concentration or the blood–CSF barrier function and therefore do not have to be related to their respective blood levels or Q_{alb} when measured in the CSF (Reiber 2001; Sussmuth et al. 2001).

Several additional factors may influence concentration of CSF proteins and have to be considered when studying CSF parameters such as (a) circadian variation, (b) volume of sampled CSF, and (c) rostrocaudal concentration gradient (Tuman and Brettschneider 2005).

In addition, posture, physical activity, circadian influence, medication, surgical intervention, intrathoracic pressure, and site of sampling may affect the CSF production rate and thereby the concentration of CSF analytes as well.

CSF levels of IL-6, TNF-alpha, and HSP72 do not change with exercise and remain below their corresponding plasma levels (Steensberg et al. 2006).

- In patients with a spinal needle placed in the lumbar region for continuous analgesia, CSF substance P increased very rapidly with surgical intervention, whereas the CSF norepinephrine concentration tended to decrease. Pregabalin at clinical doses did not modulate the spinal neurotransmitter concentrations (Buvanendran et al. 2012).

- There is a large circadian variation with nearly fourfold difference of CSF production rate between 6 p.m. (12 mL/h) and 2 a.m. (42 mL/h) as demonstrated by CSF flow analysis by MRI (Nilsson et al. 1992). Accordingly, levels of the brain-derived proteins such as tau protein and GFAP are likely to be influenced by the CSF production rate. It has been reported that the levels of specific prostaglandin-d synthase (beta-trace) in CSF, which is mainly produced by leptomeninges and glia, undergo circadian changes (Jordan et al. 2004).
- While the lumbar CSF is most prevalent in the first CSF portion, more ventricular CSF will be present when an increasing volume is sampled. Accordingly, the levels of blood-derived CSF proteins such as albumin will decrease and those of brain-derived proteins such as tau protein will increase with increasing volumes of obtained lumbar CSF (Reiber 2001; Sussmuth et al. 2001).

Serum proteins are constantly added to the descending ventricular CSF via the blood–CSF barrier, represented by the arachnoid vessels, that apparently stretches along the craniocaudal neuraxis. For this reason, under physiological conditions, there is a rising gradient of total CSF protein from ventricles (256 mg/L) and cisterna magna (316 mg/L) to the lumbar subarachnoid space (420 mg/L) (Weisner and Bernhardt 1978).

Similarly, the albumin concentration rises approximately 2.2-fold from the ventricular CSF to the lumbar CSF (Gerber et al. 1998; Reiber 2001). CNS proteins of parenchymal origin (e.g., tau protein) have a tendency to decrease, while CNS proteins of meningeal origin (e.g., beta-trace) have a rising ventriculo-lumbar concentration gradient (Tumani et al. 1999; Blödorn et al. 1999).

References

Abbott NJ, Patabendige AA, Dolman DE, Yusof SR, Begley DJ et al (2010) Structure and function of the blood-brain barrier. Neurobiol Dis 37(1):13–25

Battal B, Kocaoglu M, Bulakbasi N et al (2011) Cerebrospinal fluid flow imaging by using phase-contrast MR technique. Br J Radiol 84(1004):758–765

Blödorn B, Bruck W, Tumani H et al (1999) Expression of the beta-trace protein in human pachymeninx as revealed by in situ hybridization and immunocytochemistry. J Neurosci Res 57(5):730–734

Brettschneider J, Claus A, Kassubek J, Tumani H (2005) Isolated blood-cerebrospinal fluid barrier dysfunction: prevalence and associated diseases. J Neurol 252:1067–1073

Brinker T, Stopa E, Morrison J, Klinge P (2014) A new look at cerebrospinal fluid circulation fluids and barriers of the CNS. http://www.fluidsbarrierscns.com/content/11/1/10

Bulat M, Klarica M (2011) Recent insights into a new hydrodynamics of the cerebrospinal fluid. Brain Res Rev 2011(65):99–112

Buvanendran A, Kroin JS, Della Valle CJ, Moric M, Tuman KJ (2012) Cerebrospinal fluid neurotransmitter changes during the perioperative period in patients undergoing total knee replacement: a randomized trial. Anesth Analg 114(2):434–441

Carrion E, Hertzog JH, Medlock MD, Hauser GJ, Dalton HJ (2001) Use of acetazolamide to decrease cerebrospinal fluid production in chronically ventilated patients with ventriculopleural shunts. Arch Dis Child 84(1):68–71

Cserr HF, Harling-Berg CJ, Knopf PM (1992) Drainage of brain extracellular fluid into blood and deep cervical lymph and its immunological significance. Brain Pathol 2(4):269–276

Davson H, Hollingsworth G, Segal MB (1970) The mechanism of drainage of the cerebrospinal fluid. Brain 93(4):665–678

Deisenhammer F, Egg R, Giovannoni G, Hemmer B, Petzold A, Sellebjerg F, Teunissen C, Tumani H (2009) EFNS guidelines on disease-specific CSF investigations. Eur J Neurol 16(6):760–770

Felgenhauer K (1974) Protein size and cerebrospinal fluid composition. Klin Wochenschr 52:1158–1164

Felgenhauer K (1995) The filtration concept of the blood-CSF barrier as basis for the differentiation of CSF proteins. In: Greenwood J, Begley DJ, Segal MB (eds) New concepts of a blood-brain barrier. Plenum Press, New York, pp 209–217

Felgenhauer K, Schliep G, Rapic N (1976) Evaluation of the blood-CSF barrier by protein gradients and the humoral immune response within the central nervous system. J Neurol Sci 30:113–128

Gerber J, Tumani H, Kolenda H, Nau R (1998) Lumbar and ventricular CSF protein, leukocytes and lactate in suspected bacterial CNS infections. Neurology 51:1710–1714

Greitz D, Hannerz J (1996) A proposed model of cerebrospinal fluid circulation: observations with radionuclide cisternography. AJNR Am J Neuroradiol 17(3):431–438

Hayaishi O (2000) Molecular mechanisms of sleep-wake regulation: a role of prostaglandin D2 Philos Trans R Soc Lond B Biol Sci 355(1394):275–280

Honkanen RA, McBath H, Kushmerick C, Callender GE, Scarlata SF, Fenstermacher JD, Haspel HC (1995) Barbiturates inhibit hexose transport in cultured mammalian cells and human erythrocytes and interact directly with purified GLUT-1. Biochemistry 34(2):535–544

Iliff JJ, Wang M, Liao Y et al (2012) A paravascular pathway facilitates CSF flow through the brain parenchyma and the clearance of interstitial solutes, including amyloid beta. Sci Transl Med 4:147

Jones CF, Lee JH, Kwon BK, Cripton PA (2012) Development of a large-animal model to measure dynamic cerebrospinal fluid pressure during spinal cord injury: laboratory investigation J Neurosurg Spine 16(6):524–635

Jordan W, Tumani H, Cohrs S et al (2004) Prostaglandin D synthase (beta-trace) in healthy human sleep. Sleep 27(5):867–874

Keep RF, Ulanski LJ 2nd, Xiang J, Ennis SR, Lorris Betz A (1999) Blood-brain barrier mechanisms involved in brain calcium and potassium homeostasis. Brain Res 815(2):200–205

Link H, Tibbling G (1977) Principles of albumin and IgG analyses in neurological disorders III. Evaluation of IgG synthesis within the central nervous system in multiple sclerosis. Scand J Clin Lab Invest 37:397–401

McComb JG (1983) Recent research into the nature of cerebrospinal fluid formation and absorption. J Neurosurg 1983(59):369–383

Nagelhus EA, Ottersen OP (2013) Physiological roles of aquaporin-4 in brain. Physio Rev 93:1543–1562

Nakada T (2014) Cerebrospinal fluid physiology and movement. Croat Med J 55:328–336

Nau R, Sörgel F, Prange HW (1994) Lipophilicity at pH 7.4 and molecular size govern the entry of the free serum fraction of drugs into the cerebrospinal fluid in humans with uninflamed meninges. J Neurol Sci 122(1):61–65

Nilsson C, Stahlberg F, Thomsen C, Henriksen O, Herning M, Owman C (1992) Circadian variation in human cerebrospinal fluid production measured by magnetic resonance imaging. Am J Physiol 262:20–24

Oldendorf WH, Hyman S, Braun L, Oldendorf SZ (1972) Blood-brain barrier: penetration of morphine, codeine, heroin, and methadone after carotid injection. Science 178(4064):984–986

Oreskovic D, Klarica M (2010) The formation of cerebrospinal fluid: nearly a hundred years of interpretations and misinterpretations. Brain Res Rev 64:241–262

Quincke HI (1891) Die Lumbalpunktion des Hydrocephalus [German]. Berl Klin Wochschr 32:861–862

Reiber H (1994) Flow rate of cerebrospinal fluid (CSF)–a concept common to normal blood-CSF barrier function and to dysfunction in neurological diseases. J Neurol Sci 122:189–203

Reiber H (2001) Dynamics of brain-derived proteins in cerebrospinal fluid. Clin Chim Acta 310(2):173–186

Reiber H, Felgenhauer K (1987) Protein transfer at the blood cerebrospinal fluid barrier and the quantitation of the humoral immune response within the central nervous system. Clin Chim Acta 163:319–328

Steensberg A, Dalsgaard MK, Secher NH, Pedersen BK (2006) Cerebrospinal fluid IL-6, HSP72, and TNF-alpha in exercising humans. Brain Behav Immun 20(6):585–589

Stewart RM (1922) Critical review: the cerebrospinal fluid: its source, distribution, and circulation. J Neurol Psychopathol 3(10):144–166

Sussmuth SD, Reiber H, Tumani H (2001) Tau protein in cerebrospinal fluid (CSF): a blood-CSF barrier related evaluation in patients with various neurological diseases. Neurosci Lett 300(2):95–98

Thompson EJ, Zeman A (1992) Fluids of the brain and the pathogenesis of MS. Neurochem Res 17(9):901–905

Torbey MT, Geocadin RG, Razumovsky AY, Rigamonti D, Williams MA (2004) Utility of CSF pressure monitoring to identify idiopathic intracranial hypertension without papilledema in patients with chronic daily headache. Cephalalgia 24(6):495–502

Tourtellotte WW, Potvin AR, Baumhefner RW et al (1980) Multiple sclerosis de novo CNS IgG synthesis. Effect of CNS irradiation. Arch Neurol 37:620–624

Tumani H, Brettschneider J (2005) Brain specific proteins in CSF: factors influencing their concentration in CSF and clinical relevance. J Lab Med 29:421–428

Tumani H, Nau R, Felgenhauer K (1998) Beta-trace protein in cerebrospinal fluid: a blood-CSF barrier-related evaluation in neurological diseases. Ann Neurol 44(6):882–889

Tumani H, Shen G, Peter JB, Bruck W (1999) Glutamine synthetase in cerebrospinal fluid, serum, and brain: a diagnostic marker for Alzheimer disease? Arch Neurol 56(10):1241–1246

Urayama K (1994) Origin of lumbar cerebrospinal fluid pulse wave. Spine 19(4):441–445

Weisner B, Bernhardt W (1978) Protein fractions of lumbar, cisternal, and ventricular cerebrospinal fluid. Separate areas of reference. J Neurol Sci 37(3):205–214

Widl K, Brettschneider J, Schattauer D, Süssmuth S, Huber R, Ludolph AC, Tumani H (2007) Erythropoietin in cerebrospinal fluid: age-related reference values and relevance in neurological disease. Neurochem Res 32(7):1163–1168

Wynter WE (1891) Four cases of tubercular meningitis in which paracentesis was performed for the relief of fluid pressure. Lancet 137:981–982

Xie L, Kang H, Xu Q, Chen MJ, Liao Y, Thiyagarajan M, O'Donnell J, Christensen DJ, Nicholson C, Iliff JJ, Takano T, Deane R, Nedergaard M (2013) Sleep drives metabolite clearance from the adult brain. Science 342(6156):373–377

Yadav YR, Parihar V, Sinha M (2010) Lumbar peritoneal shunt. Neurol India 58(2):179–184

Techniques, Contraindications, and Complications of CSF Collection Procedures

Ellis Niemantsverdriet, Hanne Struyfs, Flora Duits, Charlotte E. Teunissen, and Sebastiaan Engelborghs

Contents

E. Niemantsverdriet • H. Struyfs
Reference Center for Biological Markers of Dementia (BIODEM),
University of Antwerp, Universiteitsplein 1, Antwerp BE-2610, Belgium

F. Duits
Department of Neurology and Alzheimer Center,
VU University Medical Center,
Amsterdam, The Netherlands

C.E. Teunissen
Neurochemistry Laboratory and Biobank,
Department of Clinical Chemistry,
VU University Medical Center Amsterdam,
Amsterdam, The Netherlands

S. Engelborghs (⊠)
Reference Center for Biological Markers of Dementia (BIODEM),
University of Antwerp, Universiteitsplein 1, Antwerp BE-2610, Belgium

Department of Neurology and Memory Clinic,
Hospital Network Antwerp (ZNA) Middelheim and Hoge Beuken,
Antwerp, Belgium
e-mail: Sebastiaan.Engelborghs@uantwerpen.be

© Springer International Publishing Switzerland 2015
F. Deisenhammer et al. (eds.), *Cerebrospinal Fluid in Clinical Neurology*,
DOI 10.1007/978-3-319-01225-4_4

Abstract

Lumbar puncture (LP), also known as spinal tap, is the most frequently used technique through which the restricted compartment of the subarachnoid space is accessed to sample cerebrospinal fluid. An LP can have both diagnostic and therapeutic indications. To perform an LP, the optimal length, size, and type of needle should be used, depending on the medical indication. Needles used for LP can differ in length, diameter, and design. Head-to-head studies are in favor of atraumatic-type and small-diameter needles given the lower incidence of post-lumbar puncture headache (PLPH), and consensus-based guidelines recommend to use 25G atraumatic needles.

The most important contraindication to perform an LP is a posterior fossa mass and intracranial hypertension, given the risk of central nervous system or tonsillar herniation. Other contraindications are local infections at the puncture site, congenital abnormalities, and uncorrected bleeding diathesis. The LP procedure is easy to perform by an experienced physician with proper understanding of the anatomical implications and results in low risks of complications. The most common complaint after an LP is PLPH; other infrequent complications include infections, local hematomas, pain, and local discomfort.

In conclusion, an LP is a viable therapeutic technique and a common diagnostic procedure, which, if performed correctly, has a low complication rate and a high diagnostic yield and is usually more tolerable than patients expect.

Abbreviations

AD	Alzheimer's disease
BMI	Body mass index
CNS	Central nervous system
CSF	Cerebrospinal fluid
CT	Computed tomography
G	Gauge
ICP	Intracranial pressure
JPND	The EU Joint Programme – Neurodegenerative Disease Research
LP	Lumbar puncture
MRI	Magnetic resonance imaging
PD	Parkinson's disease
PLPH	Post-lumbar puncture headache

4.1 Technique

Lumbar puncture (LP), also known as spinal tap, is an invasive technique through which the restricted compartment of the subarachnoid space is accessed to sample cerebrospinal fluid (CSF). The procedure involves introducing a needle in the spine, usually at a level below the medullary cone, and permitting access to the subarachnoid space. Another possibility to obtain CSF is to puncture at a higher level of the spine, at the cervical vertebrae (C1–C2) referred as a lateral cervical puncture, or by a suboccipital puncture that is not routinely applied.

LP has both diagnostic and therapeutic purposes. For diagnostic purposes, CSF can be analyzed for differential cell counts and cytology; biochemistry like total protein levels, protein electrophoresis, and albumin and glucose levels; as well as bacteriological or virological cultures, immunoglobulins, or disease-specific biomarkers, whereas the therapeutic indication can be either CSF removal to reduce intracranial pressure (ICP) or to gain access to the central nervous system (CNS) compartment for drug delivery, such as anesthesia or intrathecal chemotherapy. Epidural and spinal anesthesia delivery uses the same technique as diagnostic LP except that by epidural anesthesia, the needle tip is positioned in the epidural space instead of in the subarachnoid space. An LP is a viable therapeutic technique and remains a common diagnostic procedure, which, if performed correctly, has a low complication rate and a high diagnostic yield and is usually more tolerable than patients expect.

4.1.1   Procedure of LP

An LP is a stepwise procedure, from informing the patient to inserting the needle and collecting CSF. A first step is to obtain consent from the patient, whereby the physician explains the procedure and outlines the potential common complications (see Sect. 4.3). Verbal consent is often sufficient, but it is standardized in practice to obtain written consent prior to invasive procedures (Beresford 1980). Next, the equipment such as sterile gloves, sterile drape, sterile gauze dressings, antiseptic solution, eventually a local anesthetic, syringe, needles, collection tubes, and wound dressing or plaster are placed at a sterile field to avoid contamination. The physician should wash his/her hands, put on sterile gloves, and make sure all of the equipment is sterile

To start the procedure, the patient has to be positioned in either the left lateral recumbent position (for right-handed physicians) with or without knees to chest or in a sitting position. In the lateral recumbent position with knees to chest, the patient should be positioned with the back flexed forward as far as possible, and the coronal plane of the trunk should be perpendicular to the floor with one hip exactly above the other. Lumbar lordosis is overcome in this position, and the neck is maintained in the neutral position. The needle has to stay in the midline of the spine; therefore it is placed parallel to the floor. In the sitting position, the patient is positioned with the neck and back completely flexed forward as this flexion facilitates the course of the needle by widening the gap between adjacent lumbar spinal processes.

The position (recumbent or sitting up) depends on the physician, which position he or she prefers to perform the LP, and on the patient. In case of immobilized patients, being unable to sit up, the lateral recumbent position should be applied For lumbar CSF pressure measurement, patients need to be in the lateral recumbent position (Van Dellen and Bill 1978; Adams et al. 1997). Advantages of the sitting position are a higher CSF pressure and flow and thus a shorter procedure time whereas an increased risk of severe headache might be a disadvantage of sitting up (see Sect. 4.3.1) (Duits et al. submitted). Therefore, it is advised to perform LP in the lateral recumbent position, as the sitting position during LP procedure is associated with more severe headache (Engelborghs et al. submitted).

Next, the site of insertion is defined as the intersection of the line joining the most superior part of both iliac crests (Tuffier's line) and the midline at the L4 spinal process or L4/L5 interspace (Ellis and Feldman 1997; Ievins 1991). The needle is inserted at the L3/L4 or L4/L5 interspace (Abrahams and Webb 1975), as both spaces are below the level of the medullary cone (L1/L2) in the majority of adults if no other spinal malformation is present (Ellis and Feldman 1997). The L4/L5 or L5/S1 interspace should be used in children as the spinal cord ends at the L3 level. The skin of the patient should be cleaned with disinfectant, and if a local anesthetic is used, it should only be infiltrated subcutaneously because deeper structures are less sensitive to pain and an increased volume may distort the tissues.

The final step is the insertion of the needle at the superior aspect of the inferior spinal process angling the needle toward the umbilicus (15° toward the head) in case the interspace L3/L4, L4/L5, or L5/S1 is used (American Association of Clinical Anatomists EAC 1999). It is preferred to hold the bevel in the sagittal plane as this diminishes injury to the dura mater by separating its longitudinal fibers rather than cutting through them and reduces the risk of leakage of CSF after the LP. The needle passes through the supraspinal ligament that connects the tips of spinal processes and the interspinal ligaments between adjacent borders of spinal processes. In a following step when the needle gets through the ligamentum flavum, a resistance can be felt, which is referred to by the physicians as a "pop." The needle is then in the epidural space containing the internal vertebral venous plexus. A second "pop" or "give" represents penetration of the needle through the dura mater into the subarachnoid space; nevertheless, these pops cannot be felt by applying a small-gauge (G) needle. During the procedure, the stylet is removed every 2 mm interval to check for flow of CSF. When using an atraumatic needle instead of a cutting bevel needle (standard Quincke) (Quincke 1891), the technique is the same, but an introducer could be inserted into the interspinal ligament first, after which the smaller atraumatic needle is inserted through the introducer.

By an unsuccessful attempt or if the needle strikes the bone, the needle has to be withdrawn partially to the subcutaneous tissue, and the needle should be re-angled as the needle opening may be obstructed by a nerve root (Van Dellen and Bill 1978). If the attempt is still unsuccessful, it should be made sure the needle is in the midline, through re-palpation, before trying again. Multiple attempts at different sites should be avoided during the procedure, as this may cause local swelling and/or bruising and sometimes muscle spasms. Furthermore, it will obscure surface anatomical landmarks, making future attempts technically more difficult. If the LP attempt is completely unsuccessful, despite due care and advice from a colleague experienced in LP technique, fluoroscopy and ultrasound can be employed to guide the procedure (see Sect. 4.1.2.2).

Finally, in case of a successful LP, the CSF drips directly into the collection tube(s). Normal CSF is transparent and colorless ("eau de roche," according to the historical neurology textbooks). If the LP is traumatic, the collected CSF will be tinged with blood, which disappears if the CSF is collected in serial collections. Even if the CSF looks transparent and colorless, it still can contain red blood cells as the detection limit of visual inspection of CSF for blood contamination is about 0.05 % vol/vol blood (You et al. 2005). Aspirating CSF with a syringe should be avoided in the sitting position because a slight negative pressure can cause subdural hemorrhage or herniation. Aspirating CSF is probably safe in the lateral recumbent position and is only applied with small-diameter needles due to the slow flow rate; moreover, it is routinely performed in certain centers. However, active CSF withdrawal is associated with a higher risk of severe headache and should be performed with care. If a large CSF volume should be withdrawn (e.g., evacuating LP), a large needle size is preferable above active withdrawal using a syringe (Engelborghs et al. submitted). Throughout the procedure, it is essential to maintain a conversation with the patient, explain the steps, and reduce the patient's possible anxiety and discomfort. Moreover, psychological factors could play a role in the appearance of complications, and thus, patients experiencing fear before the procedure have a higher frequency of post-LP complaints (Duits et al. submitted; Alcolea et al. 2014). Routine analysis of CSF requires only 3–6 mL of fluid instead of the 30–60 mL routinely removed when the procedure was first described (Gower et al. 1987); however, the volume of CSF withdrawn is not associated with post-lumbar puncture headache (PLPH), local back pain, or other post-LP complaints (Duits et al. submitted).

CSF Pressure Measurement Pressure measurements are executed prior to CSF sampling, with a manometer connected to the end of the spinal needle once the stylet has been removed. Patients should be in the lateral recumbent position. However, if the dura can only be punctured in the sitting position, extreme care is advised in moving the patient to a lateral position, ensuring the needle is neither displaced nor broken during movement. During the pressure reading, the patient's legs should also be straightened slightly at the hips to avoid compression of the intra-abdominal cavity, which could artificially elevate CSF pressure through transmission of raised pressure within the intrathoracic cavity and consequently increase cerebral venous blood pressure. With the use of a manometer, the opening pressure is measured in terms of the height of the fluid column, in cmH_2O (Wright et al. 2012). CSF flow depends on the diameter of the needle, and normally the manometer will stabilize in a couple of minutes. To ensure peak pressure has been reached, the patient is asked to breathe quietly several times in a calm state, and the CSF level should oscillate slightly within the manometer, but not increase further. A Queckenstedt's or Valsalva maneuver should result in an increase of CSF pressure. If absent or delayed, this is indicative of spinal stenosis. Nowadays, magnetic resonance imaging (MRI) techniques have replaced these obsolete maneuvers to diagnose spinal stenosis.

4.1.2 Needle and Equipment to Perform LP

To perform an LP, the optimal length, size, and type of needle should be used, also depending on the medical indication (e.g., LP to diagnose acute bacterial meningitis vs. scheduled LP to sample CSF for biomarker analyses in case of Alzheimer's disease (AD)). Requirements include adequate flow rate, rapid and accurate transduction of CSF pressure, and minimizing traumatic taps, leakages, failures, and post-LP complications. Besides choosing the right needle, other supportive equipment can reduce failures and facilitate the procedure.

4.1.2.1 The LP Needle

Needles used for LP can differ in length, diameter, and design. Depending on the age and weight of the patient, purpose of the procedure, and minimizing discomfort and complications, a correct choice of needle should be made (Table 4.1)[1].

Length of the Needle Short needles are used for neonates and children, whereas longer spinal needles are used in adults and in obese patients. The procedure is more difficult with longer needles because the needles will typically be more flexible and consequently often divert off course during the procedure (Wright et al. 2012). Therefore, standard needles should be used where possible and, if necessary in case of a dry tap, the needle should be advanced further as required to obtain CSF.

Table 4.1 Differences with regard to needle characteristics based on systematic review conducted in April 2014

Needle	Comparison	Advantages	Disadvantages
Length	Short	Children	–
	Long	Adults or obese patients	Procedure more difficult
Diameter	Small	Less complications, pain, discomfort, blood contaminations, medication, and medical assistance	Slow flow, longer collection time, more failures, and more training/practice needed
	Large	Fast flow, shorter collection time, and less failures	More complications, large perforations, and higher risk of contaminations
Type	Cutting bevel	Feeling of penetration through skin	More complications, medication, medical assistance, and costs
	Atraumatic	Reduced complication risk and less costs, medication, medical assistance, and traumatic taps	Low CSF flow, longer collection time, more failures and attempts, and no feeling of penetration through skin

---

[1] The recommendations described are based on a systematic review conducted in April 2014. All relevant studies published between January 1970 and March 2014 were identified and included in the systematic analysis. Searches were conducted in PubMed and Google Scholar, with a filter for English and search terms in title and/or abstract: *needle* and *lumbar puncture*.

Diameter of the Needle There are many considerations to use needles with a small or a large diameter, in gauge. Small-diameter needles yield less complications after the procedure, less pain and discomfort for the patient, and lower blood patch rates as PLPH is less frequent (Hatfield et al. 2008; Lambert et al. 1997; Flaatten et al. 1998; Wilkinson and Sellar 1991; Aamodt and Vedeler 2001). Otherwise, they produce longer collection times and more failures (Tourtellotte et al. 1972; Crock et al. 2014; Ginosar et al. 2012). Another disadvantage of a smaller diameter, reported by medical staff during questionnaires in different institutions, is the need for more training during the medical education, as well as into practice to avoid the problem of failures and to increase confidence in using these needles (Tung 2013; Stendell et al. 2012; Birnbach et al. 2001; Moller et al. 2013). Considerations are vice versa for larger-bore needles.

In a total of 19 previous studies, from 1970 to 2014, different sizes of needles were compared (Table 4.2). Two study groups detected no differences in the compared needle sizes (20G vs. 22G, 23G vs. 25G) (Hammond et al. 2011; Kim and Yoon 2011); three other articles described a positive effect, such as faster collection time and less failures, when larger-bore needles were used (Ellis et al. 1992; Ready et al. 1989; Kokki and Hendolin 1996), whereas the majority of studies suggest the use of smaller-diameter needles (Hatfield et al. 2008; Lambert et al. 1997; Flaatten et al. 1998; Wilkinson and Sellar 1991; Aamodt and Vedeler 2001; Muller et al. 1994; Kleyweg et al. 1998; Vilming et al. 2001; Tourtellotte et al. 1972; Kaukinen et al. 1981; Crock et al. 2014; Lowery and Oliver 2008; Kovanen and Sulkava 1986; Palmers et al. 2002; McConaha et al. 1996; Tung 2013; Stendell et al. 2012). The articles reported a lower incidence of PLPH, low back pain and discomfort and consequently a reduced use of medical assistance and medication after the procedure, when using small-diameter needles. Needles with a smaller diameter are also normally used to reduce the risk of PLPH and to avoid blood contaminations, defined as >5/μL red blood cells in the first tube of CSF collected (Armon et al. 2005).

In diagnostic context, LPs are often performed with larger-gauge needles (20–22G), whereas for therapeutic purposes, the needles are more narrow (25–27G) (Ginosar et al. 2012; Boon et al. 2004).

Reasons for using large-bore spinal needles include the increased speed in obtaining CSF samples by passive flow and the shorter time required to equilibrate the CSF pressure, when using a manometer. For CSF pressure measurement, needles smaller than 22G (thus >22G) are not suitable. Moreover, it is not recommended to use the smallest needle available because more technical difficulties occur, leading to failures, and because the duration of the procedure will be prolonged through the slow flow with these small spine needles (Flaatten et al. 1989). On the other hand, large needles are also not preferred as they produce large dural perforations with a higher risk of PLPH and contaminations. Needles used in children are selected based on the same criteria used for adults as described above

In conclusion, a balance between the risk of PLPH, procedure duration, flow, and technical failure has to be considered for each patient individually (Turnbull

Table 4.2 Comparison between needle diameters in articles published between 1970 and 2014

Conclusion	Comparison between needle diameters (gauge)	Reasons for choosing a needle diameter	References
No difference in performance between needle sizes	20 vs. 22	= PLPH, traumatic tap incidence	Hammond et al. (2011)
	23 vs. 25	= PLPH, low back pain, attempts	Kim and Yoon (2011)
Large-bore needles are preferred	20 vs. 22	↓ Collection time, CSF pressure measurement	Ellis et al. (1992)
	22 vs. 25	↓ Leakage	Ready et al. (1989)
	25 vs. 29	↓ Collection time, failures, PLPH	Kokki and Hendolin (1996)
Small-bore needles are preferred	20 vs. 22	↓ PLPH, complaints, blood patch rates ↑ Collection time	Hatfield et al. (2008), Aamodt and Vedeler (2001), Muller et al. (1994), Kleyweg et al. (1998), Vilming et al. (2001)
	22 vs. 26	↓ PLPH, pain ↑ Practice	Wilkinson and Sellar (1991), Tourtellotte et al. (1972), Kaukinen et al. (1981)
	22 vs. 25	↓ PLPH interval, low back pain	Crock et al. (2014), Lowery and Oliver (2008)
	20 vs. 22 vs. 23	↓ PLPH	Kovanen and Sulkava (1986)
	22 vs. 24	↓ PLPH	Palmers et al. (2002)
	22 vs. 29	↓ PLPH, failures	McConaha et al. (1996)
	25 vs. 26 vs. 27	↓ PLPH, blood patch rates	Lambert et al. (1997)
	19 vs. 20 vs. 22	↓ PLPH	Flaatten et al. (1998)
	22 vs. 25 vs. 27		
Questionnaire to medical institutions, favors the small-needle type	20 vs. 22	↓ PLPH, costs	Tung (2013)
	22 vs. 24	↓ Complaints	Stendell et al. (2012)

PLPH post-lumbar puncture headache, = no difference, ↓ reduced/faster/less, ↑ more

and Shepherd 2003). The smallest needle as possible is recommended; however, longer sampling time and more failures should be taken into account for small-diameter needles, though with a reduced risk of PLPH, low back pain, and less discomfort. Nevertheless, in most centers, a 22G needle or larger needle diameter is used (Stendell et al. 2012; Birnbach et al. 2001). Once the practitioner is more confident, by often usage, the use of smaller needle types should be considered, which will lead to less failures and an easier procedure (Tung 2013).

Design of the Needle To date, different designs of needles are available; Quincke-type needles (Spinocan® and Yale™) are the standard needles with a cutting bevel and the orifice at the needle tip. Whitacre™, Sprotte®, Atraucan®, Pencan®, and Pajunk® needles are noncutting, pencil-point, or atraumatic needles (Fig. 4.1).

Cutting bevel needles are still the standard needles mostly used in practice, because of the disadvantages of the atraumatic needles, such as low CSF flow and longer sampling time, little availability of these needles, less practical experience, a high failure rate, and the fact that when using local anesthetics, due to the thick introducer needle that penetrates the skin, it cannot be felt as well as with the standard needles when the dura is penetrated (Tung 2013; Stendell et al. 2012; Birnbach et al. 2001; Moller et al. 2013; Sharma et al. 1995). Needle types were compared in 35 studies between 1970 and 2014 (Table 4.3). No difference was reported in two studies (Quincke vs. Whitacre™) by comparing transdural fluid leakage and vascular trauma associated with blood contamination in CSF (Ready et al. 1989; Knowles et al. 1999). Three studies investigated the incidence of post-LP complications, such as PLPH and low back pain, and found no differences for all comparisons (Yale™ vs. Sprotte®, Spinocan® vs. Whitacre™, Quincke vs. an atraumatic needle type) (Aamodt and Vedeler 2001; Lenaerts et al. 1993; Luostarinen et al. 2005).

Nevertheless, in the 35 published articles, most studies recommended atraumatic needles as the best needle to perform LPs, when different needle types were compared (Table 4.3) (Alcolea et al. 2014; Hatfield et al. 2008; Lambert et al. 1997; Hammond et al. 2011; Muller et al. 1994; Kleyweg et al. 1998; Lowery and Oliver 2008; Palmers et al. 2002; Braune and Huffman 1992; Ohman et al. 1995; Strupp et al. 2001;

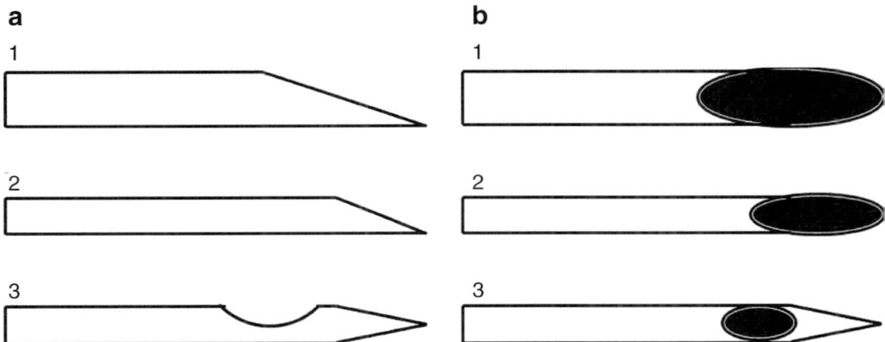

Fig. 4.1 Schematic representative of lateral (**a**) and superior (**b**) aspects of the tips of spinal needles. *1* standard large-bore beveled needle, *2* standard small-bore beveled needle, and *3* atraumatic small-bore needle

Table 4.3 Comparison between needle types in articles published between 1970 and 2014

Conclusion	Comparison between needle types	Reasons for choosing a needle type	Comments	References
Atraumatic needle favors compared to the cutting bevel needle	Quincke vs. Sprotte®	↓ PLPH, post complaints, nausea/vomiting, costs, medication, medical assistance, traumatic taps ↑ Training	Atraumatic needles less available. CSF IgM concentration is same as in serum	Hammond et al. (2011), Muller et al. (1994), Braune and Huffmann (1992), Ohman et al. (1995), Strupp et al. (2001), Tung et al. (2012), Vakharia and Lote (2012), Davis et al. (2014)
	Quincke vs. Whitacre™	↓ PLPH, post complaints, blood patch rates		Alcolea et al. (2014), Hatfield et al. (2008), Lambert et al. (1997), Pedersen (1996), Kokki et al. (1999), Lavi et al. (2006, 2007)
	Quincke vs. Sprotte® vs. Whitacre™	↓ PLPH	Minor epithelial cells, fewer and smaller cell clusters attached to needle	Puolakka et al. (2000), Quinn et al. (2013)
	Quincke vs. Spinocan® Sprotte vs. Whitacre	↓ PLPH		Carson and Serpell (1996)
	Quincke vs. Sprotte® vs. Pajunk®	↓ PLPH, ↑ failure rate		Thomas et al. (2000)
	Quincke vs. Pencan®	↓ PLPH, low back pain	Interval of PLPH is reduced	Lowery and Oliver (2008)
	Yale™ vs. Pencan®	↓ PLPH		Kokki et al. (2000)
Questionnaire to medical institutions, favors the atraumatic needle type	Quincke vs. Sprotte®	↓ PLPH, costs ↑ Practice, training		Tung (2013)

No difference in performance between needle types	Quincke vs. Whitacre™	= In RBC count, leakage		Ready et al. (1989), Knowles et al. (1999)
	Yale™ vs. Sprotte®	= PLPH, traumatic tap	Incidence of PLPH and traumatic tap is the same for both needle types	Lenaerts et al. (1993)
	Spinocan® vs. Whitacre™	= PLPH, low back pain	Incidence of PLPH and low back pain is the same for both needle types	Luostarinen et al. (2005)

PLPH post-lumbar puncture headache, *RBC* red blood cell, = no difference, ↓ reduced, ↑ more

Tung et al. 2012; Vakharia and Lote 2012; Davis et al. 2014; Pedersen 1996; Kokki et al. 1999; Lavi et al. 2007; Lavi et al. 2006; Puolakka et al. 2000; Quinn et al. 2013; Carson and Serpell 1996; Thomas et al. 2000; Kokki et al. 2000; Reynolds and O'Sullivan 1998; Dakka et al. 2011; Vidoni et al. 2014). Advantages of the atraumatic needles are a lower incidence of PLPH, low back pain, and nausea/vomiting than cutting bevel needles, which consequently reduce healthcare costs as less medication and medical assistance, such as blood patches, are needed after the procedure (Cruickshank and Hopkinson 1989). Furthermore, lower incidence in traumatic taps is described when atraumatic needles are used; however, more attempts and failures are reported for these needle types. No exact data is available concerning other post-LP complaints than PLPH, number of traumatic taps, or failures. The technical drawbacks of atraumatic needles can be overcome with more training, also within practice, and likewise, several authors conclude that the disadvantages seem less decisive if the reduced risk of PLPH and, therewith, the time and cost savings for the healthcare system are taken into account (Strupp et al. 2001; Tung et al. 2012; Linker et al. 2002; Peskind et al. 2005; Arendt et al. 2009), which especially holds true for younger patients who have a higher risk of PLPH than the elderly.

Conclusion In conclusion, head-to-head studies are in favor of atraumatic-type and small-diameter needles with regard to the lower incidence of PLPH. Recently published consensus-based recommendations for preanalytical issues on AD and Parkinson's disease (PD) CSF biomarker analysis recommend to use 25G atraumatic needles (del Campo et al. 2012). However, at least in Europe, many centers keep using small to medium cutting bevel-type needles, arguing that a higher CSF flow and, thus, shorter sampling time with a lower failure rate are important, with still very acceptable complication rates. Nevertheless, 25G atraumatic needles are recommended based on the JPND (the EU Joint Programme – Neurodegenerative Disease Research) "BIOMARKAPD" consortium on the standardization and harmonization of biomarkers for AD and PD (Engelborghs et al. submitted).

4.1.2.2 Complementary Equipment That Guide the LP Procedure

Difficulties in CSF sampling can occur, such as hemorrhagic CSF in case of a traumatic LP or a misplaced needle due to incorrect estimation of the anatomical landmarks in case of obese patients or spinal malformations. A standard LP procedure is mostly successful; nevertheless, in some patients, the execution of the technique is difficult. Alternatives to surface landmark-guided LP are fluoroscopy and ultrasound guidance (Table 4.4).

Table 4.4 Advantages and disadvantages of equipment that guide the LP procedure

Type of equipment	Advantages	Disadvantages
Fluoroscopy	Real time, less traumatic taps due to a single pass of the needle	Radiation exposure and requirement of a radiologist
Ultrasound	More certainty and no radiation	Not real time, asset is inversely related to BMI

BMI body mass index

Fluoroscopy shows the bone structures of the lumbar spine and provides real-time information about the precise position of the needle as it is being inserted (Eskey and Ogilvy 2001). During fluoroscopy, it is almost always possible to access the subarachnoid space with a single pass of the needle, whereas LPs at bedside rely on manual and mental estimation of the bone anatomy to guide the needle. While fluoroscopy is rarely needed to access the subarachnoid space with a spinal needle, it is routinely used for difficult cases in which bedside LP has failed. Traumatic taps are reduced by minimizing disruption of vascular structures, which is best accomplished by accessing the subarachnoid space with a single pass of the needle and avoiding the anterior epidural venous plexus entirely; this is easily done with the use of fluoroscopy. Disadvantages of this technique are the radiation exposure for the patient and the requirement of a radiologist to perform the procedure. To avoid these problems of fluoroscopy, ultrasound can be used to identify pertinent landmarks in those patients whose anatomical structures are difficult to palpate or whose body mass index (BMI) is in the obese category (Stiffler et al. 2007). Ultrasound may thus provide enough information to allow the physician to proceed with more certainty. However, the asset of this technique is inversely related to the patient's BMI, and ultrasound is often used before the actual LP takes place and, thus, not in real time.

4.2   Contraindications

An LP is an extremely safe procedure when performed by an experienced or properly supervised practitioner using standard methods. Nevertheless, contraindications can appear due to fluid shifts and pressure gradient changes between CNS compartments.

Lowering of the spinal compartment pressure, by removal of CSF, can cause a caudal shift of the transtentorial or tonsillar structures from their normal position, referred to as a CNS herniation (Sinclair et al. 2009). For this reason, all patients undergoing an LP have, theoretically, a risk of cerebral herniation. In patients with normal intracranial anatomy and pressure, this risk is negligible. However, by performing an LP in patients with abnormal ICP, the lumbar CSF pressure is lowered further, allowing the raised pressure compartment above the puncture site to move along the pressure gradient and consequently cause herniation. This is different from uniformly raised ICP within the whole CNS compartment, e.g., idiopathic intracranial hypertension, where no internal pressure gradient has developed and where it is safe to perform an LP.

While structural brain imaging frequently eliminates the need for diagnostic LP by providing a firm diagnosis, such as subarachnoid hemorrhage or brain tumor, indications for diagnostic LP still remain, such as suspected bacterial, viral, or carcinomatous meningitis and meningoencephalitis, suspected subarachnoid hemorrhage in case of negative structural imaging of the brain, AD and related disorders, atypical multiple sclerosis (Stangel et al. 2013), and suspected spinal cord compression from metastatic diseases requiring myelography (Gower et al. 1987; Engelborghs 2013). For these indications, drug administration, and other diagnostic purposes, the LP is contraindicated if the risk of the procedure outweighs the potential benefit. In practice, a brain computed tomography (CT) or MRI scan is always performed prior to LP if a patient is over the age of 60 years, or immunocompromised, or has a previous CNS disease, any recent seizures, reduced consciousness, papilledema, or an abnormal neurological examination. This is why, in many centers, it is routine to perform brain imaging before an LP to exclude potential risks. In some circumstances requiring urgent medical care, the physician can decide to perform a fundoscopy only in order to rule out papilledema before proceeding to LP.

The following CT criteria should be considered as a contraindication, while they can be applied for MRI imaging too. However, it should be emphasized that imaging appearances should always be put in context of the individual case (Hasbun et al. 2001; Gopal et al. 1999).

- CT evidence of unequal pressures across the falx cerebri
  Unequal supratentorial pressures are found by lateral shift of the midline structures (septum pellucidum, third ventricle, pineal gland). Asymmetry of the lateral ventricles alone is not an accurate sign, since ipsilateral ventricular dilation may occur secondary to stroke, or coaptation of a frontal horn may represent a normal anatomical variant. Result of LP of unequal supratentorial pressures would most likely lead to compression of the ipsilateral temporal lobe, leading to an uncal herniation.
- CT evidence of unequal pressures between the supratentorial and infratentorial compartments
  Two increased pressure types may be detected: the elevated pressure upward to the tentorium, pushing structures into the posterior fossa, and the elevated pressure caudal to the tentorium, pushing structures upward as well as through the foramen magnum. Decompression of the spine and posterior fossa compartments by LP may cause the medial temporal lobes to impact into the tentorial hiatus bilaterally (bilateral uncal herniation).

The most important contraindication to LP is a posterior fossa mass. Increase of pressure in this region may move the cerebellar tonsils into the region of the foramen magnum, predisposing the patient to tonsillar herniation, even when only a small amount of CSF is removed.

Other contraindications can appear at the site of the LP, such as local infections at the puncture site, congenital abnormalities, and uncorrected bleeding diathesis. Needle puncture through infected tissue prior to entry into the arachnoid space could allow infective organisms a direct route of entry into an otherwise sterile compartment. This increases the risk of CNS infection and reduces the diagnostic validity in case of suspected CNS infection. Another contraindication described is the risk of hemorrhage and spinal hematoma formation. To minimize the risk of spinal hematoma, it is recommended that prior to LP, platelet count (should be above 40×10^9/L) and coagulation status are checked and that increased bleeding risk is excluded (e.g. coagulopathy, uncorrected bleeding diathesis, anticoagulant medication). Where possible, drugs affecting coagulation should be discontinued to allow the coagulation profile to normalize to minimize hemorrhagic risks, although the risk of discontinuation and consequent risk of thrombosis need to be considered (Keeling et al. 2011). The use of antiplatelet drugs is only a very relative and weak contraindication to perform LP, and many centers perform LPs routinely in patients treated with antiplatelet drugs. Therefore, it is assumed that an LP can be safely performed in patients taking antiplatelet drugs.

4.3   Complications

The LP procedure is easy to perform by an experienced physician with proper understanding of the anatomical implications and results in low risks of complications. The most common complaint after an LP is PLPH; other infrequent complications include infections, local hematomas, pain, and local discomfort (Table 4.5). Due to precautions (like pre-LP brain imaging; see Sect. 4.2), the risk of CNS herniation is a theoretical risk. Also, the development of a post-LP subdural hematoma is extremely rare (Duffy 1969). Nevertheless, a traumatic tap, difficulties in finding landmarks, and even a successful procedure can result in an intraspinal epidermoid tumor due to introducing epithelial cells into the spinal canal because of wrong use of the stylet (McDonald and Klump 1986). Rare cases of retroperitoneal abscess produced by dural laceration in a patient with meningitis have been reported (Levine et al. 1982). Lastly, hypoxia and ventilation-perfusion mismatches due to a long period of flexion of the neck which obstructs the airway in children are reported in some rare cases (Gleason et al. 1983).

Currently, the Alzheimer's Association multicenter study on LP feasibility is running. This global and multicenter study aims to establish the incidence of PLPH and other complications in patients admitted for cognitive disturbances. The study is powered to allow evaluation of factors influencing complications, including both patient-related (age, history of headache, cognitive status, and psychological factors) and procedure-related (needle type and size, number of LP attempts, active vs. passive withdrawal of CSF, positioning of the patient during LP, local anesthesia, volume of CSF withdrawn, and bed rest after LP) factors. Preliminary data have led to consensus recommendations that are in line with those described in this chapter (Duits et al. submitted; Engelborghs et al. submitted).

Table 4.5 Prevalence of complications after LP

Complications	Prevalence (%)	References
PLPH	1–40	Strupp et al. (2001), Linker et al. (2002), Evans et al. (2000), Boonmak and Boonmak (2010)
Back pain	16	Alcolea et al. (2014)
Infection	<0.01	Baer (2006), van de Beek et al. (2010)
Spinal hematoma	<0.01	Dakka et al. (2011), Zetterberg et al. (2010)

PLPH post-lumbar puncture headache

4.3.1 Post-LP Headache

PLPH is the most common complication of LP, ranging between 1 and 40 % depending on needle type and patient population (Strupp et al. 2001; Linker et al. 2002; Evans et al. 2000; Boonmak and Boonmak 2010). In the majority of patients, the headache occurs within 3 days after the procedure, and in 66 % of patients suffering from PLPH, it starts within the first 48 h (Leibold et al. 1993). Rarely, PLPH develops either between 5 and 14 days or immediately after the LP. The location of PLPH varies, but it most commonly radiates from the frontal and occipital areas to the neck and shoulders. PLPH mostly has a moderate to severe intensity and worsens by head movement, upright posture, and Valsalva maneuvers. The pain can be relieved by lying down, which is often also recommended directly after an LP to mitigate the chance of developing a low-pressure headache. However, there is no evidence to suggest a benefit of this approach (Duits et al. submitted; Vilming et al. 1988; Dieterich and Brandt 1985; Handler et al. 1982; Winsvold et al. 2011; Arevalo-Rodriguez et al. 2013). Sometimes PLPH is accompanied by transient symptoms as nausea, vomiting, vertigo, hearing loss, tinnitus, dizziness, upper and lower limb pain, and visual disturbances.

PLPH is thought to be caused by faster leakage of CSF through the dural puncture site into the epidural and paravertebral spaces than it can be compensated by its production rate (Tourtellotte et al. 1972). Consequently, excess loss of CSF leads to intracranial hypotension and an absolute reduction of CSF volume below the cisterna magna with resultant downward movement of the brain and traction on pain-sensitive structures in the cranial cavity (Raskin 1990; Grant et al. 1991).

Risk factors for PLPH are female sex (Muller et al. 1994; Kleyweg et al. 1998; Vilming et al. 2001; Tourtellotte et al. 1972; Crock et al. 2014), younger age (<60, but not often found in children <18) (Alcolea et al. 2014; Muller et al. 1994; Dakka et al. 2011; Vidoni, et al. 2014; Zetterberg et al. 2010; Bolder 1986; Wee et al. 1996; Janssens et al. 2003), lower BMI (<25 kg/m^2) (Muller et al. 1994; Lavi et al. 2006; de Almeida et al. 2011), sitting position during LP, standard cutting bevel needle type compared to atraumatic needle of same size (see Sect. 4.1.2.1), multiple punctures, use of anticoagulants, and large needle bore (see Sect. 4.1.2.1) (Boon et al. 2004). No negative association between PLPH and cognitive dysfunction or dementia with cerebral atrophy or larger CSF spaces has been demonstrated, although PLPH occurs significantly less frequent in elderly as compared to adolescents and adults (Zetterberg et al. 2010). Three independent studies have shown that the prevalence of PLPH is systematically less than 5 % in the elderly (Zetterberg et al. 2010; Andreasen et al. 2001; Blennow et al. 1993). This suggests that PLPH is associated with factors related to aging, such as lower pain sensitivity, more rigid dural fibers or arteriosclerotic vessels, and possibly also to a lower degree of anxiety regarding the procedure. Importantly, PLPH incidence is not related to volume of CSF withdrawal (Duits et al. submitted; Grant et al. 1991; Kuntz et al. 1992).

Treatment for PLPH Conservative treatment for PLPH consists of bed rest, analgesics, and adequate hydration, as it is mostly a self-limiting headache. When conservative management fails, the aims of treatment of PLPH are to replace the lost CSF, seal the puncture site, and control the cerebral vasodilatation. Therefore, in case of persistent and severe PLPH, epidural blood patches are used with high success rates and low incidence of complications (van Kooten et al. 2008).

A blood patch consists of injecting the patient's own blood into the epidural space at the level of the original LP, where the blood will clot and occlude the perforations, preventing further CSF leak. There is no consensus on the precise volume of blood required. Likely, 20–30 mL is successful, whereas lower volumes are inadequate (Turnbull and Shepherd 2003). After injection, the blood distributes caudally and cranially and passes circumferentially around the anterior epidural space, hereby compressing the thecal space, and additionally, the blood passes out of the intervertebral foramina and into the paravertebral spaces. During the procedure, it is preferred to avoid advancing the needle through the dura, as this additional dural puncture may prolong the intracranial hypotension. If the patient describes lancinating pain of dermatomal origin, the procedure should be stopped.

Symptoms typically improve within a few hours after the blood patch is applied. Still, it is recommended that patients lie recumbent for at least 2 h before mobilizing; this is to avoid movement of the epidural blood (Martin et al. 1994). If symptoms do not improve within two days, it is likely that the procedure has failed, either due to using the wrong location, incomplete dispersing of the blood within the epidural space to the puncture site, or creating a further additional dural puncture. In such cases, MRI of the spine should be performed to ensure the correct CSF leaking site has been identified, which however may be more difficult after a blood patch.

Other therapeutic agents also exist to prevent PLPH; however, due to the lack of large, randomized, controlled clinical trials, blood patches are the gold standard (Turnbull and Shepherd 2003; van Kooten et al. 2008).

4.3.2 Infection

Post-LP infections, such as meningitis or local infections at the LP site, are uncommon. However, if infections occur, they are mostly due to accidental contamination. Potential routes of infection include from practitioner's hands, from patient's skin, or through aerosolization of organisms from the practitioner's mouth. Appropriate antimicrobial therapy depends on local hospital guidelines and should be discussed with the microbiologists.

4.3.3 Local Discomfort, Radicular Pain, and Pain Referred to the Limb

Post-LP discomfort at the puncture site is common and could be minimized by using small-diameter-bore needles and/or atraumatic needles with a single successful attempt (see Sect. 4.1.2.1) (Wright et al. 2012). Moreover, a maximum of four LP attempts is probably still acceptable (Engelborghs et al. submitted). The pain should settle promptly, within a couple of hours. However, if the pain is more severe or persistent, further investigation of possible hematoma formation (see Sect. 4.3.4) or local infection (see Sect. 4.3.2) is required. Although persistent radicular pain is infrequent, pain referred to the limb could occur if a nerve root has been damaged. By avoiding negative pressure, through withdrawal with a syringe (attached to the needle) or when an anesthetic solution is injected, the risk of nerve injury is reduced. Moreover, negative pressure may pull a spinal nerve root against the needle tip and produce paresthesia, pain, or nerve injury. Treatment for discomfort and pain depends on the severity of the complication.

4.3.4　Spinal Hematoma

A spinal hematoma occurs rarely but could cause spinal cord or cauda equina compression. The physician should be alert for the possibility of hemorrhage if post-LP the patient develops severe, persistent back pain or radicular pain, new sensory or motor symptoms, sphincter disturbance, or meningism (Sinclair et al. 2009). Spinal hematomas typically present within the first 6 h after the LP, although in 22 % of cases, it appears after 24 h. A spinal MRI scan may be indicated. Blood sampling with platelet count should be repeated, and antiplatelet or anticoagulant medications should not be restarted. Conservative treatment could be applied if the symptoms are mild and there are early signs of neurological recovery, whereas in more severe cases or when the patient deteriorates, surgical evacuation of the hematoma could be required.

4.4　　Conclusions and Recommendations

LP is a viable therapeutic technique and a common diagnostic procedure, which, if performed correctly, has a low complication rate, a high diagnostic yield, and is usually more tolerable than patients expect. The most important contraindication to perform an LP is a posterior fossa mass and intracranial hypertension, given the risk of CNS or tonsillar herniation. To perform an LP, the optimal length, size, and type of needle should be used, which may differ according to the medical indication. PLPH is the most common complication of LP, with an incidence ranging between 1 and 40 %, depending on needle type and patient population. Head-to-head studies are in favor of atraumatic and small-diameter needles, given the lower incidence of post-LP complaints. However, regardless of needle type, frequency of severe complications is very low; hence, small- to medium-diameter cutting bevel-type needles can be used with good confidence. For more detailed guidelines, we refer to the consensus-based guidelines of the JPND "BIOMARKAPD" consortium on the standardization and harmonization of biomarkers for AD and PD (Engelborghs et al. submitted).

Acknowledgments This work was supported by the University of Antwerp Research Fund; the Alzheimer Research Foundation (SAO-FRA); the Research Foundation Flanders (FWO); the Agency for Innovation by Science and Technology (IWT); the Belgian Science Policy Office

Interuniversity Attraction Poles (IAP) program; and the Flemish Government initiated Methusalem excellence grant, Belgium.

This is an EU Joint Programme – Neurodegenerative Disease Research (JPND) project, which is supported through the following funding organization under the aegis of JPND: ZonMw (the Netherlands).

References

Aamodt A, Vedeler C (2001) Complications after LP related to needle type: pencil-point versus Quincke. Acta Neurol Scand 103(6):396–398

Abrahams PH, Webb P (1975) Clinical anatomy of practical procedures. Pitman Medical, London, pp 13–15

Adams RD, Maurice V, Ropper AH (1997) Principles of neurology, 6th edn. McGraw-Hill, New York, pp 13–14

Alcolea D, Martinez-Lage P, Izagirre A, Clerigue M, Carmona-Iragui M, Alvarez RM et al (2014) Feasibility of lumbar puncture in the study of cerebrospinal fluid biomarkers for Alzheimer's disease: a multicenter study in Spain. J Alzheimers Dis 39(4):719–726

American Association of Clinical Anatomists EAC (1999) The clinical anatomy of several invasive procedures. Clin Anat 12:43–54

Andreasen N, Minthon L, Davidsson P, Vanmechelen E, Vanderstichele H, Winblad B et al (2001) Evaluation of CSF-tau and CSF-Abeta42 as diagnostic markers for Alzheimer disease in clinical practice. Arch Neurol 58(3):373–379

Arendt K, Demaerschalk BM, Wingerchuk DM, Camann W (2009) Atraumatic lumbar puncture needles: after all these years, are we still missing the point? Neurologist 15(1):17–20

Arevalo-Rodriguez I, Pedraza OL, Rodriguez A, Sanchez E, Gich I, Sola I et al (2013) Alzheimer's disease dementia guidelines for diagnostic testing: a systematic review. Am J Alzheimers Dis Other Demen 28(2):111–119

Armon C, Evans RW, Therapeutics, Technology Assessment Subcommittee of the American Academy of N (2005) Addendum to assessment: prevention of post-lumbar puncture headaches: report of the Therapeutics and Technology Assessment Subcommittee of the American Academy of Neurology. Neurology 65(4):510–512

Baer ET (2006) Post-dural puncture bacterial meningitis. Anesthesiology 105(2):381–393

Beresford HR (1980) Informed consent before lumbar puncture. N Engl J Med 303(26):1534

Birnbach DJ, Kuroda MM, Sternman D, Thys DM (2001) Use of atraumatic spinal needles among neurologists in the United States. Headache 41(4):385–390

Blennow K, Wallin A, Hager O (1993) Low frequency of post-lumbar puncture headache in demented patients. Acta Neurol Scand 88(3):221–223

Bolder PM (1986) Postlumbar puncture headache in pediatric oncology patients. Anesthesiology 65(6):696–698

Boon JM, Abrahams PH, Meiring JH, Welch T (2004) Lumbar puncture: anatomical review of a clinical skill. Clin Anat 17(7):544–553

Boonmak P, Boonmak S (2010) Epidural blood patching for preventing and treating post-dural puncture headache. Cochrane Database Syst Rev (1):CD001791

Braune HJ, Huffmann GA (1992) A prospective double-blind clinical trial, comparing the sharp Quincke needle (22G) with an "atraumatic" needle (22G) in the induction of post-lumbar puncture headache. Acta Neurol Scand 86(1):50–54

Carson D, Serpell M (1996) Choosing the best needle for diagnostic lumbar puncture. Neurology 47(1):33–37

Crock C, Orsini F, Lee KJ, Phillips RJ (2014) Headache after lumbar puncture: randomised crossover trial of 22-gauge versus 25-gauge needles. Arch Dis Child 99(3):203–207

Cruickshank R, Hopkinson J (1989) Fluid flow through dural puncture sites. Anaesthesia 44(5):415–418

Dakka Y, Warra N, Albadareen RJ, Jankowski M, Silver B (2011) Headache rate and cost of care following lumbar puncture at a single tertiary care hospital. Neurology 77(1):71–74

Davis A, Dobson R, Kaninia S, Espasandin M, Berg A, Giovannoni G et al (2014) Change practice now! Using atraumatic needles to prevent post lumbar puncture headache. Eur J Neurol 21(2):305–311

de Almeida SM, Shumaker SD, LeBlanc SK, Delaney P, Marquie-Beck J, Ueland S et al (2011) Incidence of post-dural puncture headache in research volunteers. Headache 51(10):1503–1510

del Campo M, Mollenhauer B, Bertolotto A, Engelborghs S, Hampel H, Simonsen AH et al (2012) Recommendations to standardize preanalytical confounding factors in Alzheimer's and Parkinson's disease cerebrospinal fluid biomarkers: an update. Biomark Med 6(4):419–430

Dieterich M, Brandt T (1985) Is obligatory bed rest after lumbar puncture obsolete? Eur Arch Psychiatry Neurol Sci 235(2):71–75

Duffy GP (1969) Lumbar puncture in the presence of raised intracranial pressure. Br Med J 1(5641):407–409

Duits FH, Martinez-Lage P, Paquet C, Engelborghs S, Lleo A, Hausner L et al (submitted) Performance and complications of lumbar puncture in memory clinics: results of a multicenter study. JAMA Neurol

Ellis H, Feldman S (1997) Anatomy for anesthetists, 7th edn. Blackwell Science, Oxford, pp 108–112

Ellis RW 3rd, Strauss LC, Wiley JM, Killmond TM, Ellis RW Jr (1992) A simple method of estimating cerebrospinal fluid pressure during lumbar puncture. Pediatrics 89(5 Pt 1):895–897

Engelborghs S (2013) Clinical indications for analysis of Alzheimer's disease CSF biomarkers. Rev Neurol (Paris) 169(10):709–714

Engelborghs S, Niemantsverdriet E, Struyfs H, Duits F, Teunissen C (submitted) Consensus guidelines to perform lumbar puncture for CSF sampling in neurological patients. Lancet Neurol

Eskey CJ, Ogilvy CS (2001) Fluoroscopy-guided lumbar puncture: decreased frequency of traumatic tap and implications for the assessment of CT-negative acute subarachnoid hemorrhage. AJNR Am J Neuroradiol 22(3):571–576

Evans RW, Armon C, Frohman EM, Goodin DS (2000) Assessment: prevention of post-lumbar puncture headaches: report of the therapeutics and technology assessment subcommittee of the american academy of neurology. Neurology 55(7):909–914

Flaatten H, Rodt SA, Vamnes J, Rosland J, Wisborg T, Koller ME (1989) Postdural puncture headache. A comparison between 26- and 29-gauge needles in young patients. Anaesthesia 44(2):147–149

Flaatten H, Krakenes J, Vedeler C (1998) Post-dural puncture related complications after diagnostic lumbar puncture, myelography and spinal anaesthesia. Acta Neurol Scand 98(6):445–451

Ginosar Y, Smith Y, Ben-Hur T, Lovett JM, Clements T, Ginosar YD et al (2012) Novel pulsatile cerebrospinal fluid model to assess pressure manometry and fluid sampling through spinal needles of different gauge: support for the use of a 22G spinal needle with a tapered 27G pencil-point tip. Br J Anaesth 108(2):308–315

Gleason CA, Martin RJ, Anderson JV, Carlo WA, Sanniti KJ, Fanaroff AA (1983) Optimal position for a spinal tap in preterm infants. Pediatrics 71(1):31–35

Gopal AK, Whitehouse JD, Simel DL, Corey GR (1999) Cranial computed tomography before lumbar puncture: a prospective clinical evaluation. Arch Intern Med 159(22):2681–2685

Gower DJ, Baker AL, Bell WO, Ball MR (1987) Contraindications to lumbar puncture as defined by computed cranial tomography. J Neurol Neurosurg Psychiatry 50(8):1071–1074

Grant R, Condon B, Hart I, Teasdale GM (1991) Changes in intracranial CSF volume after lumbar puncture and their relationship to post-LP headache. J Neurol Neurosurg Psychiatry 54(5):440–442

Hammond ER, Wang Z, Bhulani N, McArthur JC, Levy M (2011) Needle type and the risk of post-lumbar puncture headache in the outpatient neurology clinic. J Neurol Sci 306(1–2):24–28

Handler CE, Smith FR, Perkin GD, Rose FC (1982) Posture and lumbar puncture headache: a controlled trial in 50 patients. J R Soc Med 75(6):404–407

Hasbun R, Abrahams J, Jekel J, Quagliarello VJ (2001) Computed tomography of the head before lumbar puncture in adults with suspected meningitis. N Engl J Med 345(24):1727–1733

Hatfield MK, Handrich SJ, Willis JA, Beres RA, Zaleski GX (2008) Blood patch rates after lumbar puncture with Whitacre versus Quincke 22- and 20-gauge spinal needles. AJR Am J Roentgenol 190(6):1686–1689

Ievins FA (1991) Accuracy of placement of extradural needles in the L3-4 interspace: comparison of two methods of identifying L4. Br J Anaesth 66(3):381–382

Janssens E, Aerssens P, Alliet P, Gillis P Raes M (2003) Post-dural puncture headaches in children. A literature review. Eur J Pediatr 162(3):117–121

Kaukinen S, Kaukinen L, Kannisto K, Kataja M (1981) The prevention of headache following spinal anaesthesia. Ann Chir Gynaecol 70(3):107–111

Keeling D, Baglin T, Tait C, Watson H, Perry D, Baglin C et al (2011) Guidelines on oral anticoagulation with warfarin – fourth edition. Br J Haematol 154(3):311–324

Kim M, Yoon H (2011) Comparison of post-dural puncture headache and low back pain between 23 and 25 gauge Quincke spinal needles in patients over 60 years: randomized, double-blind controlled trial. Int J Nurs Stud 48(11):1315–1322

Kleyweg RP, Hertzberger LI, Carbaat PA (1998) Significant reduction in post-lumbar puncture headache using an atraumatic needle. A double-blind, controlled clinical trial. Cephalalgia 18(9):635–637

Knowles PR, Randall NP, Lockhart AS (1999) Vascular trauma associated with routine spinal anaesthesia. Anaesthesia 54(7):647–650

Kokki H, Hendolin H (1996) Comparison of 25 G and 29 G Quincke spinal needles in paediatric day case surgery. A prospective randomized study of the puncture characteristics, success rate and postoperative complaints. Paediatr Anaesth 6(2):115–119

Kokki H, Salonvaara M, Herrgard E, Onen P (1999) Postdural puncture headache is not an age-related symptom in children: a prospective, open-randomized, parallel group study comparing a22-gauge Quincke with a 22-gauge Whitacre needle. Paediatr Anaesth 9(5):429–434

Kokki H, Heikkinen M, Turunen M, Vanamo K, Hendolin H (2000) Needle design does not affect the success rate of spinal anaesthesia or the incidence of postpuncture complications in children. Acta Anaesthesiol Scand 44(2):210–213

Kovanen J, Sulkava R (1986) Duration of postural headache after lumbar puncture: effect of needle size. Headache 26(5):224–226

Kuntz KM, Kokmen E, Stevens JC, Miller P, Offord KP, Ho MM (1992) Post-lumbar puncture headaches: experience in 501 consecutive procedures. Neurology 42(10):1884–1887

Lambert DH, Hurley RJ, Hertwig L, Datta S (1997) Role of needle gauge and tip configuration in the production of lumbar puncture headache. Reg Anesth 22(1):66–72

Lavi R, Yarnitsky D, Rowe JM, Weissman A, Segal D, Avivi I (2006) Standard vs atraumatic Whitacre needle for diagnostic lumbar puncture: a randomized trial. Neurology 67(8):1492–1494

Lavi R, Rowe JM, Avivi I (2007) Traumatic vs. atraumatic 22 G needle for therapeutic and diagnostic lumbar puncture in the hematologic patient: a prospective clinical trial. Haematologica 92(7):1007–1008

Leibold RA, Yealy DM, Coppola M, Cantees KK (1993) Post-dural-puncture headache: characteristics, management, and prevention. Ann Emerg Med 22(12):1863–1870

Lenaerts M, Pepin JL, Tombu S, Schoenen J (1993) No significant effect of an "atraumatic" needle on incidence of post-lumbar puncture headache or traumatic tap. Cephalalgia 13(4):296–297

Levine JF, Hiesiger EM, Whelan MA, Pollock AA, Simbekoff MS, Rahal JJ Jr (1982) Pneumococcal meningitis associated with retroperitoneal abscess. A rare complication of lumbar puncture. JAMA 248(18):2308–2309

Linker G, Mirza N, Manetti G, Meyer M, Putnam K, Sunderland T (2002) Fine-needle, negative-pressure lumbar puncture: a safe technique for collecting CSF. Neurology 59(12):2008–2009

Lowery S, Oliver A (2008) Incidence of postdural puncture headache and backache following diagnostic/therapeutic lumbar puncture using a 22G cutting spinal needle, and after introduction of a 25G pencil point spinal needle. Paediatr Anaesth 18(3):230–234

Luostarinen L, Heinonen T, Luostarinen M, Salmivaara A (2005) Diagnostic lumbar puncture. Comparative study between 22-gauge pencil point and sharp bevel needle. J Headache Pain 6(5):400–404

Martin R, Jourdain S, Clairoux M, Tetrault JP (1994) Duration of decubitus position after epidural blood patch. Can J Anaesth 41(1):23–25

McConaha C, Bastiani AM, Kaye WH (1996) Significant reduction of post-lumbar puncture headaches by the use of a 29-gauge spinal needle. Biol Psychiatry 39(12):1058–1060

McDonald JV, Klump TE (1986) Intraspinal epidermoid tumors caused by lumbar puncture. Arch Neurol 43(9):936–939

Moller A, Afshari A, Bjerrum OW (2013) Diagnostic and therapeutic lumbar puncture performed safely and efficiently with a thin blunt needle. Dan Med J 60(9):A4684

Muller B, Adelt K, Reichmann H, Toyka K (1994) Atraumatic needle reduces the incidence of post-lumbar puncture syndrome. J Neurol 241(6):376–380

Ohman S, Ernerudh J, Forsberg P, Roberg M, Vrethem M (1995) Lower values for immunoglobulin M in cerebrospinal fluid when sampled with an atraumatic Sprotte needle compared with conventional lumbar puncture. Ann Clin Biochem 32(Pt 2):210–212

Palmers Y, Kuhn FP, Petersen D, De Greef D (2002) Comparison in myelography between iodixanol 270 and 320 mgI/ml and iotrolan 300 mgI/ml: a multicentre, randomised, parallel-group, double-blind, phase III trial. Eur Radiol 12(3):686–691

Pedersen ON (1996) Use of a 22-gauge Whitacre needle to reduce the incidence of side effects after lumbar myelography: a prospective randomised study comparing Whitacre and Quincke spinal needles. Eur Radiol 6(2):184–187

Peskind ER, Riekse R, Quinn JF, Kaye J, Clark CM, Farlow MR et al (2005) Safety and acceptability of the research lumbar puncture. Alzheimer Dis Assoc Dis 19(4):220–225

Puolakka R, Andersson LC, Rosenberg PH (2000) Microscopic analysis of three different spinal needle tips after experimental subarachnoid puncture. Reg Anesth Pain Med 25(2):163–169

Quincke H (1891) Die lumbarpunktion des hydrocephalus. Klin Wochenschr 28(929–33):65–68

Quinn C, Macklin EA, Atassi N, Bowser R, Boylan K, Cudkowicz M et al (2013) Post-lumbar puncture headache is reduced with use of atraumatic needles in ALS. Amyotroph Lateral Scler Frontotemporal Degener 14(7–8):632–634

Raskin NH (1990) Lumbar puncture headache: a review. Headache 30(4):197–200

Ready LB, Cuplin S, Haschke RH, Nessly M (1989) Spinal needle determinants of rate of transdural fluid leak. Anesth Analg 69(4):457–460

Reynolds F, O'Sullivan G (1998) Lumbar puncture and headache. "Atraumatic needle" is a better term than "blunt needle". BMJ 316(7136):1018

Sharma S, Gambling D, Joshi G, Sidawi J, Herrera E (1995) Comparison of 26-gauge Atraucan® and 25-gauge Whitacre needles: insertion characteristics and complications. Can J Anaesth 42(8):706–710

Sinclair AJ, Carroll C, Davies B (2009) Cauda equina syndrome following a lumbar puncture. J Clin Neurosci 16(5):714–716

Stangel M, Fredrikson S, Meinl E, Petzold A, Stuve O, Tumani H (2013) The utility of cerebrospinal fluid analysis in patients with multiple sclerosis. Nat Rev Neurol 9(5):267–276

Stendell L, Fomsgaard JS, Olsen KS (2012) There is room for improvement in the prevention and treatment of headache after lumbar puncture. Dan Med J 59(7):A4483

Stiffler KA, Jwayyed S, Wilber ST, Robinson A (2007) The use of ultrasound to identify pertinent landmarks for lumbar puncture. Am J Emerg Med 25(3):331–334

Strupp M, Schueler O, Straube A, Von Stuckrad-Barre S, Brandt T (2001) "Atraumatic" Sprotte needle reduces the incidence of post-lumbar puncture headaches. Neurology 57(12):2310–2312

Thomas SR, Jamieson DR, Muir KW (2000) Randomised controlled trial of atraumatic versus standard needles for diagnostic lumbar puncture. BMJ 321(7267):986–990

Tourtellotte WW, Henderson WG, Tucker RP, Gilland O, Walker JE, Kokman E (1972) A randomized, double-blind clinical trial comparing the 22 versus 26 gauge needle in the production of the post-lumbar puncture syndrome in normal individuals. Headache 12(2):73–78

Tung CE (2013) Education research: changing practice. Residents' adoption of the atraumatic lumbar puncture needle. Neurology 80(17):e180–e182

Tung CE, So YT, Lansberg MG (2012) Cost comparison between the atraumatic and cutting lumbar puncture needles. Neurology 78(2):109–113

Turnbull DK, Shepherd D (2003) Post-dural puncture headache: pathogenesis, prevention and treatment. Br J Anaesth 91(5):718–729

Vakharia VN, Lote H (2012) Introduction of Sprotte needles to a single-centre acute neurology service: before and after study. JRSM Short Rep 3(12):82

van de Beek D, Drake JM, Tunkel AR (2010) Nosocomial bacterial meningitis. N Engl J Med 362(2):146–154

Van Dellen JR, Bill PL (1978) Lumbar puncture – an innocuous diagnostic procedure? S Afr Med J 53(17):666–668

Van Kooten F, Oedit R, Bakker SL, Dippel DW (2008) Epidural blood patch in post dural puncture headache: a randomised, observer-blind, controlled clinical trial. J Neurol Neurosurg Psychiatry 79(5):553–558

Vidoni ED, Morris JK, Raider K, Burns JM, Alzheimer's Disease Neuroimaging I (2014) Reducing post-lumbar puncture headaches with small bore atraumatic needles. J Clin Neurosci 21(3):536–537

Vilming ST, Schrader H, Monstad I (1988) Post-lumbar-puncture headache: the significance of body posture. A controlled study of 300 patients. Cephalalgia 8(2):75–78

Vilming ST, Kloster R, Sandvik L (2001) The importance of sex, age, needle size, height and body mass index in post-lumbar puncture headache. Cephalalgia 21(7):738–743

Wee LH, Lam F, Cranston AJ (1996) The incidence of post dural puncture headache in children. Anaesthesia 51(12):1164–1166

Wilkinson AG, Sellar RJ (1991) The influence of needle size and other factors on the incidence of adverse effects caused by myelography. Clin Radiol 44(5):338–341

Winsvold BS, Hagen K, Aamodt AH, Stovner LJ, Holmen J, Zwart JA (2011) Headache, migraine and cardiovascular risk factors: the HUNT study. Eur J Neurol 18(3):504–511

Wright BL, Lai JT, Sinclair AJ (2012) Cerebrospinal fluid and lumbar puncture: a practical review. J Neurol 259(8):1530–1545

You JS, Gelfanova V, Knierman MD, Witzmann FA, Wang M, Hale JE (2005) The impact of blood contamination on the proteome of cerebrospinal fluid. Proteomics 5(1):290–296

Zetterberg H, Tullhog K, Hansson O, Minthon L, Londos E, Blennow K (2010) Low incidence of post-lumbar puncture headache in 1,089 consecutive memory clinic patients. Eur Neurol 63(6):326–330

Importance of Pre-analytical Stability for CSF Biomarker Testing

Eline A.J. Willemse and Charlotte E. Teunissen

Contents

E.A.J. Willemse
Neurochemistry Laboratory Department
of Clinical Chemistry and Alzheimer Center,
VU University Medical Center Amsterdam,
7057, Amsterdam 1007 MB, The Netherlands

C.E. Teunissen (✉)
Neurochemistry Laboratory and Biobank,
Department of Clinical Chemistry,
VU University Medical Center Amsterdam,
Amsterdam, The Netherlands
e-mail: c.teunissen@vumc.nl

© Springer International Publishing Switzerland 2015
F. Deisenhammer et al. (eds.), *Cerebrospinal Fluid in Clinical Neurology*,
DOI 10.1007/978-3-319-01225-4_5

Abstract

Variability in pre-analytical procedures is an important source of variation in laboratory medicine for diagnostics and research. The term "pre-analytical variation" is used to indicate variation in many aspects of the total biomarker analysis process, ranging from correct labeling of samples or patient misidentification, patient-related factors as dietary intake or circadian rhythm, and variation in the CSF collection processes, such as delayed processing or use of different tubes, to variation in assay performance.

We here describe pre-analytical factors that can affect CSF biomarkers and discuss the available literature. The effects of pre-analytical variability on CSF biomarker outcomes appear to differ between molecules and conditions and between laboratories. The current lack of extensive information precludes development of predictive models. Therefore, effects of pre-analytical variation need to be established in detail for every novel CSF biomarker. Moreover, quality indicators for CSF biomarkers need to be developed.

The awareness of this variation has been the basis for international consensus guidelines for pre-analytical procedures to minimize variation as presented in this chapter. These protocols have been implemented and adopted worldwide for diagnostic use of Alzheimer biomarkers and for long-term biobanking in diverse neurological diseases, including Alzheimer, multiple sclerosis, and amyotrophic lateral sclerosis.

5.1   Introduction

Pre-analytical variation can be an important source of variation in cerebrospinal fluid (CSF) biomarker analysis. In general, pre-analytical errors are known to account for 60 % of total laboratory errors (Plebani et al. 2014) and are relevant for both diagnostic and research settings. The term "pre-analytical variation" is used to indicate variation in many aspects of the total biomarker analysis process, ranging from patient-related factors and variation in the CSF collection process to variation in assay performance (Fig. 5.1). In this chapter, we describe pre-analytical factors that can affect CSF biomarkers specifically and discuss the available literature. We will expand largely on laboratory processing, to focus on CSF-specific effects and to carefully introduce the international consensus guidelines for CSF collection and biobanking. There are not many reports available in the literature addressing the effects of these issues specifically for CSF biomarkers. Nevertheless, the interest in the subject is

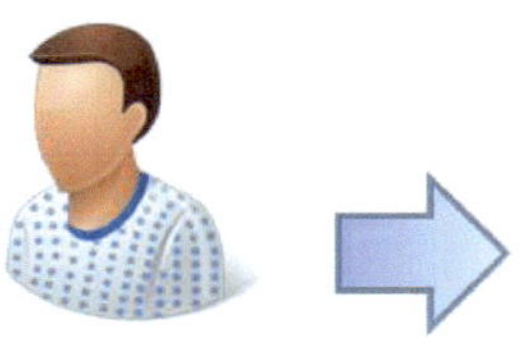
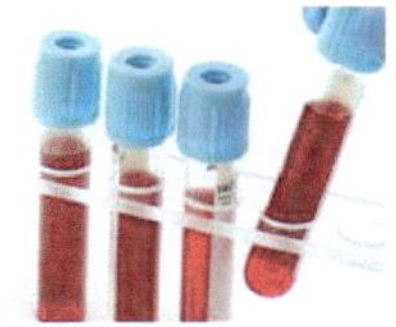

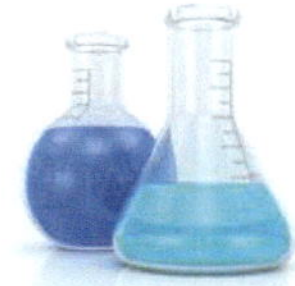

Fig. 5.1 Flowchart of pre-analytical steps in CSF analysis and common variability factors influencing outcome measures

increasing since several years due to several international initiatives to improve the (diagnostic) analysis of CSF biomarkers and long-term biobanking (del Campo et al. 2012; Otto et al. 2012; Teunissen et al. 2009, 2013, 2014; Vanderstichele et al. 2012).

To generate recommendations for pre-analytical procedures, a distinction can be made between analysis of a specific biomarker in the clinical diagnostic setting and biobanking for research purposes, where samples are usually stored to identify novel biomarkers with unknown pre-analytical specifics. To illustrate this, adding Tween-20 to a CSF sample prevents amyloid beta (Abeta)(1-42) peptides from absorbing to several lab plastic surfaces (Pica-Mendez et al. 2010). Adding Tween-20 will decrease pre-analytical variation in these samples when they are collected for amyloid determination only. On the other hand, they will be unserviceable to many other purposes, e.g., studies targeting potential new biomarkers, because Tween-20 might interact with CSF components or the assays. In biobanking practice, we therefore advise to not add any substance to CSF samples in order to avoid possible adverse effects.

Another major difference between routine analysis and biobanking for research purposes is the storage duration, which can be as short as one hour for routine tests which are often automated, including cell counts, protein concentration, and IgG index, up to 1 month for special tests as oligoclonal bands, IgG index in some settings, and Alzheimer biomarker analysis by ELISA. The value of a biobank in the research setting, in contrast, increases upon long-term follow-up of patients and when cohort sizes are allowed to increase. Thus, storage of material will be rather multiple years than months. Therefore, protocols for long-term biobanking purposes are more stringent and require storage at −80 °C.

One approach to reduce variation due to patient issues and laboratory processing is to standardize CSF collection protocols as much as possible, which has been addressed by several consortia in recent years. The current protocols are in the majority based on the initial consensus guideline of the BioMS consortium (Teunissen et al. 2009) that felt that the first step to improve the quality of biomarker studies and minimize variation between studies was to standardize the collection procedures. The most updated version of the protocol is presented in Table 5.1,

Table 5.1 Collection protocol for CSF and blood pairs for biobanking

Item no	Procedure	Ideal situation for CSF	Blood
A. Collection procedures			
1	Time of day of withdrawal and storage	Record date and time of collection	Same as for CSF
2	Preferred volume	At least 12 ml. First 1–2 ml for routine CSF assessment. Last 10 ml for biobanking	10 ml EDTA plasma, 10 ml serum
		Record volume taken and fraction used for biobanking, if applicable	
3	Location	Intervertebral space L3–L5(S1)	Venipuncture
4	If blood contamination occurred	Do not process further	Na
		Criteria for blood contamination: more than 500 red blood cells/μl	
		Record number of blood cells in diagnostic samples	
5	Type of needle	Atraumatic	Standard needles, e.g., 21–23 G
6	Type of collection tube	Polypropylene tubes, screw cap, volume >10 ml	For serum: no clotting activator or gel
			For EDTA plasma: no protease inhibitors
7	Other body fluids that should be collected simultaneously	Serum	Na
8	Other body fluids that should be collected simultaneously	Plasma: EDTA (preferred over citrate)	Na
B. Processing for storage			
9	Storage temperature until freezing	Room temperature before, during, and after centrifugation	Same as CSF
10	Centrifugation conditions	2,000 g (1,800–2,200), 10 min at room temperature. 400 g if cells are to be preserved	2,000 g (1,800–2,200), 10 min at room temperature
11	Time delay between withdrawal, processing, and freezing	Between 30 and 60 min. Max 2 h	Between 30 and 60 min. Max 2 h
		After centrifugation, samples should be aliquoted and frozen immediately, with a maximal delay of 2 h	Less than 1 h is optimal for proteomic discovery studies. Serum must clot minimal 30 min

12	Type of tube for aliquoting	Small polypropylene tubes (2 ml for routine diagnostics; 0.5 ml for biobanking) with screw caps. Record manufacturer	As CSF
13	Aliquoting	A minimum of two aliquots is recommended. The advised research sample volume of 10 ml should be enough for >10 aliquots	As CSF
14	Volume of aliquots	Minimum 0.1 ml. Depending on total volume of tube: 0.2, 0.5, and 1 ml. Preferably, the tubes are filled up to 75 % of the volume	As CSF
15	Coding	Unique codes. Freezing-proof labels. Ideally barcodes to facilitate searching, to aid in blinding the analysis, and to protect the privacy of patients	As CSF
16	Freezing temperature	−80 °C	As CSF

which includes a standardized protocol for blood collection as well. The idea behind the protocols is to standardize every aspect during the CSF process to minimize variation, even if the rationale for specific decisions cannot as yet be given due to lack of experimental data.

We used the framework of Fig. 5.1 to discuss effects of pre-analytical variation on CSF biomarker concentrations in the next paragraphs.

5.2 Patient-Related Factors

Patient misidentification or incorrect requesting are major sources of variation in laboratory settings and are not specific for CSF. These can be improved, e.g., by the introduction of electronic patient records and linkage of these systems to research databases. For example, one study reported a striking reduction of 80 % in errors, where major factors in which a reduction in errors was attained were the correct information on the sample tube (patient name, unique patient ID number, date of collection), the correct sample received, and the availability of a clinical history in primary care setting (Turner et al. 2013). The future of sample labeling in biobanking for research presumably lies in 2D barcoding, which will serve automated sample retrieving and picking, will further reduce mistakes, and facilitates research using pseudonymized samples.

5.2.1 Item 1 of Table 5.1: Time of the Day of Withdrawal and Storage

Patient-related pre-analytical factors also can influence biomarkers outcomes (Fig. 5.1). Such factors include effects of fasting, smoking, alcohol use, caffeine intake, and exercise. It is conceivable that dietary factors would primarily affect specific blood markers rather than CSF biomarkers. However, fluctuations in fatty acid amide concentrations were measured in CSF of rats between day and night, due to differences in food intake (Murillo-Rodriguez et al. 2006). Experimental evidence in humans is lacking, and where compounds, such as alcohol or smoking, have effects on neurons (Downer and Campbell 2010; Oliveira-da-Silva et al. 2009), they may also have an effect on CSF. Thus, there are limited descriptions of CSF biomarkers being affected by these lifestyle factors. However, if there are effects of smoking or drinking on CSF biomarker concentrations, it will be hard to define if these are trait markers or should be seen as direct pre-analytical confounders. For all these factors, documentation is important for long-term biobanking and future research.

Studying the effect of circadian rhythm (and fasting) of specific proteins in CSF is not easy to perform, as repeated sampling within a person needs to be performed. However, some recent reports showed fluctuations in CSF protein levels due to diurnal rhythm. For example, Kang and colleagues detected a diurnal rhythm of Abeta(1-42) levels in a group of ten healthy individuals, with a variation of 27.6 %

between morning and evening (Kang et al. 2009). A variation of 5.5–12.2 % was found in levels of Abeta(1-42), Abeta(40), Tau, and pTau, measured once per 6 h, in patients who were on CSF drainage as part of their clinical routine since they were suspected of idiopathic normal pressure hydrocephalus ($n=9$) or pseucotumor cerebri ($n=1$). This circadian variation was only slightly higher than the inter-assay coefficient of variation, and there was too much variation in rhythm between individuals to indicate a circadian fluctuation at group level (Moghekar et al. 2012). Another study from the Bateman Group reports diurnal fluctuation of amyloid CSF biomarkers (sAPPalpha, sAPPbeta, Abeta(42), and Abeta(40)) in three cohorts: a young cohort and two older cohorts, one with and one without amyloid pathology present. Amplitudes of the biomarkers were fluctuating in the range of 2–20 % over 36 h, dependent on group (diminishing with age) and specific per biomarker (Dobrowolska et al. 2014). Thus, the effects of circadian fluctuations were small since they marginally exceed the variation of the assay. The peak hours of bio-marker fluctuation could not be patterned (Dobrowolska et al. 2014), indicating that standardizing time of withdrawal will not eliminate pre-analytical variation on an individual basis.

Taken together, the only option to document this variation seems to be to drain CSF during 24 h and monitor circadian protein fluctuation per individual. This is however too time-consuming, not cost-efficient, and uncomfortable for patients to realize in practice. Given the fact that most lumbar punctures are performed during clinical work-up, it will be hard to standardize time of withdrawal. Standardizing time of withdrawal is thus not recommended, also since biomarker fluctuations differ per person and accounted so far only for minor variation in outcome, which may also be even less in the short time window of office hours. Since effects cannot be excluded for every biomarker, recording time of withdrawal is important for bio-marker development.

5.3 Laboratory Processing

In this paragraph, we discuss the guidelines for CSF processing and biobanking as presented in Table 5.1, supported by experimental research when available.

5.3.1 Item 2 of Table 5.1: Volume of Withdrawal of at Least 12 ml

The CSF volume taken can influence the concentration of biomarkers. If a small volume is taken, the CSF will reflect the composition of the lumbar dural sack, whereas large volumes may reflect the rostral spinal or even ventricular CSF. Most molecules and cell numbers are not equally distributed throughout the spinal fluid, and it is known that an increasing gradient in protein concentration from ventricular to lumbar CSF exists (Reiber 2003; Tarnaris et al. 2011). Therefore, if biomarker levels in a sample from a puncture of 2 ml are compared to that in a puncture of 15 ml, this can lead to erroneous comparisons for specific proteins.

In a recent study, CSF protein concentrations of the neuron-specific protein S100B and the neuron-specific enolase did not differ between ventricular and lumbar CSF in the same patients, though the leptomeningeal beta-trace and the blood-derived albumin did (Brandner et al. 2013). A proteomic study comparing the first and the tenth ml from one CSF withdrawal revealed only one protein, apolipoprotein C1, to be significantly increased among 41 identified masses of which 11 proteins were identified (Simonsen et al. 2010). Probably, the production location of a protein is crucial for the presence of a ventriculo-lumbar gradient in CSF (Tumani and Brettschneider 2005); however, this does not solve the uncertainty for CSF gradients being present for individual proteins, especially not if they are relatively unknown proteins. Therefore, we generally recommend to puncture a standard volume of CSF, especially for biobanking, but at least record the volume. The first 2 ml can be used for basic CSF analysis, and the remainder of the sample should be pooled before aliquoting. If this is not possible, the fraction of each portion must be recorded. Of course, a larger volume of spinal fluid will facilitate the number of possible analyses. It is well established that the volume of collected CSF does not correlate with the risk of post-lumbar puncture headache (Grant et al. 1991; Kuntz et al. 1992) (Chapter 4).

5.3.2 Item 3 of Table 5.1: Location of Puncture, L3–L5

Usually, diagnostic CSF is obtained by lumbar puncture, and the rationale for the location in relation to patient safety and to avoid discomfort is described in chapter 5. In practice, CSF will be taken only rarely from other locations than L3–L5, such as the cervical cisterns or from the lateral ventricles (e.g., ventricular drainage). Location of the puncture should thus be recorded since it matters for a few peptides (Tarnaris et al. 2011; Brandner et al. 2013) and it might affect concentrations of not yet detected CSF proteins.

5.3.3 Item 4 of Table 5.1: Removal of Bloody CSF Samples

A traumatic tap causing blood contamination of CSF occurs in about 14–20 % of standard lumbar punctures (Petzold et al. 2006). For markers that have high blood concentrations, such as coagulation factors, blood contamination can lead to false-positive results, while no effects have been reported for proteins from neuronal origin as neurofilament light and heavy chains (Koel-Simmelink et al. 2014). Vascular endothelial growth factor (VEGF) and neuron-specific enolase (NSE) are predominantly present in blood platelets and are CSF biomarker candidates for some neurological and neurodegenerative diseases. NSE levels linearly rise with increased hemolysis of both serum and CSF (Ramont et al. 2005). Also, the presence of cellular components in the CSF influences the levels of these proteins, the effect of which will be minimized by centrifugation. For example, VEGF levels remained relatively stable after spinning (Yang et al. 2011). In addition, the presence of blood proteins leads to suppressed MALDI-TOF proteomic patterns in CSF. This suppression by blood proteins is, however, highly reduced after removal of the blood cells by centrifugation of the sample prior to initial freezing and subsequent analysis (Berven et al. 2007; Jimenez et al. 2007). Recording of erythrocyte count is essential to select CSF samples appropriate for these measurements. Based on the proteomic studies, CSF samples with an erythrocyte count up to 500/μl can be included for biomarker studies, though lower percentage contamination is preferred to avoid effects on as yet unknown molecules. It is highly recommended though to spin samples to avoid blood contamination. The use of alternative markers as quality indicators to indicate hemolysis of CSF (e.g., hemoglobin alpha and beta chairs) is indicated (Jimenez et al. 2007), but thresholds remain to be defined.

5.3.4   Item 5 of Table 5.1: Use of Atraumatic Needles

There is no evidence that the type of needle for lumbar puncture influences biomarker concentrations. However, atraumatic or small-gauge needles are best tolerated by patients and are associated with a lower risk for post-lumbar puncture headache (chapter 5). An advantage of the traumatic needles is an increased CSF flow. Selecting the optimal type of needle for CSF sampling is elaborated in detail in chapter 5.

5.3.5   Item 6 of Table 5.1: Use of Polypropylene Collection Tubes

Proteins can stick to lab plastics, a characteristic that is exploited during, e.g., ELISA assays. This characteristic becomes disadvantageous though when the type of collection tube influences biomarker outcomes. Moreover, many collection tubes release polymeric components (Bowen et al. 2005) that can in some cases affect immunoassays. The Abeta(1-42) peptide in particular proves sensitive to different tubes used (Lewczuk et al. 2006; Lehmann et al. 2014; Perret-Liaudet et al. 2012; Toombs et al. 2014). The use of polypropylene tubes, with their low protein-binding potential, was proposed for collecting CSF. Actually, experimental evidence did not confirm the advantage of tubes purely composed of polypropylene (Perret-Liaudet et al. 2012), and comparing multiple polypropylene tubes did not give congruous results (Lehmann et al. 2014). Thus, harmonization of the tubes proves a worthwhile effort to reduce variation and introducing one tube type with the lowest binding capacity for universal use still lies ahead. The European JPND "BIOMARKAPD" consortium was initiated to standardize and harmonize the use of biomarkers for AD and Parkinson's disease, and it is addressing many of the before-mentioned topics. This consortium decided to use so far a Sarstedt polypropylene tube (cat nr: 62.610.018, 10 ml collection tube, round base; cat no. 62.554.502, 15 ml tube with conical base to use if a pellet is to be kept). An additional component causing variation is transferring CSF to new tubes: the more transfers, the more protein concentrations are reduced, especially for sticky peptides such as Abeta(1-42) (Toombs et al. 2014). The focus currently is on detailed examination of tube types, tube transfers, and additional elements such as tube caps in order to further optimize the recommendation of the use of specific tubes for CSF collection.

5.3.6 Items 7 and 8 of Table 5.1: Withdrawal of Serum and Plasma Linked to the CSF Sample

It is important to collect matched serum and/or plasma samples for evaluation of CSF biomarkers because the concentration of the marker in blood often influences that in CSF. Blood collection is moreover needed to calculate the IgG index for diagnostic purposes and to define the intrathecal origin of a biomarker and thus its specificity for the CNS (Deisenhammer et al. 2006). For novel biomarkers of neuronal origin, it is relevant to determine the presence of a candidate CNS marker in serum/plasma. Blood tests are ideal for monitoring biomarker concentrations over time for monitoring of disease progression or even population screening.

For work-up, vacutainer tubes that use EDTA (in dried format) are preferred over those that use citrate (in solution) because if tubes containing a standard volume of citrate solution are filled incompletely, the final biomarker concentration is diluted artificially. Serum/plasma samples should not be hemolyzed or lipemic, and a standardized blood collection protocol is also provided in Table 5.1.

5.3.7 Item 9 of Table 5.1: Storage at Room Temperature Until Spinning and Aliquoting

For CSF, there are no data available yet that support a preference for leaving the samples at either room temperature or 4 °C until processing. A direct comparison was made between neurofilament protein levels stored at room temperature or 4 °C, and no difference in protein levels was found (Koel-Simmelink et al. 2014). CSF enzymes, such as adenosine deaminase and acid sphingomyelinase, do not have a decreased enzymatic activity when stored for a maximum of 24 h at room temperature (Lu and Grenache 2012; Mühle et al. 2013). Therefore, processing at room temperature for both serum/plasma and CSF, including during and after spinning, is suitable for most studies. However, if RNA is to be sampled from CSF immune cells, the CSF should be spun immediately or stored at 4 °C until processing.

5.3.8 Item 10 of Table 5.1: Standardized Spinning Conditions

We propose to adhere to a standardized spinning protocol of 400 g for 10 min at room temperature for CSF if cells are to be collected, otherwise between 1,800 and 2,200 g (10 min at room temperature). For serum, we recommend to spin at 2,000 g for 10 min at room temperature. Not many experimental reports on this topic exist. A preliminary study showed lower concentrations of CSF protein DJ-1 with spinning at 2,000 g compared to spinning at 1,300–1,800 g; however, the effect was small and possibly due to other pre-analytical factors which differed between the experimental groups (Salvesen et al. 2014). For plasma and serum, temperature of processing is known to be critical for specific biomarkers, such as TIMP-1, probably due to degranulation of platelets at room temperature (Lomholt et al. 2007).

5.3.9 Item 11 of Table 5.1: Standardization of Time Delay Between Withdrawal, Spinning, and Freezing

Proteomic studies proved stability of CSF proteome for up to 2 h after withdrawal prior to further processing (Berven et al. 2007; Jimenez et al. 2007). Similar stability was shown for neurofilament heavy- and light-chain proteins for up to 24-h time delay between lumbar puncture and spinning, independent of the temperature as indicated at item 9 (Koel-Simmelink et al. 2014). Also after spinning, a delay of 2 h before storage did not result in changes in CSF protein profiles (Klener et al. 2014; Rosenling et al. 2011), whereas delayed storage of more than 6 h significantly changes peptide profiles (Bruegel et al. 2009). A proton nuclear magnetic resonance study showed stability of myoinositol, glucose, acetate, and alanine levels; a substantial decrease of citrate; and an increase in lactate, glutamine, creatine, and creatinine levels after a 72-h delay in processing of CSF at room temperature (Levine et al. 2000).

CSF stability studies suggest that the effect of time delay before spinning is more prominent than a delay to storing samples after centrifugation. Studies investigating delay before processing report differences in Alzheimer biomarker levels after a 24-h (Kaiser et al. 2007) or 2-day delay (Schoonenboom et al. 2005), whereas studies testing delay between processing and storage report stability after a delay of several days (Bjerke et al. 2010; Zimmermann et al. 2011) or up to 14 days (Simonsen et al. 2013). Still, Bruegel and colleagues found changes in CSF peptide profiles after 6 h of delay after spinning before storage (Bruegel et al. 2009). Despite of actual experimental data published on this subject, results thus remain discrepant. It is clear though that stability of AD biomarkers and probably many other biomarkers can be guaranteed following the proposed guideline which does not exceed a 4-h delay in total (2 before and 2 after spinning). New biomarkers should however always be tested on these aspects of stability.

5.3.10 Item 12 of Table 5.1: Use of Small Polypropylene Tubes for Aliquoting

Due to the same rationale as for CSF withdrawal (item 6), we recommend that polypropylene tubes should be used for aliquoting. Furthermore, vials with screw caps should be used for a secure sealing and should be properly closed for long-term biobanking. The proposed tube size is usually 2 ml for routine biomarkers and 0.5 ml for biobanking; however, since tubes should preferably be filled up to 75 %, other tube sizes in this range are used in practice too.

5.3.11 Item 13 of Table 5.1: Aliquoting

Freezing and thawing cycles can influence CSF biomarker concentrations, as was also shown for some specific blood biomarkers (Chaigneau et al. 2007). Studies show conflicting results in Alzheimer diagnostic CSF proteins after several freeze-thaw cycles though. One study observed a significant loss of Abeta(1-42) after one freeze-thaw cycle (Bibl et al. 2004), while others see no effects in Abeta(1-42) at all after up to three times freeze-thawing (Zimmermann et al. 2011; Simonsen et al. 2013), but rather a small decrease in Tau proteins after two to three cycles (Simonsen et al. 2013). Another study found a 20 % decrease in Abeta(1-42) after minimum three thawing cycles (Schoonenboom et al. 2005). The discrepancy in these results might lie in as yet unidentified other pre-analytical variables that differed between these studies.

Levels of several cytokines, vascular endothelial growth factor (VEGF), matrix metalloproteinase-2 (MMP-2), and neurofilament proteins were not affected by repeated freezing and thawing (Aziz et al. 1999; Koel-Simmelink et al. 2014; Sulik et al. 2008; Yang et al. 2011). Spectroscopy techniques show contradictory data too, e.g., no effects on CSF proteome profiles as determined by MALDI-MS have been observed after up to four cycles in a proteomic study (Jimenez et al. 2007). On the other hand, a Raman spectroscopy study showed a decrease in peptides, also Abeta(1-42), after one freeze-thaw cycle (Klener et al. 2014).

Altogether, freeze-thaw cycles should be avoided in principle, as data addressing this topic are available for only a few molecules and the response to freeze-thaw cycles of new molecules is not known. Thus, splitting the samples in multiple small aliquots is recommended. As indicated at item 2, the total CSF sample must be pooled before aliquoting to avoid concentration gradients.

5.3.12 Item 14 of Table 5.1: Volumes of Aliquots of 0.2, 0.5, and 1 ml (Depending on Total Volume of Tube and Minimally 0.1 ml)

Storage in small aliquots prevents CSF from degrading due to freeze-thawing. Tubes should preferably be filled up to 75 % to preserve concentration, since this could be influenced by evaporation and absorbance of CSF components to the surface of the tube wall and bottom. The true influence of both factors is under current study, but initial data show that evaporation is not relevant during 2 years of storage in at least one type of tube (del Campo et al. 2012). Preferred tube sizes are indicated at item 12.

5.3.13 Item 15 of Table 5.1: Coding and Use of Freezing-Proof Labels

All biobank samples need a unique pseudonymized coding which is coupled to a protected database providing, e.g., clinical patient information or informed consent information. Barcoded sample tubes are preferred, since it enables automation, permits double-blinded research effortlessly, and protects the privacy of the patient. Labels should be suitable for prolonged storage at −80 °C.

5.3.14 Item 16 of Table 5.1: Freezing Temperature of −80 °C

Most large proteins such as antibodies are stable at −20 °C for several months (Trendl 2000). However, epitopes of smaller molecules may change due to oxidation resulting from pH changes during storage (Poulsen et al. 2012), and this could affect protein concentration results, which depends on the particular assay used for detection. There is little published data on the effect of storage temperature on CSF constituents. Effect of storage of CSF at −20 and −80 °C on cystatin C was investigated by mass spectrometry. Cleavage of eight amino acids of this protein occurred in samples stored at −20 °C but not in samples stored at −80 °C (Berven et al. 2007; Carrette et al. 2005; Del Boccio et al. 2007; Jimenez et al. 2007). Apart from the cystatin C truncation, changes in the remainder of the low molecular weight polypeptide profile due to CSF sample storage at −20 °C for 3 months appeared to be minimal (Berven et al. 2007; Jimenez et al. 2007). Activity of secretory acid sphingomyelinase was increased when CSF samples were stored at −20 °C for 2 months compared to at −80 °C (Mühle et al. 2013), indicating that for activity of this enzyme storage at −20 °C is not sufficient. Also neuron-specific enolase is instable when CSF is stored at −20 °C (27 % concentration decrease after 1 month) and better conserved at −80 °C (22 % concentration decrease after 9 months) (Ramont et al. 2005). Oligoclonal bands in CSF may be recovered after several years of storage at −20 °C, indicating a high stability of immunoglobulins (Triendl 2000). Short-time freezing of samples at −80 or −196 °C did not change the CSF peptide profile (Bruegel et al. 2009).

There might be a beneficial effect of quick freeze-drying CSF in liquid nitrogen prior to storage at −80 °C, since the protein conformation seems less affected when compared to slow freezing at −80 °C (Klener et al. 2014). For many specific CSF markers, it is not known how freeze-drying affects their conformation and binding capacity, and it is conceivable that conformational change may be the cause of observed effects of repeated freeze-thawing. Since freeze-drying in liquid nitrogen is an expensive technique and not available in all laboratories, it is not implemented in the protocols.

Taken together, we recommend that samples should be transferred to −80 °C as soon as possible to ensure long-term stability of biomarkers. For specific biomarkers already implemented in the diagnostic work-up, such as Abeta(1-42) and oligoclonal bands, short-term storage at −20 °C will not be problematic.

5.3.15 Long-Term Storage of CSF

Long-term biobanking of human body fluids is of great importance for the discovery of novel biomarkers, but the effects of long-term storage on molecular constituents of CSF or blood are not known. There are few reports published on this, indicating stability of Abeta(1-42) and Tau proteins for at least 6 years (Schipke et al. 2011). Using an Arrhenius plot, these CSF biomarkers, and also neurofilament proteins, were predicted to be stable during storage at −80 °C (Koel-Simmelink et al. 2014; Schoonenboom et al. 2005), but real experimental evidence on this subject is lacking. Neuroactive amino acid, such as aspartate, glutamate, glycine, and taurine, concentrations can be measured reliably after up to 30 days when stored at either −20 or −80 °C, although the samples should be deproteinized and subsequently neutralized before freezing to protect from in vitro modification of amino acid concentrations in CSF (Anesi et al. 1998). The effects of long-term storage on other CSF molecules and potential beneficial effects of additives need to be established. As shown by Anesi and colleagues, additives might be necessary to detect amino acids in CSF after storage at temperatures below zero (Anesi et al. 1998). Structural changes occurring in molecules due to freezing (and thawing) and possible effects of evaporation suggest that there could indeed be changes in CSF measures after long-term storage. As this process is not yet understood, we have to settle for now with assessing long-term stability per biomarker. Hopefully, experimental data in the future will contribute to our understanding of processes during long-term storage on a molecular level since more and more samples are stored to be used for biomarker research.

5.4 Variation in Biomarker Assays

It is conceivable that a considerable part of variation in biomarker outcomes will depend on the detection method. For most proteins, more than one manufacturer provides these assays and variation may be epitope specific. For many non-standardized assays, laboratories develop their own in-house assays. Although all these assays are extensively validated, the use of different assays can lead to variations in absolute values (Malekzadeh et al. 2012) which can be problematic when replicating results of other researchers. Moreover, even using the same assays and the same samples, variation in outcomes is observed for the Alzheimer biomarkers (Mattsson et al. 2013; Teunissen et al. 2010; Sunderland et al. 2003; Verwey et al. 2009; Vos et al. 2014).

It is also possible that specific epitopes detected by an immunoassay are preserved during pre-analytical variability, while the remainder of that protein may have disappeared. These changes in proteins may remain unnotified using specific assays while they are apparent in other assays. Nevertheless, these pre-analytical effects may also not be problematic for correct diagnosis using these specific assays.

Variance while performing an ELISA thus easily occurs, e.g., due to batch variation, the lack of certified reference material, and the tendency of some proteins to aggregate during the analysis procedure (Fig. 5.1). The use of high-throughput analyzers with high precision can reduce the variation in the assays. Such tests usually only become cost-effective when a biomarker enters routine clinical practice.

5.5   Other Strategies to Solve Pre-analytical Variability: Use of Quality Markers

Another approach to solve pre-analytical variation in CSF, complementing standardization efforts, would be to use an independent sentinel molecule reflecting laboratory handlings. This molecule should be instable and ideally relates linearly to one specific pre-analytical step in the process, so that the effect of this step could be predicted by a formula. Sample quality could thus be measured according to this indicator. Presumably, a panel of sentinel molecules is required, together covering multiple laboratory steps likely causing pre-analytical variation, such as delayed storage, freeze-thaw cycles, duration of storage, temperature during transport, spinning, and storage, since they might all affect quality in a different manner. The International Society for Biological and Environmental Repositories (ISBER) Biospecimen Science working group recently reviewed the current state of this art of quality control of human biospecimens (Betsou et al. 2013), but in CSF there are no examples yet for possible quality indicators. Promising reports were published recently revealing several enzymes in blood whose levels were changed upon variation in laboratory processing, reflecting the effect of specific pre-analytical steps (Kang et al. 2013; Zander et al. 2014). These studies need replication and optimization to be implemented in the biobanking processing protocol. In CSF, the identification of such quality markers is a bit more complicated since CSF proteins are less abundant and sometimes below detection threshold and consequently fewer assays are available for screening such effects.

5.6   Conclusion and Recommendations

Pre-analytical variation is a major cause of variation in CSF biomarker outcome measures.

One may argue that CSF may be particularly prone to pre-analytical variation due to its low protein content (factor 200 lower than in blood), yet there is also a low protease activity (Berven et al. 2007; You et al. 2005).

Several studies discussed above revealed discrepant results. For example, the stability of Abeta(1-42) in CSF after spinning at room temperature was sometimes set at 3 days (Zimmermann et al. 2011), while others found a decrease after 2 days even using the same assays (Schoonenboom et al. 2005). So, even when focusing on one specific molecule, different laboratories observe different stabilities of this protein. These data leave the impression that stability is very sensitive to other handlings in the laboratory, which are not yet defined but can make the crucial difference. Or, protein changes are not detected consistently due to the use of different assays which focus on other epitopes. Due to the paucity of data on a variety of molecules, there are no predictions possible as yet.

Whereas published research on this topic is so far not extensive, the interest in the subject is currently expanding. In 2009, a recommendation protocol was established in order to standardize collection and biobanking procedures of CSF samples, to facilitate interlaboratory exchange of samples and long-term usage (Teunissen et al. 2009). Here, we updated the background information that formed the basis of this protocol and discussed recent experimental evidence. These guidelines should be used by anyone working with CSF to prevent erroneous results and to be able to exchange samples with already over 80 centers now worldwide (i.e., the participating centers of BioMS and BIOMARKAPD and ALS working group). The fact that different laboratories find discrepant results, even when investigating the same variable, emphasizes the importance of obeying these recommendations. We expect that pre-analytical variation will be better understood in the future, since the number, contents, and use of CSF biobanks are increasing, and with it the importance to control pre-analytical effects.

References

Anesi A, Rondanelli M, D'Eril GM (1998) Stability of neuroactive amino acids in cerebrospinal fluid under various conditions of processing and storage. Clin Chem 44(11):2359–2360

Aziz N et al (1999) Variables that affect assays for plasma cytokines and soluble activation markers. Clin Diagn Lab Immunol 6(1):89–95

Berven FS et al (2007) Pre-analytical influence on the low molecular weight cerebrospinal fluid proteome. Proteomics Clin Appl 1(7):699–711

Betsou F et al (2013) Identification of evidence-based biospecimen quality-control tools: a report of the International Society for Biological and Environmental Repositories (ISBER) Biospecimen Science Working Group. J Mol Diagn 15(1):3–16

Bibl M et al (2004) Cerebrospinal fluid amyloid beta peptide patterns in Alzheimer's disease patients and nondemented controls depend on sample pretreatment: indication of carrier-mediated epitope masking of amyloid beta peptides. Electrophoresis 25(17):2912–2918

Bjerke M et al (2010) Confounding factors influencing amyloid Beta concentration in cerebrospinal fluid. Int J Alzheimers Dis 2010:1–12

Bowen RAR et al (2005) Effect of blood collection tubes on total triiodothyronine and other laboratory assays. Clin Chem 51(2):424–433

Brandner S et al (2013) Neuroprotein dynamics in the cerebrospinal fluid: intraindividual concomitant ventricular and lumbar measurements. Eur Neurol 70(3–4):189–194

Bruegel M et al (2009) Standardized peptidome profiling of human cerebrospinal fluid by magnetic bead separation and matrix-assisted laser desorption/ionization time-of-flight mass spectrometry. J Proteomics 72(4):608–615

Carrette O et al (2005) Truncated cystatin C in cerebrospinal fluid: technical [corrected] artefact or biological process? Proteomics 5(12):3060–3065

Chaigneau C et al (2007) Serum biobank certification and the establishment of quality controls for biological fluids: examples of serum biomarker stability after temperature variation. Clin Chem Lab Med 45(10):1390–1395

Deisenhammer F et al (2006) Guidelines on routine cerebrospinal fluid analysis. Report from an EFNS task force. Eur J Neurol 13(9):913–922

Del Boccio P et al (2007) Cleavage of cystatin C is not associated with multiple sclerosis. Ann Neurol 62(2):201–204; discussion 205

del Campo M et al (2012) Recommendations to standardize preanalytical confounding factors in Alzheimer's and Parkinson's disease cerebrospinal fluid biomarkers: an update. Biomark Med 6:419–430

Dobrowolska JA et al (2014) Diurnal patterns of soluble amyloid precursor protein metabolites in the human central nervous system. PLoS One 9(3):e89998

Downer EJ, Campbell VA (2010) Phytocannabinoids, CNS cells and development: a dead issue? Drug Alcohol Rev 29(1):91–98

Grant R et al (1991) Changes in intracranial CSF volume after lumbar puncture and their relationship to post-LP headache. J Neurol Neurosurg Psychiatry 54(5):440–442

Jimenez CR et al (2007) Endogenous peptide profiling of cerebrospinal fluid by MALDI-TOF mass spectrometry: optimization of magnetic bead-based peptide capture and analysis of preanalytical variables. Proteomics Clin Appl 1:1385–1392

Kaiser E et al (2007) Influence of delayed CSF storage on concentrations of phospho-tau protein (181), total tau protein and beta-amyloid (1-42). Neurosci Lett 417(2):193–195

Kang J-E et al (2009) Amyloid-beta dynamics are regulated by orexin and the sleep-wake cycle. Science 326(5955):1005–1007

Kang HJ et al (2013) Identification of clinical biomarkers for pre-analytical quality control of blood samples. Biopreserv Biobank 11(2):94–100

Klener J et al (2014) Instability of cerebrospinal fluid after delayed storage and repeated freezing: a holistic study by drop coating deposition Raman spectroscopy. Clin Chem Lab Med 52(5):657–664

Koel-Simmelink MJ et al (2014) The impact of pre-analytical variables on the stability of neurofilament proteins in CSF, determined by a novel validated SinglePlex Luminex assay and ELISA. J Immunol Methods 402(1–2):43–49

Kuntz KM et al (1992) Post-lumbar puncture headaches: experience in 501 consecutive procedures. Neurology 42(10):1884–1887

Lehmann S et al (2014) Impact of harmonization of collection tubes on Alzheimer's disease diagnosis. Alzheimers Dement 10(5):S390–S394.e2

Levine J et al (2000) Stability of CSF metabolites measured by proton NMR. J Neural Transm 107(7):843–848

Lewczuk P et al (2006) Effect of sample collection tubes on cerebrospinal fluid concentrations of tau proteins and amyloid β peptides. Clin Chem 52(2):332–334

Lomholt AF et al (2007) Plasma tissue inhibitor of metalloproteinases-1 as a biological marker? Pre-analytical considerations. Clin Chim Acta 380(1–2):128–132

Lu J, Grenache DG (2012) Development of a rapid, microplate-based kinetic assay for measuring adenosine deaminase activity in body fluids. Clin Chim Acta 413(19–20):1637–1640

Malekzadeh A et al (2012) Challenges in multi-plex and mono-plex platforms for the discovery of inflammatory profiles in neurodegenerative diseases. Methods 56(4):508–513

Mattsson N et al (2013) CSF biomarker variability in the Alzheimer's Association quality control program. Alzheimers Dement 9(3):251–261

Moghekar A et al (2012) Cerebrospinal fluid abeta and tau level fluctuation in an older clinical cohort. Arch Neurol 69(2):246–250

Mühle C et al (2013) Characterization of acid sphingomyelinase activity in human cerebrospinal fluid. PLoS One 8(5):e62912

Murillo-Rodriguez E, Désarnaud F, Prospéro-García O (2006) Diurnal variation of arachidonoylethanolamine, palmitoylethanolamide and oleoylethanolamide in the brain of the rat. Life Sci 79(1):30–37

Oliveira-da-Silva A et al (2009) Increased apoptosis and reduced neuronal and glial densities in the hippocampus due to nicotine and ethanol exposure in adolescent mice. Int J Dev Neurosci 27(6):539–548

Otto M et al (2012) Roadmap and standard operating procedures for biobanking and discovery of neurochemical markers in ALS. Amyotroph Lateral Scler 13(1):1–10

Perret-Liaudet A et al (2012) Risk of Alzheimer's disease biological misdiagnosis linked to cerebrospinal collection tubes. J Alzheimers Dis 31(1):13–20

Petzold A, Sharpe LT, Keir G (2006) Review spectrophotometry for cerebrospinal fluid pigment analysis. Neurocrit Care 0961:153–162

Pica-Mendez AM et al (2010) Nonspecific binding of Aβ42 to polypropylene tubes and the effect of Tween-20. Clin Chim Acta 411(21–22):1833

Plebani M et al (2014) Harmonization of pre-analytical quality indicators. Biochem Med 24(1):105–113

Poulsen K et al (2012) Characterization and stability of transthyretin isoforms in cerebrospinal fluid examined by immunoprecipitation and high-resolution mass spectrometry of intact protein. Methods 56(2):284–292

Ramont L et al (2005) Effects of hemolysis and storage condition on neuron-specific enolase (NSE) in cerebrospinal fluid and serum: implications in clinical practice. Clin Chem Lab Med 43(11):1215–1217

Reiber H (2003) Proteins in cerebrospinal fluid and blood: barriers, CSF flow rate and source-related dynamics. Restor Neurol Neurosci 21(3–4):79–96

Rosenling T et al (2011) The impact of delayed storage on the measured proteome and metabolome of human cerebrospinal fluid. Clin Chem 57(12):1703–1711

Salvesen L et al (2014) The influence of preanalytical conditions on the DJ-1 concentration in human cerebrospinal fluid. Biomark Med 8(3):387–394

Schipke CG et al (2011) Long-term stability of Alzheimer's disease biomarker proteins in cerebrospinal fluid. J Alzheimers Dis 26(2):255–262

Schoonenboom NSM et al (2005) Effects of processing and storage conditions on amyloid beta (1-42) and tau concentrations in cerebrospinal fluid: implications for use in clinical practice. Clin Chem 51(1):189–195

Simonsen AH et al (2010) Proteomic investigations of the ventriculo-lumbar gradient in human CSF. J Neurosci Methods 191(2):244–248

Simonsen AH et al (2013) Pre-analytical factors influencing the stability of cerebrospinal fluid proteins. J Neurosci Methods 215(2):234–240

Sulik A, Wojtkowska M, Oldak E (2008) Preanalytical factors affecting the stability of matrix metalloproteinase-2 concentrations in cerebrospinal fluid. Clin Chim Acta 392(1–2):73–75

Sunderland T et al (2003) Decreased beta-amyloid1-42 and increased tau levels in cerebrospinal fluid of patients with Alzheimer disease. JAMA 289(16):2094–2103

Tarnaris A et al (2011) Rostrocaudal dynamics of CSF biomarkers. Neurochem Res 36(3):528–532

Teunissen CE et al (2009) A consensus protocol for the standardization of cerebrospinal fluid collection and biobanking. Neurology 73:1914–1922

Teunissen CE et al (2010) Standardization of assay procedures for analysis of the CSF biomarkers amyloid β(1-42), tau, and phosphorylated tau in Alzheimer's disease: report of an International workshop. Int J Alzheimers Disease Volume 2010, Article ID 635053, pp 1–6. doi:10.4061/2010/635053

Teunissen C et al (2013) Consensus definitions and application guidelines for control groups in cerebrospinal fluid biomarker studies in multiple sclerosis. Mult Scler 19:1802–1809

Teunissen CE et al (2014) Biobanking of CSF: international standardization to optimize biomarker development. Clin Biochem 47(4–5):288–292

Toombs J et al (2014) Amyloid-beta 42 adsorption following serial tube transfer. Alzheimers Res Ther 6(1):5

Triendl A (2000) Die klinische Wertigkeit des monoklonalen und biklonalen Bandenmusters in der isoelektrischen Fokussierung des Liquor cerebrospinalis. Univ., Diss, Innsbruck

Tumani H, Brettschneider J (2005) Brain specific proteins in cerebrospinal fluid (CSF): factors influencing their concentration in CSF and clinical relevance. Laboratoriumsmedizin 29(6):421–428

Turner HE et al (2013) The effect of electronic ordering on pre-analytical errors in primary care. Ann Clin Biochem 50(Pt 5):485–488

Vanderstichele H et al (2012) Standardization of preanalytical aspects of cerebrospinal fluid biomarker testing for Alzheimer's disease diagnosis: a consensus paper from the Alzheimer's Biomarkers Standardization Initiative. Alzheimers Dement 8(1):65–73

Verwey NA et al (2009) A worldwide multicentre comparison of assays for cerebrospinal fluid biomarkers in Alzheimer's disease. Ann Clin Biochem 46(Pt 3):235–240

Vos SJB et al (2014) Variability of CSF Alzheimer's disease biomarkers: implications for clinical practice. PLoS One 9(6):e100784

Yang J et al (2011) Stability analysis of vascular endothelial growth factor in cerebrospinal fluid. Neurochem Res 36(11):1947–1954

You J-S et al (2005) The impact of blood contamination on the proteome of cerebrospinal fluid. Proteomics 5:290–296

Zander J et al (2014) Effect of biobanking conditions on short-term stability of biomarkers in human serum and plasma. Clin Chem Lab Med 52(5):629–639

Zimmermann R et al (2011) Preanalytical sample handling and sample stability testing for the neurochemical dementia diagnostics. J Alzheimers Dis 25(4):739–745

Part II

Methods of CSF Analyses

Cell Count and Staining

Herwig Strik and Ingelore Nagel

6

Contents

H. Strik (✉)
Department of Neurology,
Medical School and UKGM, University of Marburg,
Marburg, Germany

Department of Neurology,
Philipps University and Hospital,
Baldinger Strasse, Marburg D-35043, Germany
e-mail: strik@med.uni-marburg.de

I. Nagel
Department of Neurology,
Medical School, University of Goettingen,
Goettingen, Germany

© Springer International Publishing Switzerland 2015
F. Deisenhammer et al. (eds.), *Cerebrospinal Fluid in Clinical Neurology*,
DOI 10.1007/978-3-319-01225-4_6

Abstract

Total cell count and differentiation of cells into their physiological and pathological forms are basic and the most valuable procedures of CSF analysis. A volume of 5–10 ml should be transferred without delay and cells separated immediately from the CSF fluid by centrifugation in order to obtain a sufficient amount of both elements for analysis. Total cell and erythrocyte count are still most accurately assessed personally in the counting chamber. After staining with the Pappenheim method, cells can be differentiated microscopically into physiological CSF cells, physiological CSF-neighbouring cells, alterations of physiological cells and pathological cells. For this purpose, good knowledge of all these cell forms is essential.

6.1 Significance of Cellular Analysis

Correct assessment of the total number and differentiation of cells is a key element of CSF diagnostics. An elevated cell count provides the most valuable information on pathological processes within the central nervous system, although normal cell counts do not completely exclude any disease. Moreover, elevated cell counts only unspecifically indicate pathological changes, because the unstained material does not allow for conclusions on the cause of pleocytosis. Therefore, in the next step, preparation and staining of the CSF sample are necessary to differentiate physiological and pathological cell types and to draw conclusions (Koelmel 2003).

CSF cells are special in that they are instable once they leave the homeostasis of the organism with constant temperature and pH. Therefore, correct sampling and processing are essential in order to obtain a high-quality sample that allows for precise evaluation (Kolmel 1977; Gondos and King 1976). In the following parts of this chapter, the necessary steps from sampling to cytological evaluation will be described.

6.2 Sampling of CSF Cells

A technically correct lumbar puncture is the first prerequisite for a good cytological assessment. In order to obtain a sufficient number of cells for a thorough cytological evaluation, 5–10 ml of CSF should be transferred to the laboratory (Grover et al. 1995). Centrifugation of the CSF separates the cells from the fluid, allowing to assess approximately 5,000 cells on the cytological slide and providing at the same time the full volume of cell-free CSF for protein analysis (Gondos and King 1976; Hansen et al. 1974; Lehmitz and Kleine 1995). Puncture of the surrounding structures can cause contamination with cartilage or bone marrow cells which can be mistaken as neoplastic by unexperienced cytologists. Long-lasting transfer to the laboratory may cause autolytic changes, because the pH of the CSF rapidly turns to basic values and cold or hot temperature outside the body additionally induces rapid cellular lysis. Fast transfer of the CSF sample to the laboratory within one hour, avoidance of cold or hot temperature and rapid procession of the cells are therefore mandatory (Koelmel 2003).

During preparation of the CSF sample, the resuspension of the sample with a special suspension-containing buffer and foetal calf serum is helpful to prevent fast deterioration of the status of the cells (Veerman et al. 1985). High protein concentration, if endogenous in the CSF or added artificially, is known to stabilise CSF cells. The application of a pH-stabilising buffer also prevents cellular autolysis.

6.3 Cell Count

The total cell count predominantly reflects the number of leucocytes. It is assessed with unstained cells, allowing to differentiate between cells with and without nucleus, corresponding to leucocytes and erythrocytes (Kleine 2003). This differentiation is essential, since erythrocytes must not be mistaken as leucocytes, which would false-positively elevate the total cell count. A further distinction of leucocytes into lymphocytes, monocytes and granulocytes is not possible, so cells lining the CSF space cannot be distinguished and will also contribute to the total number of cells counted. Also the detection of tumour cells is unreliable and can only be supposed if cells are extremely large. An exception of the rule that specific diagnoses cannot be assured with unstained CSF is the rare occurrence of cryptococcosis. These fungi have a specific appearance that is pathognomonic.

6.4 Practical Performance of Cell Count

Uncentrifuged CSF is pipetted into a Fuchs-Rosenthal counting chamber with a volume of 3.2 µl. The number of counted cells has to be divided by 3 to obtain the cell count per µL. Providing cell counts with "thirds of cells" is obsolete and may lead to confusion.

The counting chamber consists of the chamber itself that is filled with CSF and a background with a visible net which provides orientation for counting. The net consists of 16 larger squares, each of which contains 16 small squares (Fig. 5.1). The border of the squares is marked by double lines. Cells are counted within the 16 large squares at 250-fold magnification. Cells lying on the lines at the top or left will be counted; bottom or right side is not counted. Erythrocytes have to be counted separately. They can be identified through their double-ring structure without nucleus, while leucocytes contain nuclei with a visible internal structure (Fig. 5.2). Optionally, erythrocytes can be stained red to enable easier detection. A possible confounder of correct cell count may be caused by previous intrathecal treatment with liposomal cytarabinoside. These liposomes can be found within the counting chamber and up to 4 weeks after treatment and lead to erroneously elevated cell counts. Liposomes can be identified by their regular round form, small border and optically empty centre (Fig. 6.2, blue arrows).

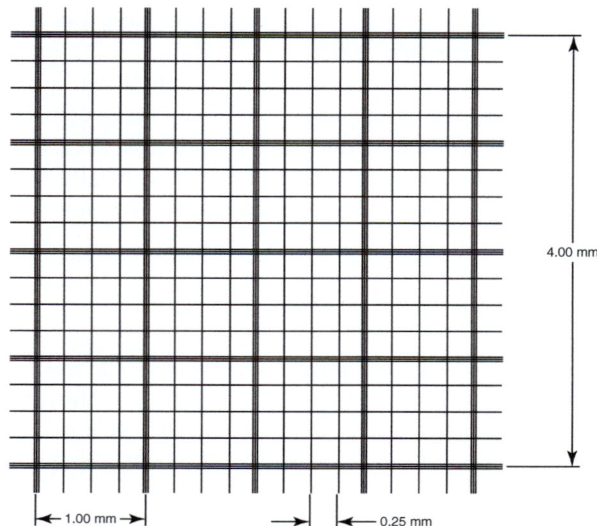

Fig. 6.1 Counting chamber. Nucleus-containing cells are counted within the *double-lined* space. Cells lying on the *upper* or *left* border are counted and on the *lower* or *right* border are not counted. The result is divided by 3 to obtain the cell count per µL

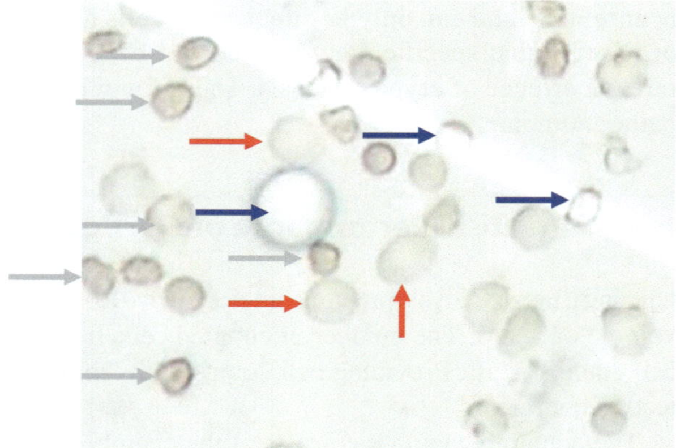

Fig. 6.2 Cell count. *Red*, erythrocyte: no nucleus, double-ring structure, *grey*, leucocyte. Irregular border of cytoplasm, inside visible structure. *Blue*, liposomes: round form, regular, slim border, optically empty

A total cell count of up to 4 cells per microlitre is normal; 5 or more is pathological. In cases of strong artificial contamination, 1 leucocyte per 1,000 erythrocytes can be subtracted from the total cell count as a rule of thumb.

Automated cell count has been propagated by several manufacturers of cytometers designed for blood cells and is used by some laboratories. These machines provide a reasonable cell count only in case of marked pleocytosis, where an exact result is less relevant. With normal cell counts or mild pleocytosis, where precise assessment is required to differentiate between normal and elevated counts, the result of automated cell counting is far less exact. Moreover, contamination with peripheral blood interferes with the results of automated cell counting. Automated analyses of CSF cell counts should therefore be regarded with caution and approved personally by an experienced technician (Strik et al. 2005; Heller et al. 2008).

6.5   Cell Differentiation

Differentiation of the different types of physiological and pathological CSF cells requires preparation and staining. Two different methods of preparation are used: sedimentation with the Sayk chamber and centrifugation with the cytospin method (Lehmitz and Kleine 1995). No clear recommendation can be made for either method, since the selection rather relies on personal preference and being familiar with one method. The sedimentation method is said to have a better efficiency of cell collection and to avoid preparation artefacts (Kolmel 1977; Gondos and King 1976). In our experience, however, cell preservation appears to be better with the cytospin method, probably because the preparation is faster and avoids autolysis (Hansen et al. 1974; Woodruff 1973). Centrifugation artefacts are rare and easy to detect and will not lead to misinterpretation. The technique of cytospin preparation is described in Fig. 6.3.

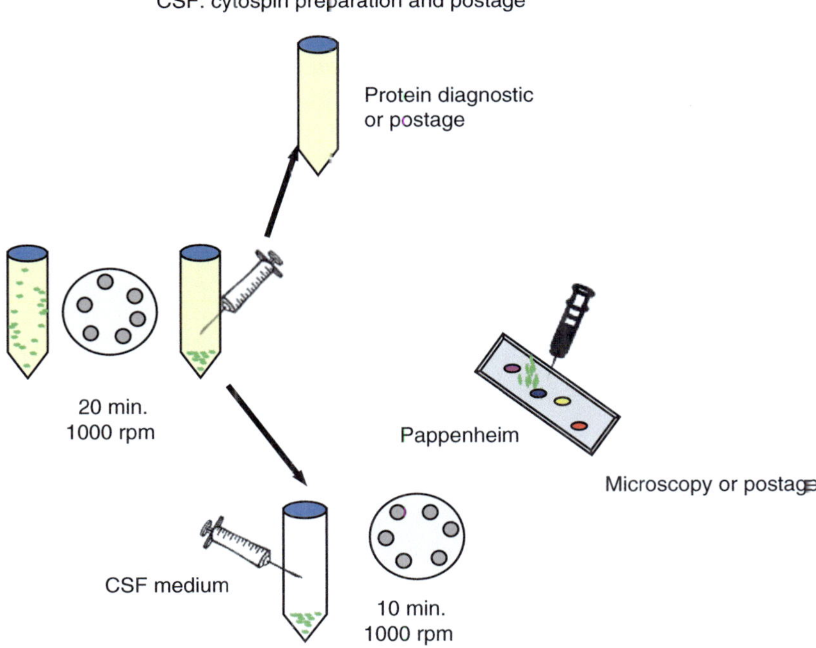

Fig. 6.3 Cytospin preparation. The CSF sample is centrifuged 20 min. with 1000 rpm. The supernatant is used for protein analysis. The remaining cells are resuspended with CSF medium containing fetal calf serum and buffer. Subsequently, the cell-containing medium is centrifuged for 10 min. at 1000 rpm on the slide. After air-drying, the preparation can be stained with May-Gruenwald – Giemsa (Pappenheim) or stored or posted for reference evaluation

Staining of the prepared cells is usually done with the Pappenheim method, a combination of May-Grünwald and Giemsa staining (Koelmel 2003). Basophilic structures are stained dark violet, eosinophilic in pink. Erythrocytes are stained in grey-shaded pink and haemosiderin in dark blue.

6.6 Physiological Cell Types

Leucocytes and monocytes (Fig. 6.4) are part of a physiological cell composition (Oehmichen 1976; Kluge et al. 2006; Worofka et al. 1997). Single polymorphonuclear, basophilic or eosinophilic granulocytes can be present. Single erythrocytes are often intermingled as a contamination artefact during lumbar puncture (Table 6.1).

Leucocytes are characteristically small to intermediate sized, approx. 1–1.5 times as large as an erythrocyte. They are round with round nuclei and have regularly shaped borders. Monocytes are more irregularly formed, often beanlike shaped, and can contain small vacuoles which are interpreted as a sign of unspecific activation. Erythrocytes are small and round and have a double-ring structure because they lack a nucleus.

Granulocytes can sporadically occur in a normal cell composition without being a sign of a pathological process. Most often, polymorphonuclear granulocytes are seen, small round cells with highly irregular, often intersected nuclei (Fig. 6.5). Less frequently, eosinophilic (Fig. 6.6) or basophilic granulocytes are found.

A normal cell composition consists primarily of lymphocytes and monocytes with a relation of 3:1–4:1 and probably single granulocytes and artificially contaminated erythrocytes.

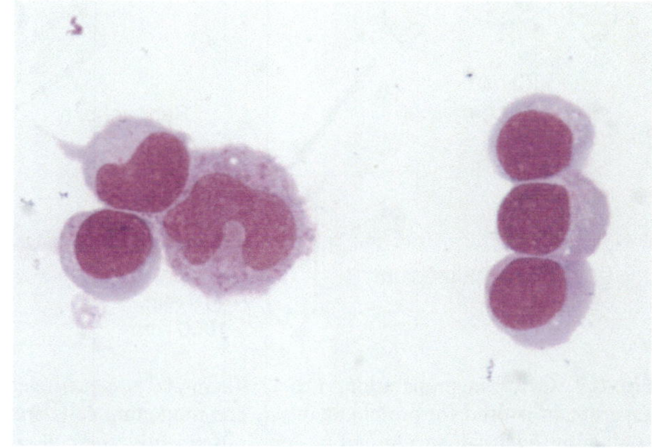

Fig. 6.4 Small- to medium-sized lymphocytes, round with thin cytoplasm (*right and lower left*) and monocytes with a broader, less homogeneous cytoplasm. Typical ratio of 2:1

Table 6.1 Cell types within the CSF

Physiological cells
Lymphocytes and monocytes, ratio 3:1–4:1
Single granulocytes or erythrocytes
Alterations of physiological cells
Lymphocytes: inflammatory changes, lymphoid cells, plasma cells
Monocytes: activated monocytes (small vacuoles), macrophages (larger vacuoles, probably visible object of phagocytosis like cells, erythrocytes, infectious agents)
Cells lining the CSF space and rarely occurring cells
Cartilage cells
Bone marrow cells
Ependymal, plexus, leptomeningeal cells
Multinucleated giant cells
Inflammatory reactions
Lymphocytic cell composition
Granulocytic cell composition
Monocytic and macrophage reaction – reparative phase
Haemorrhagic changes
Erythrophages, masked erythrophages, siderophages, haematoidin-containing macrophages
Neoplastic diseases
Neoplastic morphology (see Table 6.2)
Pigmented melanoma cells
Blast-like cells in haematological malignancy
Signet ring cells in adenocarcinoma

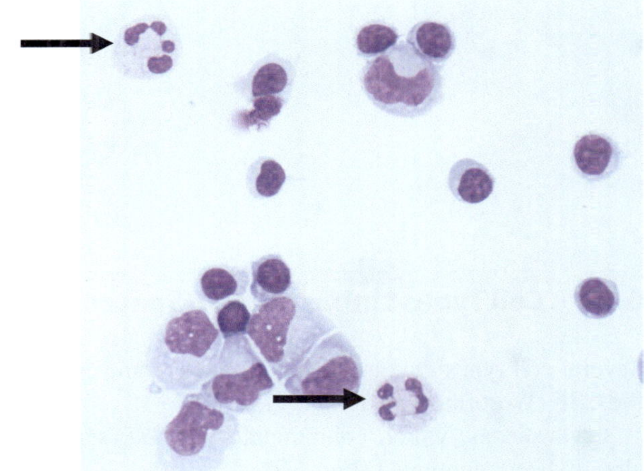

Fig. 6.5 Normal cell composition with single polymorphonuclear granulocytes (*arrows*)

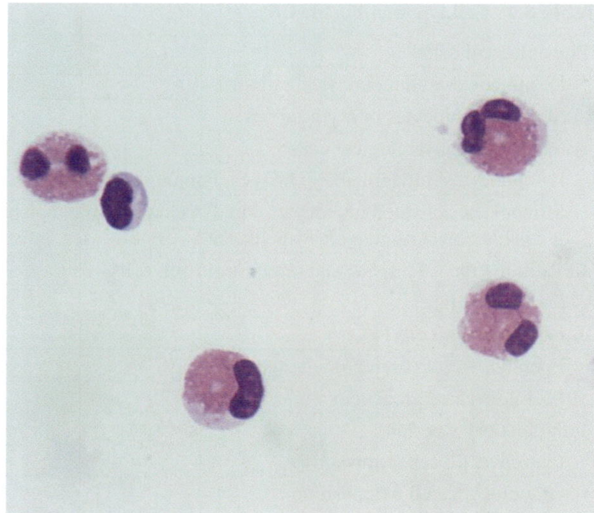

Fig. 6.6 Multiple eosinophilic granulocytes, one small lymphocyte

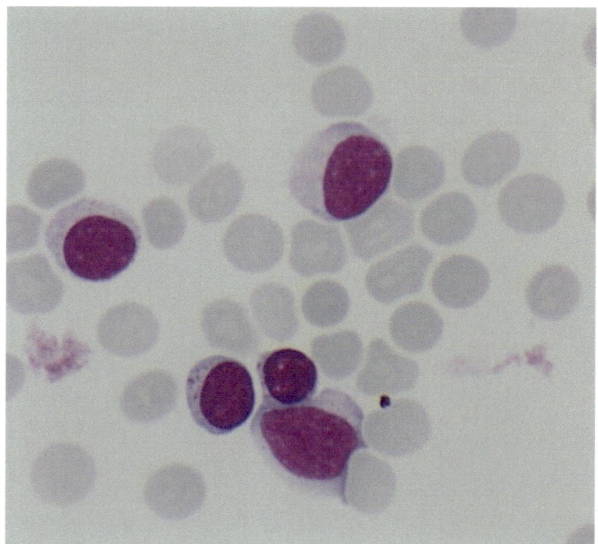

Fig. 6.7 Lymphocytes and peripheral blood. Erythrocytes are small and stain greyish-red. The absence of phagocytosis indicates that the erythrocytes result from artificial contamination

6.7   Cell Types Lining the CSF Spaces

Several cell types that are located in close vicinity to the CSF spaces can occur in the CSF (Worofka et al. 1997):

Erythrocytes, which contaminate the CSF sample during the puncture, have already been mentioned (Fig. 6.7).

Cartilage cells can be intermingled when the puncture is too deep and reaches the vertebral disk. Cartilage cells can be somewhat larger than physiological CSF cells and dark basophilic (Fig. 6.8). A less experienced cytologist may mistake these cells as malignant cells.

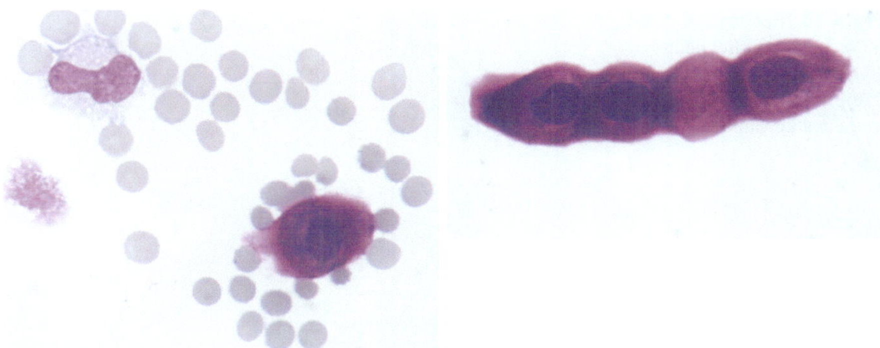

Fig. 6.8 *Left*: cartilage cell with typical dark basophilic staining of the nucleus and cytoplasm (*lower right*), monocyte (*upper left*), autolytic cell (*middle left*) and artificial blood contamination. *Right*: cartilage cells lined up

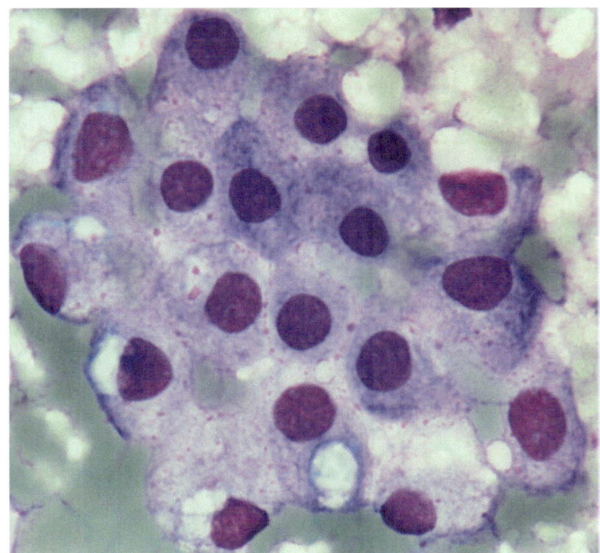

Fig. 6.9 Plexus cells with round nucleus and basophilic cytoplasm. Background of detritus with confluent erythrocytes

Bone marrow cells can contaminate the CSF during the puncture if blood-forming bone is affected. Therefore, blood precursor cells like erythroblasts or myeloblasts should be clearly identified. One hallmark to detect bone marrow contamination as opposed to malignant proliferation is the occurrence of cells from different lineages in different stages of development, while neoplastic proliferation will affect only one lineage and one certain stage of development. In case of bone marrow contamination in haematological malignancies, blasts in the CSF are not a proof of neoplastic meningitis, since artificial contamination deriving from the bone marrow cannot be differentiated from neoplastic affection of the CSF.

Other cell types that may enter the CSF space include choroid plexus (Fig. 6.9), ependymal (Fig. 6.10) and leptomeningeal cells (Fig. 6.11). Ependymal cells are up to approx. two times larger than leucocytes; their eosinophilic cytoplasm and

Fig. 6.10 Ependymal cells: large, eosinophilic, bean-shaped nucleus, loose cytoplasm. Peripheral blood in the background

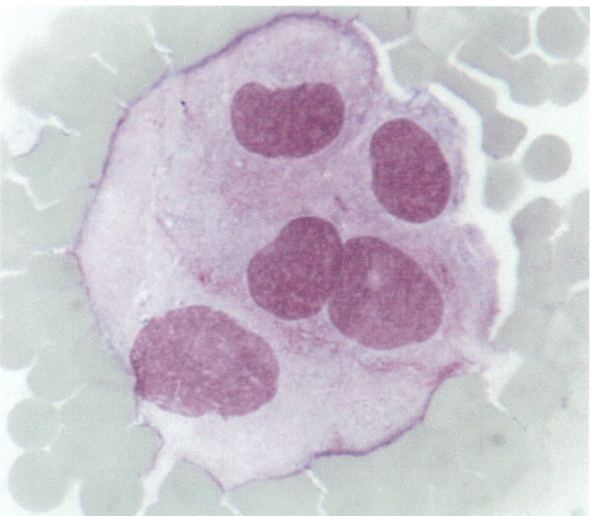

Fig. 6.11 Leptomeningeal cells. Small, beanlike shaped, always found in cellular complexes

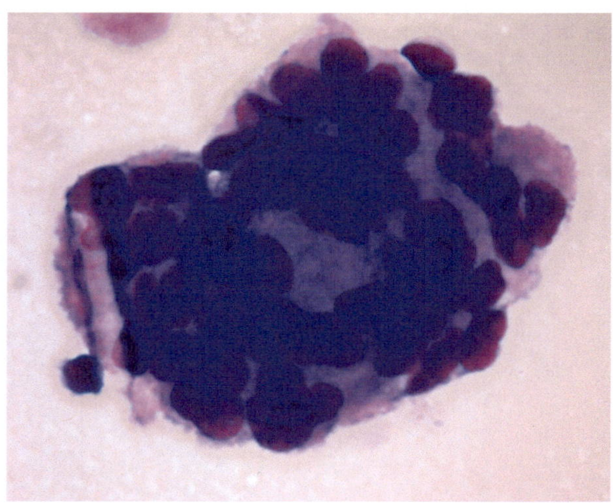

regular appearance make them relatively easy to identify. Plexus cells are relatively small, round and basophilic and usually occur in agglomerations. Leptomeningeal cells are smaller than small lymphocytes and bean shaped and always occur in agglomerations of multiple cells.

6.8   Alterations of Physiological CSF Cells

Physiological cells can modify their appearance depending on their function (Koelmel 2003; Kluge et al. 2006).

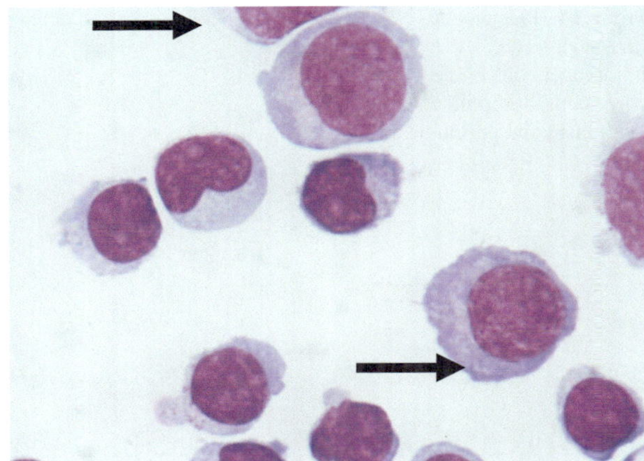

Fig. 6.12 Activated lymphocytes (*arrows*) – larger than normal lymphocytes and with more basophilic cytoplasm. The nuclear chromatin is still homogeneous and no perinuclear halo is visible, which distinguishes these cells from plasma cells

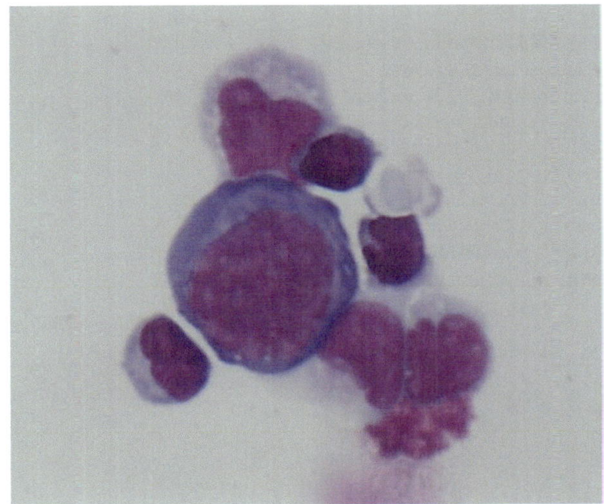

Fig. 6.13 Lymphoid cell. Large, with nucleus in the centre, basophilic cytoplasm, surrounded by small lymphocytes and monocytes

Inflammatory processes can result in activation of lymphocytes. After enlargement and more basophilic appearance of the cytoplasm (Fig. 6.12), an intermediate state of activation is a large cell with centrally positioned nucleus, the so-called lymphoid cell (Fig. 6.13). Further activation into a plasma cell results in reduced size with even more basophilic cytoplasm, eccentric nucleus with indentation and perinuclear halo (Fig. 6.14). A combination of these cells results in a typical inflammatory cell composition (Fig. 6.15).

Monocytes can be activated with small intracytoplasmic vacuoles. Macrophages, by contrast, are characterised by larger vacuoles and probably a visible object of phagocytosis (Fig. 6.16). Most often, erythrocytes or their transformation product haemosiderin or haematoidin can be observed (Fig. 6.17). Other cells can be incorporated such as lymphocytes, infectious agents like bacteria or just fatty substance.

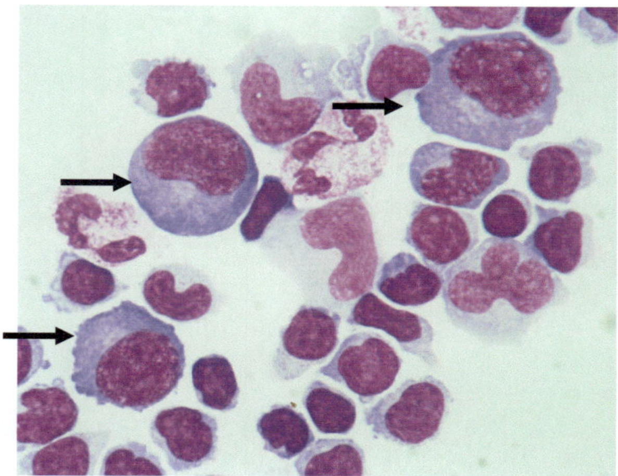

Fig. 6.14 Plasma cells (*arrows*): large, inhomogeneous nuclear chromatin, basophilic cytoplasm and perinuclear halo

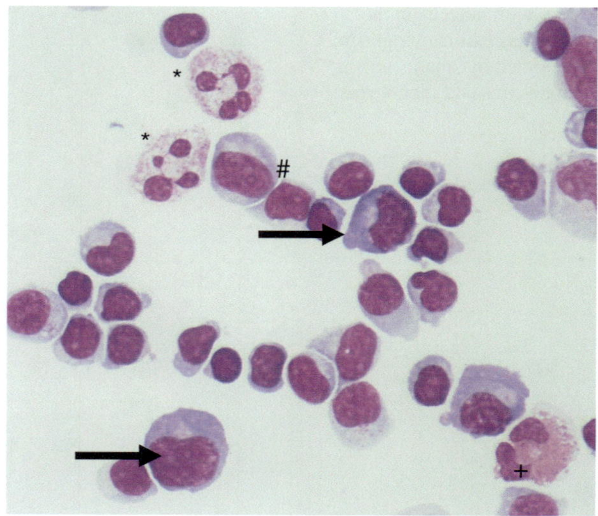

Fig. 6.15 Inflammatory cell composition in a case of neuroborreliosis. Numerous small lymphocytes, activated lymphocytes activated lymphocytes (#), monocytes, plasma cells (*arrows*), polymorphonuclear granulocytes (*) and one eosinophilic granulocyte (+)

Correspondingly, macrophages are named after the object of phagocytosis if visible, such as erythrophages, siderophages, leucophages, bacteriophages or lipophages. Most importantly, lipophages can contain very large single vacuoles and by such may appear as signet ring cells (Fig. 6.18). Cell size, appearance of the nucleus and the cellular context will give important information for the differentiation.

Cellular proliferation can occur in the case of inflammatory or reparative processes and become obvious through the appearance of mitoses. These can occur in lymphocytes and granulocytes in cases of inflammation or infection and in monocytes in the case of reparative processes in postinfectious situations, after cerebral ischaemia or trauma. Thus, the occurrence of mitoses, especially if regularly shaped,

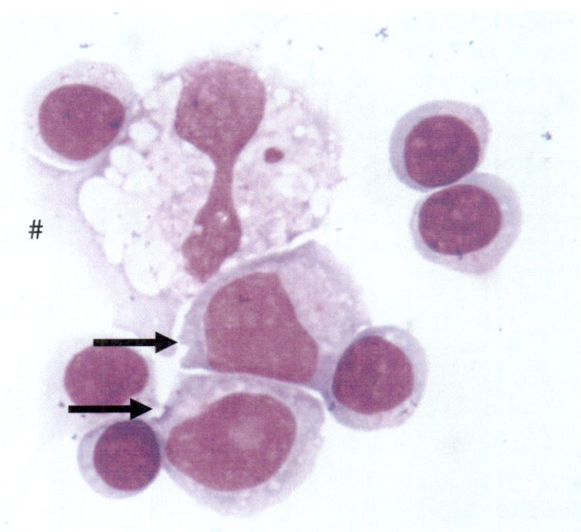

Fig. 6.16 Activated monocytes (*arrows*) – larger than the surrounding small lymphocytes, cytoplasm with single small vacuoles. Macrophage (#) – large with multiple cytoplasmic vacuoles

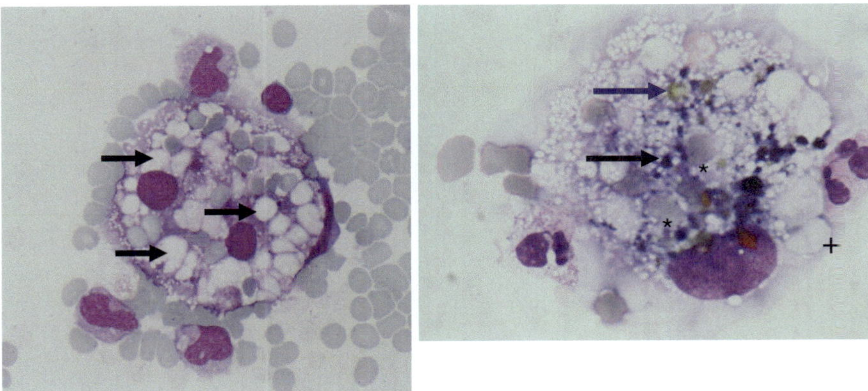

Fig. 6.17 Haemorrhage. *Left*: Huge macrophage with erythrocytes, many of them masked (*arrows*), and some leucocytes. *Right*: Macrophage containing fresh (*) and masked (+) erythrocytes, haemosiderin (*arrow*) and haematoidin (*blue arrow*)

is not necessarily a sign of malignancy (Fig. 6.19). A thorough analysis of the surrounding cell types will give important clues for the cause of cellular proliferation.

6.9 Artefacts

Several influences can alter the cellular appearance which sometimes causes difficulty to establish a reliable evaluation. Most often, autolytic changes – caused by long transportation periods, heat or cold – will change cellular morphology (Worofka

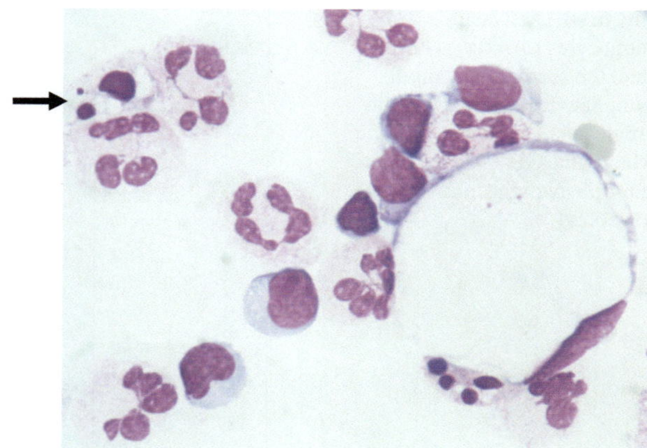

Fig. 6.18 Lipophage, pseudo-signet ring cell (*right*). Very large, eccentric nucleus, optically empty cytoplasm. Inflammatory background with granulocytes. One leucophage with fragments of a leucocyte, supposedly a lymphocyte (*arrow*)

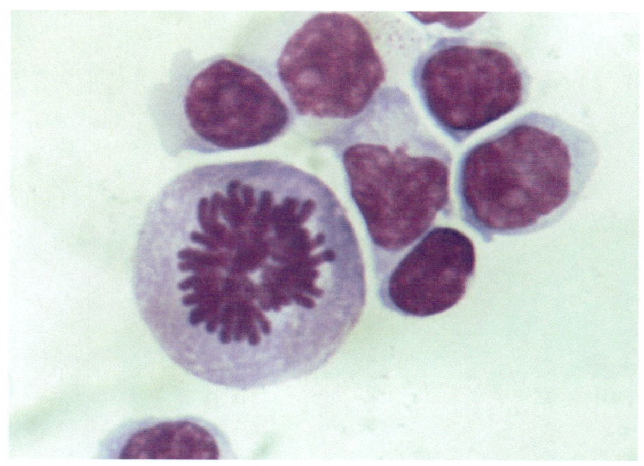

Fig. 6.19 Regular mitosis. Inflammatory proliferation in a case of neuroborreliosis

et al. 1997). It is characterised by disappearance of the borders of the nucleus and cytoplasm and fading of the staining intensity. Marked autolysis makes cytological evaluation of the cells impossible. This should be clearly communicated with the treating physician.

Centrifugation artefacts can be easily recognised by an elongation of the cytoplasm. Preservation solutions such as formalin or glutaraldehyde cause an intense shrinking of the cytoplasm which makes it impossible to further differentiate the cells. All kinds of cellular preservation should therefore be strictly avoided.

6.10 Cell Types Without Pathological Significance

Multinucleated giant cells are very rare cell types that can contain five to eight nuclei. They are assumed to develop through fusion of multiple cells and have no pathological significance (Worofka et al. 1997). Although they may appear malignant at the first glance, their singular occurrence and multiple, normal-appearing nuclei will lead to the correct diagnosis at thorough observation.

Lipophages are macrophages with large, optically empty spaces containing fatty particles. They are not associated with a specific pathology.

6.11   Inflammatory Reactions

Inflammatory alterations of CSF cells and their composition can be roughly divided into infectious and noninfectious disease and affect lymphocytes, monocytes and granulocytes. Cell composition will usually appear as mainly or exclusively lymphocytic (Fig. 6.15) in noninfectious inflammatory reactions, viral infections or Lyme borreliosis (Oehmichen 1976; Kluge et al. 2006; Worofka et al. 1997). Inflammatory alterations of lymphocyte morphology have already been described. Granulocytic reactions are typical in bacterial infections (Fig. 6.20). Predominant monocyte and macrophage reactions are seen in subacute, reparative phases of infections. A mixed-cellular picture with lymphocytes, granulocytes and monocytes/macrophages can be observed in subacute infections that develop within several days to weeks, such as listeriosis, tuberculosis or fungal infections (Fig. 6.21) (Oehmichen 1976). With inflammatory and especially infectious cellular compositions, leucophages can sometimes be found – macrophages containing lymphocytes or granulocytes. Mitoses can occur as well. Both reactions, however, can also be observed in neoplastic disease.

These rules, however, can only point towards the correct diagnosis. Only if intracellular infectious agents such as bacteria can be demonstrated, the diagnosis can be assured. Visible extracellular bacteria without signs of cellular inflammatory

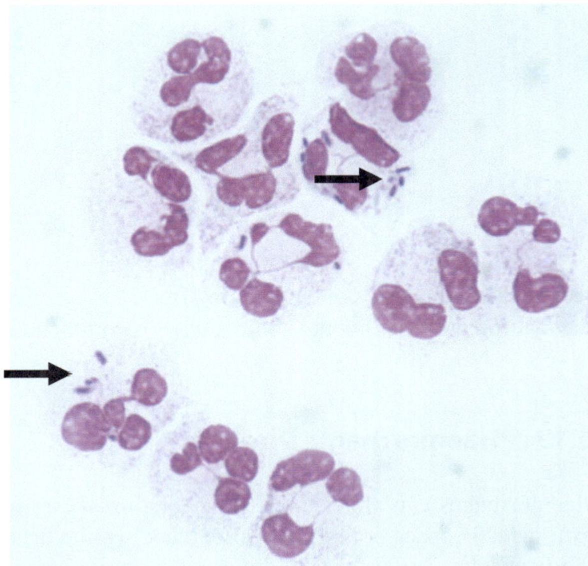

Fig. 6.20 Bacterial meningitis, *E. coli.* Polymorphonuclear granulocytes with multiple intracellular cocci (*arrows*)

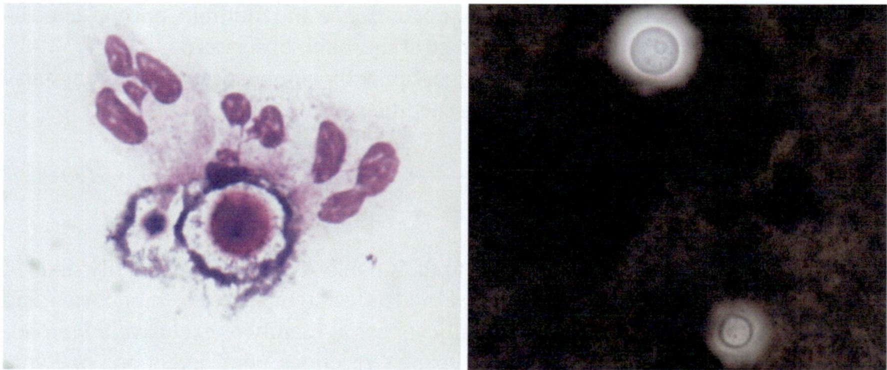

Fig. 6.21 Cryptococcal meningitis. *Left*: large cell with optically empty halo and dark rim. Second cell developing at its left. Surrounding granulocytes. *Right*: black ink preparation. The ink is kept away by the mucous rim of the cryptococci, resulting in a visible light halo

Fig. 6.22 Bacterial contamination. All bacteria (multiple *dark spots*) are located extracellularly. Monocytic predominance without inflammatory reaction

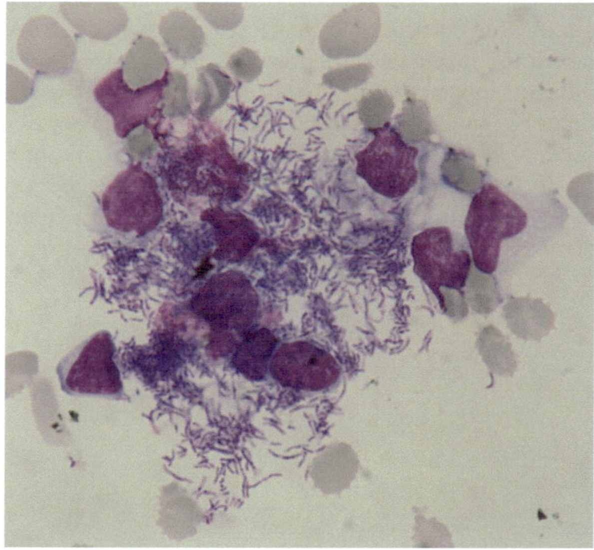

reactions are signs of contamination after CSF sampling (Fig. 6.22). The report on the cytological assessment should always recommend microbiological assessment.

6.12 Haemorrhagic Diseases

Haemorrhages can affect the CSF space directly as subarachnoid bleeding to the external CSF space or indirectly after bleeding into the brain parenchyma that enters the ventricles. In rare cases, direct intraventricular haemorrhage can occur, most probably as bleeding from the ventricular plexus.

The most important task for CSF analysis is to differentiate artificial contamination from genuine bleeding into the CSF. For this purpose, it is essential to recognise the different states of erythrocyte phagocytosis. According to the timecourse of their phagocytosis and digestion of their content, macrophages containing erythrocytes, haemosiderin and haematoidin can be observed (Fig. 6.17). Erythrophages containing normal, coloured erythrocytes are regarded as an insecure sign of haemorrhage, since it is assumed that phagocytosis may occur ex vivo in the sample containment up to 12 h after bleeding or lumbar puncture, respectively (Oehmichen 1976; Worofka et al. 1997). Colourless, so-called "masked" erythrocytes can be easily mistaken as vacuoles within the macrophage. The size and regular round shape of the erythrocytes will lead to the correct diagnosis. Masked erythrocytes are a more reliable sign of intra-CSF haemorrhage. After 24–72 h, the masked, white-appearing erythrocytes turn light and later on dark blue, as haemosiderin becomes visible. Siderophages are a secure sign of intra-CSF haemorrhage, since digestion will not reach this state ex vivo. After several weeks, haemosiderin turns into honey-yellow haematoidin crystals which are only rarely found.

6.13   Neoplastic Alterations

The differentiation of neoplastic cells from other physiological or pathological cell types remains one of the most important tasks of CSF cytology. With a frequency of 5–10 % of patients, breast and lung cancer, malignant melanoma and aggressive haematological malignancies like acute leukaemias or lymphomas most often cause tumour cell dissemination into the CSF and leptomeninges, called neoplastic meningitis. Among the primary CNS neoplasms, medulloblastomas, primitive neuroectodermal tumours (PNET) and ependymomas most frequently affect the CSF (Strik and Prommel 2010).

In general, increased total cell size, basophilic cytoplasm, nucleoli, increased size of nucleus relative to cytoplasm and deformation of total cell or nucleus are regarded as signs of malignancy (Table 6.2) (Koelmel 2003; Oehmichen 1976; Worofka et al. 1997; Bigner 1994). Mitoses often have atypical morphology with irregular chromosome composition (Fig. 6.23). Epithelial cells, usually causing neoplastic meningitis from solid tumours, often express one or several of these characteristics. Moreover, this cell type does not usually occur in the CSF. Therefore, neoplastic meningitis from solid tumours most often does not cause a major diagnostic problem. As a rule, a cytological diagnosis for certain types of malignancies is not possible, since single

Table 6.2 Classical morphological signs of malignancy

Patterns of neoplastic morphology
Increased cellular size
Increased nucleus-cell ratio
Basophilic cytoplasm
Nucleolus
Deformation of cell form
Deformation of nucleus

Fig. 6.23 Atypical mitosis with irregular chromosomes

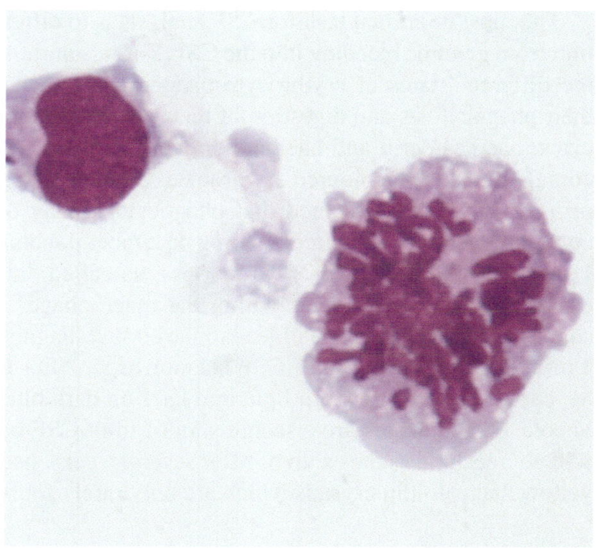

Fig. 6.24 Tumour cells in a case of malignant melanoma. Multiple times the size of the surrounding erythrocytes, eosinophilic cytoplasm, dark nucleoli and dark pigment within the cytoplasm of the upper median cell

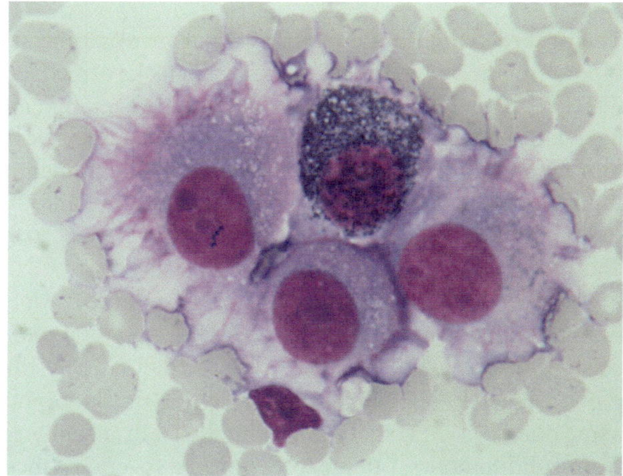

cells share morphological similarities between different tumour types. There are, however, some characteristics that may give strong evidence for certain tumours. Dark pigmentation of cells, for example, is a morphological hallmark for melanoma cells. Although pigment can sometimes be found in neoplastic meningitis from melanomas, it is rarely found, and if so, it most often stains dark blue instead of black (Fig. 6.24). This is in contrast to the appearance in histological slides and can be explained by the decreased absorption of light by the singular cells in the cytological

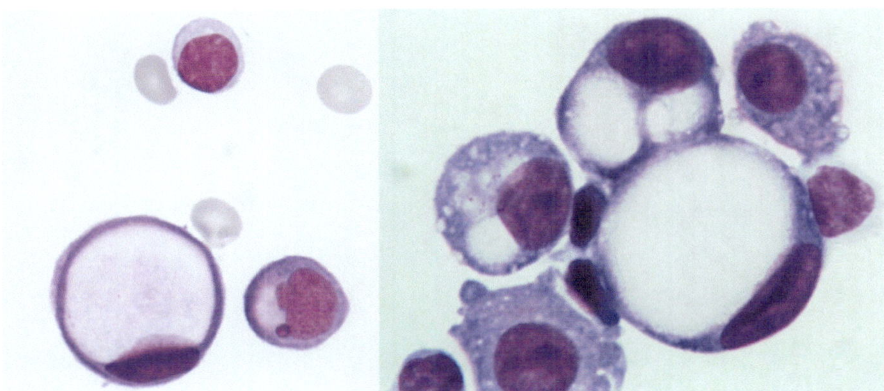

Fig. 6.25 Gastric signet cell carcinoma: malignant signet ring cells with basophilic, thick border of cytoplasm and background of large, basophilic tumour cells with vacuoles and pointed borders of the cytoplasm. Single erythrocytes and leucocytes

Table 6.3 Morphologically similar cell types that can be counfounded

Possible confounders		
Melanophages	Siderophages	Pigmented melanoma cells
Lipophages	Signet ring cells	
Cartilage cells	Multinucleated giant cells	Tumour cells
Cryptococci	Lymphocytes	
Inflammatory lymphocytes	Neoplastic lymphocytes	

preparation as compared with multiple layers of cells in a histological section. A typical sign for certain types of adenocarcinomas are signet ring cells, large cells with an optically empty centre and peripheralised nucleus (Fig. 6.25). These cells, however, can be confounded with lipophages and macrophages with a large intracytoplasmic vacuole. Markedly increased cell size, dark basophilic cytoplasm and the cellular context with surrounding tumour cells may distinguish neoplastic signet cells from lipophages (Table 6.3).

Haematological malignancies are often difficult to distinguish from nonneoplastic alterations, since lymphocytes also occur physiologically in the CSF. Long-lasting inflammatory reactions – especially of infectious origin – can lead to changes in morphology that can resemble neoplastic disease and make differentiation difficult. Very large total cell size, deep incision of the nuclei or alterations of the whole cell form (Fig. 6.26) may help to establish the diagnosis of neoplastic disease especially in B-cell lymphoma (Perske et al. 2011).

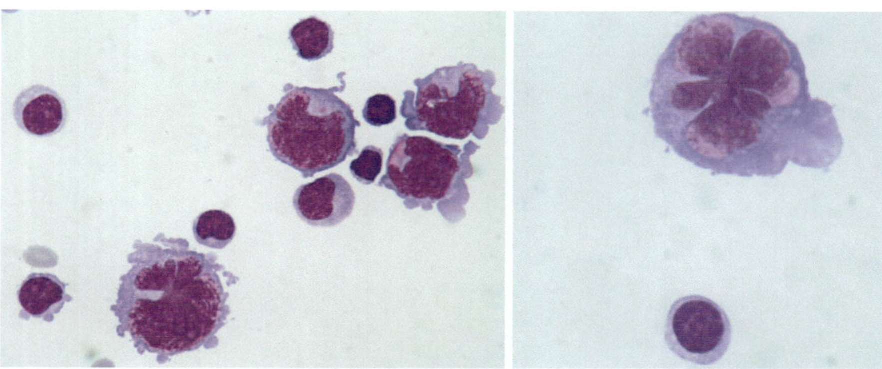

Fig. 6.26 B-cell non-Hodgkin's lymphoma. Cells are four to six times larger than the surrounding lymphocytes, nuclei have in part deep notches and the dark basophilic cytoplasm has pointed extensions

References

Bigner SH (1994) Cytopathology of the central nervous system. Edward Arnold Publishers, London

Gondos B, King EB (1976) Cerebrospinal fluid cytology: diagnostic accuracy and comparison of different techniques. Acta Cytol 20:542–547

Grover ML, Blee E, Stokes BO (1995) Effect of sample volume on cell recovery in cytocentrifugation. Acta Cytol 39:387–390

Hansen HH, Bender RA, Shelton BJ (1974) The cyto-centrifuge and cerebrospinal fluid cytology. Acta Cytol 18:259–262

Heller T, Nagel I, Ehrlich B, Bahr M, Strik H (2008) Automated cerebrospinal fluid cytology. Anal Quant Cytol Histol 30:139–144

Kleine TO (2003) Liquordiagnostik. Methoden und klinische Bedeutung. In: Zettl U, Lehmitz R, Mix E (eds) Klinische Liquordiagnostik. De Gruyter, Berlin, pp 129–130

Kluge H, Wieczorek V, Linke E, Zimmermann K, Isenmann S, Witte O (2006) Atlas of CSF cytology. Thieme, Stuttgart

Koelmel H (2003) Conventional CSF cytology. Klinische Liquordiagnostik. In: Zettl UK, Mix E, Lehmitz R (eds). Walter de Gruyter, Berlin, pp 135–160

Kolmel HW (1977) A method for concentrating cerebrospinal fluid cells. Acta Cytol 21:154–157

Lehmitz R, Kleine TO (1995) Liquorzytologie – Ausbeute, Verteilung und Darstellung von Leukozyten bei drei Sedimentationsverfahren im Vergleich zu drei Zytozentrifugen-Modifikationen. Lab Med 18:91–99

Oehmichen M (1976) Cerebrospinal fluid cytology. Thieme, Stuttgart

Perske T, Nagel I, Nagel H, Strik H (2011) CSF cytology –the ongoing dilemma to distinguish neoplastic and inflammatory lymphocytes. Diagn Cytopathol 39(8):621–6

Strik H, Prommel P (2010) Diagnosis and individualized therapy of neoplastic meningitis. Expert Rev Anticancer Ther 10:1137–1148

Strik H, Luthe H, Nagel I, Ehrlich B, Bahr M (2005) Automated cerebrospinal fluid cytology: limitations and reasonable applications. Anal Quant Cytol Histol 27:167–173

Veerman AJ, Huismans L, van Zantwijk I (1985) Storage of cerebrospinal fluid samples at room temperature. Acta Cytol 29:188–189

Woodruff KH (1973) Cerebrospinal fluid cytomorphology using cytocentrifugation. Am J Clin Pathol 60:621–627

Worofka B, Lassmann J, Bauer K, Kristoferitsch W (1997) Praktische Liquorzelldiagnostik. Springer, Wien/New York

Glucose and Lactate

Hayrettin Tumani and Harald Hegen

Contents

Abstract

Determination of the CSF/S_{Glu} ratio and/or CSF lactate concentration is part of the routine CSF work-up enabling the verification of an anaerobic glucose metabolism in the CNS. Since lactate is an end product of the anaerobic glucose metabolism and since there is an inverse relationship between CSF lactate and CSF/S_{Glu} ratio, both parameters can be used for the same diagnostic purposes. A decrease of CSF/S_{Glu} ratio and increase of CSF lactate, respectively, is found in

H. Tumani (✉)
Department of Neurology,
University of Ulm,
Ulm, Germany
e-mail: hayrettin.tumani@uni-ulm.de

H. Hegen
Department of Neurology,
University of Innsbruck,
Innsbruck, Austria

© Springer International Publishing Switzerland 2015
F. Deisenhammer et al. (eds.), *Cerebrospinal Fluid in Clinical Neurology*,
DOI 10.1007/978-3-319-01225-4_7

various neurological diseases such as bacterial and fungal meningitis or leptomeningeal metastases. In glucose transporter-1 (GLUT1) deficiency syndromes, only the CSF/S_{Glu} ratio is pathologic. A CSF/S_{Glu} ratio ≤ 0.4 (with variations depending on blood glucose concentration) and CSF lactate >3.5 mmol/L are widely accepted as pathologic.

7.1 Glucose

Glucose is actively transported from the blood into the CSF compartment by specific carrier mechanism, in the first instance GLUT1. CSF glucose concentration depends on serum concentration; therefore, it is indispensable to calculate the CSF/S_{Glu} ratio (Watson and Scott 1995; Deisenhammer et al. 2006). As already mentioned above, glucose in CSF is decreased in some neurological diseases, and one of the main diagnostic purposes of the CSF/S_{Glu} ratio is to differentiate between bacterial and viral infections of the CNS. Furthermore, pathologic CSF/S_{Glu} ratio supports diagnosis of leptomeningeal metastases or GLUT1 deficiency syndrome.

7.1.1 Preanalytics

For analysis of glucose, a pair of CSF and blood samples needs to be collected at the same time, since CSF concentration is dependent on blood concentration and requires expression as CSF/S_{Glu} ratio. Glucose in CSF samples is stable for 5 h at room temperature and for 24 h at 4 °C independent of cell counts (Dujmovic and Deisenhammer 2010). Glucose concentration in untreated serum samples decreases over time leading to a falsely increased CSF/blood ratio. Sodium fluoride-treated blood specimens remain stable for up to 3 days, whereas heparin-treated specimens tend to decline continuously. If, however, the concentration of glucose is to be measured within the first hour after sampling, use of sodium fluoride is unnecessary (Chan et al. 1989).

With regard to which blood preparation should be used, it is noteworthy that there is an average 11 % difference in glucose concentration between plasma and blood (1.11:1.0) according to the IFCC recommendations (Steffes and Sacks 2005). Plasma and blood glucose are used interchangeably with a consequent risk of misinterpretation. Serum should not be used because the glucose concentration may decrease as a result of glycolysis during its preparation (Steffes and Sacks 2005).

7.1.2 Method

Most current photometric methods to measure glucose use enzymatic conversion (e.g., hexokinase/glucose oxidase/glucose dehydrogenase) and absorbance measurements near or at 340 nm (Steffes and Sacks 2005; Thomas 2005). The concentration can also be determined by a kinetic measurement, comparing sample to a calibrator. Other methods include protein precipitation, associated with a positive bias, depending on the degree of dilution and concentration of protein. Nevertheless, all detection methods measure glucose concentration (amount of glucose per volume of sample) with sufficient trueness and precision (Steffes and Sacks 2005).

7.1.3 Reference Range

Lumbar CSF glucose levels of healthy persons are roughly 60 % of blood levels (Leen et al. 2012; Hegen et al. 2014). Reference ranges for capillary, venous, and whole blood differ. There are no sex-related differences, and reported changes of CSF/S_{Glu} ratios with age are most likely an epiphenomenon with increased serum glucose concentrations with increasing age (Hegen et al. 2014; Leen et al. 2012).

Parameter	Range
CSF glucose	2.7–4.2 (mmol/L)
Blood glucose	3.3–5.5 (mmol/L)
Glucose CSF/blood ratio	0.61–0.89
	(Cave: CSF/serum ratio may be lower than 0.5 if serum glucose concentration is >100 mg/dL) (see Fig. 7.1)

7.1.4 Interpretation

CSF/blood ratios below 0.5 are indicative of bacterial CNS infections caused by organisms such as streptococcus, meningococcus, mycobacteria, and funguses. During meningeal blastomatosis, CSF levels of glucose may also drop below this ratio of 0.5. However, in cases with increased serum glucose concentrations, the normal CSF/blood glucose ratio may drop up to below 0.4 (see Fig. 7.1a, b), and therefore an apparently decreased CSF/serum ratio may be due to a diabetic dysmetabolism which requires adjustment to avoid a misinterpretation (Hegen et al. 2014; Leen et al. 2012).

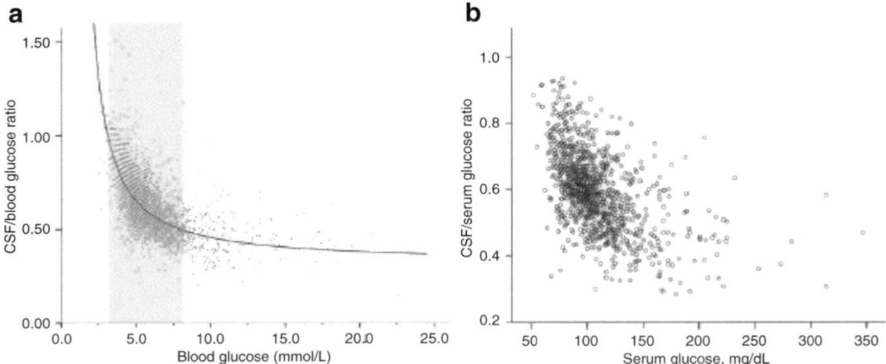

Fig. 7.1 (a) Relationship between blood glucose (mmol/L) and CSF/blood glucose ratio (Leen et al. 2012) (b) and relationship between serum glucose (mg/dL) and CSF/serum glucose ratio (Hegen et al. 2014). Due to the inverse correlation, cutoff levels for normal CSF/serum glucose ratio require adjustment to the glucose concentration in blood or serum, respectively

According to a recent study, cutoff values for normal CSF/S$_{Glu}$ ratio defined as the 5th percentile were 0.5 for patients with serum glucose concentrations <100 mg/dL, 0.4 for those with a glucose level of 100–149 mg/dL, and 0.3 for serum glucose concentrations ≥150 mg/dL (Hegen et al. 2014).

7.2 Lactate

Lactate in human brain is produced by glial cells, mainly astrocytes, and it is aerobically metabolized by neurons (Brooks 2002). Lactate in CSF is derived from the CNS and from blood. However, changes in blood concentration do not affect the CSF concentration, since the lactate transporter at the blood-brain barrier is saturated (Barros and Deitmer 2010). Therefore, when evaluating CSF concentration of lactate, knowledge of the blood level is not required.

Lactate occurs in two optical isomers, L-lactate and D-lactate. L-Lactate concentration predominates with up to 99 %; thus it is of major importance in routine CSF analysis and D-lactate has no established role in routine CSF diagnostics. L-Lactate represents the end product of the anaerobic glucose metabolism, so it can replace glucose analysis (Fig. 7.2). Elevation of lactate indicates hyperlactatemia or lactic acidosis which is an important diagnostic aspect in intensive care units.

7.2.1 Preanalytics

Stability of lactate in CSF strongly depends on the number of leukocytes, red blood cells and pathogens. Red cells in CSF cause significant increases in lactate concentrations, more so when exposed to air. This has to be considered when interpreting

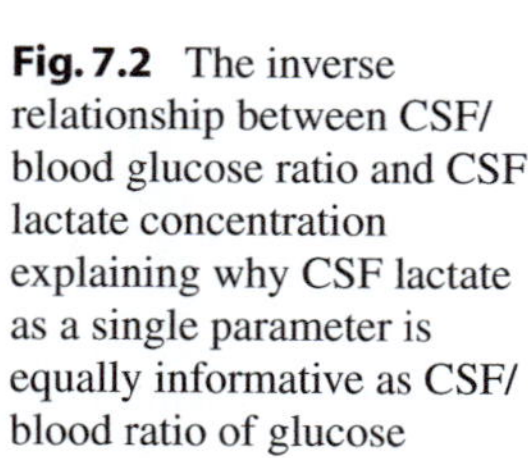

Fig. 7.2 The inverse relationship between CSF/blood glucose ratio and CSF lactate concentration explaining why CSF lactate as a single parameter is equally informative as CSF/blood ratio of glucose

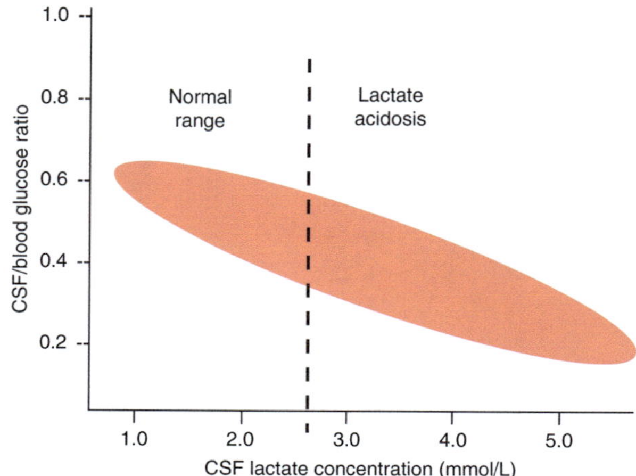

lactate in CSF contaminated by blood (Venkatesh et al. 2003). Lactate is stable at room temperature for up to 24 h independent of CSF leukocyte count without addition of sodium fluoride (Dujmovic and Deisenhammer 2010; Thomas 2005).

7.2.2 Method

Lactate is measured by enzymatic tests and photometry either using lactate dehydrogenase (conversion to pyruvate in the presence of NAD) or using lactate oxidase (conversion to pyruvate and hydrogen peroxide) (Thomas 2005).

7.2.3 Reference Range

CSF lactate concentration is age dependent with a range between 1.0 and 2.7 mmol/L (9.9–23.4 mg/dL) but not sex dependent (Zhang and Natowicz 2013).

Age (years)	L-Lactate range	
1–15	1.0–2.0 (mmol/L)	9.9–16.2 (mg/dL)
16–50	1.2–2.4 (mmol/L)	13.5–18.9 (mg/dL)
> 51	1.3–2.7 (mmol/L)	15.3–23.4 (mg/dL)

7.2.4 Interpretation

A mild to moderate lactate acidosis (2.7–3.5 mmol/L) in the CSF can be observed in many neurological diseases such as metabolic encephalopathies, autoimmune encephalitis, cerebral hemorrhage and insults, epileptic seizures, brain malignancies (glioblastoma) with a tendency for anaerobic glycolysis, viral infections (herpes viruses), Lyme neuroborreliosis, and polyradiculitis. Bacterial meningitis (pneumococcus, meningococcus, tuberculosis, listeria), cerebral metastases, neurosarcoidosis, and septic encephalopathy may be associated with severe abnormal elevations of lactate (>4.0 mmol/L).

References

Barros LF, Deitmer JW (2010) Glucose and lactate supply to the synapse. Brain Res Rev 63(1–2):149–159

Brooks GA (2002) Lactate shuttles in nature. Biochem Soc Trans 30(2):258–264

Chan AY, Swaminathan R, Cockram CS (1989) Effectiveness of sodium fluoride as a preservative of glucose in blood. Clin Chem 35(2):315–317

Deisenhammer F, Bartos A, Egg R, Gilhus NE, Giovannoni G, Rauer S, Sellebjerg F, Task Force EFNS (2006) Guidelines on routine cerebrospinal fluid analysis. Report from an EFNS task force. Eur J Neurol 13(9):913–922

Dujmovic I, Deisenhammer F (2010) Stability of cerebrospinal fluid/serum glucose ratio and cerebrospinal fluid lactate concentrations over 24 h: analysis of repeated measurements. Clin Chem Lab Med 48(2):209–212

Hegen H, Auer M, Deisenhammer F (2014) Serum glucose adjusted cut-off values for normal Cerebrospinal fluid/serum glucose ratio: implications for clinical practice. Clin Chem Lab Med 52:1335–1340

Leen WG, Willemsen MA, Wevers RA, Verbeek MM (2012) Cerebrospinal fluid glucose and lactate: age-specific reference values and implications for clinical practice. PLoS One 7(8):e42745. doi:10.1371/journal.pone.0042745

Steffes MW, Sacks DB (2005) Measurement of circulating glucose concentrations: the time is now for consistency among methods and types of samples. Clin Chem 51(9):1569–1570

Thomas L (2005) Labor und diagnose. TH Verlagsgesellschaft mbH, Frankfurt/Main

Venkatesh B, Morgan TJ, Boots RJ, Hall J, Siebert D (2003) Interpreting CSF lactic acidosis: effect of erythrocytes and air exposure. Crit Care Resusc 5(3):177–181

Watson MA, Scott MG (1995) Clinical utility of biochemical analysis of cerebrospinal fluid. Clin Chem 41(3):343–360

Zhang WM, Natowicz MR (2013) Cerebrospinal fluid lactate and pyruvate concentrations and their ratio. Clin Biochem 46(7–8):694–697

CSF Total Protein

8

Hayrettin Tumani and Harald Hegen

Contents

Abstract

The CSF total protein concentration is used in emergency diagnostics as a rough evaluation tool for the blood-CSF barrier function that may be disturbed by reduced CSF turnover occurring in different diseases such as purulent meningitis, spinal canal stenosis or polyneuroradiculitis.

The interpretation of elevated CSF protein concentration may, however, be difficult since several disease-independent factors may contribute to interindividual variability such as the individual's blood concentration, volume of sampled CSF and site of puncture in addition to intrathecally produced proteins. This shortcoming can be overcome by additional CSF analysis including albumin and immunoglobulins.

H. Tumani (✉)
Department of Neurology,
University of Ulm,
Ulm, Germany
e-mail: hayrettin.tumani@uni-ulm.de

H. Hegen
Department of Neurology,
University of Innsbruck,
Innsbruck, Austria

© Springer International Publishing Switzerland 2015
F. Deisenhammer et al. (eds.), *Cerebrospinal Fluid in Clinical Neurology*,
DOI 10.1007/978-3-319-01225-4_8

8.1   Preanalytics

For analysis of total protein, only the CSF sample is necessary. Total protein concentration is stable for at least 1 week even at room temperature(s) and when stored at fridge temperature up to a couple of months. Considerable changes due to artificial blood contamination or haemolysis are possible; for artificial blood contamination, an estimated adjustment is possible if the respective blood or serum findings are known (Reiber 1983; Reiber et al. 2003).

8.2   Method

CSF total protein is measured by turbidimetry, nephelometry and dye-binding assays. The modified dye-binding assays (e.g. biuret, pyrogallol red) have been established and validated for protein analysis in serum, but not for CSF.

The preferred method for measurement of total protein in CSF is kinetic nephelometry in 40 % trichloroacetic acid (TCA), because it is mass related and independent of the molecular form (Reiber 1983). Nephelometric two-point and turbidimetric assays with low acid concentrations are prone to instability and a tendency to flocculate. Accuracy of dye-binding reactions varies depending on the fraction of the aromatic amino acids.

A fast and simple alternative is the semiquantitative Pandy's test (phenol reaction) which can be used as a bedside test for a rough guidance in emergency conditions when quantitative techniques are not available right away (Petereit et al. 2007).

8.3   Reference Range

Concentration of total protein increases from ventricles to lumbar CSF space (Gerber et al. 1998), and it is age dependent (Breebaart et al. 1978). Therefore, reference range has to be adapted for age and site of CSF collection (Deisenhammer 2006). The ratio of ventricular to lumbar concentration of total protein is 1:2.5. Another pitfall of total protein is that upper limits of reference range highly depend on the individual protein concentration in blood and the intrathecally produced protein fraction. This might explain why several studies suggest even a higher normal cut-off, somewhere between 500 and 600 mg/L (Deisenhammer 2006).

Age (years)	Lumbar total protein range (mg/L)
Newborn	<1,700
1–15	90–350
16–60	150–450

8.4   Interpretation

Many acute inflammatory diseases of the CNS are characterized by a mild to moderate increase in total protein concentration caused either by an increased capillary permeability of the blood-CSF barrier (purulent meningitis), by disturbed elimination of CSF at the spinal radices (Guillain-Barré syndrome polyradiculitis, Lyme Neuroborreliosis) or by mechanic disturbance of CSF bulk flow (spinal canal stenosis).

Purulent meningitis is an example of severe increase of total protein (>1,000 mg/lL). Acute Lyme disease (borreliosis) and the Guillain-Barré syndrome polyradiculitis are examples for moderate (750–1,000 mg/L), and viral meningitis and polyneuropathies examples for mild abnormal elevations (500–750 mg/L).

Interpretation of total protein will be described in detail in chapters on CSF in clinical syndromes.

References

Breebaart K, Becker H, Jongebloed FA (1978) Investigation of reference values of components of cerebrospinal fluid. Journal of clinical chemistry and clinical biochemistry 16:561–565

Deisenhammer F, Bartos A, Egg R, Gilhus NE, Giovannoni G, Rauer S, Sellebjerg F, Task Force EFNS (2006) Guidelines on routine cerebrospinal fluid analysis. Report from an EFNS task force. Eur J Neurol 13(9):913–922

Gerber J, Tumani H, Kolenda H, Nau R (1998) Lumbar and ventricular CSF protein, leukocytes, and lactate in suspected bacterial CNS infections. Neurology 51(6):1710–1714

Petereit H, Sindern E, Wick M (2007) Liquordiagnostik. Leitlinien und Methodenkatalog der Deutschen Gesellschaft für Liquordiagnostik und Klinische Neurochemie. Springer Medizin Verlag, Heidelberg (see also www.dgln.de)

Reiber H (1983) Kinetics of protein agglomeration. A nephelometric method for the determination of total protein in biological samples. J Biochem Biophys Methods 7(2):153–160

Reiber H, Thompson EJ, Grimsley G, Bernardi G, Adam P, Monteiro de Almeida S, et al (2003) Quality assurance for cerebrospinal fluid protein analysis: international consensus by an Internet-based group discussion. Clin Chem Lab Med 41(3):331–337

CSF Albumin: Albumin CSF/Serum Ratio (Marker for Blood-CSF Barrier Function)

9

Hayrettin Tumani and Harald Hegen

Contents

Abstract

CSF albumin serves as an ideal parameter to evaluate the permeability of the blood-CSF barrier. The CSF/serum albumin ratio (Q-Alb) has to be used in order to correct for the individual blood concentration of albumin.

Abnormal elevations of Q-Alb occur in various disorders including inflammatory and noninflammatory neurological diseases. Mild-to-moderate elevations of Q-Alb are typical for diabetic and immune-mediated polyneuropathies or viral meningitis, while moderate-to-severe Q-Alb elevations are associated with CNS infections, immune-mediated polyradiculitis or severe spinal canal stenosis.

H. Tumani (✉)
Department of Neurology,
University of Ulm,
Ulm, Germany
e-mail: hayrettin.tumani@uni-ulm.de

H. Hegen
Department of Neurology,
University of Innsbruck,
Innsbruck, Austria

© Springer International Publishing Switzerland 2015
F. Deisenhammer et al. (eds.), *Cerebrospinal Fluid in Clinical Neurology*,
DOI 10.1007/978-3-319-01225-4_9

9.1   Introduction

Albumin is produced exclusively in the liver, so all albumin detected in the CSF originates by definition from blood. Therefore, it serves as an ideal parameter to evaluate the permeability of the blood-CSF barrier. However, for a reliable evaluation of the blood-CSF barrier integrity, CSF/serum ratio of albumin (Q-Alb) that reflects the diffusion gradient of albumin has to be used in order to correct for the individual's blood-derived fraction. An additional role of Q-Alb is that it serves as a reference for other serum proteins to allow calculation of their intrathecal synthesis, as known from the formula for IgG index (Link and Tibbling 1977; Andersson et al. 1994; Reiber 1994; Brettschneider et al. 2005).

9.2   Preanalytics

Albumin is stable in CSF for at least 1 week even at room temperature; when stored at 4 °C, several weeks up to months; and, when frozen at −20 °C, up to 2 years (Petereit et al. 2007; Thomas 2005). Considerable changes due to artificial blood contamination or haemolysis are possible.

9.3   Detection Methods

Albumin is measured immunochemically by turbidimetry or by nephelometry with a two-point or a kinetic analysis. CSF and serum samples should be analysed simultaneously in the same assay, same run and standard curve to keep the analytical variability to a minimum (Thomas 2005; Reiber et al. 2003).

9.4   Reference Intervals

An intact blood-CSF barrier in adults is associated with a CSF/serum albumin ratio of $<8 \times 10^{-3}$. The reference range is age dependent, and for individuals above 5 years, following the formula according to age has been suggested: Q-Alb = ((age in years/15) +4) × 10^{-3} (Reiber and Peter 2001). For example, the upper limit of the reference range of a 15-year-old person would be (15/15) +4 = 5 × 10^{-3}. However, this formula still returns elevated results in roughly 15 % of patients without evidence of neurological disorder (ruled out by clinical, laboratory and imaging diagnostics) (Brettschneider et al. 2005). There are several studies on normal Q-Alb that have reported higher cut-off levels (Link and

Tibbling 1977, Blennow et al. 1993). Of note, Q-Alb may be influenced by body weight or BMI, which also contributes to a large interindividual variability within a same age group (Brettschneider et al. 2005).

Age (years)	Lumbar CSF/serum ratio of albumin range ($\times 10^{-3}$)
Newborn	<28
1–15	4–5
15–60	5–8
60–90	8–10

9.5   Interpretation

A dysfunction of the blood-CSF barrier, i.e. abnormal elevation of Q-Alb, occurs in various neurological diseases of inflammatory as well as noninflammatory aetiology. While mild-to-moderate Q-Alb elevations ($8\text{–}25 \times 10^{-3}$) are seen in many diseases such as diabetic and immune-mediated polyneuropathies (PNP), viral meningitis or vertebral disc pathologies, moderate-to-severe Q-Alb elevations ($>25 \times 10^{-3}$) are associated with a purulent meningitis, acute Lyme neuroborreliosis, neurotuberculosis, immune-mediated polyradiculitis and myelitis or severe spinal canal stenosis.

Among patients with PNP, no significant correlation was found between duration of disease and extent of Q-Alb. There was also no significant difference between subtypes of PNP as classified by electroneurography or by underlying aetiology such as diabetes, vitamin B12 deficiency and others (Brettschneider et al. 2005) (Table 9.1).

Table 9.1 Spectrum of diseases associated with mild, moderate or severe Q-Alb elevations according to Brettschneider et al. 2005

Abnormal Q-Alb ranges	Neuropsychiatric diseases
$<12.5 \times 10^{-3}$	Bell's palsy, dementia, depression, idiopathic Parkinson syndrome, migraine, optic neuritis, schizophrenia, tension-type headache
$<15 \times 10^{-3}$	Amyotrophic lateral sclerosis, atypical Parkinson syndromes, diabetic polyneuropathy, epileptic seizure, ischaemic stroke, mild spinal stenosis, normal pressure hydrocephalus, transverse myelitis, viral meningitis
$<20 \times 10^{-3}$	Brain tumour, moderate spinal stenosis, viral encephalitis
$<35 \times 10^{-3}$	Guillain-Barre syndrome, CIDP, herpes simplex encephalitis
$25\text{–}100 \times 10^{-3}$	Lyme neuroborreliosis, neurotuberculosis, purulent meningitis, severe spinal stenosis, tick-borne encephalitis

References

Andersson M, Alvarez-Cermeño J, Bernardi G, Cogato I, Fredman P, Frederiksen J et al (1994) Cerebrospinal fluid in the diagnosis of multiple sclerosis: a consensus report. J Neurol Neurosurg Psychiatry 57(8):897–902

Blennow K, Fredman P, Wallin A, Gottfries CG, Karlsson I, Långström G et al (1993) Protein analysis in cerebrospinal fluid. II. Reference values derived from healthy individuals 18–88 years of age. Eur Neurol 33(2):129–133

Brettschneider J, Claus A, Kassubek J, Tumani H (2005) Isolated blood-cerebrospinal fluid barrier dysfunction: prevalence and associated diseases. J Neurol 252(9):1067–1073

Link H, Tibbling G (1977) Principles of albumin and IgG analyses in neurological disorders. III Evaluation of IgG synthesis within the central nervous system in multiple sclerosis. Scand J Clin Lab Invest 37(5):397–401

Petereit H, Sindern E, Wick M (2007) Liquordiagnostik. Leitlinien und Methodenkatalog der Deutschen Gesellschaft für Liquordiagnostik und Klinische Neurochemie. Springer Medizin Verlag, Heidelberg (see also www.dgln.de)

Reiber H (1994) Flow rate of cerebrospinal fluid (CSF)–a concept common to normal blood-CSF barrier function and to dysfunction in neurological diseases. J Neurol Sci 122(2):189–203

Reiber H, Peter JB (2001) Cerebrospinal fluid analysis: disease-related data patterns and evaluation programs. J Neurol Sci 184:101–122

Reiber H, Thompson EJ, Grimsley G, Bernardi G, Adam P, Monteiro de Almeida S et al (2003) Quality assurance for cerebrospinal fluid protein analysis: international consensus by an Internet-based group discussion. Clin Chem Lab Med 41(3):331–337

Thomas L (2005) Labor und diagnose. TH Verlagsgesellschaft mbH, Frankfurt/Main

Immunoglobulins in Cerebrospinal Fluid   10

Finn Sellebjerg

Contents

Abstract

The assessment of intrathecally synthesised immunoglobulin is an important part of routine cerebrospinal fluid (CSF) analysis. Immunoglobulins can be detected in normal CSF and are derived from plasma. The appearance of immunoglobulins in normal CSF is readily explained by size-dependent diffusion across blood-CSF barriers, and their concentrations increase with the general increase

F. Sellebjerg
Danish Multiple Sclerosis Center,
Department of Neurology Rigshospitalet, University of Copenhagen,
Copenhagen, Denmark
e-mail: sellebjerg@dadlnet.dk

© Springer International Publishing Switzerland 2015
F. Deisenhammer et al. (eds.), *Cerebrospinal Fluid in Clinical Neurology*,
DOI 10.1007/978-3-319-01225-4_10

in CSF protein concentrations observed in a wide range of neurological diseases. Therefore, methods that take the normal diffusion of immunoglobulins into account are needed for quantitative assessment of intrathecal immunoglobulin synthesis. Intrathecally synthesised immunoglobulins are usually of restricted clonality, and electrophoresis-based methods can be used for detecting this in the form of oligoclonal bands. These methods depend on comparing paired CSF and blood samples. Qualitative analyses for the assessment of intrathecally synthesised oligoclonal bands are more technically demanding, but are more sensitive for the detection of intrathecal immunoglobulin synthesis, and are less susceptible to artefacts induced by blood-CSF barrier disturbances than quantitative methods. The same general principles apply both for the detection of total intrathecal immunoglobulin synthesis and for the detection of specific antibody responses in infectious or autoimmune conditions.

10.1 Introduction

The mammalian immune system has evolved to protect against infections against a plethora of infectious agents and employs a wide range of responses to protect the host against bacterial, viral and parasitic infections. The immune system is also involved in inflammatory responses to tissue damage and in the pathogenesis of autoimmune and autoinflammatory diseases. Basically, the immune system can be divided into an innate and an adaptive part (Paul 2008). The innate immune system comprises granulocytes; mononuclear phagocytes such as monocytes, macrophages and microglia; and dendritic cells which are specialised antigen-presenting cells. These cells express a wide range of molecules including pattern recognition receptors for molecules associated with pathogens (Broz and Monack 2013). In addition, humoral factors, including pentraxins such as the acute-phase proteins C-reactive protein and serum amyloid, complement proteins, and the coagulation and kinin system are part of the innate immune system (Shishido et al. 2012).

The adaptive immune system comprises B cells and T cells, which are lymphocytes developing in the bone marrow and thymus (Paul 2008). Each newly developed B or T cell expresses a unique antigen receptor in the form of an immunoglobulin or a T-cell antigen receptor. The development of unique antigen receptors is the result of genetic recombination combined with stochastic addition of single nucleotides to the receptor-encoding DNA sequence. Developing lymphocytes undergo positive selection processes to ensure that they express functional antigen receptor molecules. This is followed by negative selection, where potentially harmful, autoreactive cells are pruned from the developing lymphocyte repertoire.

Following the activation of an antigen-specific lymphocyte in secondary lymphatic tissue, e.g. lymph node or spleen, it proliferates vigorously. This initial clonal expansion is followed by the differentiation of cells into various effector cell types and memory cells, which are long-living cells that continue to recirculate in the body or remain in peripheral tissues after the initial immune response, thus ensuring a more rapid and efficient immune response upon a second encounter with an infectious agent (Heyzer-Williams and Heyzer-Williams 2005; Sprent and Surh 2011).

10.2   The Humoral Immune Response

10.2.1 B-Cell Development and Activation

Humoral immune responses depend on the primary activation of antigen-reactive B cells, which is initiated by the binding of antigen to immunoglobulins or the B-cell surface (Harwood and Batista 2010). This activates a signalling cascade involving protein kinases, the induction of second messenger molecules and gene expression (Kurosaki et al. 2010). In addition, immunoglobulins with their bound antigen are internalised, and the antigen is processed by proteases in endosomes. This is followed by the binding of peptide fragments of the antigen to major histocompatibility class II molecules (human leucocyte antigen or HLA molecules in humans), which are subsequently expressed on the cell surface (Neefjes et al. 2011). This allows interactions between antigen-specific CD4 T cells and antigen-specific B cells, resulting in the activation of CD4 T cells with specificity for the same antigen that initially activated the B cell. A hallmark of the humoral immune response is the development of plasma cells secreting high-affinity antibodies that are class switched from the initial IgM isotype to other isotypes (see below) and the development of a long-living pool of memory B cells. Although T-cell-independent B-cell responses can provide some protection early in the course of an immune response, the development of memory B cells and plasma cells secreting high-affinity antibodies requires T-cell help (Miller et al. 1965; Vos et al. 2000). This reaction takes place in the germinal centres of secondary lymphoid organs, where targeted recombination and somatic hypermutation in the immunoglobulin genes induced by the enzyme activation-induced deaminase result in the selection of B cells producing high-affinity, class-switched antibodies (Nutt and Tarlinton 2011; Victora and Nussenzweig 2012). Based mainly on research in rodents, it was previously thought that T-cell help depends on T-helper type 2 (Th2) cells. It is now, however, widely accepted that help to B cells involves a recently discovered subtype of CD4 T cells termed follicular helper (T_{FH}) cells rather than Th2 cells (Crotty 2011; Tangye et al. 2013).

10.2.2 Immunoglobulins

Basically, immunoglobulins are composed of two heavy chain and two light chain molecules with a molecular weight of approximately 150,000 kD (Paul 2008). The heavy chains with a molecular weight of 50–70 kD are composed of four

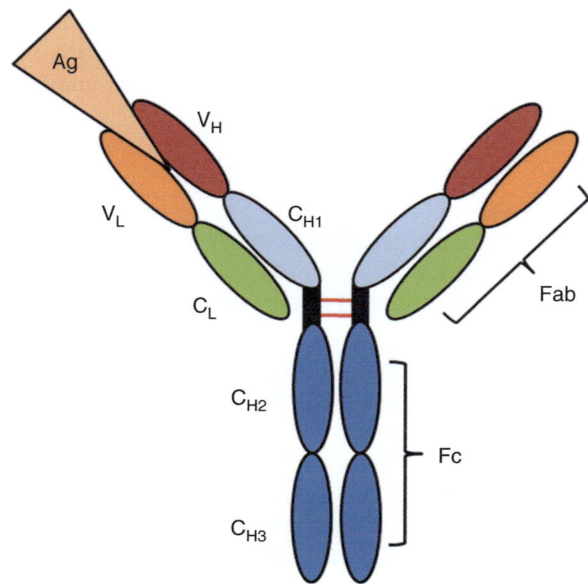

Fig. 10.1 Schematic representation of the basic structure of immunoglobulins. Immunoglobulins are composed of two heavy chains, each consisting of one variable (V_H, *red*) and three constant (C_{H1}-C_{H3}, *blue*) immunoglobulin domains and two light chains, each consisting of one variable (V_L, *orange*) and one constant (C_L) immunoglobulin domain (Paul 2008). Internally the immunoglobulin domains are stabilised by disulphide bonds. The light chain and V_H and C_{H1} domains constitute the Fab (fragment, antigen binding) part of an immunoglobulin, and the C_{H2} and C_{H3} domains from the two heavy chains form the Fc (fragment, crystallisable) part. The C_{H2} and C_{H3} domains are linked by the hinge region (*black*), and the hinge regions of the two heavy chain molecules are linked by disulphide bonds (*red*). The Fc parts of the heavy chains are glycosylated (not shown). Membrane-bound immunoglobulins have an additional, short transmembrane amino acid chain. The paratope is the distal, antigen-binding part, which consists of three hypervariable or *complementarity-determining regions (CDR1-3)* in the V_L and V_H domains. Variation in the amino acid sequence of the VL and VH chains arises from somatic recombination of V, D and J gene segments in the immunoglobulin heavy locus (*IGH*) and somatic recombination of V and J gene segments in the immunoglobulin kappa locus (*IGK*) and immunoglobulin lambda locus (*IGL*)

immunoglobulin superfamily domains linked by a hinge region, and the light chains with a molecular weight of 23 kD consist of two immunoglobulin superfamily domains (Fig. 10.1). The heavy chains specify the isotype and subclass of the immunoglobulin and are linked by disulphide bonds in the Fc (fraction, crystallisable) part of the molecule. The light chains are either kappa or lambda light chain molecules, which are linked by disulphide bonds to the other end of the heavy chain molecule, forming the Fab part (fragment, antigen binding) of the immunoglobulin. Hypervariable regions of the heavy and light chain molecules (termed complementarity-defining regions, CDR) are flanked by framework regions which together make up the antigen-binding region of the Fab part, which is also known as the paratope (Table 10.1).

Table 10.1 Immunoglobulin isoforms, subclasses and effector functions. Immunoglobulins differ in their biological function due to differences in their ability to activate the complement cascade and differences in their ability to bind to different Fc receptors on the surface of immune cells, which may have highly variable biological functions (Paul 2008)

	Fc binding	Complement activation	Biological role
IgA			Mucosal immunity (secreted)
IgA1	Yes	–	Major IgA subclass
IgA2	Yes	–	More prevalent in secreted IgA
IgD	?	–	Initial B-cell activation, role in mucosal immunity?
IgE	Yes	–	Parasite immunity, allergy
IgG			Broad role in immunity to infectious agents
IgG1	High affinity	Yes	
IgG2	Low affinity	Yes	
IgG3	High affinity	Yes	
IgG4	Intermediate	–	
IgM	Yes	Yes	Initial immune responses, natural autoantibodies

10.2.3 Plasma Cells and Plasmablasts

After activation by binding of cognate antigen to cell surface immunoglobulin, B-cell proliferation is induced, and in the absence of T-cell help, this may be sufficient to induce an antibody response, which is dominated by the secretion of IgM antibodies by plasmablasts. Plasmablasts are B cells that have developed into a phenotype where they retain some B-cell surface markers, but also secrete immunoglobulins (Heyzer-Williams and Heyzer-Williams 2005; Kurosaki et al. 2010). Such T-cell-independent immune responses can be induced by multivalent antigens, e.g. bacterial surface antigens, and elicit initial antibody responses which provide some protection until high-affinity, class-switched T-cell-dependent antibody responses have evolved (Berland and Wortis 2002; Mebius and Kraal 2005).

T-cell-dependent antibody responses develop in germinal centres in secondary lymphatic tissues and involve interactions between antigen-specific T_{FH} cells, B cells and follicular dendritic cells (FDCs) (Victora and Nussenzweig 2012). FDCs are specialised stroma cells that express antigen complexed with complement or immunoglobulins on their surface in the follicular area of secondary lymphoid organs. FDCs are important for the selection of high-affinity, mutated immunoglobulin-expressing B cells (Gonzalez et al. 2011). The interaction between antigen-specific T_{FH} and B cells induces the expression of the enzyme activation-induced deaminase (AID) in B cells. This results in class switch recombination from the initial expression of IgM and IgD to other immunoglobulin isotypes. The precise class switch undertaken is influenced by cytokines present in the environment with, e.g. transforming growth factor-β (TGF-β) inducing class switching to IgA and Th2 cytokines inducing class switching to IgE (Fagarasan et al. 2010). Furthermore, AID induces somatic hypermutation in the variable region of immunoglobulin genes. This stochastic reaction results in the chance generation of B cells expressing immunoglobulin genes, which show increased affinity for antigen (Heyzer-Williams and Heyzer-Williams 2005). Such high-affinity antibody-secreting cells are selected by poorly understood processes and differentiate either to plasma cells or to long-living memory B cells, which are able to generate a swift antibody response upon re-exposure to the same antigen.

10.3   B Cells and Immunoglobulins in the Central Nervous System

10.3.1 CNS Immunoprivilege and B-Cell Responses

The CNS is conventionally considered an immunoprivileged organ (Carson et al. 2006). The presence of a blood-brain barrier, the lack of a conventional lymphatic drainage system and the sparseness of conventional antigen-presenting cells do, indeed, impose constraints on intrathecal immune responses. B-cell responses are, however, readily induced in the CNS and may be of a similar or even higher magnitude than systemic responses to the same antigen (Gordon et al. 1992). Interestingly, it is possible to induce antibody responses to myelin basic protein (MBP) infused into the CSF, and this results in the subsequent protection against experimental autoimmune encephalomyelitis induced by MBP (Harling-Berg et al. 1991). It appears that the administration of antigen to the CSF is especially immunogenic and the induction of an intrathecal antibody response is associated with the development of a clonally restricted, specific antibody response as assessed by analysis for oligoclonal bands (Harling-Berg et al. 1989; Knopf et al. 1995).

10.3.2 Quantitative Assessment of Intrathecal Immunoglobulin Synthesis

Normal CSF contains low concentrations of all immunoglobulins. Immunoglobulins in normal CSF derive from passive diffusion across the blood-CSF barriers (Thompson 1988). Diffusion is size-dependent, and the CSF-plasma concentration quotient for various proteins correlates negatively with the size of the individual molecules (Felgenhauer et al. 1976; Felgenhauer and Renner 1977). The CSF-plasma concentration quotient for albumin (Q_{alb}) is commonly used as a measure of barrier integrity and is used to correct for general blood-CSF protein transfer in formulae for the quantitative assessment of intrathecal immunoglobulin synthesis. The size selectivity of the blood-CSF barriers may, however, become disturbed in disease states, leading to erroneous results when the Qalb is used for correction, especially for larger molecules such as IgA and IgM (Thompson 1988).

There is a close relationship between the Q_{alb} and the CSF-plasma concentration quotient for IgG (Q_{IgG}) in control subjects (Delpech and Lichtblau 1972; Ganrot and Laurell 1974). This relationship led to the development of the IgG index, which is Q_{IgG}/Q_{alb}, for the assessment of intrathecal IgG synthesis (Link and Tibbling 1977). The IgG index assumes that there is a linear relationship between the Qalb and the

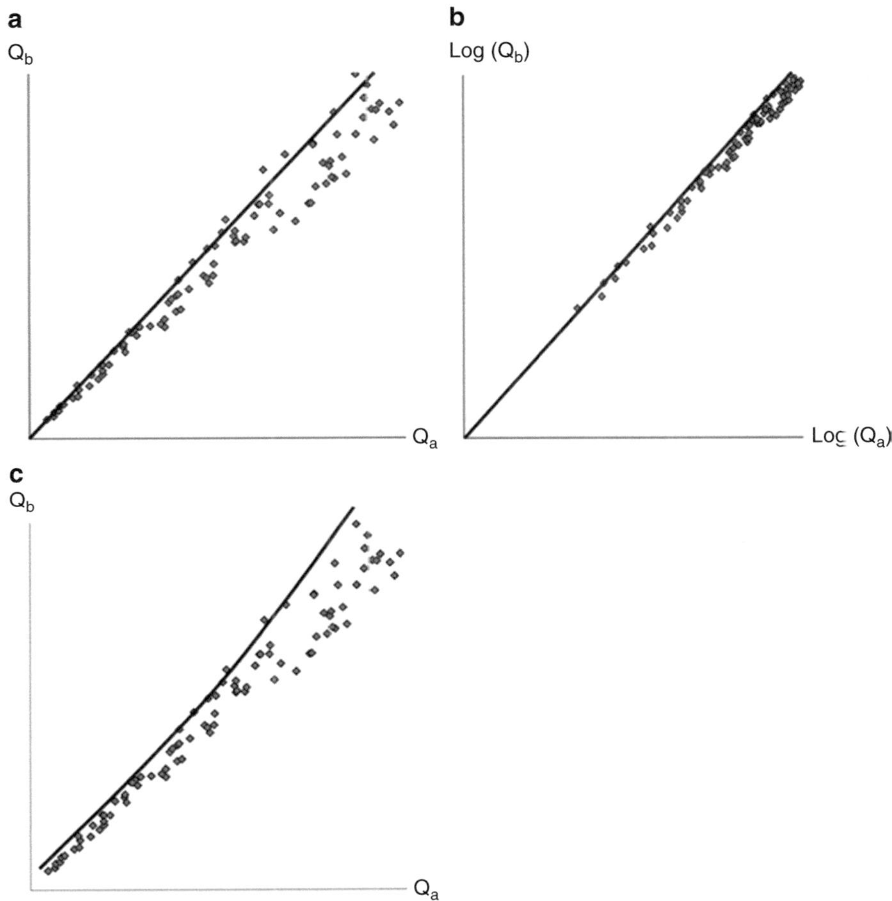

Fig. 10.2 Graphic representation of the consequence of measuring inaccuracy for the use of intrathecal immunoglobulin synthesis formulae (see text for discussion). (**a**) models a linear relationship, e.g., (**b**) a double-logarithmic relatoinship, and (**c**) a hyperbolic relationship between the CSF-plasma quotient of a reference protein (**a**) and an immunoglobulin of interest (**b**)

QIgG. This has, however, been questioned by other researchers, who argue that CSF bulk flow is the major determinant of the CSF protein content and that the diffusion theory indicates that the relationship between the Qalb and the QIgG is better explained by a hyperbolic formula (Reiber 1994). Hyperbolic formulae have also been developed for assessing intrathecal synthesis of IgA and IgM (Reiber 1994).

The hyperbolic model is not universally accepted as other researchers have reported that the relationship between the Qalb and the QIgG is linear in a double logarithmic plot and that there is no statistical evidence suggesting that a hyperbolic formula provides a better fit for the data (Öhman 1994). The relationship observed in double logarithmic plots led to the development of the extended IgG index (Öhman et al. 1989) and was later developed into similar extended indices for IgA and IgM (Öhman et al. 1993).

The extended index model is, indeed, the expected model if a linear relationship between the Qalb and the QIgG is assumed, but measuring inaccuracy is also taken into

Table 10.2 Selected formulae for assessment of intrathecal immunoglobulin synthesis

Conventional immunoglobulin indices (Delpech and Lichtblau 1972; Ganrot and Laurell 1974; Link and Tibbling 1977; Lolli et al. 1989)		
IgG index $= Q_{IgG}/Q_{alb}$	IgA index $= Q_{IgA}/Q_{alb}$	IgM index $= Q_{IgM}/Q_{alb}$

Extended immunoglobulin indices (Öhman et al. 1989, 1993). Values for parameter a are IgG, $a = 1.12$; IgA, $a = 1.15$; IgM, $a = 1.9$

Extended Ig index $= Q_{Ig}/Q_{alb}{}^{a}$

Hyperbolic immunoglobulin formulae (Reiber 1994). Hyperbolic 99 % upper reference limits for immunoglobulin quotients are calculated from the Q_{alb} (IgG: $a = 0.93$, $b = 6 \times 10^{-6}$, $c = 1.7 \times 10^{-3}$; IgA: $a = 0.77$, $b = 2.3 \times 10^{-5}$, $c = 3.1 \times 10^{-3}$; IgM: $a = 0.67$, $b = 1.2 \times 10^{-4}$, $c = 7.1 \times 10^{-3}$)

Upper limit of $Q_{Ig} = a \sqrt{(Q_{alb}{}^{2} + b)} + c$

account (Fig. 10.2). If there is no inaccuracy in the measurements, a linear formula such as the IgG index is well suited to establish increased levels of IgG synthesis. Some measuring inaccuracy is, however, unavoidable, and if the same relative measuring inaccuracy applies both for the Qalb and the QIgG at high and low values, this will result in increased variability in the relationship at higher levels. Thus, the linear formula (the IgG index) will tend to give false-positive results at higher Qalb values (Fig. 10.2a), whereas the formulae based on non-linear relationships, i.e. the extended index (Fig. 10.2b) and hyperbolic formula (Fig. 10.2c), are less prone to this error. Indeed, extended immunoglobulin indices and hyperbolic formulae perform better than conventional indices for the quantitative assessment of intrathecal immunoglobulin synthesis (Öhman et al. 1989, 1993; Sellebjerg et al. 1996). None of the formulae are comparable to the detection of oligoclonal bands for the assessment of intrathecal IgG synthesis (Öhman et al. 1992; Sellebjerg et al. 1996). There may, however, be a role for the assessment of intrathecal IgA and IgM synthesis in the diagnosis of infectious diseases in the nervous system (Deisenhammer et al. 2006).

The passive diffusion of immunoglobulins from plasma into the CSF should also be considered when specific antibodies are investigated in patients with CNS infections. Simply calculating an antibody index by comparing the concentration of the specific antibody in CSF and plasma to the CSF and plasma concentrations of IgG is usually sufficient, and similar methods can be applied for the analysis of specific IgM antibodies (Deisenhammer et al. 2006). The application of antibody indices has been used for many antigens, but the results should be interpreted with caution as some patients with MS also show intrathecal synthesis of several virus-specific antibodies, mostly directed against measles, rubella and varicella-zoster virus, the so-called MRZ reaction (Table 10.2) (Felgenhauer and Reiber 1992).

10.3.3 Qualitative Assessment of Immunoglobulin Synthesis

The detection of clonally restricted, intrathecally synthesised IgG is a hallmark of multiple sclerosis and is observed in more than 90 % of patients with MS (Freedman et al. 2005). IgG oligoclonal bands can, however, also be observed in other diseases

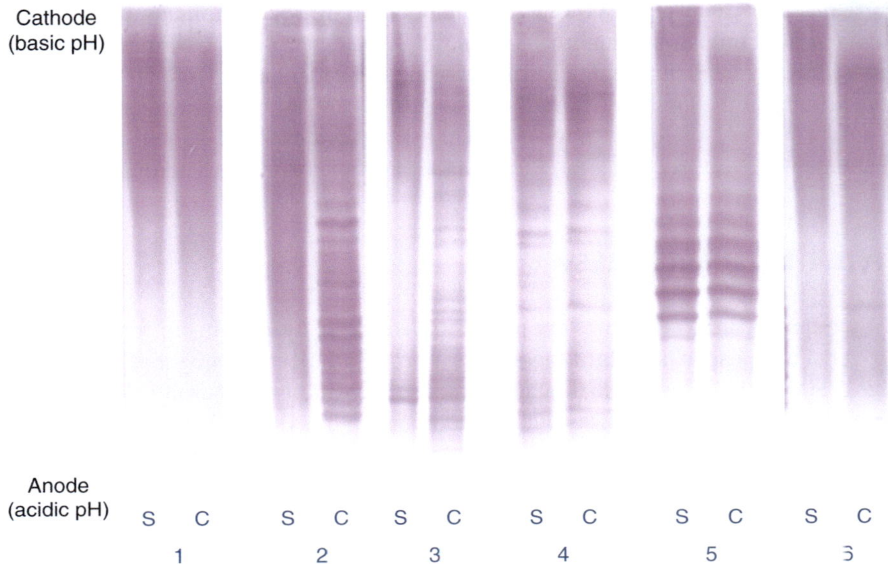

Fig. 10.3 Isoelectric focusing patterns (immunostaining for IgG) showing *1* normal (polyclonal) serum (*S*) and CSF (*C*) (no intrathecal IgG synthesis), *2* normal serum and oligoclonal CSF (intrathecal oligoclonal IgG synthesis present), *3* oligoclonal serum and CSF with additional bands in CSF not present in serum (intrathecal oligoclonal IgG synthesis present), *4* identical oligoclonal bands in serum and CSF (mirror pattern, no intrathecal IgG synthesis), *5* paraprotein (monoclonal) resolving in several adjacent bands with a similar pattern in serum and CSF (no intrathecal oligoclonal IgG synthesis), *6* normal serum and single band in CSF (equivocal pattern not considered to represent intrathecal oligoclonal IgG synthesis) (Figure supplied by Poul Erik Hyldgaard Jensen, Neuroimmunology Laboratory, Danish Multiple Sclerosis Center, Rigshospitalet, University of Copenhagen)

(Kostulas et al. 1987; McLean et al. 1990). An account of the development of oligoclonal band analyses is given in the chapter on the history of the CSF earlier in this book. Briefly, it is recommended that oligoclonal bands are analysed by isoelectric focusing followed by immunochemical detection of IgG (Keir et al. 1990). The simultaneous analysis of the CSF and serum with similar amounts of IgG being analysed is mandatory in order to distinguish between CSF bands resulting from local synthesis and bands derived from plasma (Fig. 10.3).

It is generally recommended that five different patterns are distinguished: normal pattern, paraprotein, oligoclonal IgG bands only in the CSF, oligoclonal IgG synthesis with identical bands in the CSF and plasma and systemic IgG synthesis with additional bands only in the CSF (Andersson et al. 1994). The latter two patterns are observed in many infectious and inflammatory diseases, whereas the majority of MS patients have IgG oligoclonal bands only in the CSF.

Isoelectric focusing has also been used for the analysis of other immunoglobulin isoforms and for detection of intrathecal synthesis of free immunoglobulin light chains, but these analyses are not in routine use (Deisenhammer et al. 2006; Freedman et al. 2005).

Isoelectric focusing followed by immunoblotting to membranes coated with antigen from infectious agents can be helpful in the diagnosis of CNS infections, but is technically challenging. Interestingly, using methods that provide an estimate of the affinity of the antibody, it has been suggested that antibodies against viral antigens in MS are of low affinity compared to antibodies to the same antigens in patients with viral encephalitis (Luxton et al. 1995; Luxton and Thompson 1990).

10.3.4 Intrathecal IgM Synthesis

Monomers of IgM molecules are joined in pentamers by J chains to form secreted IgM but may also exist as IgM monomers. The high molecular weight of pentameric IgM (900,000 kD) means that quantitative assessment of intrathecal IgM synthesis is especially prone to artefacts due to alterations in blood-CSF barriers. Intrathecal IgM synthesis is observed in MS and infectious and other inflammatory diseases (Öhman et al. 1993; Sellebjerg et al. 1996). The analysis of IgM oligoclonal bands is technically challenging but is less prone to artefacts than quantitative analysis, and it has been suggested that the presence of IgM oligoclonal bands in MS associated with disease activity and a poor prognosis (Sharief and Thompson 1991, 1992; Villar et al. 2002, 2003). Interestingly, intrathecally secreted IgM in the CSF is derived from cells carrying somatic hypermutations, suggesting that they may be derived from an intrathecal germinal centre-like reaction (Beltran et al. 2014).

10.3.5 Intrathecal IgG Synthesis

The major indication for assessing intrathecal IgG synthesis is for the diagnosis of MS (Deisenhammer et al. 2006; Freedman et al. 2005). Intrathecal IgG synthesis is, however, observed in a wide variety of inflammatory diseases and infections, and the IgG index or IgG oligoclonal band analysis is often used to screen for inflammatory CNS diseases. Due to its higher sensitivity and specificity, oligoclonal band analysis is the preferred method for assessment of intrathecal IgG synthesis. The IgG oligoclonal bands observed in MS are synthesised by local plasmablasts and plasma cells and have accumulated somatic mutations, suggesting that they represent high-affinity antibodies, but the antigenic target of these antibodies is unknown (Obermeier et al. 2008, 2011). Interestingly, similar clones have been observed among circulating B cells in MS patients (Palanichamy et al. 2014).

10.3.6 Intrathecal IgA Synthesis

IgA is mainly secreted as a dimer, and upon addition of the secretory component, it is excreted from mucosal surfaces where it has an important role in mucosal immune responses (Holmgren and Czerkinsky 2005). The IgA1 subclass accounts for the majority of circulating and secreted IgA (Delacroix et al. 1982). The IgA2 subclass is more prevalent in secreted IgA. IgA can also be produced intrathecally. However, when intrathecally produced, it is not associated with the secretory component (Woo et al. 1993), and monomeric IgA is produced in substantial amounts during an intrathecal antiviral immune response (Öhman et al. 1995). The class switch to IgA production is directed by TGF-β, and mice with selective deficiency of TGF-β in B cells show a complete absence of IgA in plasma (Cazac and Roes 2000; van Vlasselaer et al. 1992). Interestingly, the endogenous production of TGF-β in B cells contributes to class switching to IgA in human B cells (Zan et al. 1998).

Most studies addressing intrathecal synthesis of IgA have used quantitative methods. Intrathecal synthesis of IgA is less prevalent than intrathecal IgG synthesis but has been reported to occur commonly in patients with bacterial meningitis, including neurotuberculosis (Felgenhauer and Schadlich 1987; Lolli et al. 1989; Sellebjerg et al. 1996). Interestingly, two studies have demonstrated that intrathecal IgA synthesis as assessed by extended immunoglobulin indices is associated with a less severe disease course in patients with MS. The first study showed that the quantitatively assessed intrathecal IgA synthesis correlated negatively with the CSF concentration of MBP as biomarker of demyelination (Sellebjerg et al. 1998). The second study found a relationship between intrathecal IgA synthesis and overall mortality (Vrethem et al. 2004). It is tempting to speculate that this might relate to an immunoregulatory effect of the IgA isotype shift factor TGF-β or IgA itself (Fagarasan et al. 2010).

10.3.7 Intrathecal IgE Synthesis

Only few studies have investigated IgE in the CSF, and at present the assessment of intrathecal IgE synthesis has no role in routine CSF diagnostics. IgE is secreted as a monomer and is involved in the host response against parasitic infections and allergic reactions. The isotype shift to IgE and the IgG4 subclass is associated with Th2 immune responses, and in multiple sclerosis (MS) there is predominantly intrathecal synthesis of the Th1-associated IgG1 subclass, whereas IgE indices are reduced (Greve et al. 2001). Conversely, in patients with eosinophilic meningitis due to infection with the nematode *Angiostrongylus cantonensis*, intrathecal synthesis of IgE is prominent, consistent with the known role of Th2 immune responses in parasitic infections (Padilla-Docal et al. 2008). Such patients do, however, also show evidence of intrathecal synthesis of other immunoglobulins than IgE (Dorta-Contreras et al. 2005).

10.3.8 Intrathecal IgD Synthesis

The biological role of IgD in immune responses is poorly understood. IgD is coexpressed with IgM on the surface of naïve B cells, and IgD or IgM signalling is involved in initial B-cell activation (Harwood and Batista 2010). Only a small proportion of B cells do, however, undergo somatic hypermutation and class switching for the development of IgD-secreting plasma cells. IgD may have a role in mucosal immunity in the airways, providing a link between innate and adaptive immune responses by binding to basophilic granulocytes (Chen et al. 2009). In one study using immunoglobulin indices to compare intrathecal synthesis of IgG, IgM, IgA and IgD, increased IgG index values were more commonly increased in MS than in patients with other inflammatory diseases, whereas the latter patient group more commonly showed increased IgA index, IgD index and IgM index values than did patients with MS (Lolli et al. 1989). In other studies, IgD oligoclonal bands were found mainly in patients with demyelinating diseases, infections and tumours (Mavra et al. 1992, 1999).

Conclusions

The analysis of intrathecal immunoglobulin synthesis is important for the diagnosis of multiple sclerosis and other inflammatory neurological diseases. The analysis of IgG is most widely used, and it is recommended that this is done by isoelectric focusing with specific immunochemical detection of IgG bands. For quantitative analysis, the IgG index is often used, but non-linear formulae such as hyperbolic formulae and extended indices are better suited, especially for the analysis of IgA and IgM and when there is an impairment of the blood-CSF barrier function independent of its cause.

References

Andersson M, Varez-Cermeno J, Bernardi G et al (1994) Cerebrospinal fluid in the diagnosis of multiple sclerosis: a consensus report. J Neurol Neurosurg Psychiatry 57:897–902

Beltran E, Obermeier B, Moser M et al (2014) Intrathecal somatic hypermutation of IgM in multiple sclerosis and neuroinflammation. Brain 137:2703–2714

Berland R, Wortis HH (2002) Origins and functions of B-1 cells with notes on the role of CD5. Annu Rev Immunol 20:253–300

Broz P, Monack DM (2013) Newly described pattern recognition receptors team up against intracellular pathogens. Nat Rev Immunol 13:551–565

Carson MJ, Doose JM, Melchior B et al (2006) CNS immune privilege: hiding in plain sight. Immunol Rev 213:48–65

Cazac BB, Roes J (2000) TGF-beta receptor controls B cell responsiveness and induction of IgA in vivo. Immunity 13:443–451

Chen K, Xu W, Wilson M et al (2009) Immunoglobulin D enhances immune surveillance by activating antimicrobial, proinflammatory and B cell-stimulating programs in basophils. Nat Immunol 10:889–898

Crotty S (2011) Follicular helper CD4 T cells (TFH). Annu Rev Immunol 29:621–663

Deisenhammer F, Bartos A, Egg R et al (2006) Guidelines on routine cerebrospinal fluid analysis. Report from an EFNS task force. Eur J Neurol 13:913–922

Delacroix DL, Dive C, Rambaud JC et al (1982) IgA subclasses in various secretions and in serum. Immunology 47:383–385

Delpech B, Lichtblau E (1972) Immunochemical estimation of IgG and albumin in cerebrospinal fluid. Clin Chim Acta 37:15–23

Dorta-Contreras AJ, Noris-Garcia E, Escobar-Perez X et al (2005) IgG1, IgG2 and IgE intrathecal synthesis in Angiostrongylus cantonensis meningoencephalitis. J Neurol Sci 238:65–70

Fagarasan S, Kawamoto S, Kanagawa O et al (2010) Adaptive immune regulation in the gut: T cell-dependent and T cell-independent IgA synthesis. Annu Rev Immunol 28:243–273

Felgenhauer K, Reiber H (1992) The diagnostic significance of antibody specificity indices in multiple sclerosis and herpes virus induced diseases of the nervous system. Clin Investig 70:28–37

Felgenhauer K, Renner E (1977) Hydrodynamic radii versus molecular weights in clearance studies of urine and cerebrospinal fluid. Ann Clin Biochem 14:100–104

Felgenhauer K, Schadlich HJ (1987) The compartmental IgM and IgA response within the central nervous system. J Neurol Sci 77:125–135

Felgenhauer K, Schliep G, Rapic N (1976) Evaluation of the blood-CSF barrier by protein gradients and the humoral immune response within the central nervous system. J Neurol Sci 30: 113–128

Freedman MS, Thompson EJ, Deisenhammer F et al (2005) Recommended standard of cerebrospinal fluid analysis in the diagnosis of multiple sclerosis: a consensus statement. Arch Neurol 62:865–870

Ganrot K, Laurell CB (1974) Measurement of IgG and albumin content of cerebrospinal fluid, and its interpretation. Clin Chem 20:571–573

Gonzalez SF, Degn SE, Pitcher LA et al (2011) Trafficking of B cell antigen in lymph nodes. Annu Rev Immunol 29:215–233

Gordon LB, Knopf PM, Cserr HF (1992) Ovalbumin is more immunogenic when introduced into brain or cerebrospinal fluid than into extracerebral sites. J Neuroimmunol 40:81–87

Greve B, Magnusson CG, Melms A et al (2001) Immunoglobulin isotypes reveal a predominant role of type 1 immunity in multiple sclerosis. J Neuroimmunol 121:120–125

Harling-Berg C, Knopf PM, Merriam J et al (1989) Role of cervical lymph nodes in the systemic humoral immune response to human serum albumin microinfused into rat cerebrospinal fluid. J Neuroimmunol 25:185–193

Harling-Berg CJ, Knopf PM, Cserr HF (1991) Myelin basic protein infused into cerebrospinal fluid suppresses experimental autoimmune encephalomyelitis. J Neuroimmunol 35:45–51

Harwood NE, Batista FD (2010) Early events in B cell activation. Annu Rev Immunol 28: 185–210

Heyzer-Williams LJ, Heyzer-Williams MG (2005) Antigen-specific memory B cell development. Annu Rev Immunol 23:487–513

Holmgren J, Czerkinsky C (2005) Mucosal immunity and vaccines. Nat Med 11:S45–S53

Keir G, Luxton RW, Thompson EJ (1990) Isoelectric focusing of cerebrospinal fluid immunoglobulin G: an annotated update. Ann Clin Biochem 27(Pt 5):436–443

Knopf PM, Cserr HF, Nolan SC et al (1995) Physiology and immunology of lymphatic drainage of interstitial and cerebrospinal fluid from the brain. Neuropathol Appl Neurobiol 21:175–180

Kostulas VK, Link H, Lefvert AK (1987) Oligoclonal IgG bands in cerebrospinal fluid. Principles for demonstration and interpretation based on findings in 1114 neurological patients. Arch Neurol 44:1041–1044

Kurosaki T, Shinohara H, Baba Y (2010) B cell signaling and fate decision. Annu Rev Immunol 28:21–55

Link H, Tibbling G (1977) Principles of albumin and IgG analyses in neurological disorders. III. Evaluation of IgG synthesis within the central nervous system in multiple sclerosis. Scand J Clin Lab Invest 37:397–401

Lolli F, Halawa I, Link H (1989) Intrathecal synthesis of IgG, IgA, IgM and IgD in untreated multiple sclerosis and controls. Acta Neurol Scand 80:238–247

Luxton RW, Thompson EJ (1990) Affinity distributions of antigen-specific IgG in patients with multiple sclerosis and in patients with viral encephalitis. J Immunol Methods 131:277–282

Luxton RW, Zeman A, Holzel H et al (1995) Affinity of antigen-specific IgG distinguishes multiple sclerosis from encephalitis. J Neurol Sci 132:11–19

Mavra M, Luxton R, Keir G et al (1992) Oligoclonal immunoglobulin D in the cerebrospinal fluid of neurologic patients. Neurology 42:1244–1245

Mavra M, Drulovic J, Levic Z et al (1999) CNS tumours: oligoclonal immunoglobulin D in cerebrospinal fluid and serum Acta Neurol Scand 100:117–118

McLean BN, Luxton RW, Thompson EJ (1990) A study of immunoglobulin G in the cerebrospinal fluid of 1007 patients with suspected neurological disease using isoelectric focusing and the Log IgG-Index. A comparison and diagnostic applications. Brain 113(Pt 5):1269–1289

Mebius RE, Kraal G (2005) Structure and function of the spleen. Nat Rev Immunol 5:606–616

Miller JF, De Burgh PM, Grant GA (1965) Thymus and the production of antibody-plaque-forming cells. Nature 208:1332–1334

Neefjes J, Jongsma ML, Paul P et al (2011) Towards a systems understanding of MHC class I and MHC class II antigen presentation. Nat Rev Immunol 11:823–836

Nutt SL, Tarlinton DM (2011) Germinal center B and follicular helper T cells: siblings, cousins or just good friends? Nat Immunol 12:472–477

Obermeier B, Mentele R, Malotka J et al (2008) Matching of oligoclonal immunoglobulin transcriptomes and proteomes of cerebrospinal fluid in multiple sclerosis. Nat Med 14:688–693

Obermeier B, Lovato L, Mentele R et al (2011) Related B cell clones that populate the CSF and CNS of patients with multiple sclerosis produce CSF immunoglobulin. J Neuroimmunol 233: 245–248

Öhman S (1994) Points of view concerning the diffusion theory for blood-CSF barrier function and dysfunction. J Neurol Sci 126:240–245

Öhman S, Forsberg P, Nelson N et al (1989) An improved formula for the judgement of intrathecally produced IgG in the presence of blood brain barrier damage. Clin Chim Acta 181: 265–272

Öhman S, Ernerudh J, Forsberg P et al (1992) Comparison of seven formulae and isoelectrofocusing for determination of intrathecally produced IgG in neurological diseases. Ann Clin Biochem 29(Pt 4):405–410

Öhman S, Ernerudh J, Forsberg P et al (1993) Improved formulae for the judgement of intrathecally produced IgA and IgM in the presence of blood CSF barrier damage. Ann Clin Biochem 30(Pt 5):454–462

Öhman S, Ernerudh J, Roberg M et al (1995) Determination of total and herpes simplex virus specific monomeric and dimeric IgA in serum and cerebrospinal fluid by ultracentrifugation. Ann Clin Biochem 32(Pt 6):550–556

Padilla-Docal B, Dorta-Contreras AJ, Bu-Coifiu-Fanego R et al (2008) Intrathecal synthesis of IgE in children with eosinophilic meningoencephalitis caused by Angiostrongylus cantonensis. Cerebrospinal Fluid Res 5:18

Palanichamy A, Apeltsin L, Kuo TC et al (2014) Immunoglobulin class-switched B cells form an active immune axis between CNS and periphery in multiple sclerosis. Sci Transl Med 6: 248ra106

Paul WE (2008) Fundamental immunology. Lippincott, Williams & Wilkins, Philadelphia

Reiber H (1994) Flow rate of cerebrospinal fluid (CSF)–a concept common to normal blood-CSF barrier function and to dysfunction in neurological diseases. J Neurol Sci 122:189–203

Sellebjerg F, Christiansen M, Rasmussen LS et al (1996) The cerebrospinal fluid in multiple sclerosis. Quantitative assessment of intrathecal immunoglobulin synthesis by empirical formulae. Eur J Neurol 3:548–559

Sellebjerg F, Christiansen M, Nielsen PM et al (1998) Cerebrospinal fluid measures of disease activity in patients with multiple sclerosis. Mult Scler 4:475–479

Sharief MK, Thompson EJ (1991) Intrathecal immunoglobulin M synthesis in multiple sclerosis. Relationship with clinical and cerebrospinal fluid parameters. Brain 114(Pt 1A):181–195

Sharief MK, Thompson EJ (1992) Distribution of cerebrospinal fluid oligoclonal IgM bands in neurological diseases: a comparison between agarose electrophoresis and isoelectric focusing. J Neurol Sci 109:83–87

Shishido SN, Varahan S, Yuan K et al (2012) Humoral innate immune response and disease. Clin Immunol 144:142–158

Sprent J, Surh CD (2011) Normal T cell homeostasis: the conversion of naive cells into memory-phenotype cells. Nat Immunol 12:478–484

Tangye SG, Ma CS, Brink R et al (2013) The good, the bad and the ugly – TFH cells in human health and disease. Nat Rev Immunol 13:412–426

Thompson EJ (1988) The CSF proteins a biochemical approach. Elsevier, Amsterdam

van Vlasselaer P, Punnonen J, de Vries JE (1992) Transforming growth factor-beta directs IgA switching in human B cells. J Immunol 148:2062–2067

Victora GD, Nussenzweig MC (2012) Germinal centers. Annu Rev Immunol 30:429–457

Villar LM, Masjuan J, Gonzalez-Porque P et al (2002) Intrathecal IgM synthesis predicts the onset of new relapses and a worse disease course in MS. Neurology 59:555–559

Villar LM, Masjuan J, Gonzalez-Porque P et al (2003) Intrathecal IgM synthesis is a prognostic factor in multiple sclerosis. Ann Neurol 53:222–226

Vos Q, Lees A, Wu ZQ et al (2000) B-cell activation by T-cell-independent type 2 antigens as an integral part of the humoral immune response to pathogenic microorganisms. Immuno Rev 176:154–170

Vrethem M, Fernlund I, Ernerudh J et al (2004) Prognostic value of cerebrospinal fluid IgA and IgG in multiple sclerosis. Mult Scler 10:469–471

Woo AH, Cserr HF, Knopf PM (1993) Elevated cerebrospinal fluid IgA in humans and rats is not associated with secretory component. J Neuroimmunol 44:129–135

Zan H, Cerutti A, Dramitinos P et al (1998) CD40 engagement triggers switching to IgA and IgA2 in human B cells through induction of endogenous TGF-beta: evidence for TGF-beta but not IL-10-dependent direct S mu → S alpha and sequential S mu → S gamma, S gamma → S alpha DNA recombination. J Immunol 161:5217–5225

Detection of Infectious Agents

Annette Spreer

Contents

Abstract

Cerebrospinal fluid (CSF) analysis is of utmost importance to establish an early diagnosis of central nervous system (CNS) infections and to start appropriate therapy. Besides the basic diagnostics containing CSF white cell count, lactate concentration and protein analysis, substantial efforts have to be made to identify and characterise the causing pathogen. Decisive methods are bacterial and fungal staining, microbiological culture methods, antigen and serologic testings including the determination of pathogen-specific intrathecal immunoglobulin synthesis and nucleic acid amplification methods. As preanalytic requirements and the choice of analytical methods depend on the suspicion of bacterial, fungal or viral CNS infections, a close communication between the laboratory and the clinician is important.

A. Spreer
Department of Neurology,
University Medical Centre Göttingen, University Göttingen,
Göttingen, Germany
e-mail: aspreer@med.uni-goettingen.de

© Springer International Publishing Switzerland 2015
F. Deisenhammer et al. (eds.), *Cerebrospinal Fluid in Clinical Neurology*,
DOI 10.1007/978-3-319-01225-4_11

"

In search for viral, bacterial or parasitic agents of CNS infection, the examination of cerebrospinal fluid is of particular importance. It is the treating physician who hypothesises the CNS infection prior to further diagnostic procedures, and it is the clinician's hypothesis that triggers the preanalytic and analytic process and the special diagnostic assays of CSF analysis.

In suspected acute infections, direct methods of pathogen detection are important; CSF specimens require immediate processing as well as prompt reporting of results of Gram stain or of other direct tests as cryptococcal antigen test. In subacute or chronic infections, indirect serological methods are relevant diagnostic tools. In search for bacterial, fungal and parasitic agents, the direct microscopy and bacteriological culture methods are of outstanding importance; in case of suspected viral CNS infection, the direct detection of viral genome by polymerase chain reaction is often the method of choice. Therefore, a close communication between the laboratory physicians and the clinicians improve early and goal-directed diagnostic measures and early confirmation of diagnoses.

11.1 Sampling and Transport of CSF for Microbiological Examination

CSF sampled to detect bacterial, fungal or viral infectious agents has to be drawn under sterile conditions. Prior to puncture, the skin has to be disinfected thoroughly to avoid nosocomial infection of the patient and to avoid contamination of the sample with resident dermal bacteria (e.g. coagulase-negative staphylococci). In general, 10 ml should be drawn for CSF analysis; in case of suspected tuberculous meningitis, larger volumes and repeated punctures are recommended. Gram stain and routine culture may require only 1–2 ml of CSF; however, if fungal or mycobacterial infection is suspected, larger volumes increase the likelihood of successful culture. Thus, a recommended minimal sample volume for bacteriological–mycological examination is 5 ml, for virological examinations 2 ml and for suspected tuberculosis 10–15 ml (Wildemann et al. 2006; Kennedy and Fallon 1979).

CSF for bacterial culture should not be centrifuged and should be transported at room temperature as soon as possible to the microbiological laboratory. Transport time should not take longer than 30 min. Beyond the common causative agents of bacterial meningitis, especially meningococci and *H. influenza* are fastidious organisms. In infections with these organisms, high or low temperatures and long storage time in nutrient-poor culture medium (as it is cerebrospinal fluid) can decrease bacterial cell viability and sensitivity of microbiological culture methods. Pneumococci and *Listeria monocytogenes* are more resistant to low temperature and can still be grown despite storage at 4 °C for several hours. If these requirements of transport conditions are not realisable, it is recommended to transport a part of CSF after addition into an aerobic blood culture flask (Nau 2005).

On the other hand, CSF sampled for supposed acute viral meningoencephalitis should be analysed for viral DNA or RNA by PCR. For this purpose, the PCR is optimally run on freshly obtained and non-centrifugal CSF samples. The decline in sensitivity has not been studied in detail. The stability of RNA viruses is less than that of DNA viruses. In general, it is recommended to store CSF for PCR analysis at 4 °C or −20°, and it should be analysed within few days (Debiasi and Tyler 2004).

11.2 Staining and Microscopy

Preparation of CSF cytospins, cell sedimentation or at least smears should be a routine part of CSF analysis. The morphological detection of infectious agents in stained cytological preparations allows nearly immediate diagnosis of bacterial and fungal CNS infection (Fig. 11.1).

In acute bacterial meningitis, Gram staining of CSF preparations allows rapid diagnosis in 60–90 % of cases. However, the sensitivity varies between the pathogen species between 90 % in pneumococcal meningitis and <50 % in CNS infection with *Listeria monocytogenes* (Tunkel and Scheld 2005). Likewise, sensitivity depends on the preparation and staining technique. Cytocentrifuge preparations

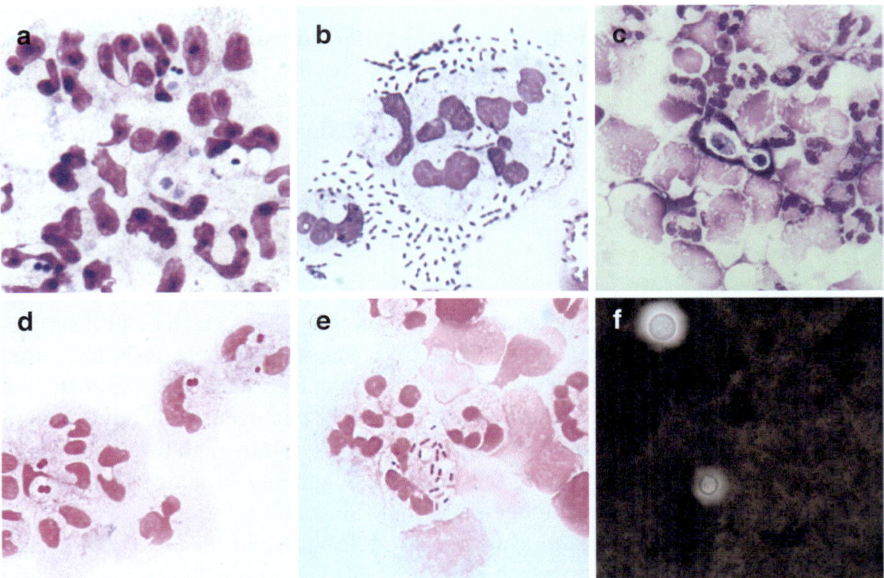

Fig. 11.1 Examples of stainings visualising meningitis-causing agents. *Upper panel*: May–Grünwald–Giemsa-stained cytospin for cytological differentiation of CSF cells can already visualise bacteria or fungi, and thorough inspection is mandatory: (**a**) mostly intracellularly located diplococci, culturally confirmed *Neisseria meningitides*; (**b**) extracellularly located diplococcic, culturally confirmed *Streptococcus pneumonia*; (**c**) budding yeast surrounded by a capsule, culturally confirmed *Cryptococcus neoformans*. *Lower panel*: Pathogen-specific staining for further characterisation: (**d**) Gram-negative, mostly intracellularly located diplococci, culturally confirmed *Neisseria meningitides* (same patient as *upper panel* **a**); (**e**) Gram-positive bacilli, culturally confirmed *Listeria monocytogenes*; (**f**) Indian ink visualising the capsule of *Cryptococcus neoformans* in CSF (same patient as *upper panel* **c**) (Special thanks to Ingelore Nagel for images and continuous support)

showed greater sensitivity in comparison to smears after conventional centrifugation (Chapin-Robertson et al. 1992). Low bacterial CSF load, of course, results in lower sensitivity than high bacterial load; microscopical detection can be achieved in samples with bacterial cell counts below $<10^3$ CFU/ml (colony-forming units per ml) in 25 %, in samples with $>10^5$ CFU/ml in 97 % (La Scolea and Dryja 1984). After onset of antibiotic treatment, sensitivity of Gram-stained smear is reduced to 40–60 %, and sensitivity of cultural detection is reduced to less than 50 %. In children, effective antibiotic treatment results in sterilisation of initially positive CSF cultures after 24–36 h (Bonadio 1992). Due to this reason, it should never be missed to draw blood cultures and in suspected meningococcal meningitis also pharyngeal swabs and samples of petechial skin lesions prior to start of antibiotic treatment.

In suspected tuberculous meningitis, CSF cell sediment should be analysed after Ziehl–Neelsen staining with a low sensitivity of about 30 % (Erdem et al. 2013), but the sensitivity can be increased by repeated lumbar punctures for CSF analysis (Kennedy and Fallon 1979).

Fungal CNS infections occur in Europe mainly in immunocompromised patients with especial importance of the yeasts *Cryptococcus* and *Candida* and the mould *Aspergillus*. Meningitis due to *Cryptococcus neoformans* is one of the most frequent opportunistic infections in patients with impaired cellular immunity. Sensitivity of microscopic detection of cryptococci after CSF staining with Indian ink or May–Grünwald–Giemsa is with 80–90 % high (Zhang et al. 2014; Saha et al. 2009); cultural methods and antigen detection in CSF and serum are important, too (Perfect 2005; Marchetti et al. 2012).

11.3 Antigen Tests

Detection of antigens of pathogenic agents within the CSF can be a helpful supplement for diagnosing bacterial and fungal CNS infections. These tests are based upon the principle to detect antigens by antibody-coated latex particles that will agglutinate with specimens containing the respective pathogens. The advantage of these tests is the rapid procedure and result. Sensitivity is only high in case of a high pathogen load in the CSF, and by this way, the sensitivity of antigen tests is not superior to microscopy after pathogen-specific CSF staining.

Bacterial antigen tests are available to detect *Streptococcus pneumoniae*, *Neisseria meningitidis* (serotypes A, B, C, Y, W135), group B streptococci and *Escherichia coli* K1. There is a certain benefit of bacterial antigen tests to confirm diagnosis and bacterial species in case of antibiotic pretreatment that lowers the sensitivity of bacterial culture; the method should be used in sense of confirmation and not exclusion. As the diagnostic value of bacterial antigen tests has been questioned repeatedly, there are no clear recommendations (Tunkel et al. 2004) and many laboratories have discontinued the use of the bacterial antigen tests. In any case, additional routine microbiological analyses including microscopy and cultural methods are mandatory.

In contrast, in the diagnosis of cryptococcal meningitis, the use of cryptococcal antigen test is clearly recommended in addition to staining and fungal culture (Portegies et al. 2004; Arendt 2012). The test detects polysaccharide antigens of the encapsulated yeast *Cryptococcus neoformans* in serum and CSF (Bennett et al. 1964), and its sensitivity is very high (in CSF 95–99 %) in comparison to fungal culture.

11.4 Microbiological Culture

Microbial cultures are the gold standard to determine the pathogenic agent in bacterial or fungal CNS infection. Beyond the determination of the type of organism, it allows the detection and quantification of the strain-specific susceptibility to antibiotic or antifungal drugs.

Most bacteria that cause acute meningitis grow well on solid or fluid culture media like blood and chocolate agar or tryptic soy broth, unless they have been damaged by antibiotic intervention (Gill et al. 2005). Selective culture media are, for example, Sabouraud agar suitable for the cultivation and differentiation of fungi or Löwenstein–Jensen medium, specially used for culture of *Mycobacterium*.

CSF specimens drawn for suspected acute bacterial meningitis will be cultivated for at least 72 h at 35–37 °C and in CO_2-enriched aerobic atmosphere. Other suspected CNS infections, as fungal or tuberculous meningitis, require different and specialised growth media and conditions (selective media, special temperatures, longer cultivation time). Therefore, it is of outstanding importance that the treating physician informs the microbiological laboratory about the suspected diagnosis.

In any case of suspected bacterial meningitis, it should be kept in mind to draw specimens for aerobic and anaerobic blood cultures prior to antibiotic treatment.

11.5 Molecular Assays

Amplification techniques such as those using PCR provide increased sensitivity and specificity with short processing time because of the rapid and extensive amplification of target nucleic acid. They are method of choice in the diagnosis of numerous viral CNS infections and improve the diagnosis of bacterial, tuberculous and parasitic infections and can detect, for example, *herpes simplex* virus (HSV) DNA by amplification of below ten copies DNA per ml. Due to the high sensitivity of PCR, care must be taken to avoid contamination with other templates and amplicons that may be present in the laboratory environment; thus, strict intra-laboratory quality standards are necessary to ensure accurate results. In addition to the high clinical utility of PCR in identifying aetiologic agents of CNS disease, also quantification of viral load to monitor duration and adequacy of antiviral drug therapy (e.g. HIV) is routinely used.

In most PCR protocols and assays, DNA or RNA is extracted from a sample volume of about 100–200 µl (Debiasi and Tyler 2004). For CSF analysis in suspected tuberculous meningitis, relevant larger sample volumes up to volumes >6 ml CSF are recommended (Thwaites et al. 2004).

In general, endogenous polymerase inhibitors are much less commonly present in CSF than in other body fluids or tissues. Nevertheless, false-negative results also occur in CSF analysis. Factors, which might contribute to low sensitivity, include low viral load, delay in CSF processing or rapid clearance due to robust host neutralising antibody response. False-negative results may also occur in the presence of endogenous polymerase inhibitors; especially haeme products from artificial blood contamination may inhibit the PCR, and this should be kept in mind in case of unexpected negative results as in suspected herpes simplex encephalitis (Debiasi and Tyler 2004).

Important applications of PCR-based CSF analytics are suspected herpes simplex encephalitis caused by HSV-1 or less common HSV-2, CNS infections by varicella zoster virus (VZV), Epstein–Barr virus (EBV), cytomegalovirus (CMV), enteroviruses or the polyomavirus JC virus causing progressive multifocal leukoencephalopathy (PML).

In herpes simplex encephalitis, the sensitivity of PCR-based assays is above 95 % with likewise high specificity of 99 %. HSV DNA can still be detected after onset of antiviral treatment for at least 5–7 days. In this early stage of the disease, serological assays to detect intrathecal antibody synthesis against HSE are not of clinical relevance. However, within the first 72 h of herpes simplex encephalitis, false-negative results occur. In well-founded clinical suspicion of herpes simplex encephalitis, antiviral treatment must not be interrupted because of a negative PCR result. Negative results should be interpreted with particular caution, if the CSF specimen was sanguineous or xanthochrome (Tyler 2004; Steiner et al. 2012).

Also diagnostic of bacterial CNS infections is improved by PCR methods. The availability of results (within 8–24 h) is faster in comparison to conventional culture methods, for which results usually are not available for 48 h. Real-time multiplex PCR methods detect *H. influenzae*, *N. meningitidis*, *S. pneumoniae* and *L. monocytogenes* with high sensitivity (87–100 %) and specificity (98–100 %) (Chaudhuri et al. 2008). PCR methods are of special interest in specimen with delayed processing time or sampling after onset of antibiotic treatment, in which sensitivity of microscopy and bacterial culture decreases. In cases of uncommon or unsuspected bacterial agents, broad-range bacterial PCR assays can be useful in detecting the bacterial gene coding for the 16S ribosomal ribonucleic acid, followed by DNA sequencing for species identification (Greisen et al. 1994; Srinivasan et al. 2012). In suspected neurotuberculosis, PCR assays are supplemental diagnostic tools, especially due to the rapid availability of results in comparison to the long duration of cultivation of up to 6 weeks. But the reported sensitivities of PCR-based tests for *Mycobacterium tuberculosis* in CSF samples range from 46 to 66 % and specificities from 97 to 99 %. Thus, results must be interpreted with caution (Steiner et al. 2012).

11.6 Serology

Besides the methods for direct detection of pathogens, serological tests play an important in role in diagnosing and confirming CNS infections. Serological tests to identify pathogen-directed antibodies in serum and CSF are especially important in subacute or chronic infectious diseases, as, for example, neuroborreliosis or the second phase of the biphasic presenting tick-borne encephalitis. In contrast to the acute infections in bacterial meningitis and herpes simplex encephalitis, clinical signs of CNS involvement present weeks after infection.

For example, neuroborreliosis is diagnosed by the combination of typical neurological symptoms, parameter of acute meningeal inflammation within the CSF (pleocytosis, blood–CSF barrier dysfunction) and *Borrelia burgdorferi*-specific antibodies produced intrathecally. Serological evidence of intrathecal immune response by detection of *B. burgdorferi*-specific IgG and IgM antibody index (AI) values is gold standard in the diagnosis of neuroborreliosis and has a sensitivity of 80 % (duration of infection <6 weeks) to nearly 100 % (>6 weeks). Due to its low sensitivity of only 10–30 %, *B. burgdorferi* PCR is not of significant clinical relevance and should be limited on very early stages of disease or in patients with immunosuppression (Mygland et al. 2009).

Tick-borne encephalitis (TBE) is a characteristic biphasic febrile illness, involving the central nervous system with symptoms of meningitis, encephalitis or meningoencephalitis. After an asymptomatic incubation period between 7 and 14 days, an initial phase of fever and non-specific symptoms occurs. After about 1 week of remission, CNS affection occurs in 10–30 % of patients. CSF analysis reveals signs of acute viral infection with pleocytosis, blood–CSF barrier dysfunction and intrathecally produced antibodies against TBE virus by detection of TBEV-specific antibody index values (Holzmann 2003).

11.6.1 Detection of Antigen-Specific Intrathecal Immune Response

Intrathecal synthesis of total IgG, IgA and IgM can be detected by immunonephelometric determination of the CSF-to-serum ratios of IgG, IgA, IgM and albumin and plotting IgG, IgA and IgM ratios versus albumin ratio according to the nomogram of Reiber and Felgenhauer (Reiber and Felgenhauer 1987) (see also Chap. 10)

To detect a pathogen-specific intrathecal antibody synthesis, calculation of antigen-specific antibody index (AI) values is commonly used (Reiber and Lange 1991). The determination of specific antibody index values allows detecting a pathological, brain-derived fraction of specific antibodies in CSF, not deriving from serum by flow-depended diffusion via the "blood–CSF barrier". Species-specific immunoglobulins deriving from serum enter the CSF at equal proportion as total immunoglobulin of the same isotype (Fig. 11.2a). Therefore, the quotient of

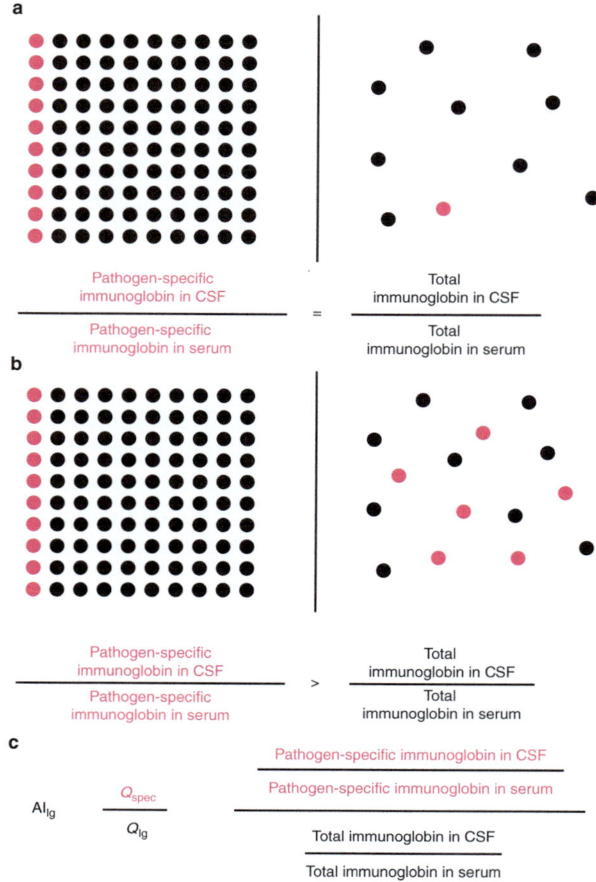

Fig. 11.2 Schematic diagram of antigen-specific antibody index calculation. (**a**) Species-specific immunoglobulins deriving from serum enter the CSF at equal proportion as total immunoglobulin of the same isotype; this results in equality of the quotient of pathogen-specific immunoglobulin concentration in CSF divided by pathogen-specific immunoglobulin concentration of in serum (Q_{spec}) and the quotient of total immunoglobulin concentration in CSF divided by total immuno-globulin concentration in serum (Q_{Ig}). (**b**) In case of intrathecal immunoglobulin synthesis, the pathogen-specific antibody concentration ratio (Q_{spec}) increases in relation to the total antibody concentration ratio (Q_{Ig}) resulting in elevated antibody index values above 1. (**c**) Equation for calculation of antigen-specific antibody index (AI) if QIg < QLim

arbitrary or absolute concentration of pathogen-specific immunoglobulin in CSF divided by concentration of pathogen-specific immunoglobulin in serum (Q_{spec}) has to be the same as the quotient of total immunoglobulin concentration in CSF divided by total immunoglobulin concentration in serum (Q_{Ig}). As the antibody index is the ratio of Q_{spec} divided by Q_{Ig} (Fig. 11.2c), the resulting antibody index is 1. In case of intrathecal immunoglobulin synthesis (Fig. 11.2b), the pathogen-specific antibody concentration ratio (Q_{spec}) increases in relation to the total antibody concentration ratio (Q_{Ig}) resulting in elevated antibody index values above 1.

In practice, absolute or arbitrary concentration units of species-specific antibodies are determined with respect to a standard curve, for example, derived from twofold serial dilutions of a positive standard serum pool or (if available) commercial standard samples. The CSF and serum pair of a patient has to be essentially analysed in the same run of the same analytical test system (e.g. the same plate of an ELISA), and CSF and serum samples should be diluted to yield concentrations that are located in similar parts of the standard curve. Q_{spec} will be related to either the total immunoglobulin quotient ($Q_{Ig\ total}$ = total immunoglobulins in CSF: total immunoglobulins in serum) ($Q_{spec}/Q_{Ig\ total}$), or in cases with a local IgG or IgM synthesis (IgIF >0 %), Q_{spec} is related to the limiting IgG or IgM quotient (Q_{Lim}) (Q_{spec}/Q_{Lim}) (Reiber and Lange 1991; Kaiser and Lucking 1993). The antibody index value mostly is defined as pathologic (i.e. indicating the synthesis of antibodies against the specific pathogen within the CNS), when it is ≥ 1.5).

Table 11.1 Examples of agents and diagnostic methods in CNS infections

Infectious agent	Clinical presentation and hints	Diagnostic methods
Bacteria		
Streptococcus pneumoniae	Ambulant acquired purulent meningitis	**Microscopy (Gram-positive extracellular diplococcus)**, **culture**, antigen test, PCR (specific, multiplex or broad-range 16S RNA)
Neisseria meningitides	Ambulant acquired purulent meningitis, petechial skin lesions	**Microscopy (Gram-negative intracellular diplococcus)**, **culture**, antigen test, PCR (specific, multiplex or broad-range 16S RNA)
Haemophilus influenzae	Ambulant acquired purulent meningitis, rare since implementation of vaccination	**Microscopy (Gram-negative extracellular coccobacillus)**, **culture**, antigen test, PCR (specific, multiplex or broad-range 16S RNA)
Listeria monocytogenes	Ambulant acquired purulent meningoencephalitis, predisposing immunosuppressive factors or age, pregnancy	**Microscopy (Gram-positive bacillus)**, **culture**, PCR (specific, multiplex or broad-range 16S RNA)

(continued)

Table 11.1 (continued)

Infectious agent	Clinical presentation and hints	Diagnostic methods
Escherichia coli K1	Purulent meningitis in neonates	**Microscopy (Gram-negative bacillus)**, **culture**, antigen test, PCR (specific or broad-range 16S RNA)
Staphylococcus aureus and other staphylococci	Nosocomial infections, predisposing immunosuppressive factors, brain abscess	**Microscopy (Gram-positive, extracellular cocci)**, **culture**, PCR (specific or broad-range 16S RNA)
Enterobacteriaceae or Pseudomonas aeruginosa	Nosocomial infections, predisposing immunosuppressive factors, brain abscess	**Microscopy (Gram-negative bacilli)**, **culture**, PCR (specific or broad-range 16S RNA)
Borrelia burgdorferi	Lymphocytic meningoradiculitis, facial nerve palsy, rarely encephalomyelitis, medical history or risk of tick bite	**Serology, antigen-specific antibody index** (PCR very early in disease)
Treponema pallidum	Medical history of syphilis	**Serology, antigen-specific antibody index**
Mycobacterium tuberculosis	Basal meningitis, medical history of extracerebral tuberculosis	**Microscopy (Ziehl–Neelsen staining), culture (long cultivation time), specific PCR (variable sensitivity), large sample volumes**
Viruses		
Herpes simplex virus (HSV) 1, 2	Sporadic focal necrotising encephalitis, meningitis, neonatal sepsis	**PCR (in acute infection)**, antigen-specific antibody index (>2 weeks after onset of symptoms)
Varicella zoster virus (VZV)	Radiculitis, facial nerve palsy, meningitis, myelitis, vasculitis, encephalitis	**PCR, antigen-specific antibody index**
Epstein–Barr virus (EBV)	Meningoencephalitis in immunocompromised patients, association with primary CNS lymphoma	**PCR**, antigen-specific antibody index
Cytomegalovirus (CMV)	Necrotising encephalitis in immunocompromised patients, polyradiculomyelitis, retinitis	**PCR**, antigen-specific antibody index
Enteroviruses (Coxsackie virus, echovirus, enterovirus)	Meningitis, encephalitis, neonatal sepsis syndrome, extracerebral manifestations	**Group-specific PCR**
Poliovirus	Poliomyelitis, meningitis, encephalitis	**PCR, virus isolation (cell culture), serology**, poliovirus neutralisation test

(continued)

Table 11.1 (continued)

Infectious agent	Clinical presentation and hints	Diagnostic methods
JC polyomavirus	Progressive multifocal leukoencephalopathy in immunocompromised patients	**PCR**, brain biopsy (serology for risk estimation)
Tick-borne encephalitis virus (FMSE, RSSE)	Tick-borne encephalitis, medical history or risk of tick bite in endemic areas of Europe and Asia	**Serology, antigen-specific antibody index** (exceptionally PCR in immunocompromised patients or vaccine failure)
Human immunodeficiency virus (HIV)	HIV dementia, myelopathy, neuropathy, myopathy, immunosuppression	**Serology, PCR, antigen-specific antibody index**
Mumps virus	Meningitis, parotitis	**Serology, PCR**, antigen-specific antibody index
Measles virus	Acute encephalitis, SSPE, skin rash	**Serology, antigen-specific antibody index**, PCR
Fungi		
Aspergillus fumigatus	Immunocompromised patients	**Culture**, antigen test, broad-range PCR (18S RNA), brain biopsy
Candida albicans	Immunocompromised patients	**Culture**, antigen test, broad-range PCR (18S RNA)
Cryptococcus neoformans	Immunocompromised patients	**Culture, microscopy (Indian ink staining), antigen test**
Parasites		
Toxoplasma gondii	Reactivation in immunocompromised patients, prenatal infection	**PCR, antigen-specific antibody index**

List of some frequent agents of CNS infections in Europe with selected remarks to clinical findings and typical diagnostic methods (predominantly used methods or methods of choice are marked in bold)

References

Arendt G (2012) Diagnostik und Therapie HIV-1-assoziierter neurologischer Erkrankungen. In: Diener HC, Weima C (eds) Leitlinien für Diagnostik und Therapie in der Neurologie. Thieme, Stuttgart, p

Bennett JE, Hasenclever HF, Tynes BS (1964) Detection of cryptococcal polysaccharide in serum and spinal fluid: value in diagnosis and prognosis. Trans Assoc Am Physicians 77:145–150

Bonadio WA (1992) The cerebrospinal fluid: physiologic aspects and alterations associated with bacterial meningitis. Pediatr Infect Dis J 11:423–431

Chapin-Robertson K, Dahlberg SE, Edberg SC (1992) Clinical and laboratory analyses of cytospin-prepared Gram stains for recovery and diagnosis of bacteria from sterile body fluids. J Clin Microbiol 30:377–380

Chaudhuri A, Martinez-Martin P, Kennedy PG et al (2008) EFNS guideline on the management of community-acquired bacterial meningitis: report of an EFNS Task Force on acute bacterial meningitis in older children and adults. Eur J Neurol 15:649–659

Debiasi R, Tyler K (2004) Molecular methods for diagnosis of viral encephalitis. Clin Microbiol Rev 17:903–925

Erdem H, Ozturk-Engin D, Elaldi N et al (2013) The microbiological diagnosis of tuberculous meningitis: results of Haydarpasa-1 study. Clin Microbiol Infect 20:O600–608

Gill VJ, Fedorko DP, Witebsky FG (2005) Clinical microbiology. In: Mandell GL, Bennett JE, Dolin R (eds) Principles and practice of infectious diseases. Elsevier, Philadelphia, pp 203–241

Greisen K, Loeffelholz M, Purohit A et al (1994) PCR primers and probes for the 16S rRNA gene of most species of pathogenic bacteria, including bacteria found in cerebrospinal fluid. J Clin Microbiol 32:335–351

Holzmann H (2003) Diagnosis of tick-borne encephalitis. Vaccine 21(Suppl 1):S36–S40

Kaiser R, Lucking CH (1993) Intrathecal synthesis of specific antibodies in neuroborreliosis. Comparison of different ELISA techniques and calculation methods. J Neurol Sci 118:64–72

Kennedy DH, Fallon RJ (1979) Tuberculous meningitis. JAMA 241:264–268

La Scolea LJ Jr, Dryja D (1984) Quantitation of bacteria in cerebrospinal fluid and blood of children with meningitis and its diagnostic significance. J Clin Microbiol 19:187–190

Marchetti O, Lamoth F, Mikulska M et al (2012) ECIL recommendations for the use of biological markers for the diagnosis of invasive fungal diseases in leukemic patients and hematopoietic SCT recipients. Bone Marrow Transplant 47:846–854

Mygland A, Ljostad U, Fingerle V et al (2009) EFNS guidelines on the diagnosis and management of European Lyme neuroborreliosis. Eur J Neurol 17(8–16):e11–e14

Nau R (2005) Liquordiagnostik bei bakteriellen ZNS-Erkrankungen. In: Zettl U, Lehmitz R, Mix E (eds) Klinische Liquordiagnostik. Walter de Gruyter, Berlin, pp 301–316

Perfect J (2005) Cryptococcus neoformans. In: Mandell GL, Bennett JE, Dolin R (eds) Principles and practice of infectious diseases. Elsevier, Philadelphia, pp 2997–3011

Portegies P, Solod L, Cinque P et al (2004) Guidelines for the diagnosis and management of neurological complications of HIV infection. Eur J Neurol 11:297–304

Reiber H, Felgenhauer K (1987) Protein transfer at the blood cerebrospinal fluid barrier and the quantitation of the humoral immune response within the central nervous system. Clin Chim Acta 163:319–328

Reiber H, Lange P (1991) Quantification of virus-specific antibodies in cerebrospinal fluid and serum: sensitive and specific detection of antibody synthesis in brain. Clin Chem 37:1153–1160

Saha DC, Xess I, Biswas A et al (2009) Detection of Cryptococcus by conventional, serological and molecular methods. J Med Microbiol 58:1098–1105

Srinivasan L, Pisapia JM, Shah SS et al (2012) Can broad-range 16S ribosomal ribonucleic acid gene polymerase chain reactions improve the diagnosis of bacterial meningitis? A systematic review and meta-analysis. Ann Emerg Med 60:609–620 e602

Steiner I, Schmutzhard E, Sellner J et al (2012) EFNS-ENS guidelines for the use of PCR technology for the diagnosis of infections of the nervous system. Eur J Neurol 19:1278–1291

Thwaites G, Caws M, Chau T et al (2004) Comparison of conventional bacteriology with nucleic acid amplification (amplified mycobacterium direct test) for diagnosis of tuberculous meningitis before and after inception of antituberculosis chemotherapy. J Clin Microbiol 42:996–1002

Tunkel A, Scheld W (2005) Acute meningitis. In: Mandell GL, Bennett JE, Dolin R (eds) Principles and practice of infectious diseases. Elsevier, Philadelphia, pp 1083–1125

Tunkel AR, Hartman BJ, Kaplan SL et al (2004) Practice guidelines for the management of bacterial meningitis. Clin Infect Dis 39:1267–1284

Tyler KL (2004) Herpes simplex virus infections of the central nervous system: encephalitis and meningitis, including Mollaret's. Herpes 11(Suppl 2):57A–64A

Wildemann B, Geiss H, Schnitzler P (2006) Erregerdiagnostik. In: Wildemann B, Oschmann P, Reiber H (eds) Neurologische Labordiagnostik. Thieme, Stuttgart, pp 59–68

Zhang M, Li J, Lin H et al (2014) Diagnostic value of cytological and microbiological methods in cryptococcal meningitis. Genet Mol Res 13:9253–9261

Immunohistochemistry

12

Romana Höftberger, Simone Mader, and Markus Reindl

Contents

Abstract

Several autoantibodies associated with neurological diseases of the central nervous system have been described in the last decade. The clinical symptoms and disorders associated with these autoantibodies are diverse, including limbic

R. Höftberger
Institute of Neurology, Medical University of Vienna,
Vienna, Austria
e-mail: romana.hoeftberger@meduniwien.ac.at

S. Mader
Center for Autoimmune and Musculoskeletal Diseases,
The Feinstein Institute for Medical Research, Manhasset, NY, USA
e-mail: smader@nshs.edu

M. Reindl (✉)
Clinical Department of Neurology, Medical University of Innsbruck,
Innsbruck, Austria
e-mail: markus.reindl@i-med.ac.at

© Springer International Publishing Switzerland 2015
F. Deisenhammer et al. (eds.), *Cerebrospinal Fluid in Clinical Neurology*,
DOI 10.1007/978-3-319-01225-4_12

encephalitis and demyelinating diseases. The autoantibodies target neuronal and glial channels, channel-associated proteins, and surface receptors, and their detection is strongly dependent on the usage of high-affinity immunoassays. Immunohistochemistry and immunofluorescence techniques are used to detect a certain staining pattern on brain tissue (tissue-based assays), or cells are used expressing autoantigens (cell-based assays) that reflects the presence of a specific antibody in serum or cerebrospinal fluid of patients. Tissue-based assays use frozen brain slides of rodents or primates, and immunolabeling is performed on cryostat sections. Epitopes of intracellular antigens need retrieval techniques using perfusion and chemical fixation of brains, whereas epitopes of surface antigens require the use of fresh brains that are post-fixed. Cell-based assays use mammalian cells transfected with a plasmid encoding the specific antigen for the detection of antibodies. Antibodies can recognize conformational epitopes, and assays are highly specific. Anti-neuronal antibodies associated with autoimmune encephalitis are directed against intracellular (e.g., Hu, Yo, Ri) or surface antigens (e.g., NMDAR, LGI1, CASPR2) and are usually detected by a combination of tissue- and cell-based assays. Among the antibodies to glial autoantigens, aquaporin-4 antibodies have emerged as sensitive and specific biomarkers for neuromyelitis optica, and antibodies to the myelin oligodendrocyte glycoprotein are associated with a subset of predominantly pediatric demyelinating diseases. These antibodies are usually detected by cell-based assays.

In the past years several novel autoantibody-associated neurological diseases of the central nervous system (CNS) have been described, and further specific antibodies are identified every year (Lancaster and Dalmau 2012; Reindl et al. 2013; Vincent et al. 2011; Wildemann and Jarius 2013; Wingerchuk et al. 2007). These autoantibodies target neuronal and glial channels, channel-associated proteins, and surface receptors and can only be detected using high-affinity immunoassays. The clinical symptoms and disorders associated with these autoantibodies are diverse, including limbic encephalitis and demyelinating diseases such as neuromyelitis optica (NMO) or acute disseminated encephalomyelitis (ADEM). In this chapter we will give an overview on these autoantibodies and the immunological methods used for their detection.

12.1 Detection of Anti-neuronal Antibodies

12.1.1 Introduction

Immunohistochemistry has an essential role in the diagnosis of anti-neuronal antibodies. The technique is applied to detect a certain staining pattern that reflects the presence of a specific antibody in serum and/or CSF of the patient. Several aspects should be taken into consideration in the interpretation of the results: (1) the currently available conventional test systems and commercial kits are optimized to detect already known and well-characterized antibodies, while novel antibodies might be missed; (2) labeling may sometimes be absent in serum, while CSF gives strong results and vice versa; and (3) immunohistochemistry is an excellent diagnostic tool, but the results should always be interpreted in context with the clinical presentation of the patient.

There is a rapid advance in the identification of new antigens that play a role in autoimmune encephalitis, and the number of anti-neuronal antibodies that can be identified with immunohistochemistry is growing. Currently, the antibodies are classified according to the localization of the targeted antigen in antibodies against intracellular antigens (e.g., Hu, Yo, Ri) and antibodies targeting surface antigens (e.g., NMDAR, LGI1, CASPR2) (Graus et al. 2010). This chapter aims to summarize the principles of the methodology and to describe the specific immunohistochemical staining patterns of the currently known antibodies relevant to diagnosis. Aspects relating to specific disorders will be described in the chapter by Titulaer.

12.1.2 Methods for Immunohistochemistry

Immunohistochemistry is used to visualize and localize a certain binding pattern either on brain tissue (tissue-based assay) or on cell lines, transfected with a particular antigen (cell-based assay). The principle of the technique is the specific affinity of the patient's antibody for its antigen.

12.1.2.1 Tissue-Based Assay

The tissue-based assay uses brains either of rodents or primates that are frozen, and immunolabeling is performed on cryostat sections. The epitopes of intracellular antigens need retrieval techniques using perfusion and fixation of brains with paraformaledehyde. In contrast, the epitopes of surface antigens require the use of fresh brains (not perfused) that are only post-fixed. Sections pretreated for the detection of intracellular antigens are usually obtained from the cerebellum, whereas surface antigens are analyzed in the hippocampus. Tissue-based assays can be made in-house, but they are also commercially available.

12.1.2.2 Cell-Based Assay

The cell-based assay uses mammalian cells (e.g., human embryonic kidney cells HEK293) that are transfected with a plasmid encoding the specific antigen and is used for the detection of antibodies against surface antigens. Non-transfected cells are used as controls. With this technique, the antibodies can recognize a conformational epitope, and the tests are thus highly specific. Most cell-based assays currently used for the diagnosis are formalin-fixed and can be stored until required. However, some antibodies may only give satisfactory results with live cell staining, which is time effective and requires cell culture facilities in the laboratory.

To visualize the patient's antibodies, a secondary antibody against human immunoglobulin is applied (indirect detection method) that either detects a specific immunoglobulin class (IgG, IgA, IgM) or recognizes all classes. The secondary antibody may be subsequently conjugated either with an avidin-biotin-peroxidase method (tissue-based assays) or fluorochromes (cell-based assays and tissue-based assay; for tissue-based assays, it is a matter of personal preference to either use peroxidase or fluorochrome).

12.1.3　Immunohistochemical Staining Patterns of Anti-neuronal Antibodies

The number of anti-neuronal antibodies that are detectable by immunohistochemistry is constantly increasing and summarized in Table 12.1.

12.1.3.1　Antibodies Targeting Intracellular Antigens

All antibodies targeting intracellular antigens are paraneoplastic except anti-GAD65 antibodies, anti-Homer3, and anti-AK5. The detection of these antibodies confirms the immune-mediated origin of the neurological disorder and is helpful in tumor search. The following immunohistochemical staining patterns can be observed:

Hu antibodies (type 1 anti-neuronal nuclear autoantibodies, ANNA1) and *Ri antibodies* (type 2 anti-neuronal nuclear antibodies, ANNA2) label nuclei and cytoplasm of neurons in cerebrum, cerebellum, and brain stem; nucleoli are spared (Fig. 12.1a). In the peripheral nervous system, Hu-antibodies stain the myenteric plexus, while Ri-antibodies do not. Both antibodies bind to neuron specific RNA-binding proteins with wide distribution in the nervous system (Graus et al. 2001; Pittock et al. 2003). *Anti-Yo antibodies* (*PCA1*) label the cytoplasm of Purkinje cells and some stellate and basket cells in the molecular layer of the cerebellum (Fig. 12.1b). The antibodies recognize the cerebellar degeneration–related protein 2 (CDR-2), a Purkinje cell protein that is involved in signal transduction and gene transcription. *Anti-CV2 antibodies* (CRMP5) label oligodendrocytes in the white matter of cerebellum, brainstem, and spinal cord (Fig. 12.1c). The antibodies target a cytoplasmic protein of the collapsin response mediator protein family with a potential role in synaptic events (Honnorat et al. 1996). *Anti-amphiphysin antibodies* show a synaptic staining of the molecular and granular cell layer of the cerebellar cortex, and midbrain, the Purkinje cells are unstained (Pittock et al. 2005). Amphiphysin is a synaptic vesicle protein that is important for vesicle membrane recycling after depolarization. *Anti-Ma1/2 antibodies* show a dot-like staining pattern that is found in the nuclei and cytoplasm of large neurons of the brainstem and hippocampus (Fig. 12.1d). The Ma protein family concentrates in interchromatin granule clusters and coiled bodies in nuclei and cytoplasm and is involved in transcription and pre-mRNA processing (Rosenfeld et al. 2001). *Anti-PKCγ* (protein kinase Cγ), *anti-ARHGAP26* (rhoGTPase-activating protein 26), and *anti-CARPVIII antibodies* (carbonic anhydrase-related protein VIII) label the cytoplasm, axons, and dendrites of Purkinje cells (Fig. 12.1e). The antibodies recognize the respective intracellular proteins that are all specific for Purkinje cells (Doss et al. 2014; Hoftberger et al. 2013a, 2014). *Anti-SOX1 antibodies* (anti-glial nuclear antibody, AGNA) label the nuclei of Bergmann glia of the cerebellum (Fig. 12.1f). SOX1

Table 12.1 Clinical symptoms and associated malignancies of anti-neuronal antibodies (Dalmau and Rosenfeld 2014; Graus et al. 2010)

Intracellular antigen	Associated tumor	Clinical symptoms
Hu (ANNA1)	SCLC	Encephalomyelitis, PCD, LE, brainstem encephalitis
Ri (ANNA2)	Breast, SCLC	Brainstem encephalitis, opsoclonus myoclonus
Yo (PCA1)	Ovary, breast	PCD
CV2 (CRMP5)	SCLC, thymoma	Encephalomyelitis, Chorea, PCD, LE
Amphiphysin	SCLC, breast	SPS, myelopathy and myoclonus, encephalomyelitis
MA-1/2	Testicular seminoma, NSCLC	LE, brainstem encephalitis
PKCγ	Adenocarcinoma	PCD
ARHGAP26	Ovary	PCD
CARPVIII	Ovary, melanoma	PCD
SOX1 (AGNA)	SCLC	LEMS, PCD
ZIC4	SCLC	Cerebellar ataxia
GAD65	–	SPS, cerebellar ataxia, LE
Homer3	–	Cerebellar ataxia
AK5	–	LE
Surface antigens		
NMDAR	Ovarian teratoma (58 % in patients >18 years)	Encephalitis
LGI1		LE, tonic seizures
CASPR2	Thymoma (38 %)	LE, Morvan syndrome
AMPAR	SCLC, breast, thymoma (60 %)	LE, psychosis
GABA$_B$R	SCLC (50 %)	LE, ataxia
GABA$_A$R	–	Status epilepticus, seizures, encephalitis
mGluR1	M. Hodgkin	Cerebellar ataxia
mGluR5	M. Hodgkin	Ophelia syndrome
DPPX (Kv4.1)	–	Hallucinations, agitation, myoclonia, tremor, seizures, diarrhea
Iglon5	–	NREM/REM parasomnia, sleep apnea, and brainstem dysfunction
GlyR	Lung cancer	PERM, SPS
D2R	–	Basal ganglia encephalitis, Sydenham's chorea
VGCC	SCLC	LEMS, PCD
DNER (TR)	M. Hodgkin	PCD

Abbreviations: *ANNA* anti-neuronal nuclear antibody, *PCA* Purkinje cell autoantibody, *CRMP* collapsin response mediator protein, *PKCγ* protein kinase C gamma, *ARGHAP26* rhoGTPase-activating protein 26, *CARPVIII* carbonic anhydrase-related protein VIII, *AGNA* anti-glial nuclear antibody, *ZIC4* zinc-finger protein 4, *GAD65* glutamic acid decarboxylase 65, *AK5* adenylate kinase 5, *NMDAR* N-methyl-D-aspartate receptor, *LGI1* leucine-rich glioma-inactivated 1, *CASPR2* contactin-associated protein-like 2, *AMPAR* amino-3-hydroxy-5-hydroxy-5-methyl-4-isoxazolepropionic acid receptor, *GABA A/B R* gamma-aminobutyric acid A/B receptor, *mGluR1/5* metabotropic glutamate receptor type 1/5, *DPPX* dipeptidyl-peptidase-like protein-6, *GlyR* Glycine receptor, *D2R* dopamine 2 receptor, *VGCC* P/Q type calcium channel, *DNER* delta/notch-like epidermal growth factor-related receptor, *SCLC* small-cell lung cancer, *NSCLC* non-small-cell lung cancer, *PCD* paraneoplastic cerebellar degeneration, *LE* limbic encephalitis, *SPS* stiff-person syndrome, *PERM* progressive encephalomyelitis with rigidity and myoclonus, *LEMS* Lambert-Eaton myasthenic syndrome

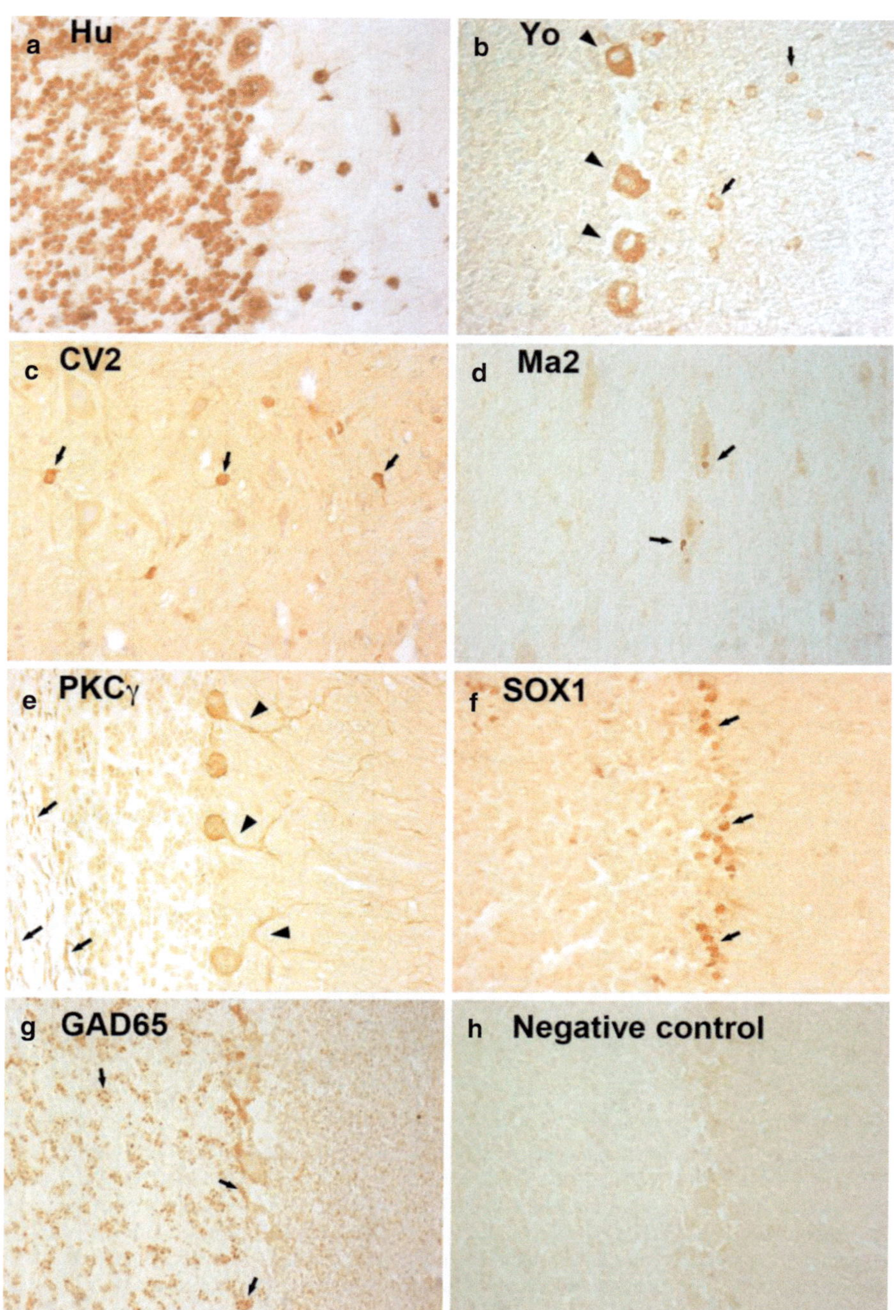
a Hu
b Yo
c CV2
d Ma2
e PKCγ
f SOX1
g GAD65
h Negative control

belongs to a family of transcription factors that is expressed in the developing brain (Graus et al. 2005). *Anti-ZIC-antibodies* (zinc-finger proteins) label the granule cell layer of the cerebellum and less intensively the cytoplasm of Purkinje cells. ZIC proteins play a role in cerebellar development, and the antibodies target a conserved zinc-finger domain that is common in different ZIC proteins (Bataller et al. 2002). *Anti-GAD65 antibodies* (glutamic acid decarboxylase 65 antibodies) label axonal terminals in the molecular layer, at the base of Purkinje cells, and rosettes of axonal terminals in the glomeruli of the granular layer of the cerebellum (Fig. 12.1g) (Solimena et al. 1990). GAD65 is the brain-specific isoform of GAD and the rate-limiting enzyme for the synthesis of the transmitter gamma-aminobutyric acid (GABA). *Anti-Homer3 antibodies* show an intense labeling of the molecular layer of the cerebellum and weaker reactivity with the cytoplasm of Purkinje cells. Homer 3 interacts with the metabotropic glutamate receptor type 1 (mGluR1) and enables clustering of the receptor (Hoftberger et al. 2013c). *Anti-adenylate kinase 5 (AK5) antibodies* react with the cytoplasm of neurons in cerebrum, cerebellum, and brain stem; nuclei are spared. The protein AK5 is neuron specific and involved in metabolic processes and RNA/DNA synthesis (Tuzun et al. 2007). *Anti-Tr antibodies* label the Purkinje cell cytoplasm and show a dot-like staining pattern in the molecular layer of the cerebellum. The antigen was initially described intracellular but was recently identified as delta/notch-like epidermal growth factor-related receptor (DNER) (De Graaff et al. 2012).

12.1.3.2 Antibodies Targeting Surface Antigens

The association of antibodies targeting surface antigens with malignancy is less consistent. The detection of these antibodies is important because patients usually respond to immunotherapy. Both serum and CSF should be tested, and it is reasonable to follow an algorithmic diagnostic approach (Fig. 12.2):

A first screening should be performed by a tissue-based assay optimized for surface receptor antibodies, where most of the antibodies show a characteristic

Fig. 12.1 Staining pattern of antibodies targeting intracellular antigens. (**a**) Anti-Hu-antibodies show an intensive labeling of cytoplasm and nuclei of Purkinje and granule cells. (**b**) Anti-Yo antibodies label the cytoplasm of Purkinje cells (*arrow heads*) and stellate and basket cells in the molecular layer (*arrows*). (**c**) Anti-CV2-antibodies mark a subgroup of oligodendrocytes in the brainstem (*arrows*). (**d**) Anti-Ma2-antibodies show a dot-like staining pattern in large neurons of the brainstem (*arrows*). (**e**) Anti-PKC-antibodies label the cytoplasm, axons (*arrows*), and dendrites (*arrow heads*) of Purkinje cells. (**f**) Anti-SOX1-antibodies stain the nuclei of Bergmann glia in the cerebellum (*arrows*). (**g**) Anti-GAD65-antibodies show a rosette-like staining pattern in the granular layer of the cerebellum and a dot-like staining of the base of Purkinje cells (*arrows*). (**h**) Serum of a healthy individual remains negative. Magnification: (**a–h**) ×400

Fig. 12.2 Algorithmic approach for the diagnosis of antibodies targeting surface antigens. *Abbreviations*: *CBA* cell-based assay, *Gly R* Glycine receptor, *D2 R* Dopamine 2 receptor, *VGCC* P/Q type calcium channel

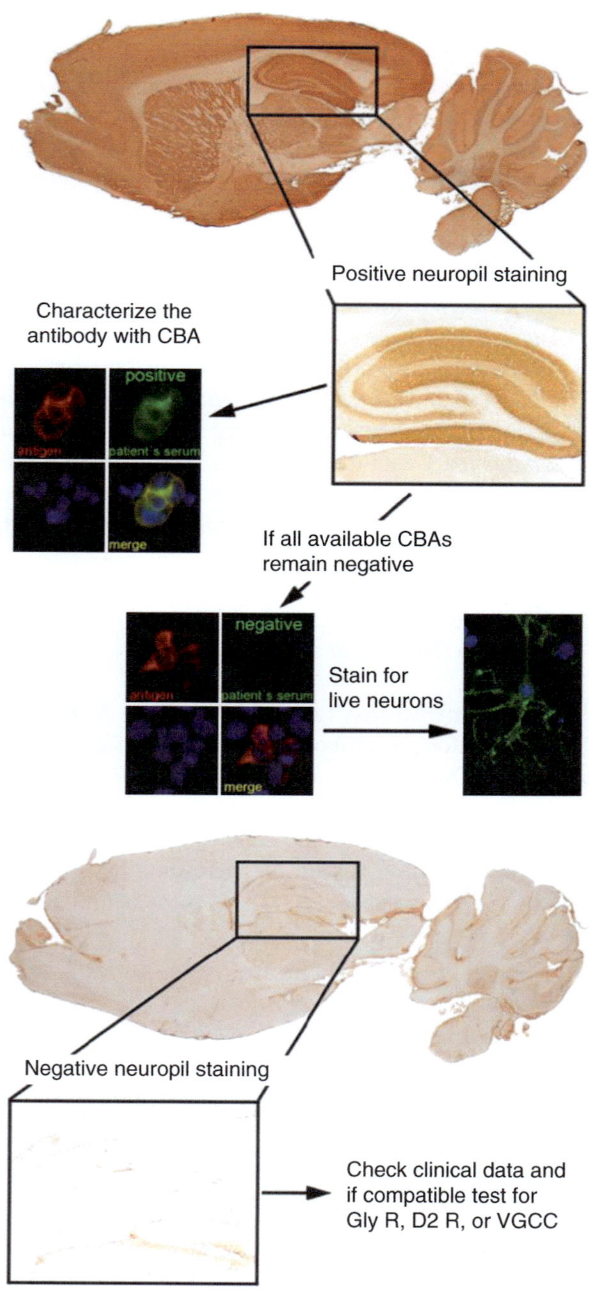

neuropil staining pattern in the hippocampus. In case of a positive result, the sample should be tested on a cell-based assay that specifically expresses the antigen of interest (e.g., NMDAR, GABA(B)R, AMPAR). If all currently available cell-based assays remain negative, the sample should be stained on live hippocampal neurons. A positive result confirms that the patient's antibody recognizes a surface receptor antigen, and the technique can be used for characterizing the novel antibody by immunoprecipitation. Glycinreceptor (GlyR) antibodies, dopamin2 receptor (D2R) antibodies, and P/Q type calcium channel (VGCC) antibodies are not detectable by immunohistochemistry and have to be tested either directly by a cell-based assay (GlyR antibodies, D2R antibodies) or by radioimmunoassay (VGCC antibodies).

12.2 Detection of Anti-glial Antibodies

As mentioned above, various anti-neuronal antibodies have been described in the past few years. In contrast, the role of antibodies to glial antigens for the pathogenesis and diagnosis of inflammatory demyelinating CNS diseases is still unclear, except for antibodies to astrocytic aquaporin-4 (AQP4) in NMO. Evidence for a role of antibodies and B-cells in demyelinating diseases comes from neuropathological investigations (Lassmann et al. 2007), the effect of B-cell directed therapies (Hauser et al. 2008; Keegan et al. 2005; Krumbholz et al. 2012) and the finding of intrathecal immunoglobulin (Ig)G antibody production, dominance of B-cells and oligoclonal IgG bands in the CSF (Cepok et al. 2001; Freedman et al. 2005; Krumbholz et al. 2012; Kuenz et al. 2008; Reindl et al. 2006). Various myelin and non-myelin antigens were suspected as targets for humoral immune reactions in demyelinating diseases (Krumbholz et al. 2012; Reindl et al. 2006). Recently, antibodies to aquaporin-4 (AQP4) have emerged as sensitive and specific biomarkers for NMO (Wingerchuk et al. 2007), and antibodies to the myelin oligodendrocyte glycoprotein (MOG) are associated with a subset of predominantly pediatric demyelinating diseases (Reindl et al. 2013).

12.2.1 Antibodies to Astrocytic Aquaporin-4 (AQP4) in NMO Spectrum Disorders

So far NMO is the only disease among the spectrum of inflammatory demyelinating diseases, which was proven to be antibody mediated. In 2004 Lennon and colleagues identified an autoantibody targeting the astrocytic water channel protein aquaporin-4 (AQP4) as a highly sensitive and specific biomarker for NMO (Lennon et al. 2004), which was included into the diagnostic criteria of NMO (Wingerchuk et al. 2006) and helped to define NMO spectrum disorders (NMOSD) (Wingerchuk et al. 2007). Moreover, recent studies have also confirmed that AQP4-IgG are not only important diagnostic biomarkers but are also relevant in the pathogenesis of NMO by direct transfer of pathology by human AQP4-IgG antibodies to rodents

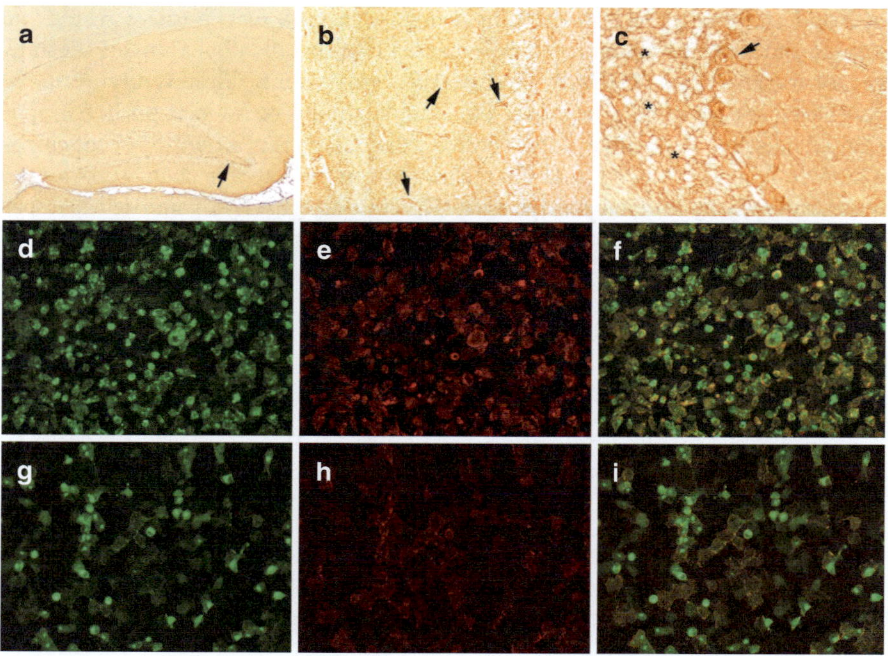

Fig. 12.3 Staining pattern of AQP4 antibodies on a tissue-based assay optimized for surface receptor antibodies. (**a**) Anti-AQP4-antibodies show a mild neuropil staining pattern in the hippocampus with a stronger laminar staining in the subgranular zone (*arrow*) and (**b**) labeling of the glia limitans perivascularis in the entire brain (*arrows*). (**c**) The cerebellum shows a marked reticular staining of the granular layer (*asterisks*) with basket-shaped processes around Purkinje cell bodies (*arrow*). (**d–f**) Cell-based assay for AQP4 antibodies. AQP4-EmGFP expressing HEK cells are shown in *green* (**d**), bound serum AQP4 IgG antibodies in *red* (**e**), and the colocalization of serum autoantibody binding and AQP4-EmGFP expression in *yellow* (**f**). (**g–i**) Cell-based assay for MOG antibodies. MOG-EmGFP expressing HEK cells are shown in *green* (**g**), bound serum MOG-IgG antibodies in *red* (**h**), and the colocalization of serum autoantibody binding and MOG-EmGFP expression in *yellow* (**i**). Magnification: **a**, ×20; **b**, ×100; **c**, ×200; **d** and 2, ×200

(Bennett et al. 2009; Bradl et al. 2009; Saadoun et al. 2010), thus fulfilling Witebsky's criteria for autoimmune diseases (Witebsky et al. 1957).

AQP4-IgG antibodies were first discovered by Vanda Lennon using an indirect immunofluorescence assay with a composite substrate of mouse tissue (Lennon et al. 2004). After this discovery, various assays with different sensitivity and specificity have been developed, including tissue-based and cell-based assays (Chan et al. 2010; De Vidi et al. 2011; Fazio et al. 2009; Granieri et al. 2012; Hoftberger et al. 2013b; Iorio et al. 2013; Isobe et al. 2012; Jarius et al. 2007, 2008, 2010b; Jiao et al. 2013; Lennon et al. 2005; Mader et al. 2010; Marignier et al. 2013; Matsuoka et al. 2007; Mckeon et al. 2009; Paul et al. 2007; Pisani et al. 2013; Takahashi et al. 2006, 2007; Waters et al. 2008, 2012). Pictures from tissue- and cell-based assays for AQP4-IgG are shown in Fig. 12.3.

Multicenter studies comparing different assays for AQP4-IgG detection showed the highest sensitivity and specificity for cell-based assays (Waters et al. 2012).

Recently, we have compared 21 different AQP4-IgG assays from 15 European laboratories in 101 NMOSD patients and 92 controls for the ERAENET ERARE project EDEN in 2013, and the results indicated that cell-based assays expressing the M23 AQP4 isoform in human cells yielded the highest sensitivity and specificity. Consensus on AQP4-IgG detection method has been established, and cell-based assays should be used for the detection of AQP4 IgG in serum samples. AQP4-IgG are found in 60–95 % of patients who are positive for the diagnostic criteria for NMO (Wingerchuk et al. 2006), and the specificity of the assays used is 90–100 %. Like with most other autoantibodies, the prevalence of AQP4-IgG is higher in female patients (Trebst et al. 2014). Although in most patients AQP4-IgG remain detectable despite immunosuppressive treatment, antibody testing should be performed on samples taken prior to treatment commencement (Jarius et al. 2008; Trebst et al. 2014). According to recent guidelines of the German Neuromyelitis Optica Study Group (NEMOS) AQP4-IgG test results should either be confirmed using a second, methodologically independent assay with high sensitivity and specificity, or testing should be repeated (Trebst et al. 2014).

The diagnostic value of AQP4-Ab in the CSF is controversial because most studies indicate that AQP4-IgG are produced peripherally without clear evidence of intrathecal synthesis (Dujmovic et al. 2011; Jarius et al. 2010a; Takahashi et al. 2007). Only two studies reported the presence of CSF AQP4-IgG in a small number of AQP4-IgG seronegative patients (Klawiter et al. 2009; Long et al. 2013).

12.2.2 Antibodies to the Myelin Oligodendrocyte Glycoprotein (MOG) in Demyelinating Diseases

Antibodies to MOG were extensively analyzed in the past 20 years and results indicated a possible role in MS pathogenesis. Cell-based assays turned out to be of major importance for detecting MOG-specific serum autoantibodies and helped to (re)define the spectrum of MOG autoantibody-associated demyelinating diseases (Reindl et al. 2013). The autoantigen MOG makes up a small part of the myelin sheath and is expressed on the surface of the myelin sheath and plasma membrane of oligodendrocytes (Brunner et al. 1989). In addition MOG is a CNS-specific protein (Brunner et al. 1989), which belongs to the highly conserved immunoglobulin superfamily (Pham-Dinh et al. 1993). The presence of MOG antibodies in CNS demyelinating disease has been controversially described over the last decade of years (Krumbholz et al. 2012; Reindl et al. 2006). This is mainly due to the fact that the detection of conformational dependent anti-MOG antibodies depends on the antigen preparation and detection system. Former studies used Western blot or ELISA assays which do not represent the correct conformation and glycosylation of MOG. A successful detection of conformational MOG-IgG antibodies depends on fluid-phase and cell-based assays. O'Connor and colleagues developed a radioimmunoassay (RIA) and were the first to detect conformational dependent anti-MOG antibodies in a cohort of patients with acute disseminated encephalomyelitis (ADEM) but only rarely in adult onset MS

(O'connor et al. 2007). This finding was confirmed by several groups using cell-based assays. Despite the reproducible detection of MOG-IgG antibodies in pediatric ADEM patients, all studies showed a variable degree of MOG-IgG detection in CNS demyelinating diseases and controls (Brilot et al. 2009; Di Pauli et al. 2011; Gredler et al. 2013; Hacohen et al. 2014; Kitley et al. 2012, 2014; Lalive et al. 2011; Mader et al. 2011; Mayer et al. 2013; Mclaughlin et al. 2009; Probstel et al. 2011; Rostasy et al. 2012, 2013; Sato et al. 2014; Selter et al. 2010; Titulaer et al. 2014; Woodhall et al. 2013). The clinical spectrum of MOG-IgG-associated CNS demyelinating diseases is broad, with a higher frequency of MOG-IgG found in pediatric patients with ADEM, CIS, MS, monophasic and recurrent optic neuritis and myelitis, NMO, and patients with NMDAR-encephalitis and demyelination. These differences could be due to variations in methodology, antigen, titer cutoff levels, and age differences of patients, emphasizing the need for a standardized method as well as cutoff values (Reindl et al. 2013). Most groups use a cell-based assay with human MOG transfected cells, and they detect bound antibodies by immunofluorescence or FACS. We have developed a cell-based immunofluorescence assay using living HEK cells transfected with MOG which is labeled with a fluorescence protein on the C terminus (Di Pauli et al. 2011). Like most other groups, we implemented a high titer cutoff value at 1:160 as the antibodies at lower titers can also be found in controls, indicating a more unspecific immune reaction at lower titer levels.

Longitudinal analysis using cell-based assays showed a decrease of serum MOG-IgG titers in monophasic ADEM patients compared to persisting MOG-IgG in ongoing diseases (Di Pauli et al. 2011; Probstel et al. 2011). Recent studies indicate that MOG-IgG are also present in 20–40 % of AQP4-IgG negative adult and pediatric NMO cases (Gredler et al. 2013; Hacohen et al. 2014; Kitley et al. 2012, 2014; Mader et al. 2011; Mayer et al. 2013; Rostasy et al. 2012, 2013; Sato et al. 2014; Woodhall et al. 2013). These MOG-IgG-positive patients often present with a severely disabling clinical phenotype at onset but have a good recovery and outcome, a higher prevalence in male patients and a younger age at onset.

There is only limited data available concerning conformational dependent anti-MOG antibodies in the CSF of patients with ADEM, CIS, or MS. So far MOG-IgG-positive NMOSD patients have not been tested for CSF MOG-IgG. We analyzed MOG antibodies in matched serum and CSF samples of 33 patients with ADEM, CIS, and MS (Di Pauli et al. 2011). Out of 12 MOG-IgG-seropositive patients, we detected MOG-IgG in the CSF of seven patients, who all had serum MOG-IgG titers of 1:640 and above (Di Pauli et al. 2011), whereas none of the MOG-IgG seronegative patients and controls turned out to be MOG-IgG positive in the CSF. Therefore, our data indicate a mainly peripheral production of MOG-IgG as the majority of CSF MOG-IgG-positive ADEM patients had significantly less OCB and lower IgG indices compared to CSF MOG-IgG-seronegative patients (Di Pauli et al. 2011). Overall the findings of MOG antibodies in the CSF of patients with high titer serum MOG antibodies are similar to the findings shown with CSF AQP4 antibodies in AQP4-IgG-seropositive NMOSD.

References

Bataller L, Wade DF, Fuller GN et al (2002) Cerebellar degeneration and autoimmunity to zinc-finger proteins of the cerebellum. Neurology 59:1985–1987

Bennett JL, Lam C, Kalluri SR et al (2009) Intrathecal pathogenic anti-aquaporin-4 antibodies in early neuromyelitis optica. Ann Neurol 66:617–629

Bradl M, Misu T, Takahashi T et al (2009) Neuromyelitis optica: pathogenicity of patient immunoglobulin in vivo. Ann Neurol 66:630–643

Brilot F, Dale RC, Selter RC et al (2009) Antibodies to native myelin oligodendrocyte glycoprotein in children with inflammatory demyelinating central nervous system disease. Ann Neurol 66:833–842

Brunner C, Lassmann H, Waehneldt TV et al (1989) Differential ultrastructural localization of myelin basic protein, myelin/oligodendroglial glycoprotein, and 2′,3′-cyclic nucleotide 3′-phosphodiesterase in the CNS of adult rats. J Neurochem 52:296–304

Cepok S, Jacobsen M, Schock S et al (2001) Patterns of cerebrospinal fluid pathology correlate with disease progression in multiple sclerosis. Brain 124:2169–2176

Chan KH, Kwan JS, Ho PW et al (2010) Aquaporin-4 autoantibodies in neuromyelitis optica spectrum disorders: comparison between tissue-based and cell-based indirect immunofluorescence assays. J Neuroinflammation 7:50

Dalmau J, Rosenfeld MR (2014) Autoimmune encephalitis update. Oncol, Neuro

De Graaff E, Maat P, Hulsenboom E et al (2012) Identification of delta/notch-like epidermal growth factor-related receptor as the Tr antigen in paraneoplastic cerebellar degeneration Ann Neurol 71:815–824

De Vidi I, Boursier G, Delouche N et al (2011) Strategy for anti-aquaporin-4 auto-antibody identification and quantification using a new cell-based assay. Clin Immunol (Orlando, Fla) 138:239–246

Di Pauli F, Mader S, Rostasy K et al (2011) Temporal dynamics of anti-MOG antibodies in CNS demyelinating diseases. Clin Immunol 138:247–254

Doss S, Numann A, Ziegler A et al (2014) Anti-Ca/anti-ARHGAP26 antibodies associated with cerebellar atrophy and cognitive decline. J Neuroimmunol 267:102–104

Dujmovic I, Mader S, Schanda K et al (2011) Temporal dynamics of cerebrospinal fluid anti-aquaporin-4 antibodies in patients with neuromyelitis optica spectrum disorders. J Neuroimmunol 234:124–130

Fazio R, Malosio ML, Lampasona V et al (2009) Antiacquaporin 4 antibodies detection by different techniques in neuromyelitis optica patients. Mult Scler (Houndmills, Basingstoke, England) 15:1153–1163

Freedman MS, Thompson EJ, Deisenhammer F et al (2005) Recommended standard of cerebrospinal fluid analysis in the diagnosis of multiple sclerosis: a consensus statement. Arch Neurol 62:865–870

Granieri L, Marnetto F, Valentino P et al (2012) Evaluation of a multiparametric immunofluorescence assay for standardization of neuromyelitis optica serology. PLoS One 7:e38896

Graus F, Keime-Guibert F, Rene R et al (2001) Anti-Hu-associated paraneoplastic encephalomyelitis: analysis of 200 patients. Brain 124:1138–1148

Graus F, Vincent A, Pozo-Rosich P et al (2005) Anti-glial nuclear antibody: marker of lung cancer-related paraneoplastic neurological syndromes. J Neuroimmunol 165:166–171

Graus F, Saiz A, Dalmau J (2010) Antibodies and neuronal autoimmune disorders of the CNS. J Neurol 257:509–517

Gredler V, Mader S, Schanda K et al (2013) Clinical and immunological follow-up of B-cell depleting therapy in CNS demyelinating diseases. J Neurol Sci 328:77–82

Hacohen Y, Absoud M, Woodhall M et al (2014) Autoantibody biomarkers in childhood-acquired demyelinating syndromes: results from a national surveillance cohort. J Neurol Neurosurg Psychiatry 85:456–461

Hauser SL, Waubant E, Arnold DL et al (2008) B-cell depletion with rituximab in relapsing-remitting multiple sclerosis. N Engl J Med 358:676–688

Hoftberger R, Kovacs GG, Sabater L et al (2013a) Protein kinase Cgamma antibodies and paraneoplastic cerebellar degeneration. J Neuroimmunol 256:91–93

Hoftberger R, Sabater L, Marignier R et al (2013b) An optimized immunohistochemistry technique improves NMO-IgG detection: study comparison with cell-based assays. PLoS One 8

Hoftberger R, Sabater L, Ortega A et al (2013c) Patient with homer-3 antibodies and cerebellitis. JAMA Neurol 70:506–509

Hoftberger R, Sabater L, Velasco F et al (2014) Carbonic Anhydrase-Related Protein VIII antibodies and paraneoplastic cerebellar degeneration. Neuropathol Appl Neurobiol 40:650–653

Honnorat J, Antoine JC, Derrington E et al (1996) Antibodies to a subpopulation of glial cells and a 66 kDa developmental protein in patients with paraneoplastic neurological syndromes. J Neurol Neurosurg Psychiatry 61:270–278

Iorio R, Fryer JP, Hinson SR et al (2013) Astrocytic autoantibody of neuromyelitis optica (NMO-IgG) binds to aquaporin-4 extracellular loops, monomers, tetramers and high order arrays. J Autoimmun 40:21–27

Isobe N, Yonekawa T, Matsushita T et al (2012) Quantitative assays for anti-aquaporin-4 antibody with subclass analysis in neuromyelitis optica. Mult Scler (Houndmills, Basingstoke, England) 18:1541–1551

Jarius S, Franciotta D, Bergamaschi R et al (2007) NMO-IgG in the diagnosis of neuromyelitis optica. Neurology 68:1076–1077

Jarius S, Aboul-Enein F, Waters P et al (2008) Antibody to aquaporin-4 in the long-term course of neuromyelitis optica. Brain 131:3072–3080

Jarius S, Franciotta D, Paul F et al (2010a) Cerebrospinal fluid antibodies to aquaporin-4 in neuromyelitis optica and related disorders: frequency, origin, and diagnostic relevance. J Neuroinflammation 7:52

Jarius S, Probst C, Borowski K et al (2010b) Standardized method for the detection of antibodies to aquaporin-4 based on a highly sensitive immunofluorescence assay employing recombinant target antigen. J Neurol Sci 291:52–56

Jiao Y, Fryer JP, Lennon VA et al (2013) Updated estimate of AQP4-IgG serostatus and disability outcome in neuromyelitis optica. Neurology 81:1197–1204

Keegan M, Konig F, Mcclelland R et al (2005) Relation between humoral pathological changes in multiple sclerosis and response to therapeutic plasma exchange. Lancet 366:579–582

Kitley J, Woodhall M, Waters P et al (2012) Myelin-oligodendrocyte glycoprotein antibodies in adults with a neuromyelitis optica phenotype. Neurology 79:1273–1277

Kitley J, Waters P, Woodhall M et al (2014) Neuromyelitis optica spectrum disorders with aquaporin-4 and myelin-oligodendrocyte glycoprotein antibodies: a comparative study. JAMA Neurol 71:276–283

Klawiter EC, Alvarez E 3rd, Xu J et al (2009) NMO-IgG detected in CSF in seronegative neuromyelitis optica. Neurology 72:1101–1103

Krumbholz M, Derfuss T, Hohlfeld R et al (2012) B cells and antibodies in multiple sclerosis pathogenesis and therapy. Nat Rev Neurol 8:613–623

Kuenz B, Lutterotti A, Ehling R et al (2008) Cerebrospinal fluid B cells correlate with early brain inflammation in multiple sclerosis. PLoS One 3:e2559

Lalive PH, Hausler MG, Maurey H et al (2011) Highly reactive anti-myelin oligodendrocyte glycoprotein antibodies differentiate demyelinating diseases from viral encephalitis in children. Mult Scler 17:297–302

Lancaster E, Dalmau J (2012) Neuronal autoantigens–pathogenesis, associated disorders and antibody testing. Nat Rev Neurol 8:380–390

Lassmann H, Bruck W, Lucchinetti CF (2007) The immunopathology of multiple sclerosis: an overview. Brain Pathol 17:210–218

Lennon VA, Wingerchuk DM, Kryzer TJ et al (2004) A serum autoantibody marker of neuromyelitis optica: distinction from multiple sclerosis. Lancet 364:2106–2112

Lennon VA, Kryzer TJ, Pittock SJ et al (2005) IgG marker of optic-spinal multiple sclerosis binds to the aquaporin-4 water channel. J Exp Med 202:473–477

Long Y, Qiu W, Lu Z et al (2013) Clinical features of Chinese patients with multiple sclerosis with aquaporin-4 antibodies in cerebrospinal fluid but not serum. J Clin Neurosci 20:233–237

Mader S, Lutterotti A, Di Pauli F et al (2010) Patterns of antibody binding to aquaporin-4 isoforms in neuromyelitis optica. PLoS One 5:e10455

Mader S, Gredler V, Schanda K et al (2011) Complement activating antibodies to myelin oligodendrocyte glycoprotein in neuromyelitis optica and related disorders. J Neuroinflammation 8:184

Marignier R, Bernard-Valnet R, Giraudon P et al (2013) Aquaporin-4 antibody-negative neuromyelitis optica: distinct assay sensitivity-dependent entity. Neurology 80:2194–2200

Matsuoka T, Matsushita T, Kawano Y et al (2007) Heterogeneity of aquaporin-4 autoimmunity and spinal cord lesions in multiple sclerosis in Japanese. Brain 130:1206–1223

Mayer MC, Breithaupt C, Reindl M et al (2013) Distinction and temporal stability of conformational epitopes on myelin oligodendrocyte glycoprotein recognized by patients with different inflammatory central nervous system diseases. J Immunol 191:3594–3604

Mckeon A, Fryer JP, Apiwattanakul M et al (2009) Diagnosis of neuromyelitis spectrum disorders: comparative sensitivities and specificities of immunohistochemical and immunoprecipitation assays. Arch Neurol 66:1134–1138

Mclaughlin KA, Chitnis T, Newcombe J et al (2009) Age-dependent B cell autoimmunity to a myelin surface antigen in pediatric multiple sclerosis. J Immunol 183:4067–4076

O'connor KC, Mclaughlin KA, De Jager PL et al (2007) Self-antigen tetramers discriminate between myelin autoantibodies to native or denatured protein. Nat Med 13:211–217

Paul F, Jarius S, Aktas O et al (2007) Antibody to aquaporin 4 in the diagnosis of neuromyelitis optica. PLoS Med 4:e133

Pham-Dinh D, Mattei MG, Nussbaum JL et al (1993) Myelin/oligodendrocyte glycoprotein is a member of a subset of the immunoglobulin superfamily encoded within the major histocompatibility complex. Proc Natl Acad Sci U S A 90:7990–7994

Pisani F, Sparaneo A, Tortorella C et al (2013) Aquaporin-4 autoantibodies in Neuromyelitis Optica: AQP4 isoform-dependent sensitivity and specificity. PLoS One 8:e79185

Pittock SJ, Lucchinetti CF, Lennon VA (2003) Anti-neuronal nuclear autoantibody type 2: paraneoplastic accompaniments. Ann Neurol 53:580–587

Pittock SJ, Lucchinetti CF, Parisi JE et al (2005) Amphiphysin autoimmunity: paraneoplastic accompaniments. Ann Neurol 58:96–107

Probstel AK, Dornmair K, Bittner R et al (2011) Antibodies to MOG are transient in childhood acute disseminated encephalomyelitis. Neurology 77:580–588

Reindl M, Khalil M, Berger T (2006) Antibodies as biological markers for pathophysiological processes in MS. J Neuroimmunol 180:50–62

Reindl M, Di Pauli F, Rostasy K et al (2013) The spectrum of MOG autoantibody-associated demyelinating diseases. Nat Rev Neurol 9:455–461

Rosenfeld MR, Eichen JG, Wade DF et al (2001) Molecular and clinical diversity in paraneoplastic immunity to Ma proteins. Ann Neurol 50:339–348

Rostasy K, Mader S, Schanda K et al (2012) Anti-myelin oligodendrocyte glycoprotein antibodies in pediatric patients with optic neuritis. Arch Neurol 69:752–756

Rostasy K, Mader S, Hennes E et al (2013) Persisting myelin oligodendrocyte glycoprotein antibodies in aquaporin-4 antibody negative pediatric neuromyelitis optica. Mult Scler 19: 1052–1059

Saadoun S, Waters P, Bell BA et al (2010) Intra-cerebral injection of neuromyelitis optica immunoglobulin G and human complement produces neuromyelitis optica lesions in mice. Brain 133:349–361

Sato DK, Callegaro D, Lana-Peixoto MA et al (2014) Distinction between MOG antibody-positive and AQP4 antibody-positive NMO spectrum disorders. Neurology 82:474–481

Selter RC, Brilot F, Grummel V et al (2010) Antibody responses to EBV and native MOG in pediatric inflammatory demyelinating CNS diseases. Neurology 74:1711–1715

Solimena M, Folli F, Aparisi R et al (1990) Autoantibodies to GABA-ergic neurons and pancreatic beta cells in stiff-man syndrome. N Engl J Med 322:1555–1560

Takahashi T, Fujihara K, Nakashima I et al (2006) Establishment of a new sensitive assay for anti-human aquaporin-4 antibody in neuromyelitis optica. Tohoku J Exp Med 210:307–313

Takahashi T, Fujihara K, Nakashima I et al (2007) Anti-aquaporin-4 antibody is involved in the pathogenesis of NMO: a study on antibody titre. Brain 130:1224–1234

Titulaer MJ, Hoftberger R, Iizuka T et al (2014) Overlapping demyelinating syndromes and anti-NMDA receptor encephalitis. Neurol, Ann

Trebst C, Jarius S, Berthele A et al (2014) Update on the diagnosis and treatment of neuromyelitis optica: recommendations of the Neuromyelitis Optica Study Group (NEMOS). J Neurol 261:1–16

Tuzun E, Rossi JE, Karner SF et al (2007) Adenylate kinase 5 autoimmunity in treatment refractory limbic encephalitis. J Neuroimmunol 186:177–180

Vincent A, Bien CG, Irani SR et al (2011) Autoantibodies associated with diseases of the CNS: new developments and future challenges. Lancet Neurol 10:759–772

Waters P, Jarius S, Littleton E et al (2008) Aquaporin-4 antibodies in neuromyelitis optica and longitudinally extensive transverse myelitis. Arch Neurol 65:913–919

Waters PJ, Mckeon A, Leite MI et al (2012) Serologic diagnosis of NMO: a multicenter comparison of aquaporin-4-IgG assays. Neurology 78:665–671

Wildemann B, Jarius S (2013) The expanding range of autoimmune disorders of the nervous system. Lancet Neurol 12:22–24

Wingerchuk DM, Lennon VA, Pittock SJ et al (2006) Revised diagnostic criteria for neuromyelitis optica. Neurology 66:1485–1489

Wingerchuk DM, Lennon VA, Lucchinetti CF et al (2007) The spectrum of neuromyelitis optica. Lancet Neurol 6:805–815

Witebsky E, Rose NR, Terplan K et al (1957) Chronic thyroiditis and autoimmunization. J Am Med Assoc 164:1439–1447

Woodhall M, Coban A, Waters P et al (2013) Glycine receptor and myelin oligodendrocyte glycoprotein antibodies in Turkish patients with neuromyelitis optica. J Neurol Sci 335:221–223

Methods for Biomarker Analysis

Diego Franciotta, Massimo Alessio, Livia Garzetti, and Roberto Furlan

Contents

Abstract

Neuroinflammatory disorders such as multiple sclerosis (MS) encountered a therapeutic revolution in the last 20 years and have raised hope also for neurodegenerative diseases affecting especially the elderly population in western countries. Biomarkers, especially those from the field of neuroimaging, were decisive in accelerating drug development and optimization of treatments. Neuroimaging,

D. Franciotta
Laboratory of Neuroimmunology,
IRCCS, National Institute of Neurology "C. Mondino",
Pavia, Italy

M. Alessio
Proteome Biochemistry,
San Raffaele Scientific Institute,
Milan, Italy

L. Garzetti • R. Furlan (✉)
Division of Neuroscience,
Institute of Experimental Neurology, San Raffaele Scientific Institute,
Milan, Italy
e-mail: furlan.roberto@hsr.it

© Springer International Publishing Switzerland 2015
F. Deisenhammer et al. (eds.), *Cerebrospinal Fluid in Clinical Neurology*,
DOI 10.1007/978-3-319-01225-4_13

however, may be not sufficient in the case of neurodegeneration, where structural alterations accumulate at a very low rate over several years. To capture this slow evolution, biomarkers in the cerebrospinal fluid appear as a very plausible candidate. We will review here, in general terms, the state of the art in the field biomarkers in the CSF with a special focus on the application of "omics" platforms.

13.1 Introduction

The availability of reliable biomarkers is a cornerstone of the up-to-date medicine. However, it may happen that new biomarkers prove weak, whereas old, consistent ones are downgrading. For instance, the analysis of the cerebrospinal fluid (CSF) has considerably lost relevance in the revised diagnostic criteria for multiple sclerosis (Polman et al. 2011). For decennia, oligoclonal IgG bands in the CSF have been one major supporting diagnostic criterion for multiple sclerosis (Freedman et al. 2005), and their down qualification has raised a certain debate (Siritho and Freedman 2009; Galea et al. 2011). This appears paradoxical if one considers that huge investments have been made by the academy but especially by the industry to find new biomarkers in the CSF in the last few years (over 3,000 papers published in the last 5 years). This great effort has yielded an enormous list of candidate bio-markers for neurological disorders, of which only few have reached the bedside. The difficulty to translate this enormous amount of data into useful tools for the clinical neurologist is due to several problems. The first is the relatively poor meth-odological quality of most studies. The general impression is that in several cases, the isolated finding of the involvement of a certain pathway during disease, lacking mechanistic insight, is reported by authors as a potential biomarker, to pretend a more focused aim to a study with limited ambition. Secondly, pre-analytical errors, which account for the most part of the analytical errors (Plebani et al. 2014) and affect many different aspects (comparable sample selection in multicentric studies, time to processing, sample storage, etc.), are rarely considered. The third most common error is that many studies are designed to answer a clinically irrelevant question (such as distinguishing established AD from healthy donors), rarely addressing the real diagnostic dilemma (e.g., comparing the many different condi-tions leading to mild cognitive decline). This approach is preliminary and useful for the selection of candidate biomarkers, requiring validation studies on appropri-ate case series.

On the other hand, the development of technologies able to perform unbiased analysis of nucleic acids, proteins, lipids, and metabolites has provided powerful tools to identify potential biomarkers in the CSF, and these technologies have been applied and are currently applied to this kind of investigations. As for other biologi-cal fluids, the enormous amount of data generated by these technologies represents a challenge that needs complex statistical and bioinformatics analyses. The general concept, in fact, is that for most multifactorial diseases, to find a pattern or signa-ture, possibly of different molecular nature, will be more likely than the golden bullet, the perfect biomarker. Thus, new approaches such as neural networks and machine learning are increasingly used for data mining.

This field of investigation on the CSF topic has already changed the way we approach cognitive decline and the differential diagnosis of Alzheimer's disease (AD). In this disease, lumbar puncture was rarely performed (and mostly by mistake), while today, CSF biomarkers, such as low beta-amyloid 1–42, elevated protein tau, and phosphorylated protein tau, are routinely used also in prodromal AD (Ritchie et al. 2014) to help diagnosis or to confirm diagnosis in later stages. Despite the final validation of these CSF biomarkers, especially in combination with other markers such as neuroimaging pictures and psychological tests (Filippi et al. 2013), is still missing (Ferreira et al. 2014), they are cost-effective in identifying AD among MCI patients (Nazco et al. 2014). CSF biomarkers in AD are also aimed at capturing phenomena that associate with underlying pathogenetic mechanisms, such as neuroinflammation (Alcolea et al. 2014) and structural damage (Fortea et al. 2014), and, possibly, at monitoring disease progression in clinical trials (Dumurgier et al. 2014). CSF biomarkers have been linked to cognitive performance also during aging (Li et al. 2014), thus becoming, in perspective, a monitoring that will be proposed to the general elderly population to predict cognitive decline. We can only expect that extensive evaluation of currently used biomarkers in MCI/AD patients over the next years, with accumulation of further experience, and possibly the identification of new biomarkers will most likely yield more accurate diagnostic and prognostic information in the future (Lista et al. 2014).

While CSF beta-amyloid 1–42, protein tau, and phosphorylated protein tau are routinely tested in most neurology departments for the differential diagnosis between AD and other forms of dementia, the field is moving forward also in other neurodegenerative disorders. In Parkinson's disease (PD), for example, the evaluation of AD biomarkers appears to be useful to predict the occurrence of associated dementia (Alves et al. 2014; Siderowf and Logroscino 2014), rather than to discriminate PD with cognitive onset from AD (Vranová et al. 2014). In PD, investigations on several CSF biomarkers, including synuclein, are ongoing but are far from being conclusive or clinically validated (Parnetti et al. 2014; Malek et al. 2014).

In several other neurological disorders such as infections (Fraisier et al. 2014; Cassol et al. 2014), spinal cord injury (Pouw et al. 2014), amyotrophic lateral sclerosis (Tortelli et al. 2014), and stroke (Hjalmarsson et al. 2014), investigations are actually in progress, revealing the enormous interest in finding new ways to stratify neurological disorders, especially in view of forthcoming clinical trials. A very interesting field, characterized by a reappreciation of possible organic causes, is psychiatry. As a result of such reappreciation, CSF biomarkers are, of course, matter of intense investigation. While a neuroimmunological pathophysiology is evident in the multifaceted psychiatric manifestations of limbic encephalitis, characterized by the presence in the CSF of specific antibodies, such as anti-NMDA-R, anti-VGKC, anti-glycine, etc., in mood disorders, organic causes are less evident. Depression, bipolar disorder, and other major psychoses have been linked to altered innate immunity (Bergink et al. 2014). Major depression seems currently the most promising disease to be characterized by CSF abnormalities: protein profiles (Woods et al.

2014), choroidal gene expression (Turner et al. 2014), neurofilaments (Jakobsson et al. 2014), and cytokines (Kern et al. 2014) are all examples of potential CSF biomarkers that have been investigated and proposed as biomarkers.

The development of more potent technological platforms, the identifications in relatively recent years of new entities in molecular and cellular biology, such as miRNA and microvesicles, both promising categories of biomarkers, increase the expectation that in the near future, clinicians will have refined tools to diagnose neurological and psychiatric disorders, foresee disease evolution, plan therapy, and monitor outcomes. But, as stated above, the field is invaded by relatively low-quality literature, and the issue that only a very limited number of apparently promising biomarkers undergo proper clinical validation still remains. Is this shortcoming unavoidable? Not necessarily. Over a decennium ago, this same concern resulted in the development, during a consensus meeting, of a checklist and a generic flow diagram for studies of diagnostic accuracy called the STARD initiative (Bossuyt et al. 2003). Over the years, this checklist has been published in numerous medicine journals and has been implemented by many editors. Nevertheless, a minority of biomarker studies, even among those cited in the present chapter, do adhere to these guidelines. Implementation of these guidelines is mandatory, in our opinion, to strengthen studies and focus investments on solid results. Further, clinical validation of biomarkers needs large cohorts that are difficult to put together in single centers, not mentioning that the challenge of the slight differences in terms of clinical classification, processing, and storage of samples constitutes a necessary test for biomarkers that aim at being employed in daily clinical practice. To this respect, it is noteworthy to mention the publication of a consensus protocol for the collection and storage of CSF aimed at minimizing preclinical errors, standardize procedures, and allowing, therefore, biomarker validation studies on large number of relatively homogeneous samples (Tumani et al. 2009; Teunissen et al. 2009). In the following paragraphs, we will discuss the main findings and the major technical difficulties in the CSF biomarkers research that exploits various approaches such as proteomic analysis, gene expression studies, and characterization of miRNA.

13.2 Proteomics Analysis of CSF

Different methodological approaches can be used for the analysis of the CSF's protein content. The most frequently used techniques are addressed to perform the total differential protein expression analysis comparing two or more experimental conditions or group of samples. Quantitative proteomics measures the relative or absolute protein abundance or specific post-translation modifications (van Gool and Hendrickson 2012; Craft et al. 2013) and is nowadays principally based on mass spectrometry approaches, even though classical gel-based analyses (namely, 2-dimensional electrophoresis and 2-dimensional differential fluorescence gel electrophoresis) are still largely used. Gel-based methodologies are limited in the number and in the specific type of protein that can be resolved, while the tandem mass spectrometry approaches coupled with liquid chromatography (LC-MS/MS) are able to resolve without limitation thousands of proteins (Yuan and Desiderio 2005a; Huang et al. 2007b). The relative quantitation of protein expression is typically reported as a fold change and can be obtained by label-based or label-free methods, while absolute quantitation can be determined by addition in the samples of internal stable-isotopic standards (see Craft et al. (2013) for a detailed methodological review).

Using these approaches, CSF studies have been conducted in several neurological diseases including neurodegenerative diseases, in particular in Alzheimer (see Liu et al. (2014) for review) (Lista et al. 2014), in psychosis (Huang et al. 2007a), multiple sclerosis (Stoop et al. 2010b; Lourenco et al. 2011), amyotrophic lateral sclerosis (Conti et al. 2008), brain injury (Conti et al. 2004), peripheral neuropathies (Conti et al. 2005), etc. (see Craft et al. (2013) for a review). However, the biological implications and the relevance of the proposed biomarker of many of the published studies remain to be clearly established.

In addition to the analysis of differential protein expression level, some interesting results have been obtained, investigating specific post-translation modifications promoted by the pathological conditions that can be used as putative source of biomarker discovery. In fact, in several neurological diseases characterized by the presence of neuroinflammation or oxidative stress conditions, like in the case of some neurodegenerative disease, oxidative modifications of the CSF protein have been investigated as acidification of the protein isoelectric point (Olivieri et al. 2011) or as increase in protein carbonylation (Olivieri et al. 2011; Iannaccone et al. 2013), protein nitration (Castegna et al. 2003), protein thiol group modifications (S-cysteinylation, S-glutathionylation, S-nitrosylation) (Nakamura et al. 2013; Poulsen et al. 2014), and protein deamidation (Barbariga et al. 2014) the latest reflecting accelerated protein aging under pathological conditions. Furthermore, the protein phosphorylation, the most common post-translational modification for the reversible regulation of protein function, has also been investigated (Yuan and Desiderio 2003).

An alternative proteomics approach for CSF investigation might be the serological proteome analysis (SERPA) (De Monte et al. 2008; Privitera et al. 2013) that exploits the presence of autoantibodies in some neurological disease like multiple sclerosis (Menon et al. 2011). In the SERPA approach, the autoantibodies present in the CSF of the patients are used to screen the proteome of the patient resolved by 2-dimensional electrophoresis in order to identify putative autoantigen/s. The presence and the titer of specific autoantibodies might be considered itself a putative biomarker.

Regardless of the type of the methodological approaches used, the biological and chemical features of the CSF made necessary the introduction in the experimental pipeline of sample preprocessing steps to improve the quality of the results. For example, for the gel-based approaches, the high salt concentration (>150 mM) and the relative low protein concentration (0.2–0.7 mg/ml) require the introduction of desalting and protein concentration steps that can be performed by ultrafiltration, dialysis, and protein precipitation (Yuan and Desiderio 2005a). Another technical problem for CSF proteins is the wide dynamic range (several orders of magnitude) of some specific protein concentration that causes difficulties in the detection of low-abundant proteins. Therefore, very abundant proteins like albumin, immunoglobulin, transthyretin, etc. can be eliminated by affinity chromatography removal or by CSF sample pre-fractionation (Yuan and Desiderio 2005a). Protein pre-fractionation can be achieved by standard biochemical methods that exploit different biochemical features of the protein like hydrophobicity, size, charge, etc. (Zhang et al. 2005; Yuan and Desiderio 2005a). The most popular techniques used for CSF protein fractionation are the reversed-phase solid-phase extraction (Yuan and Desiderio 2005b) and liquid- or semi-solid-phase isoelectric focusing that allow protein separation on a solid pH gradient and a protein recovery in liquid phase. These kinds of approaches allow the separation and concentration of low-abundant proteins, but generate for each CSF sample a large number of fractions that must be analyzed.

Some other warning rises for specific post-translation modification analysis like in the case of oxidative modifications; in fact, the risk of artifactual modification does exist due to the ex vivo protein oxidation fostered by the experimental conditions or by sample storage conditions (Olivieri et al. 2011; Poulsen et al. 2014). In our experience, we avoid experimental oxidation by storing the sample and performing the experiments under nitrogen-conditioned atmosphere (Olivieri et al. 2011; Barbariga et al. 2014). In the case of protein deamidation, for example, it is mandatory to set up a different protocol for tryptic digestion necessary for mass spectrometry analysis because the standard conditions used (ammonium bicarbonate buffer at pH 8.5, at 37 °C) are the ideal conditions to promote very strong in vitro deamidation (Barbariga et al. 2014). Thus, for every kind of analysis, methods for simple, robust, and reproducible inhibition of artificial modifications should be developed.

Other general critical points that must be taken into consideration are the risk of CSF contamination by blood proteins that may occur during sample collection, the interindividual variation of the specific protein concentration (Stoop et al. 2010a; Perrin et al. 2013), and the age-related changes in protein relative abundance (Zhang et al. 2005) that might dramatically affect the outcome of the analyses.

In conclusion, the proteomics approaches may offer very interesting input for CSF biomarker discovery; however, in order to transform this vast experimental effort in meaningful information, there is still a need for standardization of methods and experimental design.

13.3 mRNA in the CSF

Gene expression studies are possible in the CSF only if examined mRNA is cell associated or if it is protected from degradation, i.e., it is packaged in extracellular membrane vesicles (EMVs). In the last years, EMVs and their content have gained attention as potential biomarkers also in clinical neurosciences (Borgiani et al. 2012; Rao et al. 2013). There are two main populations of EMVs, exosomes (50–80 nm in diameter, of intracellular origin) and shed vesicles or ectosomes

(200–2,000 nm in diameter, budding from plasma membrane). For biomarker studies, this difference is not only relevant for biological reasons, but because, despite a certain loss, exosomes survive freeze and thawing, shed vesicles/ectosomes don't. In practical terms, archival CSF samples, stored frozen, are inadequate for shed vesicles/ectosomes analysis. Further, processing and storage of CSF determine what kind of molecules, formerly packaged into EMVs, are detectable in cell-free CSF. Nevertheless, the content, especially RNA species of EMVs, is considered a very promising biomarker (Ratajczak et al. 2006; Valadi et al. 2007; Deregibus et al. 2007; Skog et al. 2008; Hong et al. 2009; Choi et al. 2013a, b). To date, around 50 high-throughput extracellular vesicles (EVs) transcriptomic studies based on micro-array and next-generation sequencing have been published (Choi et al. 2013a). However, these studies are controversial. It has been described in several different systems that mRNAs and miRNAs are packaged into EVs. Several studies have reported that specific mRNA is enriched into EVs by means of sorting a specific mRNA present in the cell cytoplasm (Valadi et al. 2007; Deregibus et al. 2007; Palanisamy et al. 2010). Also, Hong and Skog have demonstrated that the mRNA content of EVs reflects the cellular mRNA of the cell of origin. In contrast, they demonstrated that EVs and their original cells have a similar number of mRNA, and some vesicular RNAs were relatively enriched (Skog et al. 2008; Hong et al. 2009; Choi et al. 2013a).

Discordant results emerging among these transcriptomic studies have been affected by non-vesicular RNAs, degraded RNAs, or bovine serum-derived EVs contamination. To avoid this contamination, EVs purification requires critical steps such as RNase digestion and differential centrifugation EVs isolation using swinging bucket rotor (Choi et al. 2013a; Cvjetkovic et al. 2014). Thus, EVs isolation protocols affect the yield and purity of EVs RNA.

We have previously described that microvesicles (MVs) of myeloid origin in the cerebrospinal fluid (CSF) are a marker of microglia/macrophage activation (Verderio et al. 2012). Starting with the hypothesis that MVs content reflects processes ongoing in pathologically relevant cell types and may be a useful biomarker in several pathological processes, we performed in vitro and in vivo mRNA studies in MVs from classically M1- and alternatively M2-activated macrophages. Because the number of myeloid MVs in the CSF does not allow collecting enough material for transcriptome analysis, we performed mRNA studies in murine macrophages.

In accordance to previous reports (Valadi et al. 2007; Skog et al. 2008; Pegtel et al. 2011; Chen et al. 2012), our microarray data indicate that MVs content is not the mere sampling of mRNAs present in the cell cytoplasm: a specific set of transcripts are enriched in MVs as compared to parental cells. Furthermore, there is certain number of transcripts that are packaged into MVs regardless of activation state and type. Both M1 and M2 activation, however, induce the expression and sorting into MVs of specific transcripts. We validated by real-time RT-PCR typical M1 and M2 markers, identified as enriched in MVs by the microarray analysis. To perform RT-PCR assays, we had to overcome the lack of a validated housekeeping gene for MVs. Using bioinformatic tools and assessing stability and expression levels, we identified PSAP, a known marker of extracellular membrane vesicles

(Shan 2011), as a reliable housekeeping gene for myeloid MVs (Garzetti et al. 2013). All these studies have demonstrated that mRNAs associated to MVs reflect the functional phenotype of parental cells. Thus, for neurological disorders characterized by microglial activation, the idea will be to exploit these data to identify biomarkers able to measure microglia activation and activation type.

13.4   miRNAs in the CSF

Among noncoding RNAs, miRNAs are short RNA molecules that, through regulation of translation of messenger RNAs into proteins, control all cellular processes, including cell cycle, differentiation, functional phenotype, etc. (Cech and Steitz 2014). The discovery that miRNAs can be detected in biological fluids has made the obvious candidates as biomarkers. In biological fluids, miRNAs are more stable than expected, because they are complexed with proteins or encapsulated in extracellular membrane vesicles (EMVs). Their detection, upon purification of total RNA or using techniques specific for short RNA species, is performed using RT-PCR, deep sequencing, or microarrays. Advantages and pitfalls of these approaches are not the topic of this chapter. The experience accumulated in the field of oncology, which has pioneered the use of miRNAs as biomarkers, can be useful to evaluate promises and pitfalls of this research topic (Jarry et al. 2014).

Most of the studies in the CSF deal with the search for miRNAs able to identify AD patients. The design of all reports is of little clinical relevance, comparing already diagnosed, frankly demented AD patients either with healthy donors or with nondemented patients affected by other neurological disorders. Mild cognitive decline and different types of dementia, whose differential diagnosis represents the real challenge for the clinical neurologist, are never investigated, as also a possible prognostic value. Reproducibility of results is also disappointing. Out of 60 miRNAs identified in one small study (10 demented AD patients vs. 10 nondemented controls) (Cogswell et al. 2008), none was shared by the others, although some miRNAs were found significantly altered at least in two studies. The only miRNA found altered in three reports, hsa-miR-146a, was detected as decreased in two studies (Kiko et al. 2013; Müller et al. 2014) and elevated in another (Alexandrov et al. 2012). The only study trying to validate a single miRNA in two independent cohorts identified a decreased miRNA that has not been identified in the other investigations (Frigerio et al. 2013). Patient selection and stratification, preclinical errors, technical issues, all may have contributed to contradictory results. Despite short RNAs are the most abundant RNA species in the CSF (Pogue et al. 2014), still their purification and analysis using different techniques may lead to incoherent results. Most of the studies use commercial kits designed for small RNA species for extraction and RT-PCR, either candidate miRNAs or cards encompassing assays for most known miRNAs. Quantification using microarrays for miRNA is certainly less reliable and may explain some contradiction in reports. The most robust approach, deep sequencing, is rarely used also because of relatively high costs as compared to RT-PCR and microarrays, although costs should be calculated also taking in account reliability of results.

The situation, both for patient selection and for technical hurdles, is slightly better in the only other CNS pathology where more than one report is available, namely, brain tumors. Three reports agree that hsa-miR21 is elevated in the CSF of patients with glioblastoma in comparison with brain metastasis (Baraniskin et al. 2011b; Teplyuk et al. 2012; Akers et al. 2013); however, the same miRNA is elevated also in the main CNS brain tumor that goes in differential diagnosis with glioblastoma, primitive B-cell lymphoma (Baraniskin et al. 2011a).

Pioneering, preliminary studies are available in other neurological disorders. In multiple sclerosis (MS), Hagikia and colleagues preliminarily identified miRNAs able to differentiate MS patients from those affected by other neurological disorders and MS patients with different disease courses (Haghikia et al. 2012). After the identification of miRNA binding TDP-43, a gene involved in familial amyotrophic lateral sclerosis (ALS), Freischmidt and coworkers measured five of them as being dysregulated also in the CSF of sporadic ALS (Freischmidt et al. 2013). A pilot study has identified that a certain number of miRNAs have been found in the CSF associated to HIV infection and to HIV encephalitis (Pacifici et al. 2013). Finally, miRNAs specific to psychoses have been identified in the CSF of a very small cohort of psychiatric patients in comparison with healthy donors using microarrays (Gallego et al. 2012).

Conclusions

CSF is a difficult specimen to obtain; very few longitudinal studies are allowed; it can be easily contaminated by blood; it has peculiar matrix effects altering the detection of molecules. Nevertheless, it holds an enormous potential as source of biomarkers for neurological disorders. The application of the powerful technologies of the current "omics" era, now also encompassing lipids, metabolites, etc., calls for the prompt identification of such biomarkers. The field needs however a strengthening of research criteria, at all levels: clinical inclusion and stratification criteria, proper control groups, adequate sample size, standardization of processing, storage, measurements, and statistical or bioinformatics analysis. Existing guidelines are adequate, but need to be implemented by editors and reviewers, granting agencies to favor that the current huge effort on biomarker research in the CSF results in clinically useful tools supporting the development of new treatments for neurological diseases.

References

Akers JC, Ramakrishnan V, Kim R et al (2013) miR-21 in the extracellular vesicles (EVs) of cerebrospinal fluid (CSF): a platform for glioblastoma biomarker development. PLoS One 8:e78115. doi:10.1371/journal.pone.0078115.s009

Alcolea D, Carmona-Iragui M, Suárez-Calvet M et al (2014) Relationship between β-secretase. Inflammation and core cerebrospinal fluid biomarkers for Alzheimer's disease. J Alzheimers Dis. doi:10.3233/JAD-140240

Alexandrov PN, Dua P, Hill JM et al (2012) microRNA (miRNA) speciation in Alzheimer's disease (AD) cerebrospinal fluid (CSF) and extracellular fluid (ECF). Int J Biochem Mol Biol 3:365–373

Alves G, Lange J, Blennow K et al (2014) CSF Aβ42 predicts early-onset dementia in Parkinson disease. Neurology 82:1784–1790. doi:10.1212/WNL.0000000000000425

Baraniskin A, Kuhnhenn J, Schlegel U et al (2011a) Identification of microRNAs in the cerebrospinal fluid as marker for primary diffuse large B-cell lymphoma of the central nervous system. Blood 117:3140–3146. doi:10.1182/blood-2010-09-308684

Baraniskin A, Kuhnhenn J, Schlegel U et al (2011b) Identification of microRNAs in the cerebrospinal fluid as biomarker for the diagnosis of glioma. Neuro Oncol 14:29–33. doi:10.1093/neuonc/nor169

Barbariga M, Curnis F, Spitaleri A et al (2014) Oxidation-induced structural changes of ceruloplasmin foster NGR motif deamidation that promotes integrin binding and signaling. J Biol Chem 289:3736–3748. doi:10.1074/jbc.M113.520981

Bergink V, Gibney SM, Drexhage HA (2014) Autoimmunity, inflammation, and psychosis: a search for peripheral markers. Biol Psychiatry 75:324–331. doi:10.1016/j.biopsych.2013.09.037

Borgiani B, Colombo E, Furlan R (2012) Microvesicles: novel biomarkers for neurological disorders. Front Physiol 3:1–6. doi: 10.3389/fphys.2012.00063/abstract

Bossuyt PM, Reitsma JB, Bruns DE et al (2003) The STARD statement for reporting studies of diagnostic accuracy: explanation and elaboration. Clin Chem 49:7–18

Cassol E, Misra V, Dutta A et al (2014) Cerebrospinal fluid metabolomics reveals altered waste clearance and accelerated aging in HIV patients with neurocognitive impairment. AIDS. doi:10.1097/QAD.0000000000000303

Castegna A, Thongboonkerd V, Klein JB et al (2003) Proteomic identification of nitrated proteins in Alzheimer's disease brain. J Neurochem 85:1394–1401

Cech TR, Steitz JA (2014) The noncoding RNA revolution— trashing old rules to forge new ones. Cell 157:77–94. doi:10.1016/j.cell.2014.03.008

Chen X, Liang H, Zhang J et al (2012) Secreted microRNAs: a new form of intercellular communication. Trends Cell Biol 22:125–132. doi:10.1016/j.tcb.2011.12.001

Choi D-S, Kim D-K, Kim Y-K, Gho YS (2013a) Proteomics, transcriptomics and lipidomics of exosomes and ectosomes. Proteomics 13:1554–1571. doi:10.1002/pmic.201200329

Choi D-S, Lee J, Go G et al (2013b) Circulating extracellular vesicles in cancer diagnosis and monitoring: an appraisal of clinical potential. Mol Diagn Ther 17:265–271. doi:10.1007/s40291-013-0042-7

Cogswell JP, Ward J, Taylor IA et al (2008) Identification of miRNA changes in Alzheimer's disease brain and CSF yields putative biomarkers and insights into disease pathways. J Alzheimers Dis 14:27–41

Conti A, Sanchez-Ruiz Y, Bachi A et al (2004) Proteome study of human cerebrospinal fluid following traumatic brain injury indicates fibrin(ogen) degradation products as trauma-associated markers. J Neurotrauma 21:854–863. doi:10.1089/0897715041526212

Conti A, Ricchiuto P, Iannaccone S et al (2005) Pigment epithelium-derived factor is differentially expressed in peripheral neuropathies. Proteomics 5:4558–4567. doi:10.1002/pmic.200402088

Conti A, Iannaccone S, Sferrazza B et al (2008) Differential expression of ceruloplasmin isoforms in the cerebrospinal fluid of amyotrophic lateral sclerosis patients. Proteomics Clin Appl 2:1628–1637. doi:10.1002/prca.200780081

Craft GE, Chen A, Nairn AC (2013) Recent advances in quantitative neuroproteomics. Methods 61:186–218. doi:10.1016/j.ymeth.2013.04.008

Cvjetkovic A, Lötvall J, Lässer C (2014) The influence of rotor type and centrifugation time on the yield and purity of extracellular vesicles. J Extracell Vesicles. doi:10.3402/jev.v3.23111

De Monte L, Sanvito F, Olivieri S et al (2008) Serological immunoreactivity against colon cancer proteome varies upon disease progression. J Proteome Res 7:504–514. doi:10.1021/pr070360m

Deregibus MC, Cantaluppi V, Calogero R et al (2007) Endothelial progenitor cell derived microvesicles activate an angiogenic program in endothelial cells by a horizontal transfer of mRNA. Blood 110:2440–2448. doi:10.1182/blood-2007-03-078709

Dumurgier J, Laplanche J-L, Mouton-Liger F et al (2014) The screening of Alzheimer's patients with CSF biomarkers, modulates the distribution of APOE genotype: impact on clinical trials. J Neurol 261:1187–1195. doi:10.1007/s00415-014-7335-6

Ferreira D, Perestelo-Pérez L, Westman E et al (2014) Meta-review of CSF core biomarkers in Alzheimer's disease: the state-of-the-art after the new revised diagnostic criteria. Front Aging Neurosci 6:47. doi:10.3389/fnagi.2014.00047

Filippi M, Canu E, Agosta F (2013) The role of amyloid-β, tau, and apolipoprotein E epsilon4 in Alzheimer disease: how is the team playing? AJNR Am J Neuroradiol 34:511–512. doi:10.3174/ajnr.A3295

Fortea J, Vilaplana E, Alcolea D et al (2014) Cerebrospinal fluid β-amyloid and phospho-tau biomarker interactions affecting brain structure in preclinical Alzheimer disease. Ann Neurol. doi:10.1002/ana.24186

Fraisier C, Papa A, Granjeaud S et al (2014) Cerebrospinal fluid biomarker candidates associated with human WNV neuroinvasive disease. PLoS One 9:e93637. doi:10.1371/journal.pone.0093637

Freedman MS, Thompson EJ, Deisenhammer F et al (2005) Recommended standard of cerebrospinal fluid analysis in the diagnosis of multiple sclerosis: a consensus statement. Arch Neurol 62:865–870. doi:10.1001/archneur.62.6.865

Freischmidt A, Ller KM, Ludolph AC, Weishaupt JH (2013) Systemic dysregulation of TDP-43 binding microRNAs in amyotrophic lateral sclerosis. Acta Neuropathol Commun 1(1):1. doi:10.1186/2051-5960-1-42

Frigerio CS, Lau P, Salta E et al (2013) Reduced expression of hsa-miR-27a-3p in CSF of patients with Alzheimer disease. Neurology 81:2103–2106

Galea I, Freedman MS, Thompson EJ (2011) Cerebrospinal fluid analysis in the 2010 revised McDonald's multiple sclerosis diagnostic criteria. Ann Neurol 70:183. doi:10.1002/ana.22466, author reply 183–184

Gallego JA, Gordon ML, Claycomb K et al (2012) In vivo microRNA detection and quantitation in cerebrospinal fluid. J Mol Neurosci 47:243–248. doi:10.1007/s12031-012-9731-7

Garzetti L, Menon R, Finardi A et al (2013) Activated macrophages release microvesicles containing polarized M1 or M2 mRNAs. J Leukoc Biol. doi:10.1189/jlb.0913485

Haghikia A, Haghikia A, Hellwig K et al (2012) Regulated microRNAs in the CSF of patients with multiple sclerosis: a case–control study. Neurology 79:2166–2170. doi:10.1212/WNL.0b013e3182759621

Hjalmarsson C, Bjerke M, Andersson B et al (2014) Neuronal and glia-related biomarkers in cerebrospinal fluid of patients with acute ischemic stroke. J Cent Nerv Syst Dis 6:51–58. doi:10.4137/JCNSD.S13821

Hong BS, Cho J-H, Kim H et al (2009) Colorectal cancer cell-derived microvesicles are enriched in cell cycle-related mRNAs that promote proliferation of endothelial cells. BMC Genomics 10:556. doi:10.1186/1471-2164-10-556

Huang JT, Leweke FM, Tsang TM et al (2007a) CSF metabolic and proteomic profiles in patients prodromal for psychosis. PLoS One 2:e756. doi:10.1371/journal.pone.0000756

Huang JT, McKenna T, Hughes C et al (2007b) CSF biomarker discovery using label-free nano-LC-MS based proteomic profiling: technical aspects. J Sep Sci 30:214–225

Iannaccone S, Cerami C, Alessio M et al (2013) In vivo microglia activation in very early dementia with Lewy bodies, comparison with Parkinson's disease. Parkinsonism Relat Disord 19:47–52. doi:10.1016/j.parkreldis.2012.07.002

Jakobsson J, Bjerke M, Ekman CJ et al (2014) Elevated concentrations of neurofilament light chain in the cerebrospinal fluid of bipolar disorder patients. Neuropsychopharmacology. doi:10.1038/npp.2014.81

Jarry J, Schadendorf D, Greenwood C et al (2014) ScienceDirect. Mol Oncol 8:819–829. doi:10.1016/j.molonc.2014.02.009

Kern S, Skoog I, Börjesson-Hanson A et al (2014) Higher CSF interleukin-6 and CSF interleukin-8 in current depression in older women. Results from a population-based sample. Brain Behav Immun. doi:10.1016/j.bbi.2014.05.006

Kiko T, Nakagawa K, Tsuduki T et al (2013) MicroRNAs in plasma and cerebrospinal fluid as potential markers for Alzheimer s disease. J Alzheimers Dis 39:253–259. doi:10.3233/JAD-130932

Li G, Millard SP, Peskind ER et al (2014) Cross-sectional and longitudinal relationships between cerebrospinal fluid biomarkers and cognitive function in people without cognitive impairment from across the adult life span. JAMA Neurol 71:742–751. doi:10.1001/jamaneurol.2014.445

Lista S, Zetterberg H, Dubois B et al (2014) Cerebrospinal fluid analysis in Alzheimer's disease: technical issues and future developments. J Neurol 261:1234–1243. doi:10.1007/s00415-014-7366-z

Liu Y, Qing H, Deng Y (2014) Biomarkers in Alzheimer's disease analysis by mass spectrometry-based proteomics. Int J Mol Sci 15:7865–7882. doi:10.3390/ijms15057865

Lourenco AS, Baldeiras I, Graos M, Duarte CB (2011) Proteomics-based technologies in the discovery of biomarkers for multiple sclerosis in the cerebrospinal fluid. Curr Mol Med 11:326–349

Malek N, Swallow D, Grosset KA et al (2014) Alpha-synuclein in peripheral tissues and body fluids as a biomarker for Parkinson's disease – a systematic review. Acta Neurol Scand. doi:10.1111/ane.12247

Menon KN, Steer DL, Short M et al (2011) A novel unbiased proteomic approach to detect the reactivity of cerebrospinal fluid in neurological diseases. Mol Cell Proteomics 10(M110):000042. doi:10.1074/mcp.M110.000042

Müller M, Kuiperij HB, Claassen JA et al (2014) Neurobiology of aging. Neurobiol Aging 35:152–158. doi:10.1016/j.neurobiolaging.2013.07.005

Nakamura T, Tu S, Akhtar MW et al (2013) Aberrant protein s-nitrosylation in neurodegenerative diseases. Neuron 78:596–614. doi:10.1016/j.neuron.2013.05.005

Nazco CV, Pérez LP, Molinuevo JL et al (2014) Cost-effectiveness of the use of biomarkers in cerebrospinal fluid for Alzheimer's disease. J Alzheimers Dis. doi:10.3233/JAD-132216

Olivieri S, Conti A, Iannaccone S et al (2011) Ceruloplasmin oxidation, a feature of Parkinson's disease CSF, inhibits ferroxidase activity and promotes cellular iron retention. J Neurosci 31:18568–18577. doi:10.1523/JNEUROSCI. 3768-11.2011

Pacifici M, Delbue S, Ferrante P et al (2013) Cerebrospinal fluid miRNA profile in HIV-encephalitis. J Cell Physiol 228:1070–1075. doi:10.1002/jcp.24254

Palanisamy V, Sharma S, Deshpande A et al (2010) Nanostructural and transcriptomic analyses of human saliva derived exosomes. PLoS One 5:e8577. doi:10.1371/journal.pone.0008577

Parnetti L, Farotti L, Eusebi P et al (2014) Differential role of CSF alpha-synuclein species, tau, and Aβ42 in Parkinson's disease. Front Aging Neurosci 6:53. doi:10.3389/fnagi.2014.00053

Pegtel DM, van de Garde MDB, Middeldorp JM (2011) Viral miRNAs exploiting the endosomal-exosomal pathway for intercellular cross-talk and immune evasion. Biochim Biophys Acta 1809:715–721. doi:10.1016/j.bbagrm.2011.08.002

Perrin RJ, Payton JE, Malone JP et al (2013) Quantitative label-free proteomics for discovery of biomarkers in cerebrospinal fluid: assessment of technical and inter-individual variation. PLoS One 8:e64314. doi:10.1371/journal.pone.0064314

Plebani M, Sciacovelli L, Aita A et al (2014) Quality indicators to detect pre-analytical errors in laboratory testing. Clin Chim Acta 432:44–48. doi:10.1016/j.cca.2013.07.033

Pogue AI, Hill JM, Lukiw WJ (2014) MicroRNA (miRNA): sequence and stability, viroid-like properties, and disease association in the CNS. Brain Res 1584:73–9. doi: 10.1016/j.brainres.2014.03.042

Polman CH, Reingold SC, Banwell B et al (2011) Diagnostic criteria for multiple sclerosis: 2010 revisions to the McDonald criteria. Ann Neurol 69:292–302. doi:10.1002/ana.22366

Poulsen K, Bahl JM, Simonsen AH et al (2014) Distinct transthyretin oxidation isoform profile in spinal fluid from patients with Alzheimer's disease and mild cognitive impairment. Clin Proteomics 11:12. doi:10.1186/1559-0275-11-12

Pouw MH, Kwon BK, Verbeek MM et al (2014) Structural biomarkers in the cerebrospinal fluid within 24 h after a traumatic spinal cord injury: a descriptive analysis of 16 subjects. Spinal Cord 52:428–433. doi:10.1038/sc.2014.26

Privitera D, Corti V, Alessio M et al (2013) Proteomic identification of aldolase A as an autoantibody target in patients with atypical movement disorders. Neurol Sci 34:313–320. doi:10.1007/s10072-012-0996-y

Rao P, Benito E, Fischer A (2013) MicroRNAs as biomarkers for CNS disease. Front Mol Neurosci 6:39. doi:10.3389/fnmol.2013.00039

Ratajczak J, Miekus K, Kucia M et al (2006) Embryonic stem cell-derived microvesicles reprogram hematopoietic progenitors: evidence for horizontal transfer of mRNA and protein delivery. Leukemia 20:847–856. doi:10.1038/sj.leu.2404132

Ritchie C, Smailagic N, Noel-Storr AH et al (2014) Plasma and cerebrospinal fluid amyloid beta for the diagnosis of Alzheimer's disease dementia and other dementias in people with mild cognitive impairment (MCI). Cochrane Database Syst Rev 6:CD008782. doi: 10.1002/14651858. CD008782.pub4

Shan L (2011) CellVue Maroon–labeled saposin C-dioleylphosphatidylserine nanovesicles. Molecular Imaging and Contrast Agent Database (MICAD)

Siderowf A, Logroscino G (2014) β-Amyloid in CSF: a window into Parkinson disease dementia. Neurology 82:1758–1759. doi:10.1212/WNL.0000000000000437

Siritho S, Freedman MS (2009) The prognostic significance of cerebrospinal fluid in multiple sclerosis. J Neurol Sci 279:21–25. doi:10.1016/j.jns.2008.12.029

Skog J, Würdinger T, Van Rijn S et al (2008) Glioblastoma microvesicles transport RNA and proteins that promote tumour growth and provide diagnostic biomarkers. Nat Cell Biol 10:1470–1476. doi:10.1038/ncb1800

Stoop MP, Coulier L, Rosenling T et al (2010a) Quantitative proteomics and metabolomics analysis of normal human cerebrospinal fluid samples. Mol Cell Proteomics 9:2063–2075. doi:10.1074/mcp.M900877-MCP200

Stoop MP, Singh V, Dekker LJ et al (2010b) Proteomics comparison of cerebrospinal fluid of relapsing remitting and primary progressive multiple sclerosis. PLoS One 5:e12442. doi:10.1371/journal.pone.0012442

Teplyuk NM, Mollenhauer B, Gabriely G et al (2012) MicroRNAs in cerebrospinal fluid identify glioblastoma and metastatic brain cancers and reflect disease activity. Neuro Oncol 14:689–700. doi:10.1093/neuonc/nos074

Teunissen CE, Petzold A, Bennett JL et al (2009) A consensus protocol for the standardization of cerebrospinal fluid collection and biobanking. Neurology 73:1914–1922. doi:10.1212/WNL.0b013e3181c47cc2

Tortelli R, Copetti M, Ruggieri M et al (2014) Cerebrospinal fluid neurofilament light chain levels: marker of progression to generalized amyotrophic lateral sclerosis. Eur J Neurol. doi:10.1111/ene.1242

Tumani H, Hartung H-P, Hemmer B et al (2009) Cerebrospinal fluid biomarkers in multiple sclerosis. Neurobiol Dis 35:117–127. doi:10.1016/j.nbd.2009.04.010

Turner CA, Thompson RC, Bunney WE et al (2014) Altered choroid plexus gene expression in major depressive disorder. Front Hum Neurosci. doi:10.3389/fnhum.2014.00238/abstract

Valadi H, Ekström K, Bossios A et al (2007) Exosome-mediated transfer of mRNAs and microRNAs is a novel mechanism of genetic exchange between cells. Nat Cell Biol 9:654–659. doi:10.1038/ncb1596

van Gool AJ, Hendrickson RC (2012) The proteomic toolbox for studying cerebrospinal fluid. Expert Rev Proteomics 9:165–179. doi:10.1586/epr.12.6

Verderio C, Muzio L, Turola E et al (2012) Myeloid microvesicles are a marker and therapeutic target for neuroinflammation. Ann Neurol 72:610–624. doi:10.1002/ana.23627

Vranová HP, Hényková E, Kaiserová M, et al (2014) Tau protein, beta-amyloid$_{1-42}$ and clusterin CSF levels in the differential diagnosis of Parkinsonian syndrome with dementia. J Neurol Sci 343:120–4. doi: 10.1016/j.jns.2014.05.052

Woods AG, Iosifescu DV, Darie CC (2014) Biomarkers in major depressive disorder: the role of mass spectrometry. Adv Exp Med Biol 806:545–560. doi:10.1007/978-3-319-06068-2_27

Yuan X, Desiderio DM (2003) Proteomics analysis of phosphotyrosyl-proteins in human lumbar cerebrospinal fluid. J Proteome Res 2:476–487

Yuan X, Desiderio DM (2005a) Proteomics analysis of human cerebrospinal fluid. J Chromatogr B Analyt Technol Biomed Life Sci 815:179–189. doi:10.1016/j.jchromb.2004.06.044

Yuan X, Desiderio DM (2005b) Human cerebrospinal fluid peptidomics. J Mass Spectrom 40:176–181. doi:10.1002/jms.737

Zhang J, Goodlett DR, Peskind ER et al (2005) Quantitative proteomic analysis of age-related changes in human cerebrospinal fluid. Neurobiol Aging 26:207–227. doi:10.1016/j.neurobiolaging.2004.02.012

Part III

CSF in Clinical Syndromes

Acute Infectious Diseases

14

Erich Schmutzhard and Bettina Pfausler

Contents

E. Schmutzhard (✉) • B. Pfausler
Neurocritical Care Unit, Department of Neurology,
Innsbruck Medical University,
Innsbruck, Austria
e-mail: erich.schmutzhard@i-med.ac.at

© Springer International Publishing Switzerland 2015
F. Deisenhammer et al. (eds.), *Cerebrospinal Fluid in Clinical Neurology*,
DOI 10.1007/978-3-319-01225-4_14

Abstract

Acute infectious diseases of the nervous system are potentially life threatening, inherently carrying a high long-term morbidity and mortality. Therefore, the earliest possible diagnosis is absolutely essential. Examination of cerebrospinal fluid frequently leads the way towards correct diagnosis and allows for focused antimicrobial and adjunctive therapy. This chapter deals with acute infectious diseases of the nervous system, diagnostic procedures being indispensable. Encephalitis, meningitis, poliomyelitis and polyradiculoneuritis are the most important clinical/neurological entities in case of viral infection. It is the acute bacterial meningitis for which the earliest possible diagnosis carries the most important prognostic implication. For this disease, the appropriate examination of the cerebrospinal fluid (including glucose, cell count, lactate) is of utmost importance. Besides antimicrobial chemotherapy, the best possible adjunctive therapies are essential for acute bacterial meningitis. Fungal, protozoal and helminthic infections of the central nervous system are detailed with respect to diagnostic aspects and therapeutic implications (e.g. eosinophilic meningitis, radiculitis, etc.); for some of these diseases, e.g. cerebral malaria, a normal CSF leads the way to correct diagnosis in a patient with severe impairment of consciousness, high fever and history of exposure to *Plasmodium falciparum*, thereby easily mistaken for viral encephalitis or acute bacterial meningitis.

14.1   Introduction

Virtually every pathogen can cause disease of the nervous system if it succeeds to traverse the blood-brain barrier (Brouwer et al. 2013a). Besides its inherent pathogenicity, being responsible for the type of disease, the acuteness of disease and the course of disease, but also the anatomical predilection and the anatomically affected region and the systemic as well as the local immune response play a decisive role for clinical presentation, neurological signs and symptoms and eventually the course of disease and prognosis. i.e. morbidity and mortality.

History, epidemiologic features, initial presenting signs and symptoms as well as peracute, acute or subacute evolution of the initial disease are – in a reasonable number of cases – highly suggestive for a suspected pathogen, thus allowing best possible emergency management. As in sepsis syndrome, the earliest possible maximal focused therapy has the most important impact on morbidity and mortality, proven both in acute bacterial meningitis and in sepsis syndrome. Each subchapter contains a short review of epidemiology; discusses etiologic agents, clinical features, diagnostic procedures, in particular, imaging, CSF changes and microbiological findings; discusses specific peculiarities and differential diagnoses; and summarises specific and adjunctive therapies, prognosis and potential preventive measures.

14.2   Acute Viral Diseases of the Nervous System

14.2.1 Introduction

Each part of the central and peripheral nervous system, even arteries and muscles, may be the target of viral pathogens. Therefore, viruses may cause a wide range of clinical signs and symptoms, as listed in Table 14.1. Viruses may behave differently in the state of immunosuppression or immunocompromise potentially leading to more acute or progressive disease, as seen in progressive multifocal leucoencephalopathy or EBV-associated lymphoproliferative disease. Besides this, post- or

Table 14.1 Clinical features in viral disease of the nervous system (any of any combination is possible) (Cree 2014; Handique and Handique 2011; Nigrovic 2013; Putz et al. 2013; Ross 2014; Roman 2014)

Meningitis
Encephalitis
Encephalopathy
Myelitis
Myelopathy
Radiculitis
Radiculoneuritis
Cranial neuritis
Meningovasculitis
Myositis (not discussed in this chapter)

parainfectious and post-paravaccinal diseases of the central (and also peripheral) nervous system as well as secondary encephalopathy – as seen in influenza virus infection – may be the cause of an even potentially life-threatening disease (Handique and Handique 2011). These secondary diseases of the nervous system are not dealt with in this chapter. Most viruses have specific predilections, causing meningitis or encephalitis or myelitis or any type of combination of the clinical features, listed in Table 14.1.

14.2.2 Epidemiology

Many of the viruses causing acute disease of the nervous system can be acquired worldwide, e.g. measles, mumps, coxsackievirus, echovirus, enterovirus, herpesviridae, HIV, lymphocytic choriomeningitis virus, papovavirus, etc. Some of the viruses, in particular those which are acquired by mosquito bite or tick bite, show a clear-cut regional or continental occurrence, e.g. tick-borne encephalitis virus, West Nile virus, Japanese encephalitis virus or other arboviruses. Other viruses which have been the aim of eradication campaigns occur only in well-circumscribed regions, e.g. poliomyelitis virus, enterovirus 68–71, Nipah virus or Zika virus, occurring in certain tropical areas both as epidemics and endemically. Besides the geographic distribution of these various viruses, the way of transmission may play an important epidemiological role (Handique and Handique 2011; Lyons and McArthur 2013). Due to various programmes of eradicating viral diseases by global vaccination campaigns as for measles, mumps and poliomyelitis or regional campaigns to prevent diseases like Japanese encephalitis or tick-borne encephalitis, a changing epidemiology requires the best possible and regular flow of information, i.e. an international surveillance system.

14.2.3 Pathogenesis and Pathophysiology

Tables 14.2a, 14.2b and 14.2c list the more important viral causes of acute meningitis, encephalitis, myelitis or any combination of these; in rare cases, meningovasculitis, encephalomyelitis or radiculomyelitis may be caused.

The route of infection differs greatly: enteroviridae being transmitted via the faeco-oral route, arboviruses – as the name arthropod-borne viruses indicates – are transmitted by mosquitoes or ticks and herpesviridae and most of the other viruses are transmitted via droplet infection, by direct contact and/or exchange of body fluids.

14.2.4 Clinical Features

14.2.4.1 Viral Meningitis

The term viral meningitis (lymphocytic/aseptic meningitis used as synonym) is a syndrome with the triad of fever, headache and stiff neck associated with

Table 14.2a Viral causes of meningitis (Franzen-Rohl et al. 2008; Handique and Handique 2011; Huang and Shih 2014; Nicolasora and Kaul 2008; Nigrovic 2013; Putz et al. 2013)

Enteroviridae
Coxsackieviruses A and B
Echoviruses
Enteroviruses (Pomar et al. 2013; Pcstels and Birbeck 2013; Putz et al. 2013; Rodgers 2010)
In rare cases: poliomyelitis virus
Arboviruses
Tick-borne encephalitis virus
West Nile virus
Japanese encephalitis virus
St. Louis encephalitis virus
La Crosse virus
Western equine encephalitis virus
Colorado tick fever virus
Dengue viruses
Zika viruses
Herpesviridae
Herpes simplex virus type 2 (in particular relapsing meningitis – Mollaret meningitis)
Epstein-Barr virus
Varicella zoster virus
Human herpes virus 6 (potentially also 7 and 8)
Human immunodeficiency virus (after acute infection)
Mumps virus
Lymphocytic choriomeningitis virus
Adenoviruses
Arenaviruses
Filoviridae
Rubella

photophobia and possibly signs and symptoms of the autonomic nervous system. It is associated with cerebrospinal fluid lymphocytic pleocytosis. A viral meningitis might evolve into a meningoencephalitis, myelitis, etc.; in these cases, the prognosis is determined by the encephalitic, radiculitic or myelitic part of the disease. A viral meningitis in its pure form has virtually zero mortality and an extremely low long-term morbidity.

14.2.4.2 Viral Encephalitis

The typical clinical presentation of encephalitis is an acute, sometimes subacute condition of fever, headache (frequently holocranial sometimes hemicranial), increasing behavioural abnormalities, mental disturbances, focal or generalised seizure activity, focal or generalised neurological deficits (aphasia, hemiparesis) and

Table 14.2b Viral causes of encephalitis (De Souza and Madhusudana 2014; Handique and Handique 2011; Kant Upadhyay 2013; Lyons and McArthur 2013; Mann et al. 2013; Misra et al. 2014; Moritani et al. 2014; Nicolasora and Kaul 2008; Ross 2014; Rudolph et al. 2014; Tyler 2014)

Arboviruses
Tick-borne encephalitis virus
Powassan virus
Colorado tick fever virus
West Nile virus
La Crosse virus
St. Louis encephalitis virus
Japanese encephalitis virus
Yellow fever
Dengue virus
Equine encephalitis viruses
Adenoviruses
Herpesviridae
Herpes simplex 1
Herpes simplex 2 (in neonates)
Varicella zoster virus
Epstein-Barr virus
Cytomegalovirus (rare in immune competent)
Enteroviruses
Nipah virus
Zika virus
Measles virus
Rubella virus (very rare)
Filoviridae (very rare encephalitis, more frequent intracranial haemorrhage)
Rabies viruses

Table 14.2c Viral causes of myelitis (direct viral invasion) (Cree 2014; Roman 2014)

Poliomyelitis viruses
West Nile virus
Tick-borne encephalitis virus
Japanese encephalitis virus
Chikungunya virus (mainly myelo-radiculitic form)
Rabies viruses (dumb rabies: radiculomyelitis)

increasing qualitative and quantitative impairment of consciousness. It must be, however, noted that the clinical presentation also depends, at least to some extent, on the specific virus. Arboviruses, in particular Japanese encephalitis virus, West Nile virus and tick-borne encephalitis virus, may manifest with a predominating basal ganglia syndrome, tremor, bradykinesia and rigidity being the most important signs and symptoms. The course of the disease might evolve into a status epilepticus, a condition which carries a very high morbidity and acute mortality. In encephalitis, focal and/or generalised seizures may occur in up to 60 % of the cases

(Handique and Handique 2011; Lyons and McArthur 2013; Misra et al. 2014; Nicolasora and Kaul 2008; Ross 2014; Rudolph et al. 2014).

14.2.4.3 Viral Myelitis

A direct invasion of viruses into the myelon is rather typical for enteroviruses (Huang and Shih 2014), frequently causing a well-circumscribed myelitis within the grey matter of the myelon, i.e. a poliomyelitic course of disease. Besides enteroviruses (poliomyelitis viruses, enterovirus 69–71), West Nile viruses and tick-borne encephalitis virus may also cause a poliomyelitic course of disease. Rare cases of "poliomyelitis" have been described in Chikungunya virus and in Japanese encephalitis. Completely different – from a direct viral invasion into the myelon – is the post- or parainfectious myelitis which frequently presents as a transverse myelitis (Cree 2014; Roman 2014; Tyler 2014).

14.2.5 Diagnostic Features

History of exposure (mumps, measles) and the clinical syndrome of the respective infectious disease (again mumps, measles or varicella, shingles, etc.) are – in case the patients develop signs and symptoms of acute meningitis – highly suggestive of the aetiology of meningitic disease. In pure meningitis, neuroimaging neither is indicated nor carries a chance of suggestive findings. However, if the viral meningitis progresses to meningoencephalitis or meningoencephalomyelitis or if the presenting features suggest encephalitis or myelitis, neuroimaging is essential, both in ascertaining and confirming the neurological syndrome and being helpful in establishing the appropriate diagnosis and prognosis. The most important is neuroimaging – if possible, at any rate, nuclear magnetic resonance imaging – in case of meningoencephalitis, since certain patterns of affection within the brain frequently allow the best possible "guess" in attributing the disease to a certain virus family (Table 14.3).

Electroencephalography is indicated in case of encephalitic signs and symptoms, with or without epileptic features. Both epilepsy-specific EEG changes and focal or diffuse abnormalities are clearly associated with a malfunction of the cortical areas, thereby allowing to objectivise the clinical syndrome of an encephalitis. In case of myelitis, somatosensory-evoked potentials and motor-evoked potentials help to classify an incomplete poliomyelitic or transverse myelitis course of disease, both allowing early diagnosis and accompanying ascertainment of the clinical course.

Table 14.3 Virus-specific typical localisation in neuroimaging (Gupta et al. 2012)

Flaviviruses: basal ganglia, thalami
Enteroviruses: thalami
Herpes simplex type 1: fronto-temporo-basal
Rabies: brainstem, initially in particular medulla oblongata

14.2.6 Non-CSF Laboratory Analyses

In viral CNS disease, the extra CSF laboratory values do not usually yield a specific result. It is essential to point towards the capacity of a wide range of viruses to involve – beside the meninges – also other organs, like the liver, kidney, etc. Therefore, minor laboratory signs of hepatic or renal involvement might easily underline the viral pathogenesis. However, only Epstein-Barr virus or cytomegalovirus clearly and regularly affect the kidney and/or liver so that the aetiological involvement of one of these viruses might correctly be surmised. Leucocyte count, C-reactive protein or procalcitonin do not show a clear pattern in the case of viral meningitis. In contrast to this, the differential count frequently shows a relative lymphocytosis; in case of Epstein-Barr-virus or cytomegalovirus infection, monocytes predominate differential white blood cell count.

14.2.7 Cerebrospinal Fluid (CSF)

In many cases of viral meningitis, in the earliest hours of the disease, a mixed or even predominantly polymorphonuclear leucocytosis in the CSF might be found. However, this is rapidly followed (within 12–24 h) by a predominance of the lymphocytes and monocytes. The CSF glucose and the CSF/serum glucose ratio are normal, and in the case of viral meningitis, CSF protein is only mildly elevated and CSF lactate normal. The microbiological diagnostic studies in a patient with viral meningitis or encephalitis are shown in Table 14.4.

14.2.8 Differential Diagnosis

Table 14.5 lists nonviral causes of lymphocytic/aseptic meningitis syndrome, a disease which might be mistaken for a viral CNS infection.

14.2.9 Therapeutic Management

14.2.9.1 Antiviral Therapies

If diagnosed early enough, enteroviral meningitis can be treated with pleconaril 200 mg t.i.d. for 1 week, herpes simplex virus type 2 meningitis with acyclovir 1,000 mg daily for 10 days and varicella zoster virus meningitis with acyclovir 2–3 g daily for 5 days, and a patient with acute HIV meningitis should receive a combination therapy (2 nucleoside analogue reverse transcriptase inhibitors or a non-nucleoside reverse transcriptase inhibitor combined with 2 nucleoside analogues). Every patient with signs and symptoms of viral encephalitis receives acyclovir intravenously (10 mg/kg b.w. t.i.d.). If the clinical course and both the neuroimaging/EEG and the CSF PCR clearly exclude HSV1 aetiology, acyclovir is stopped and either another specific treatment, if indicated, or at least symptomatic therapy is initiated.

Table 14.4 Diagnostic studies for microbiological/serological studies

Enteroviruses including poliomyelitis
CSF viral culture
CSF RT-PCR
Throat and stool culture
Arboviruses
CSF IgM antibody-capture ELISA
CSF PCR West Nile virus
Paired acute and convalescent sera[a]
Herpes simplex virus (HSV)
CSF PCR HSV DNA
Genital lesions
Epstein-Barr virus
Serology
Heterophilic antibodies
Antiviral capsid antigen (VCA) titres of 1:320 or higher
EBV VCA IgM antibodies
Absence of anti-EBNA IgG antibodies
CSF PCR EBV DNA
Human immunodeficiency virus (HIV)
CSF PCR HIV-1 RNA
Anti-HIV-1 IgG in CSF
CSF viral culture
Varicella zoster virus (VZV)
CSF PCR VZV DNA
CSF VZV IgG antibodies (serum/CSF ratio)
CSF VZV IgM antibodies
HHV-6
Isolation of virus in CSF culture
Plus
Paired acute and convalescent sera[a]
Lymphocytic choriomeningitis virus
Herpes simplex virus 2
Cultures are positive for herpes simplex virus 2 in the majority of cases of meningitis associated with primary genital herpes, but they rarely are positive in recurrent episodes
Paired acute and convalescent sera mumps
Paired acute and convalescent sera[a]

Modified according to Brouwer et al. (2013), Franzen-Rohl et al. (2008), Nigrovic (2013), Putz et al. (2013), Ross (2014)

CSF cerebrospinal fluid, *PCR* polymerase chain reaction, *RT-PCR* reverse transcription-polymerase chain reaction

[a]Fourfold or greater increase in IgG between acute and convalescent sera

Table 14.5 Nonviral causes of acute lymphocytic/aseptic meningitis syndrome

Infectious causes
Trypanosoma cruzi
Cysticercus cellulosae
Larva migrans
Cryptococcus neoformans
Coccidioides immitis
Histoplasma capsulatum
Sporothrix schenckii
Mycobacterium tuberculosis
Mycoplasma pneumoniae
Rickettsia spp.
Bartonella henselae
Anaplasma spp.
Treponema pallidum
Borrelia burgdorferi
Noninfectious causes
Sarcoidosis
Leptomeningeal carcinomatosis
Lymphoma
Wegener granulomatosis
Behcet's disease
Systemic lupus erythematosus
Drugs
Nonsteroidal anti-inflammatory agents
Sulphonamides
Intravenous immunoglobulins
OKT3 antibodies
Isoniazid

Table adapted according to Auriel et al. (2014), Blasi et al. (2009), Greenblatt et al. (2013), Putz et al. (2013), Ross (2014)

Patients with viral meningitis do not need specific antiviral therapy; however, the best possible symptomatic care, e.g. analgesics, anti-emetics, etc., is essential. Clinical observation supplements the acute care. Specific antivirals or the administration of hyperimmunoglobulins is not recommended in a case with pure viral meningitis (De Souza and Madhusudana 2014; Nigrovic 2013; Putz et al. 2013; Ross 2014).

14.2.9.2 Symptomatic/Adjunctive Therapies

Every patient with a potentially life-threatening course of encephalitis and/or myelitis must be managed in an (neuro) ICU. If intracranial pressure is suspected, the placement of an ICP probe is indispensable; if ICP remains elevated or cerebral perfusion pressure is dangerously low (<50 mmHg), immediate follow-up neuroimaging is mandatory.

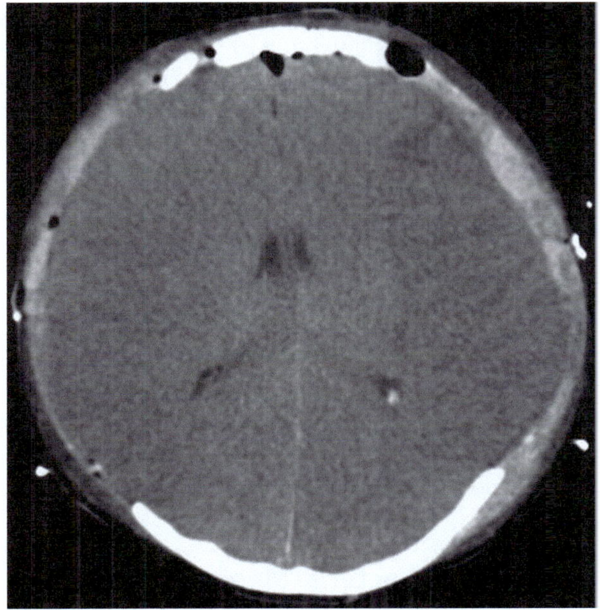

Fig. 14.1 Epstein-Barr virus encephalitis with life-threatening diffuse brain oedema, successful bilateral decompressive craniectomy

Encephalitic brain oedema may be diffuse or focal; however, anti-oedematous therapy with corticosteroids or osmotherapy is still a matter of discussion. No prospective randomised trials with respect to corticosteroids or osmotherapy exist for viral encephalitides. A small group of patients with severe viral encephalitis and hyperpyrexia may benefit from therapeutic hypothermia or, at least, therapeutic normothermia, i.e. targeted temperature management or decompressive craniectomy (Fig. 14.1).

Isolated seizures, a common finding in encephalitis, need to be treated as any other symptomatic epileptic seizure. In the case of refractory status epilepticus, barbiturates may be considered; however, this group of drugs should only be given in encephalitic patients if an ICP monitoring probe is in place and the patient is on continuous EEG monitoring (Edberg et al. 2011).

14.2.10 Prognosis

Short-term and long-term prognosis in a patient with pure lymphocytic, viral meningitis is good, long-term mortality virtually zero and long-term morbidity also very low. In encephalitis and encephalomyelitis, long-term morbidity and mortality is definitely much higher than in pure meningitis. Without treatment, herpes simplex virus type 1 encephalitis carries a mortality rate of 70 %, the European tick-borne encephalitis or myelitis carries a mortality rate of up to 10 %, and the far eastern variant of TBE (Russian spring summer time encephalitis) has a mortality rate similar to Japanese encephalitis (30 %). Patients who survive an encephalitis or a myelitis have a likelihood of >10 % to suffer from severe neurological long-term sequelae, paraplegia or tetraplegia and epilepsy as well as focal or diffuse encephalopathies being the major long-term sequelae in patients with severe encephalitis and/or myelitis (Nigrovic 2013; Putz et al. 2013; Ross 2014; Zhang et al. 2014).

14.2.11 Prophylaxis

The avoidance of exposure to the various pathogenic agents (by avoiding areas of increased risk of transmission) and exposure to vectors in the case of arboviruses and the avoidance of close contacts in the case of droplet-, faeco-oral route of infection (mumps, measles, enteroviruses, etc.) are the most important steps of prevention. When available, active immunisation is a highly efficacious way to avoid the respective viral CNS disease (TBE, Japanese encephalitis, measles, mumps, poliomyelitis etc.).

14.3 Acute Bacterial Meningitis

14.3.1 Introduction

Acute bacterial meningitis is one of the most important acute inflammatory diseases of the central nervous system, early diagnosis and immediate initiation of the best possible empirical therapy being extremely important in reducing morbidity and the still high mortality. Despite improvements in antimicrobial chemotherapy over the past decades, neurological sequelae and mortality still remain unacceptably high for which mainly intracranial complications are responsible. The earliest possible recognition of such intracranial complications, e.g. diffuse brain oedema, status epilepticus, meningovasculitis leading to stroke, sinus or intracranial venous thrombosis, hydrocephalus, pyocephalus, is needed to allow – equally important – the earliest possible adequate adjunctive therapeutic measures. Only very recently, neurocritical care measures, by means of invasive intracranial pressure monitoring, have been shown to lead to an improvement of mortality in comatose patients with acute bacterial meningitis (from 30 to 10 %). Therefore, the earliest possible diagnosis, earliest possible specific and adjunctive therapeutic measures as well as monitoring and management in an intensive care unit setting are, besides prevention, the essential clue to further improve morbidity and mortality in acute bacterial meningitis.

14.3.2 Epidemiology

Worldwide, the incidence of acute bacterial meningitis is estimated to be 5–10 cases per 100,000 persons/year. These figures have changed dramatically throughout the past decade, in particular after the introduction of *Haemophilus influenzae* type B vaccine and the growing number of persons at risk who receive the appropriate polyvalent pneumococcal vaccine. Since the immunogenicity and safety of the multicomponent recombinant meningococcal serogroup B vaccine has been shown, the European Medicines Agency (EMA) issued an approval of this vaccine in January 2013. Serogroup B meningococci being responsible for more than 60 % of meningococcal diseases in central European countries, the other third mostly being caused by serogroup C meningococci (Bijlsma et al. 2014), it seems reasonable to assume that within the coming years, acute bacterial meningitis due to the "common pathogenic agents", i.e. pneumococci and meningococci, will become rare events, the incidence dropping well below 1/100,000/year, as has been seen in the 1990s in Europe or a decade later in African countries for *Haemophilus influenzae* type B meningitis. Due to the demographic development and the fact that the ageing population will suffer more and more from various co-morbidities, enhancing the risk of either hitherto unusual or even unknown pathogenic agents leading to bacteraemia (e.g. Gram negatives, anaerobes, etc.), it might be assumed that in the future years, both community-acquired meningitis due to unusual bacterial pathogens and nosocomial bacterial meningitis in the case of invasive therapeutic or monitoring procedures (external ventricular drain, intracranial pressure probe, other monitoring probes, more invasive neurosurgical procedures, etc.) will replace the so far common and well-known pathogenic agents, in particular pneumococci and meningococci (Bhimraj 2012; Kasanmoentalib et al. 2013; Pomar et al. 2013). In the so-called meningitis belt – Sub-Saharan Africa, Arab Peninsula and northern part of India and Pakistan – meningococci still are the cause of epidemics, incidence rates being as high as 1,000/100,000/year in such an epidemic setting. However, even in sub-Saharan Africa, a change of epidemiology has been seen, these meningococcal epidemics moving from the immediate semiarid area of the Sahel zone towards the southern countries, extending towards Angola, Mozambique or Namibia.

Specific attention has to be paid to the development of antibiotic resistance, which has been shown, in particular, to be the case for *Streptococcus pneumoniae* (pneumococci), becoming more and more prevalent in Asia, the USA and in certain European countries. Almost 20 years ago, already a third of cases of pneumococcal meningitides in the USA were caused by organisms not susceptible to penicillin, in European countries (Spain, France, Hungary, etc.) penicillin resistance rates even reaching more than 50 %. Very rare cases of penicillin resistance strains of *Neisseria meningitidis* (meningococci) have been reported so far. Besides this, age and seasonality and the place of acquiring the meningitis (community acquired versus nosocomial) are important epidemiological features in acute bacterial meningitis. Neonates and young children show a completely different pattern of pathogenic agents as do children and adolescents; these, again, show a different distribution of pathogenic agents compared to elderly and old patients. It is mainly age but also other predisposing factors like immunocompromised state, e.g. traumatic brain injury, preceding parameningeal infection (sinusitis, otitis, mastoiditis) which predispose patients to pneumococcal meningitis (Fig. 14.2). Neurosurgical interventions, open traumatic brain injury and invasive monitoring devices carry a high risk (up to 3 %/day) for nosocomial meningitis, caused by staphylococci or Gram negatives.

Fig. 14.2 Frontal sinusitis extending towards the meninges, causing pneumococcal meningitis with subdural empyema

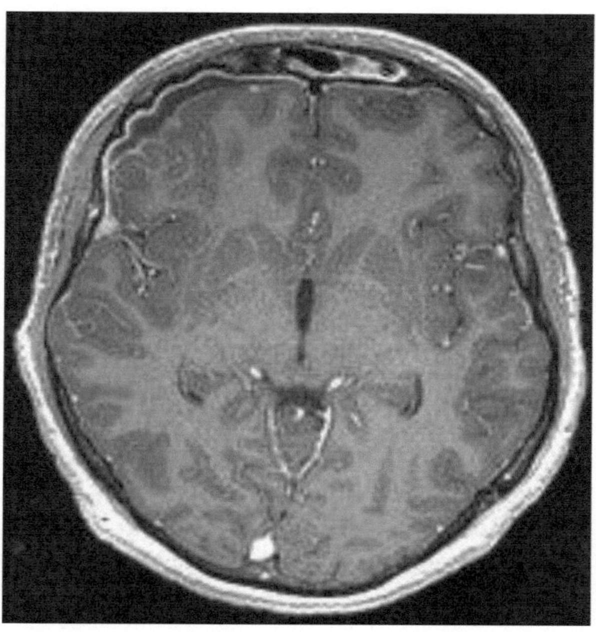

Community-acquired meningitis is usually caused by pneumococci or meningococci; in neonates, however, group B streptococci, *Listeria* spp. and Gram negatives are most frequently seen. In the elderly, potentially immunocompromised patients, pneumococci, *Listeria* spp. and Gram negatives are the major causative agents for bacterial meningitis. In nosocomial meningitis (hospital-acquired meningitis), staphylococci or streptococci other than *S. pneumoniae* and, in particular, Gram-negative rods (e.g. *Enterobacter* spp., *Klebsiella* spp., *Escherichia coli*, *Pseudomonas aeruginosa* or Acinetobacter spp.) are the most frequently seen pathogenic agents.

14.3.3 Pathogenesis and Pathophysiology

Table 14.6a lists the most common pathogens of bacterial meningitis with respect to age and Table 14.6b with respect to predisposing conditions (the latter in adults) (Roos and van de Beek 2010; Sellner et al. 2010).

Any bacterial pathogen which succeeds to cross the blood-brain barrier has the potential to cause acute bacterial meningitis. This sequence of events eventually leads to bacterial meningitis: colonisation of the host mucosal epithelium, successfully overcoming the local (mucosal) immune mechanisms (e.g. with the help of viral pharyngitis, laryngitis, rhinitis), invasion (and survival) within the intravascular space, arrival at the choroid plexus with successful crossing/penetration of the blood-brain barrier and, finally, survival and multiplication within the CSF. Replication and autolysis of bacteria lead to the release of bacterial cell wall components into the CSF, which is the most powerful stimulus to provoke the release of proinflammatory host factors (Mook-Kanamori et al. 2014; Sellner et al. 2010). Experimental and clinical studies have helped specify the complex

Table 14.6a Most common pathogens in acute bacterial meningiti

Age	Most common bacteria
<1 month	Gram-negative Enterobacteriaceae
	Streptococcus agalactiae (group B streptococci)
	Listeria monocytogenes
1 year – 12 months	*S. pneumoniae, N. meningitidis, H. influenzae* type B, *S. agalactiae, E. coli*
1 year – 18 years	*N. meningitidis, H. influenza* type B, *S. pneumoniae*
19–50 years	*S. pneumoniae, N. meningitidis*
>50 years	*S. pneumoniae, Listeria monocytogenes*, Enterobacteriaceae, *N. meningitidis*

Table 14.6b Acute bacterial meningitis: predisposing factor

Predisposing factor in adults	Typical pathogen
Healthy, immunocompetent (community acquired)	*S. pneumonia, N. meningitidis, L. monocytogenes*
Nosocomial (hospital acquired, post-neurosurgical, posttraumatic brain injury, device related (e.g. external ventricular drainage, etc.))	*Staphylococci*, Enterobacteriaceae, *Pseudomonas aeruginosa*
Shunt infection	*Staphylococcus epidermidis, Staphylococcus aureus*, Enterobacteriaceae, *Pseudomonas aeruginosa*
Immunosuppressed patients	*Listeria monocytogenes*, Enterobacteriaceae, *Pseudomonas aeruginosa*, pneumococci
Old/elderly patients	*Listeria monocytogenes*, pneumococci, Enterobacteriaceae

pathogenic network in bacterial meningitis. Part of this network are cytokines (interleukin 1β, interleukin 6, tumour necrosis factor-α), chemokines, reactive oxygen species and reactive nitrogen intermediates (Mook-Kanamori et al. 2014; Sellner et al. 2010). Such chemotactic factors, and induced adhesion molecules, mediate the massive influx of leucocytes into the CSF (Sellner et al. 2010). It is this complex pathogenic network which contributes to CNS complications and brain damage, as there is hydrocephalus, meningovasculitis, venous/sinus thrombosis, brain oedema and eventually increased intracranial pressure. Besides these intracranial pathophysiological processes, in many cases, life-threatening systemic signs and symptoms can be attributed to related septicaemia, septic shock and even Waterhouse-Friderichsen syndrome. Bilateral adrenal haemorrhage, as typically seen in Waterhouse-Friderichsen syndrome, is thought to be rather a terminal phenomenon than the immediate cause of a potentially fatal adrenal insufficiency. Patients with meningococcal septicaemia, with overwhelming pneumococcal sepsis syndrome (in splenectomised patients) (Adriani et al. 2013), and patients with accompanying Gram-negative sepsis syndrome are highly likely to develop multiorgan failure, including shock, coagulopathy, kidney and liver failure, myocardial failure, pericarditis, arthritis, intestinal failure and metabolic derangement including SIADH, hyperglycaemia, etc. All these aspects contribute to morbidity and mortality.

14.3.4 Clinical Features

Typically, acute bacterial meningitis presents with headache, fever, photophobia, vomiting and malaise, neck stiffness and, eventually, qualitative and/or quantitative impairment of consciousness and seizures (Bhimraj 2012). In the very old and in the very young as well as the deeply comatose patient, neck stiffness may be very mild or even absent. Almost every patient (>95 %) with acute bacterial meningitis complains at least of two of the four symptoms: headache, fever, neck stiffness and qualitative/quantitative impairment of consciousness. The potentially life-threatening clinical signs and symptoms can evolve very rapidly within few hours, thus, rendering the disease a true neurological emergency. It is the earliest possible diagnosis with the earliest possible initiation of antimicrobial chemotherapy and the necessary initiation of adjunctive therapeutic measures that are the most important factors in reducing morbidity and mortality. Purpura fulminans (on presentation) is typical for meningococcal meningitis and sepsis syndrome but can also be seen in staphylococcal or pneumococcal disease. About 10 % of meningococcal infection shows a fulminant meningococcal septicaemia (Waterhouse-Friderichsen syndrome) which is characterised by septic shock, large petechial haemorrhages, multiorgan failure and disseminated intravascular coagulation (Fig. 14.3a–d). Such petechiae need to be differentiated from Osler's spots (typically located on the fingers and toes) which are highly suggestive of infective endocarditis. In up to 15 %

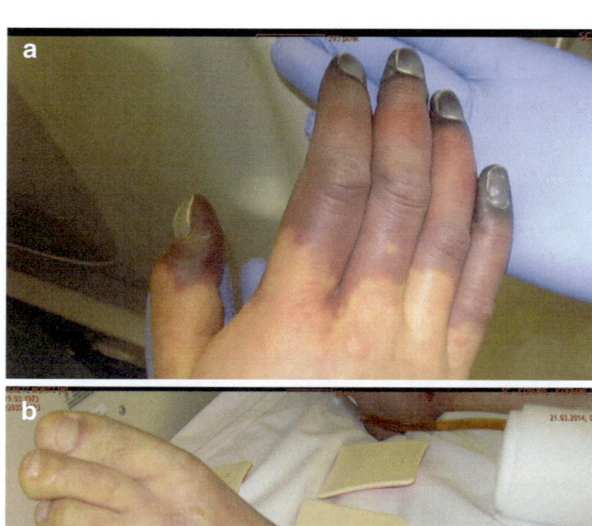

Fig. 14.3 (**a–d**) Meningococcal meningitis and meningococcal sepsis syndrome, purpura fulminans (**a**, **b**, day 3 after onset; **c**, **d**, day 19 after onset)

Fig. 14.3 (continued)

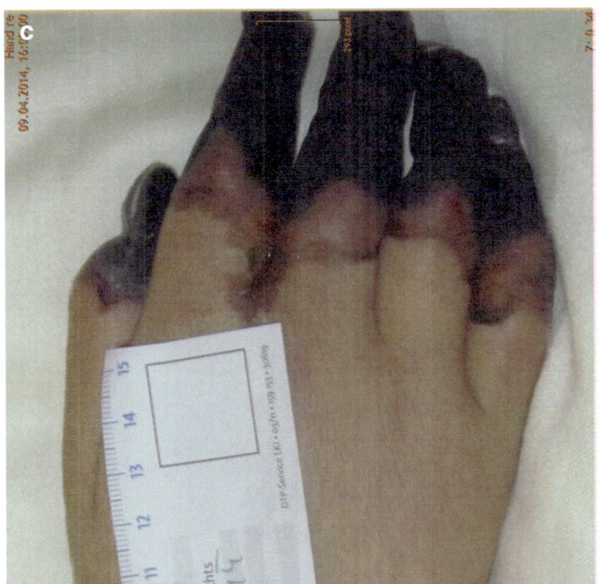

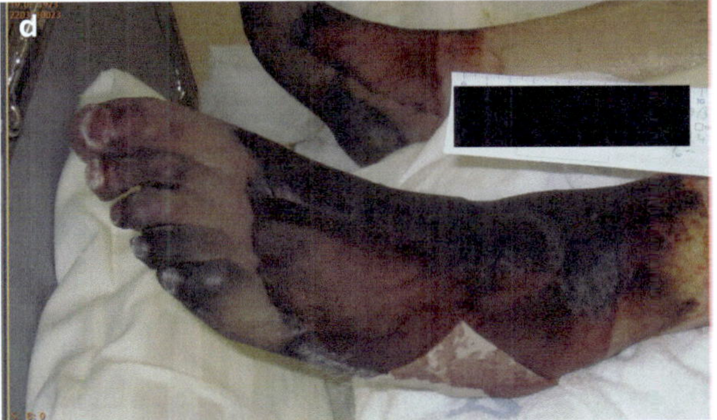

of patients with bacterial meningitis, focal neurological signs and symptoms may be found, suggesting brain abscess, subdural or epidural empyema, stroke or venous thrombosis (Alvis Miranda et al. 2013). Cranial nerve involvement is seen in approximately 10 % of patients with acute bacterial meningitis; seizures occur in up to a third of these patients.

The course of meningococcal disease is frequently characterised by sepsis syndrome and septic shock, whereas the course of pneumococcal meningitis more often is characterised by intracranial complications.

Posttraumatic bacterial meningitis is often clinically indistinguishable from community-acquired meningitis. Therefore, in any traumatic brain injury patient, fever, deterioration of consciousness and impairment of vital function may indicate the advent or the presence of acute nosocomial meningitis. The presence of a CSF leak clearly supports the notion of a nosocomial meningitis which might, however, be hard to detect.

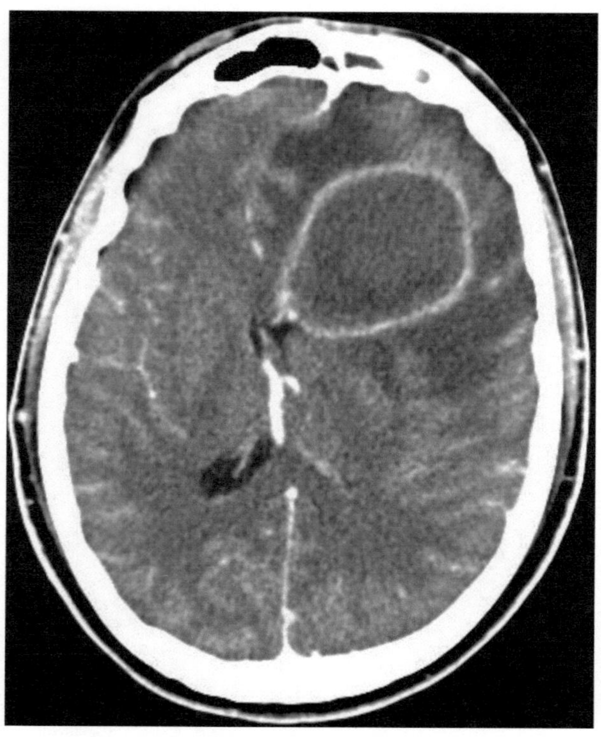

Fig. 14.4 Patient with clinical signs and symptoms of acute bacterial meningitis and left frontal focal signs – acute bacterial meningitis + frontal abscess

An infected permanent cerebrospinal fluid shunt usually causes a more insidious onset of disease with low-grade fever and with features typical for shunt malfunction, like headache, vomiting and impaired consciousness. Fever, usually a sign of CNS infection, is frequently absent in shunt infections. It should be noted that the peripheral part of the shunt may be infected without causing signs and symptoms of meningitis. Shunts draining into the venous system might produce a right-sided infective endocarditis; infection of shunts draining into the peritoneal cavity may produce focal or even diffuse peritonitis (Aftab and Shoaib 2013).

14.3.5 Diagnostic Features

The history, in particular the presence of predisposing factors or meningococcal disease in contact persons, the typical signs and symptoms of acute bacterial meningitis and/or sepsis syndrome are highly suggestive for the disease. The positive proof of the diagnosis can only be done by examining the cerebrospinal fluid. Every patient with suspected bacterial meningitis needs a spinal tap (Glimåker et al. 2013b); however, before that, neuroimaging is indicated if the patient shows impairment of consciousness and/or focal neurological signs and symptoms (Brouwer et al. 2014) (Fig. 14.4). In such a case, the administration of the first dose of the empirical antibiotic must never be delayed simply because of waiting for the

Table 14.7 Emergency algorithm for a patient with suspected acute bacterial meningitis (Bhimraj 2012; Brouwer et al. 2012; Glimåker et al. 2013a; Heckenberg et al. 2014; Roos and van de Beek 2010)

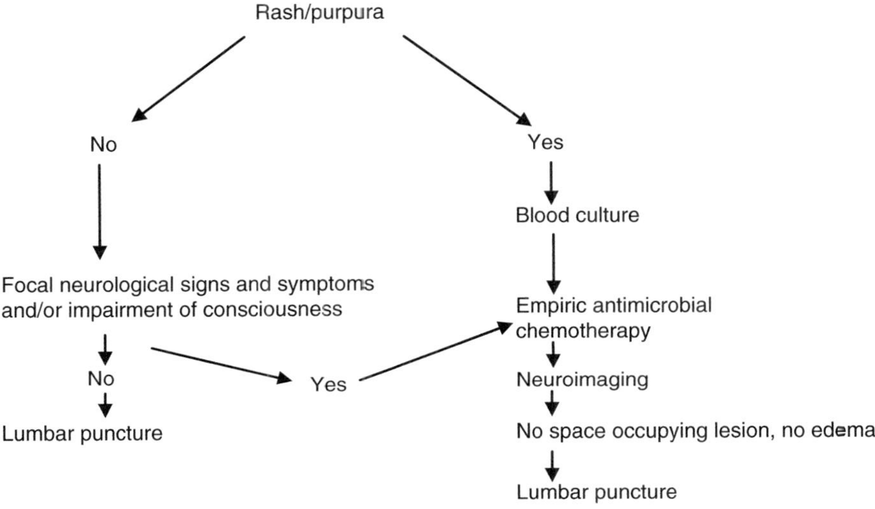

neuroimaging. The very simple algorithm shown in Table 14.7 allows the best possible emergency care management of a patient with bacterial meningitis.

14.3.6 Non-CSF Laboratory Analyses

In acute bacterial meningitis, septic shock is reflected by deranged laboratory parameters indicating multiple organ failure, in particular coagulation, kidney and/or liver failure. Typically, leucocyte count, C-reactive protein and, slightly later, procalcitonin are highly elevated.

14.3.7 Cerebrospinal Fluid (CSF)

With a pathological CSF analysis, it is important to discriminate between viral meningitis and the potentially life-threatening bacterial meningitis. The CSF in bacterial meningitis typically shows polymorphonuclear leucocytosis, decreased glucose concentration, in particular, markedly decreased CSF/serum glucose ratio, increased protein concentration and, most sensitively, increased CSF lactate. More than 90 % of patients with acute bacterial meningitis show a CSF pleocytosis of more than 1,000/μl: only in the very old or immunocompromised patient the leucocyte count in the CSF might be low or even very low. With the normal CSF glucose concentration being approximately 60–70 % of the serum glucose, any CSF/serum glucose ratio below 0.4 is considered indicative of acute bacterial meningitis (Glimåker et al. 2013a; Hasbun et al. 2013; Heckenberg et al. 2014; Roos and van de Beek 2010; Welch and Hasbun 2010).

CSF Gram stain, CSF PCR and CSF culture are essential components for diagnosing acute bacterial meningitis. Gram staining of CSF permits a rapid identification of the pathogens with a sensitivity of up to 90 % and a specificity even beyond 90 %. If a patient has received antibiotics prior to the lumbar puncture, CSF culture will yield a positive result in 40–50 %, whereas CSF Gram stain and CSF PCR still show a positive result in up to 90 %. Latex particle agglutination tests for detecting antigens of the various pathogenic agents do not increase the diagnostic yield and are no longer advised. It is in particular the PCR which has proven to add to the diagnostic accuracy, in particular if antibiotics have already been administered. Nevertheless, culture of the CSF is and will remain the golden standard for diagnosing acute bacterial meningitis, and the lumbar puncture is obligatory (in the sequence of events according to Table 14.7). Blood culture, culture from parameningeal foci and skin biopsy cultures may add to the diagnostic yield (Welch and Hasbun 2010).

14.3.8 Differential Diagnosis

A subacute course of tuberculous meningitis, as seen in patients on immunosuppressive therapies, fungal meningitis, fulminant meningitis due to free-living amoebae, carcinomatous meningitis, infective endocarditis with septic embolism (Fernández Guerrero et al. 2012; Ferro and Fonseca 2014) and parameningeal purulent infectious foci such as spinal/intracranial epidural abscess or subdural empyema and brain abscess need to be considered in the differential diagnostic discussion (Bijlsma et al. 2013; Brouwer et al. 2013a; Greenblatt et al. 2013). Similarly, sinus or intracranial venous thrombosis, subarachnoid haemorrhage and even severe migraine might be on the list of differential diagnoses.

14.3.9 Therapeutic Management

In every patient with acute bacterial meningitis, immediate diagnosis and immediate initiation of the best possible empirical antibiotic therapy are essential to reduce morbidity and mortality (Deghmane et al. 2009; Forestier 2009; Klein et al. 2009; Pines 2008; Roos and van de Beek 2010; Tessier and Scheid 2010). Table 14.8 shows the proposed algorithm, which aims to reduce both unnecessary delay of empirical antibiotic therapy and the risk of secondary damage due to herniation, brain abscess rupture etc.

It is the age which determines the likelihood of the pathogens causing bacterial meningitis, thus guiding the empirical antimicrobial therapy. Table 14.9 lists the empirical antimicrobial chemotherapy according to the age (and, hence, the most likely and most common pathogen in the respective age group).

Table 14.8   Algorithm of therapeutic management in acute bacterial meningitis (Bhimraj 2012; Brouwer et al. 2013b; Klein et al. 2009; Pines 2008; Roos and van de Beek 2010; Tessier and Scheid 2010)

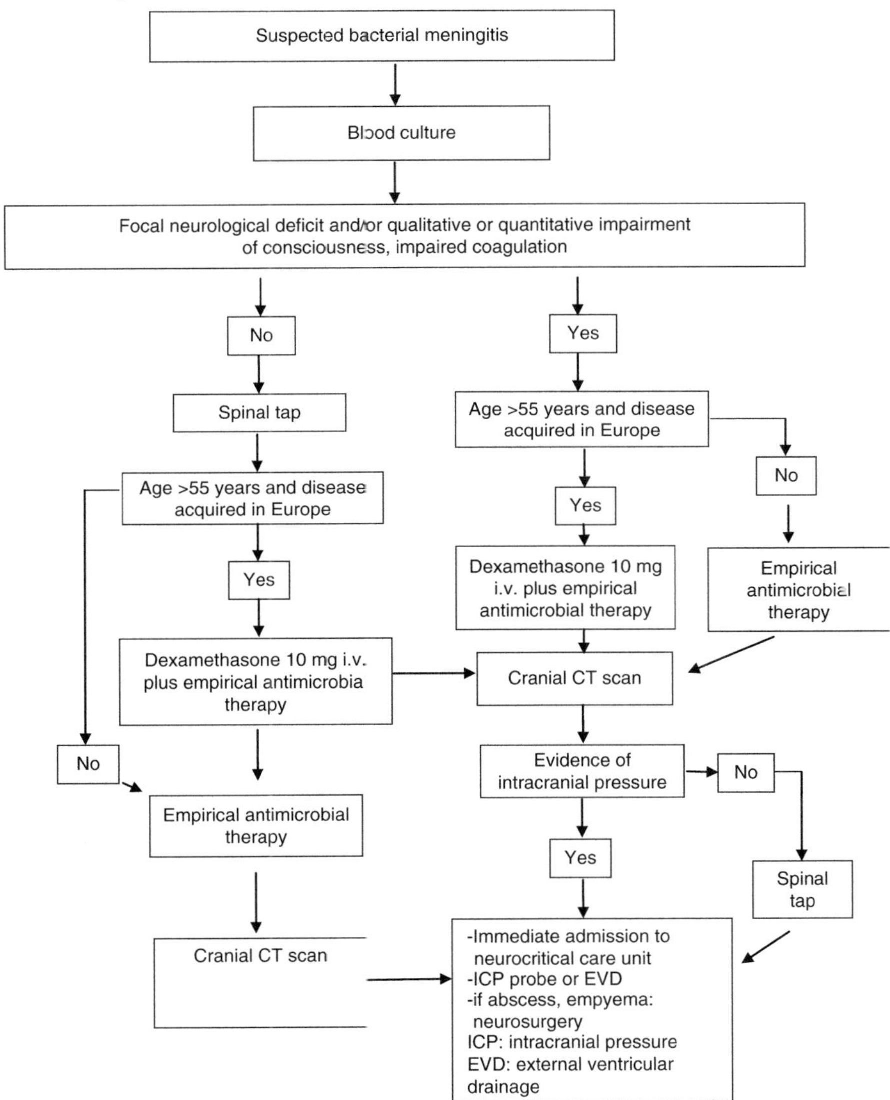

Table 14.10 lists the initial semiempirical antibiotic therapy for acute bacterial meningitis depending on the predisposing factors and the predisposing clinical condition.

If, by Gram stain PCR or culture, the pathogen finally has been determined, a de-escalation of the antimicrobial chemotherapy is recommended. Those antimicrobial chemotherapeutic agents which should be used in patients with bacterial meningitis and defined pathogen are listed in Table 14.11.

Table 14.9 Empirical antimicrobial chemotherapy according to the age group (Bhimraj 2012; Roos and van de Beek 2010; Tessier and Scheid 2010)

Age	Typical microorganisms	Recommended antibiotic regimen
<1 month	Gram-negative Enterobacteriaceae	Cefotaxime plus ampicillin
	(*E. coli, Klebsiella, Enterobacter, Proteus*)	Ampicillin plus
	S. agalactiae	Aminoglycoside
1–23 months	*S. pneumoniae, N. meningitidis, S. agalactiae, H. influenzae, E. coli*	Ceftriaxone (plus vancomycin)
2–50 years	*N. meningitidis, S. pneumoniae*	Ceftriaxone (plus vancomycin)
>50 years	*S. pneumoniae, N. meningitidis, Listeria monocytogenes,* Enterobacteriaceae	Ceftriaxone (plus vancomycin) plus ampicillin

Table 14.10 Initial empirical antibiotic therapy for bacterial meningitis in adults (Bhimraj 2012; Roos and van de Beek 2010; Tessier and Scheid 2010)

Clinical condition	Typical pathogens	Recommended antibiotics
Immunocompetent, community acquired	*S. pneumoniae, N. meningitidis* *L. monocytogenes*	Ceftriaxone (plus vancomycin) plus ampicillin
Nosocomial (e.g. post-neurosurgical or posttraumatic brain injury) ventriculitis, meningitis shunt infection	Staphylococci, Enterobacteriaceae, *P. aeruginosa, S. epidermidis,* *S. aureus,* Enterobacteriaceae, *P. aeruginosa*	Ceftazidime (or meropenem) plus vancomycin
		Ceftazidime (or meropenem) plus vancomycin
Immunosuppressed or older patients (T-cell immunodeficiency)	*L. monocytogenes,* Enterobacteriaceae, *P. aeruginosa,* pneumococci	Ceftazidime plus vancomycin plus ampicillin

Nosocomial meningitis, ventriculo-meningitis or ventriculitis need to be treated according to the local (hospital based) resistance pattern of the most likely pathogens, e.g. *Staphylococcus epidermidis, Staphylococcus aureus* and *Enterobacteriaceae.* In such a clinical setting, either third (fourth)-generation cephalosporin or meropenem in combination with vancomycin or fosfomycin is recommended. Intraventricular vancomycin may be used for catheter (EVD)-associated ventriculitis caused by staphylococci. Linezolid has an antimicrobial efficacy similar to vancomycin or teicoplanin and shows a good blood-brain barrier penetration (Roos and van de Beek 2010; van de Beek et al. 2010).

Whether antimicrobial chemotherapy should be given as a bolus or in a continuous infusion is still a matter of discussion, most recent studies point towards the superiority of continuous administration (at least over a period of 2–4 h given by means of an injection pump) (Roos and van de Beek 2010; van de Beek et al. 2010).

The duration of antibiotic therapy is determined by the causative agent: meningococci need a minimum of 5 days, pneumococci most likely 10–14 days and

Table 14.11 Recommended antibiotics for treatment of bacterial meningitis (Bhimraj 2012; Roos and van de Beek 2010; Tessier and Scheid 2010; Thwaites 2014)

Causative organism	Drugs of choice	Alternatives
N. meningitidis	Penicillin G	Ceftriaxone (or cefotaxime), ampicillin, rifampin
S. pneumoniae, penicillin susceptible	Penicillin G (or ampicillin)	Ceftriaxone (or cefotaxime)
S. pneumoniae, penicillin tolerant (MIC 0,1–1 mg/ml)	Ceftriaxone (or cefotaxime)	Meropenem, cefepime
S. pneumoniae, penicillin resistant (MIC 1 mg/ml)	Ceftriaxone + vancomycin or ceftriaxone + rifampin	Meropenem, cefepime
H. influenzae group B streptococci	Ceftriaxone (or cefotaxime)	Ampicillin plus chloramphenicol
	Penicillin G (± gentamicin)	Ceftriaxone, ampicillin (plus gentamicin), vancomycin
Gram-negative Enterobacteriaceae (e.g. *Klebsiella*, *E. coli*, *Proteus*)	Ceftriaxone (or cefotaxime)	Meropenem, cefepime, aminoglycoside
Pseudomonas aeruginosa	Ceftazidime (± gentamicin)	Meropenem, cefepime
Staphylococci (methicillin susceptible)	Nafcillin	Fosfomycin, vancomycin (or flucloxacillin)
Staphylococci (methicillin resistant)	Vancomycin	Trimethoprim-sulfamethoxazole, rifampin, linezolid
Listeria monocytogenes	Ampicillin (± gentamicin)	Trimethoprim-sulfamethoxazole, meropenem
Bacteroides fragilis	Metronidazole	Meropenem, clindamycin

MIC minimal inhibitory concentration

Listeria spp. and Gram negatives for a minimum of 3 weeks (Roos and van de Beek 2010; Tessier and Scheid 2010; van de Beek et al. 2010).

14.3.10 Adjunctive Therapies

Accompanying meningovasculitis leading to stroke, diffuse brain oedema and hydrocephalus, pyocephalus, empyema and brain abscess, sinus or intracranial venous thrombosis are the most frequent intracranial complications and need to be monitored, actively looked for and managed within a neurocritical care unit (Edberg et al. 2011; Glimåker et al. 2014). Very recently, it has been shown that in case of impaired consciousness, the placement of an intracranial pressure monitoring probe and external ventricular drainage may reduce mortality from 30 to 10 % (Glimåker et al. 2014). Therefore, every patient with acute bacterial meningitis and impaired consciousness needs to be monitored for intracranial pressure in a specialised neurocritical care unit. The diffuse brain oedema does not respond to osmotherapy (Ajdukiewicz et al. 2011;

Wall et al. 2013). In the case of therapy-refractory elevated ICP (i.e. nonresponding to deepening of analgosedation, cautious hyperventilation, external ventricular drainage), second-tier management strategies need to be employed; they may include therapeutic hypothermia, barbiturate coma and even decompressive craniotomy (Mourvillier et al. 2013; Nau et al. 2013; Wall et al. 2013).

14.3.11 Prevention

In patients/subjects having had close (kissing mouth) contact with patients with meningococcal disease or *H. influenzae* type B meningitis, chemotherapeutic prophylactic therapy with rifampicin (600 mg p.i.d., for 2 days) or ciprofloxacin (500 mg once) is recommended.

For *H. influenzae* type B, all important serogroups of *Streptococcus pneumoniae* and, by now, all important serogroups of *Neisseria meningitidis*, active immunisation is available (Roos and van de Beek 2010).

14.3.12 Prognosis

By employing both the quickest possible and the best possible antimicrobial chemotherapy, the mortality rate of patients with pure acute bacterial meningitis should be below 10 %, even if the initial clinical situation is dangerously bad (GCS <8). However, in the case of pre-existing immunocompromised conditions (e.g. splenectomy), pneumococcal meningitis might evolve into an overwhelming pneumococcal sepsis syndrome, and in up to 50 % of the patients with serogroup B or serogroup C meningococcal disease, the course of the disease is characterised by a sepsis syndrome with impairment of the adrenal function, coagulopathy, multiorgan failure and necrosis of the extremities, in the worst case being purpura fulminans (Waterhouse-Friderichsen syndrome), a condition which still has a very high morbidity and mortality (up to 50 %).

The most common long-term sequela in bacterial meningitis is hearing impairment. Consequences of ischaemic stroke, increased intracranial pressure and sinus thrombosis might cause diffuse or focal neurological long-term damage (including epileptic seizures) (Roos and van de Beek 2010).

14.4 Acute Fungal Infections of the Central Nervous System

14.4.1 Introduction

Over the last few decades, fungal infections of the central nervous system have been increasingly diagnosed. This is due to increased awareness, advances in neuroimaging, microbiological and molecular biological diagnostic techniques and the rapid expansion of patients being immunocompromised or immunosuppressed and may

Table 14.12 Central nervous system in invasive fungal disease (Gullo et al. 2013; Lahoti and Berger 2013; Murthy and Sundaram 2014)

Fungi	Neurological presentation	Predisposing condition
Candida spp.	Meningitis, (micro-)abscesses	Long-term hospitalisation, long-term antibacterial chemotherapy, critical care patient
Cryptococcus neoformans spp.	Subacute, chronic meningitis, hydrocephalus, rarely cryptococcoma	HIV and other cellular-derived immunocompromised state
Aspergillus spp.	Meningovasculitis, brain abscess	Immunocompromised state, e.g. s.p. organ transplantation
Histoplasma spp.	Meningitis, granuloma	Geographic exposure, Latin America, Southern USA
Blastomyces spp.	Granuloma, meningitis	Geographic exposure, HIV, Africa, USA-Mississippi valley
Zygomycetes	Meningitis, granuloma, in particular, rhinocerebral form, meningovasculitis	Immunosuppression diabetes mellitus, in particular, diabetic ketoacidosis renal failure, severe burns and penetrating injuries
Coccidioides immitis	Meningitis, rarely meningovasculitis	Geographic exposure (southern USA, Mexico, South America)

even be iatrogenically caused. It is mainly the latter condition which has led to a sharp increase in systemic fungal infection, frequently associated with central nervous system involvement. The type of central nervous system involvement is listed in Table 14.12.

14.4.2 Epidemiology

An immunocompromised state might be caused by HIV infection, organ transplantation, immunosuppressive chemotherapy, chronic corticosteroid therapy, malignancies in particular chemotherapy of malignant diseases, and other chronic conditions, in particular autoimmune diseases. However, several fungal pathogens may also be seen in fully immunocompetent patients, in particular *Coccidioides immitis* causing acute or subacute meningitis, *Histoplasma* spp. causing meningitis or granuloma and *Cryptococcus* spp. causing mainly basally accentuated meningitis. In few patients, even aspergillus granuloma or abscess formation has been seen in immunocompetent individuals (Gullo et al. 2013; Lahoti and Berger 2013; Murthy and Sundaram 2014; Pappas 2013).

14.4.3 Aetiology and Pathogenesis

The fungal pathogens, causing acute-subacute infection of the central nervous system, are listed in Table 14.12. Fungi are saprophytic organisms, found almost everywhere in soil, vegetation, skin and faeces of mammals or birds. It is usually the route via inhalation into the lung which allows entrance of fungal spoors into the body, colonising the mucosae. Secondarily, fungi spread to the lung but also haematogeneously to other organs, e.g. central nervous system. However, CNS invasion can also be by direct extension from neighbouring structures such as paranasal sinuses, pharynx or middle ear.

14.4.4 Clinical Features

Table 14.12 lists the most important clinical features of fungal infection: acute-subacute (also chronic) meningitis, granuloma formation, meningovasculitis and even spinal cord involvement. Of specific note is the rhinocerebral form in case of colonised paranasal sinuses by Zygomycetes. It is the focal destructive process which involves the orbit, eye, optic nerve and frontobasal brain, even involving the sinus cavernosus, eye and regional blood vessels causing blindness by central retinal artery thrombosis. Moulds, in particular, *Aspergillus* but also Zygomycetes, are the major cause of cerebrovascular fungal diseases causing stroke syndrome. Fungal mycotic aneurysmal subarachnoid haemorrhage is rarely seen but typically associated with very poor outcome. In rare cases spinal syndromes have been reported, either due to focal granuloma or epidural abscess or involvement of spinal arteries (Gullo et al. 2013; Lahoti and Berger 2013; Murthy and Sundaram 2014).

14.4.5 Diagnostic Features

It is mainly the history, the presence of predisposing factors (immunocompromised state) and geographic exposure which should draw the attention, in association with specific clinical features, towards a possible fungal aetiology (Jarvis et al. 2013; Murthy and Sundaram 2014).

14.4.6 CSF

Whereas in cryptococcal meningitis, a lymphocytic pleocytosis is typically found; a mixture of neutrophils and monocytes predominates in candida infection, blastomycosis, histoplasmosis and, also, *Aspergillus* spp. infection. However, the latter frequently shows a predominantly neutrophilic pleocytosis, which is also seen in coccidioides meningitis; this fungal pathogen, however, is frequently associated with CSF eosinophilia. Patients who are immunocompromised/immunosuppressed frequently show a very low level of pleocytosis; in the acute – subacute – course of the disease, the CSF glucose may be mildly decreased; CSF protein is definitely increased. Cryptococci can be found by India ink preparation. Cryptococcal antigen assays, *Histoplasma* antigen detection in the CSF and complement fixation antigen assays are positive in more than 80 % of cases of active cryptococcal, *Histoplasma* or coccidioidal meningeal infection (Murthy and Sundaram 2014; Yansouni et al. 2013).

14.4.7 Serum Antigens and Antibodies

Serum antigen determination for *Cryptococcus* (Jarvis et al. 2013) or *Histoplasma* antigen has a specificity of more than 98 %, while the sensitivity is rather low in HIV-negative patients (Jarvis et al. 2013; Murthy and Sundaram 2014).

14.4.8 Fungus-Specific Markers

1,3-beta-d-glucan is a cell wall component of fungi and has been used as a diagnostic adjuvant in invasive fungal infections. It serves as a preliminary screening tool in the case of invasive fungal disease; however, it needs to be noted that 1,3-beta-d-glucan is always negative in infection by Zygomycetes. Other rather unspecific fungal antigens include mannan (*Candida* spp.), galactomannan (*Aspergillus* spp.) and galactoxylomannan (*Cryptococcus* spp.). These molecules are cell wall polysaccharides which are released by the fungi during growth. The most intriguing aspect is that these circulating molecules can be detected up to 1 week before the development of clinical signs and symptoms of systemic fungal disease. Sensitivity (for the galactomannan test) has been reported to be almost 90 % with a specificity of >98 % (Murthy and Sundaram 2014; Yansouni et al. 2013).

14.4.9 Microbiological/Mycological Diagnosis

Fungal cultures are time consuming and laborious; for this reason, molecular biologic-based methods offer a highly specific and rather sensitive way to diagnose within a shorter time. Detection of fungal DNA by means of PCR allows a microbiologically based decision for the initiation of antifungal chemotherapy (Murthy and Sundaram 2014).

14.4.10 Neuroimaging, Histology

Neuroimaging will confirm the clinically suspected neurological features as there are basal meningitis, meningovasculitis, hydrocephalus and, in particular, granuloma formation. It is mainly the latter which will guide the decision to do biopsy, thereby allowing best possible confirmation diagnosis.

Table 14.13 Therapy in CNS mycoses (Jarvis et al. 2013; Katchanov et al. 2014; Murthy and Sundaram 2014)

Fungal pathogen	Antifungal agent
Aspergillus spp.	Amphotericin B (liposomal amphotericin B), voriconazole, posaconazole, Caspofungin
Candida spp.	Amphotericin B, fluconazole, voriconazole, caspofungin, anidulafungin, flucytosine
Cryptococcus spp.	Combination therapy: amphotericin B and 5-flucytocine; fluconazole
Coccidioides spp.	Liposomal amphotericin
Blastomyces spp.	Liposomal amphotericin, ketoconazole (non-immunocompromised)
Histoplasma spp.	Liposomal amphotericin, amphotericin B lipid complex, ketoconazole (non-immunocompromised)
Zygomycetes	Liposomal amphotericin, amphotericin B lipid complex

14.4.11 Therapy

Both the earliest possible initiation of antifungal therapy and the earliest possible reversal of the underlying host immunodeficiency are the cornerstones of treatment of CNS fungal infection. However, inflammatory responses triggered off by rapid improvement of the immune status can lead to localised and systemic reactions which are termed immune reconstitution inflammatory syndrome (IRIS), transitorily aggravating and deteriorating the neurological signs and symptoms.

Table 14.13 lists those antifungal agents which should be used if the specific diagnosis of CNS mycosis has been confirmed.

In rhinocerebral zygomycosis, neuroimaging is essential. Besides antifungal therapy, aggressive surgical debridement of necrotic tissue is required.

14.4.12 Prognosis

Prognosis depends on the underlying immunocompromised condition, earliest possible diagnosis, initiation of therapy and earliest possible recognition of immune reconstitution syndrome.

14.5 Protozoal Infection and Infestation of the Nervous System

14.5.1 Introduction

Protozoa and metazoa (mainly helminths) can directly or indirectly cause severe impairment of central nervous system function (Abdel Razek et al. 2011; Kristensson et al. 2013). Amoebae, *Toxoplasma gondii* and *Trypanosoma* spp. may readily invade the central nervous system causing abscess formation, acute meningoencephalitis, granuloma formation or chronic encephalitis, whereas *Babesia* spp. and *Plasmodium*

Table 14.14 Protozoal infections of the CNS (Abdel Razek et al. 2011; Schmutzhard and Helbok 2014)

Pathogenic agent	Pathogenetic mechanism, neurological syndrome	Geographic distribution
Free-living amoebae	Granuloma, fulminant meningitis	Temperate climate zones
Babesia divergens	Anaemia-hypoxic encephalopathy	Only in splenectomised, USA, Europe
Entamoeba histolytica	Brain abscess	Tropical/subtropical areas
Plasmodium falciparum	Cerebral malaria (impairment of microcirculation)	Tropical regions, mainly Sub-Saharan Africa, Papua New Guinea, Solomon Islands
Toxoplasma gondii	Granuloma, encephalitis (immunocompromised state – HIV)	Worldwide
Trypanosoma brucei rhodesiense/gambiense	Subacute/chronic encephalitis	Tropical Africa
Trypanosoma cruzi	Subacute meningitis and myocarditis	Latin America

falciparum cause potentially life-threatening CNS disease via indirect affection of the brain (Aird et al. 2014; Hawkes et al. 2013; Ho 2014; Ioannidis et al. 2014).

14.5.2 Epidemiology

Table 14.14 lists the protozoa which have the capacity to cause neurologic disease, the neurological syndrome, the pathogenetic mechanisms and the geographic distribution.

14.5.3 Clinical Features

It is mainly the history, in particular the history of exposure, as well as the predisposing underlying condition (HIV, etc.) which directs the differential diagnostic consideration towards protozoal disease. Babesiosis and, in particular, the much more frequent cerebral malaria show normal CSF; diagnosis is made in such patients by means of blood film examination showing intraerythrocytic ring forms in Giemsa stain. Cerebral malaria with multiorgan failure due to *Plasmodium falciparum* infection is a further typical hallmark of this life-threatening disease (Ho 2014; Ioannidis et al. 2014; Masocha and Kristensson 2012; Pittella 2013; Sondgeroth et al. 2013). *Entamoeba histolytica* brain abscess is only seen in patients suffering from concomitant liver abscess. Free-living amoeba (in particular *Naegleria fowleri*), occurring worldwide, invades the human host through the mouth/nasal mucosa via the olfactory route (when water enters the nostrils or the mouth) and causes a fulminant purulent meningitis, rapidly progressing to coma and death. It is the acute purulent, bacterial meningitis which is the major differential diagnosis. Therefore, such a fulminant frequently fatal disease is to be suspected when the patient reports a history of exposure to fresh water (jumping into swimming pools, etc.) in summertime.

Subacute meningitis due to *Trypanosoma cruzi* infection is to be suspected after exposure to the transmitting vector (reduviid bugs) in Latin America. Frequently, this meningitis is associated with myocarditis. Very rarely, *Trypanosoma brucei rhodesiense* presents as subacute encephalitis; typically, the course of the disease in sleeping sickness is chronic, i.e. over weeks and months.

14.5.4 Diagnostic Features

It is mainly the history which draws the attention towards this type of diseases. Detailed consultation of a tropical medical specialist is advised. Depending on the type of the disease, neuroimaging (Jayakumar et al. 2013), microbiological and molecular biological techniques are indicated. CSF examination shows an extremely broad variety of changes, ranging from a mild IgM increase and mild pleocytosis in sleeping sickness towards a purulent CSF with thousands of polymorphonuclear neutrophils per µl, high CSF protein and low CSF glucose (in purulent meningitis due to free-living amoebae) or having virtually normal CSF as seen in *Toxoplasma gondii*, cerebral malaria or infection by *Babesia* spp.

14.5.5 Therapy

In those protozoal diseases which show an acute or even peracute course of disease, the earliest possible diagnosis and the quickest possible initiation of specific antiprotozoal therapy are essential. In patients with purulent meningitis due to free-living amoebae (*Naegleria fowleri*), immediate initiation of amphotericin B combined with intravenous miconazole or – alternatively – amphotericin B combined with rifampicin is absolutely essential. Miconazole, however, should never be combined with rifampicin. A similarly dramatic course of disease may be seen in cerebral malaria; in such a suspected patient, immediate initiation of intravenous artesunate (if not available, intravenous quinine) is the cornerstone of therapy. Adjunctive therapeutic measures include ICU management and recognition and therapy of complications (e.g. hydrocephalus, brain oedema, etc.).

14.6   Helminthic Infections and Infestations of the Central Nervous System

14.6.1 Introduction and Epidemiology

Helminths and arthropods are metazoa which can have the capacity to penetrate the blood-brain barrier, thus invading intracranial structures.

Table 14.15 Larvae migrantes of the CNS (Finsterer and Auer 2013; Schmutzhard and Helbok 2014)

Species	Geographic distribution	Neurological features
Angiostrongylus cantonensis and *Angiostrongylus costaricensis*	Meningitis, cranial nerve involvement	East Asia, Central America
Gnathostoma spinigerum	Meninges, spinal cord, nerve roots, brain	South East Asia, in rare cases in Eastern Africa
Strongyloides stercoralis	In immunocompromised (HIV): hyperinfection syndrome accompanied with purulent Gram-negative meningitis and sepsis syndrome	Worldwide
Toxocara canis and *Toxocara cati*	Rarely focal neurological signs and symptoms, vasculitis, typically ocular larva migrans	Worldwide
Trichinella spp.	Myositis, rarely encephalitis	Worldwide

Most helminthoses of the central nervous system cause a subacute or chronic disease. They may invade in various stages of development into the brain or spinal cord causing focal or generalised neurological signs and symptoms. *Echinococcus* spp., *Paragonimus* spp., *Schistosoma* spp. and *Cysticercus cellulosae* may cause space-occupying lesions, eventually leading to increased intracranial pressure, epileptic seizures or focal and diffuse encephalopathy (Abdel Razek et al. 2011; Chai 2013; Coyle 2013; Del Brutto 2014; Finsterer and Auer 2013; McConkey et al. 2013; Nicoletti 2013; Petri and Hague 2013; Postels and Birbeck 2013; Rodgers 2010; Schmutzhard and Helbok 2014; Singh et al. 2013; Sondgeroth et al. 2013; Tudisco et al. 2013).

14.6.2 Clinical Features

The infestation with larvae of certain nematodes, as *Angiostrongylus* spp., *Gnathostoma spinigerum*, *Strongyloides stercoralis*, *Trichinella spiralis* and *Toxocara* spp., usually causes a syndrome called larva migrans visceralis. On their route through the body of the host, they may invade the central nervous system causing an eosinophilic meningitis, radiculitis, cranial nerve neuritis, myelitis and even encephalitis and, in rare cases, subarachnoid haemorrhage. The hallmark of these diseases is a high-grade eosinophilia in the peripheral blood and the CSF. In rare cases, haemorrhage in the CSF may be seen (mainly in *Gnathostoma spinigerum* infestation). Table 14.15 lists those nematodes which are frequently seen as the cause of eosinophilic CNS infection, their geographic distribution and the typical neurological involvement

The fish tapeworm, *Diphyllobothrium latum*, may cause a subacute syndrome of folic acid deficiency, thereby leading to the neurological syndrome of myelopathy, neuropathy and even encephalopathy. *Diphyllobothrium latum* has been reported from Europe, East Asia and Latin America and is acquired by ingestion of raw freshwater fish (Schmutzhard and Helbok 2014).

14.6.3 Diagnostic Features

The direct visualisation of the causative pathogen (e.g. migrating larva) confirms the diagnosis (Tudisco et al. 2013); in the case of eosinophilic meningitis or meningoradiculitis, the history (geographic exposure ingestion of suspected food) guides the differential diagnosis. Serological examination might be helpful to confirm the diagnosis (Rodriguez et al. 2012; Schmutzhard and Helbok 2014; Singh et al. 2013). Neuroimaging may also aid in the diagnosis (Abdel Razek et al. 2011; Lerner et al. 2012; MacLean et al. 2013; McConkey et al. 2013; Petri and Hague 2013; Pittella 2013).

14.6.4 Therapy

Although for those worms/larvae causing acute CNS disease the best possible anthelmintic therapy has not been evaluated in prospective and randomised studies, azole therapies (in particular albendazole) have been used and have been shown to reduce clinical signs and symptoms and the duration of the disease and to lower the frequency of long-term sequelae.

References

Abdel Razek AA, Watcharakorn A, Castillo M (2011) Parasitic diseases of the central nervous system. Neuroimaging Clin N Am 21:815–841

Adriani KS, Brouwer MC, van der Ende A, van de Beek D (2013) Bacterial meningitis in adults after splenectomy. Mayo Clin Proc 88:571–578

Aftab K, Shoaib M (2013) Nosocomial bacterial meningitis – prevention rather than cure! J Pak Med Assoc 63(7):945

Aird WC, Mosnier LO, Fairhurst RM (2014) Plasmodium falciparum picks (on) EPCR. Blood 123:163–167

Ajdukiewicz KM, Cartwright KE, Scarborough M, Mwambene JB, Goodson P, Molyneux ME et al (2011) Glycerol adjuvant therapy in adults with bacterial meningitis in a high HIV seroprevalence setting in Malawi: a double-blind, randomised controlled trial. Lancet Infect Dis 11:293–300

Alvis Miranda H, Castellar-Leones SM, Elzain MA, Moscote-Salazar LR (2013) Brain abscess: current management. J Neurosci Rural Pract 4:67–81

Auriel E, Regev K, Korczyn AD (2014) Nonsteroidal anti-inflammatory drugs exposure and the central nervous system. Handb Clin Neurol 119:577–584

Bhimraj A (2012) Acute community-acquired bacterial meningitis in adults: an evidence-based review. Cleve Clin J Med 79:393–400

Bijlsma MW, Brouwer MC, van de Beek D (2013) Prognostic risk score for pleocytosis with a negative gram stain: valid but of limited utility in bacterial meningitis patients. Mayo Clin Proc 88:421

Bijlsma MW, Brouwer MC, van den Kerkhof H, Knol MJ, van de Beek D, van der Ende A (2014) No evidence of clusters of serogroup C meningococcal disease in the Dutch MSM community. J Infect 68:296–297

Blasi F, Tarsia P, Aliberti S (2009) Chlamydophila pneumoniae. Clin Microbiol Infect 15(1):29–35

Brouwer MC, Thwaites GE, Tunkel AR, van de Beek D (2012) Dilemmas in the diagnosis of acute community-acquired bacterial meningitis. Lancet 380:1684–1692

Brouwer MC, Jim KK, Benschop KS, Benschop KS, Wolthers KC, van der Ende A, de Jong MD, van de Beek D (2013a) No evidence of viral coinfection in cerebrospinal fluid from patients with community-acquired bacterial meningitis. J Infect Dis 208(1):182–184

Brouwer MC, McIntyre P, Prasad K, van de Beek D (2013) Corticosteroids for acute bacterial meningitis. Cochrane Database Syst Rev 6:CD004405

Brouwer MC, Coutinho JM, van de Beek D (2014) Clinical characteristics and outcome of brain abscess: systematic review and meta-analysis. Neurology 4(82):806–813

Chai JY (2013) Paragonimiasis. Handb Clin Neurol 114:283–296

Coyle CM (2013) Schistosomiasis of the nervous system. Handb Clin Neurol 114:271–281

Cree BA (2014) Acute inflammatory myelopathies. Handb Clin Neurol 122:613–667

De Souza A, Madhusudana SN (2014) Survival from rabies encephalitis. J Neurol Sci 339:8–14

Deghmane AE, Alonso JM, Taha MK (2009) Emerging drugs for acute bacterial meningitis. Expert Opin Emerg Drugs 14:381–393

Del Brutto OH (2014) Neurocysticercosis. Handb Clin Neurol 121:1445–1459

Edberg M, Furebring M, Sjölin J, Enblad P (2011) Neurointensive care of patients with severe community-acquired meningitis. Acta Anaesthesiol Scand 55:732–739

Fernández Guerrero ML, Álvarez B, Manzarbeitia F, Renedo G (2012) Infective endocarditis at autopsy: a review of pathologic manifestations and clinical correlates. Medicine (Baltimore) 91:152–164

Ferro JM, Fonseca AC (2014) Infective endocarditis. Handb Clin Neurol 119:75–79

Finsterer J, Auer H (2013) Parasitoses of the human central nervous system. J Helminthol 87:257–270

Forestier E (2009) Managing adult patients with acute community-acquired meningitis presumed of bacterial origin. Med Mal Infect 39:606–614

Franzen-Rohl E, Larsson K, Skoog E, Tiveljung-Lindell A, Grillner L, Aurelius E et al (2008) High diagnostic yield by CSF-PCR for entero- and herpes simplex viruses and TBEV serology in adults with acute aseptic meningitis in Stockholm. Scand J Infect Dis 40:914–921

Glimåker M, Johansson B, Bell M, Ericsson M, Bläckberg J, Brink M et al (2013a) Early lumbar puncture in adult bacterial meningitis – rationale for revised guidelines. Scand J Infect Dis 45:657–663

Glimåker M, Lindquist L, Sjölin J, Working Party of the Swedish Infectious Disease Society for Bacterial CNS Infections (2013b) Lumbar puncture in adult bacterial meningitis: time to reconsider guidelines? BMJ 346:f361

Glimåker M, Johansson B, Halldorsdottir H, Wanecek M, Elmi-Terander A, Ghatan PH et al (2014) Neuro-intensive treatment targeting intracranial hypertension improves outcome in severe bacterial meningitis: an intervention-control study. PLoS One 9(3):e91976

Greenblatt D, Krupp LB, Belman AL (2013) Parainfectious meningo-encephalo-radiculo-myelitis (cat scratch disease, Lyme borreliosis, brucellosis, botulism, legionellosis, pertussis, mycoplasma). Handb Clin Neurol 112:1195–1207

Gullo FP, Rossi SA, Sardi Jde C, Teodoro VL, Mendes-Giannini MJ, Fusco-Almeida AM (2013) Cryptococcosis: epidemiology, fungal resistance, and new alternatives for treatment. Eur J Clin Microbiol Infect Dis 32:1377–1391

Gupta RK, Soni N, Kumar S, Khandelwal N (2012) Imaging of central nervous system viral diseases. J Magn Reson Imaging 35:477–491

Handique SK, Handique SK (2011) Viral infections of the central nervous system. Neuroimaging Clin N Am 21:777–794

Hasbun R, Bijlsma M, Brouwer MC, Khoury N, Hadi CM, van der Ende A et al (2013) Risk score for identifying adults with CSF pleocytosis and negative CSF Gram stain at low risk for an urgent treatable cause. J Infect 67:102–110

Hawkes M, Elphinstone RE, Conroy AL, Kain KC (2013) Contrasting pediatric and adult cerebral malaria: the role of the endothelial barrier. Virulence 4:543–555

Heckenberg SG, Brouwer MC, van de Beek D (2014) Bacterial meningitis. Handb Clin Neurol 121:1361–1375

Ho M (2014) EPCR: holy grail of malaria cytoadhesion? Blood 123:157–159

Huang PN, Shih SR (2014) Update on enterovirus 71 infection. Curr Opin Virol 5C:98–104

Ioannidis LJ, Nie CQ, Hansen DS (2014) The role of chemokines in severe malaria: more than meets the eye. Parasitology 141(5):602–613

Jarvis JN, Harrison TS, Lawn SD, Meintjes G, Wood R, Cleary S (2013) Cost effectiveness of cryptococcal antigen screening as a strategy to prevent HIV-associated cryptococcal meningitis in South Africa. PLoS One 8(7):e69288

Jayakumar PN, Chandrashekar HS, Ellika S (2013) Imaging of parasitic infections of the central nervous system. Handb Clin Neurol 114:37–64

Kant Upadhyay R (2013) Biomarkers in Japanese encephalitis: a review. Biomed Res Int 2013:591290

Kasanmoentalib ES, Brouwer MC, van de Beek D (2013) Update on bacterial meningitis: epidemiology, trials and genetic association studies. Curr Opin Neurol 26:282–288

Katchanov J, Kleist MV, Arastéh K, Stocker H (2014) Time-to-amphotericin B' in cryptococcal meningitis in a European low-prevalence setting: analysis of diagnostic delays. QJM 107: 799–803

Klein M, Pfister HW, Leib SL, Koedel U (2009) Therapy of community-acquired acute bacterial meningitis: the clock is running. Expert Opin Pharmacother 10(16):2609–2623

Kristensson K, Masocha W, Bentivoglio M (2013) Mechanisms of CNS invasion and damage by parasites. Handb Clin Neurol 114:11–22

Lahoti S, Berger JR (2013) Iatrogenic fungal infections of central nervous system. Curr Neurol Neurosci Rep 13(11):399

Lerner A, Shiroiski MS, Zee CS, Law M, Go JL (2012) Imaging of neurocysticercosis. Neuroimaging Clin N Am 22(4):659–676

Lyons J, McArthur J (2013) Emerging infections of the central nervous system. Curr Infect Dis Rep 15(6):576–582

MacLean L, Myburgh E, Rodgers J, Price HP (2013) Imaging African trypanosomes. Parasite Immunol 35(9–10):283–284

Mann BR, McMullen AR, Swetnam DM, Barrett AD (2013) Molecular epidemiology and evolution of West Nile virus in North America. Int J Environ Res Public Health 10(10):5111–5129

Masocha W, Kristensson K (2012) Passage of parasites across the blood-brain barrier. Virulence 3(2):202–212

McConkey GA, Martin HL, Bristow GC, Webster JP (2013) Toxoplasma gondii infection and behavior – location, location, location? J Exp Biol 216(1):113–119

Misra UK, Kalita J, Bhoi SK (2014) Spectrum and outcome predictors of central nervous system infections in a neurological critical care unit in India: a retrospective review. Trans R Soc Trop Med Hyg 108(3):141–146

Mook-Kanamori BB, Brouwer MC, Geldhoff M, Ende AV, van de Beek D (2014) Cerebrospinal fluid complement activation in patients with pneumococcal and meningococcal meningitis. J Infect 68:542–547

Moritani T, Capizzano A, Kirby P, Policeni B (2014) Viral infections and white matter lesions. Radiol Clin North Am 52(2):355–382

Mourvillier B, Tubach F, van de Beek D, Garot D, Pichon N, Georges H et al (2013) Induced hypothermia in several bacterial meningitis: a randomized clinical trial. JAMA 310(20): 2174–2183

Murthy JM, Sundaram C (2014) Fungal infections of the central nervous system. Handb Clin Neurol 121:1383–1401

Nau R, Djukic M, Spreer A, Eiffert H (2013) Bacterial meningitis: new therapeutic approaches. Expert Rev Anti Infect Ther 11(10):1079–1095

Nicolasora N, Kaul DR (2008) Infectious disease emergencies. Med Clin North Am 92(2): 427–441

Nicoletti A (2013) Toxocariasis. Handb Clin Neurol 114:217–228

Nigrovic LE (2013) Aseptic meningitis. Handb Clin Neurol 112:1153–1156

Pappas PG (2013) Lessons learned in the multistate fungal infection outbreak in the United States. Curr Opin Infect Dis 26(6):545–550

Petri WA, Hague R (2013) Entamoeba histolytica brain abscess. Handb Clin Neurol 114: 147–152

Pines JM (2008) Timing of antibiotics for acute, severe infections. Emerg Med Clin North Am 26(2):245–257

Pittella JE (2013) Pathology of CNS parasitic infections. Handb Clin Neurol 114:65–88

Pomar V, Benito N, Lopoez-Contreras J, Coll P, Gurgui M, Domingo P (2013) Spontaneous gram-negative bacillary meningitis in adult patients: characteristics and outcome. BMC Infect Dis 13:451

Postels DG, Birbeck GL (2013) Cerebral malaria. Handb Clin Neurol 114:91–102

Putz K, Havani K, Zar FA (2013) Meningitis. Prim Care 40(3):707–726

Rodgers J (2010) Trypanosomiasis and the brain. Parasitology 137(14):1995–2006

Rodriguez S, Wilkins P, Domy P (2012) Immunological and molecular diagnosis of cysticercosis. Pathog Glob Health 106(5):286–298

Roman GC (2014) Tropical myelopathies. Handb Clin Neurol 121:1521–1548

Roos KL, van de Beek D (2010) Bacterial meningitis. Handb Clin Neurol 96:51–63

Ross KL (2014) Encephalitis. Handb Clin Neurol 121:1377–1381

Rudolph KE, Lessler J, Moloney RM, Kimush B, Cummings DA (2014) Incubation periods of mosquito-Borne Viral Infections: a systematic review. Am J Trop Med Hyg 90:882–891

Schmutzhard E, Helbok R (2014) Rickettsiae, protozoa, and opisthokonta/metazoa. Handb Clin Neurol 121:1403–1443

Sellner J, Täuber MG, Leib SL (2010) Pathogenesis and pathophysiology of bacterial CNS infections. Handb Clin Neurol 96:1–16

Singh G, Burneo JG, Sander JW (2013) From seizures to epilepsy and its substrates: neurocysticercosis. Epilepsia 54(5):783–792

Sondgeroth KS, McElwain TF, Allen AJ, Chen AV, Lau AO (2013) Loss of neurovirulence is associated with reduction of cerebral capillary sequestration during acute Babesia bovis infection. Parasit Vectors 18(6):181

Tessier JM, Scheid WM (2010) Principles of antimicrobial therapy. Handb Clin Neurol 96:17–29

Thwaites GE (2014) Brain infections in 2013: good drugs and bad bugs. Lancet Neurol 13(1): 20–21

Tudisco JB, Fumeaux C, Petignat PA (2013) Eosinophilic meningitis, a very rare entity in Europe. Rev Med Suisse 9(406):2082, 2084–2087

Tyler KL (2014) Current developments in understanding of West Nile virus central nervous system disease. Curr Opin Neurol 27(3):342–348

van de Beek D, Drake JM, Tunkel AR (2010) Nosocomial bacterial meningitis. N Engl J Med 362(2):146–154

Wall EC, Ajdukiewicz KM, Heyderman RS, Garner P (2013) Osmotic therapies added to antibodies for acute bacterial meningitis. Cochrane Database Syst Rev 3:CD008806

Welch H, Hasbun R (2010) Lumbar puncture and cerebrospinal fluid analysis. Handb Clin Neurol 96:31–49

Yansouni CP, Bottieau E, Lutumba P, Winkler AS, Lynen L, Büscher P (2013) Rapid diagnostic tests for neurological infections in central Africa. Lancet Infect Dis 13(6):546–558

Zhang Y, Wang Z, Chen H, Chen Z, Tian Y (2014) Antioxidants: potential antiviral agents for Japanese encephalitis virus infection. Int J Infect Dis 24:30–36

Chronic Infectious Inflammatory Diseases of the Central Nervous System

15

Pille Taba and Irja Lutsar

Contents

P. Taba, MD, PhD (✉)
Department of Neurology and Neurosurgery,
University of Tartu, Puusepa 8 – H452,
Tartu 51014, Estonia
e-mail: Pille.Taba@kliinikum.ee

I. Lutsar, MD, PhD
Department of Microbiology,
University of Tartu,
Tartu, Estonia

© Springer International Publishing Switzerland 2015
F. Deisenhammer et al. (eds.), *Cerebrospinal Fluid in Clinical Neurology*,
DOI 10.1007/978-3-319-01225-4_15

Abstract

Chronic infections of the central nervous system (CNS) tend to progress over months or years. The incubation period is usually considerably longer than that of acute infections. Chronic infections of the CNS could be triggered by persistence of infecting organisms in the brain or spinal cord causing direct tissue damage (e.g. neurosyphilis, CNS tuberculosis) or by the host immunological response in the absence of continuing infection. Often both factors are involved. Onset of symptoms is usually subacute, and CSF findings include predominantly lymphocytic pleocytosis and elevated protein and sometimes decreased glucose level. Several CNS-prone microorganisms are difficult to eradicate from CNS, and confirmation of diagnosis may be challenging, but it is critical for prognosis. Infecting organisms are rarely detected in the CSF by classical culture methods. The methods used for diagnosis are either serological tests of blood or CSF (e.g. HIV, Lyme borreliosis, syphilis) or detection of nucleic acids in the CSF (Table 15.1). CNS inflammation is confirmed by the CSF examination that may need repeated examinations. In infections associated with the persistence of microorganisms, long-term antibacterial therapy is recommended (syphilis, TBE, toxoplasmosis, Lyme borreliosis). In diseases in which host immunological response plays a predominant role, the treatment of chronic CNS infection is usually symptomatic.

Abbreviations

ADA	Adenosine deaminase
AIDS	Acquired immunodeficiency syndrome

CATT	Card agglutination test for trypanosomiasis
CJD	Creutzfeldt–Jakob disease
CNS	Central nervous system
CSF	Cerebrospinal fluid
CXCL	Chemokine ligand
DNA	Deoxyribonucleic acid
EIA	Treponemal enzyme immunoassay
ELISA	Enzyme-linked immunosorbent assay
FTA	Fluorescent treponemal antibody
FTA-abs	Fluorescent treponemal antibody absorption
HIV	Human immunodeficiency virus
IgG	Immunoglobulin G
IgM	Immunoglobulin M
IGRA	Interferon-gamma release assays
IP-10	Interferon protein 10
ITPA	Intrathecal *Treponema pallidum* antibody
JCV	JC virus/John Cunningham virus
MCP-1	Monocyte chemokine protein 1
MHA-TP	Microhaemagglutination for *Treponema pallidum*
MMP-9	Matrix metallopeptidase 9
MODS	Microscopic observation drug susceptibility
MRI	Magnetic resonance imaging
NAAT	Nucleic acid amplification tests
NFL	Neuronal injury neurofilament
NSE	Neuron-specific enolase
PCR	Polymerase chain reaction
PML	Progressive multifocal leucoencephalopathy
PrP	Prion protein
RNA	Ribonucleic acid
RPR	Rapid plasma regain
RT-PCR	Real-time polymerase chain reaction
SSPE	Subacute sclerosing panencephalitis
sVCAM-1	Soluble vascular adhesion molecule 1
TBE	Tick-borne encephalitis
TBEV	Tick-borne encephalitis virus
TIMP-1	Tissue inhibitor of metalloproteinases 1
TNFα	Tumour necrosis factor alpha
TPHA	*Treponema pallidum* haemagglutination
TPPA	*Treponema pallidum* particle agglutination
VDRL	Venereal disease research laboratory
WBC	White blood cell
WHO	World Health Organisation
β2M	Beta-2-microglobulin

Table 15.1 Summary of chronic CNS infections: the diagnostic tools and CSF findings

Disease	Causative agent	Primary diagnostic tests[a]	Cerebrospinal fluid				Other markers
			Infecting organism	WBC	Protein	Presence of antibodies	
HIV infection	HIV-1, HIV-2	Specific antibodies in serum	HIV RNA	↑ Lymphocytes	NA	NA	↑ Neopterin
				CD4+ cells			↑ CCL2, CXCL10, β2M, TNFα, sCD14, sCD163, sVCAM-1, MMP-9, TIMP-1
				CD8+ cells			
Neurosyphilis	*Treponema pallidum*	Non-treponemal and specific treponemal antibodies in CSF	RT-PCR (sensitivity of 50 %)	↑ Lymphocytes	↑ Protein	Non-treponemal (VDRL, PRP) and specific treponemal antibodies (TPHA)	↑ CXCL13?
		CSF pleocytosis and protein					
CNS tuberculosis	*Mycobacterium tuberculosis*	CSF pleocytosis, ↑protein	CSF acid-fast bacilli	↑ Lymphocytes	↑ Protein >1 g/L	Insufficient data	Mildly ↓ glucose
		↓ Glucose					
		CSF culture	Positive culture	10–1,500 cells			
		CSF acid-fast bacilli					↑ ADA?
		Skin test	PCR				
		IGRA					

Chronic neuroborreliosis	*Borrelia burgdorferi sensu lato*	CSF pleocytosis	Positive culture 10–17 %	↑ Lymphocytes <1,000 cells	↑ Protein 1–3 g/L	IgM and IgG antibodies	↓ glucose
		Specific antibodies in CSF	Positive PCR 10–30 %			CSF/serum optical density ratio >1.3	↑ IL-4, IL-5, IL-6, IL-8, IL-10, IL-12, IL-18, IFN-γ
							↑ CXCL13?
Tick-borne encephalitis (chronic form)	TBE virus	CSF pleocytosis	NA	↑ Lymphocytes <1,000 cells	↑ Protein	NA	Poorly studied
		Specific antibodies in serum					
Creutzfeldt-Jakob disease (sporadic)	Unknown	EEG with periodic sharp wave complexes	NA	Typically normal	Typically normal	NA	14-3-3 protein
		14-3-3 protein in CSF					Tau protein?
		MRI					
Variant Creutzfeldt-Jakob disease	BSE prion	Neuropathological changes	NA	Typically normal	Typically normal	NA	NA
		EEG normal					
		MRI findings					
Progressive multifocal leucoencephalopathy	JC virus	PCR of CSF	PCR	Normal	↑ Protein	Insufficient data	NA
		MRI findings	Cell culture				
		Brain biopsy and electron microscopy	Immunochemistry				
			Electron microscopy				
Subacute sclerosing panencephalitis	Measles virus (*Rubeola*)	Specific antibodies in CSF	NA	↑ Lymphocytes	Normal or ↑ protein	Anti-measles antibodies	Insufficient data
		EEG					
		MRI findings					

(continued)

Table 15.1 (continued)

Disease	Causative agent	Primary diagnostic tests[a]	Cerebrospinal fluid				
			Infecting organism	WBC	Protein	Presence of antibodies	Other markers
Toxoplasmosis	*Toxoplasma gondii*	CSF pleocytosis	Tachyzoites in ventricular CSF extremely rare	↑ Lymphocytes	↑ Protein	50 % of patients have antibodies	Poorly studied
		Specific antibodies in CSF	Positive PCR 0–100 %			Good sensitivity, poor specificity to distinguish between acute, chronic and past infection	
		MRI findings					
Sleeping sickness (African trypanosomiasis)	*Trypanosoma brucei gambiense*	CATT for screening (*T. b. gambiense*)	Giemsa staining	↑ lymphocytes 100–300 cells	↑ protein	IgM antibodies – need for further validation	Poorly studied
	Trypanosoma brucei rhodesiense	Giemsa staining of blood or lymph nodes or bone marrow or CSF	Native CSF – motile trypanosomes				
Nipah encephalitis	Nipah virus	RT-PCR of CSF	RT-PCR	↑ Lymphocytes	↑ Protein	Poorly studied	Poorly studied
		IgM and IgG antibodies	Cell culture				
		MRI findings					
Mollaret meningitis	Not known	Typical Mollaret cells in CSF	NA	Mild ↑ lymphocytes	↑ Protein	NA	Poorly studied
	HHV-2 proposed						

Abbreviations: *RT-PCR* real-time PCR, *IL* interleukin, *TBE* tick-borne encephalitis, *BSE* bovine spongiform encephalopathy, *IGRA* interferon-gamma release assays, *CATT* card agglutination test for trypanosomiasis (*T. b. gambiense*)
[a]Does not include clinical findings

15.1   Human Immunodeficiency Virus (HIV) Infection

15.1.1 Clinical Background

Approximately 35 million people were living with human immunodeficiency virus (HIV) in the world in 2012, with 2.5 million new cases occurring each year (WHO 2014a). The HIV is a double-stranded enveloped RNA virus belonging to the family of retroviruses. Two subtypes HIV-1 and HIV-2 exist of which HIV-1 in far the most common. HIV is a direct cause of acquired immunodeficiency syndrome (AIDS), a condition in which progressive failure of the immune system allows life-threatening opportunistic infections and cancers to appear. At present, with almost 30 different antiretroviral agents registered, the number of AIDS cases has dropped in developed countries, but the HIV epidemic still has a major impact on the human health in Sub-Saharan Africa and some areas of the former Soviet Union (UNAIDS 2013: www.unaids.org last accessed 21.09.2014) *Fehler! Hyperlink-Referenz ungültig.* The effective treatment has turned HIV into a chronic disease with the life expectancy approaching population norms for patients who comply with an appropriate antiretroviral treatment. Still specific populations, such as men who have sex with men in industrialised countries, intravenous drug users in the former Soviet Union areas, and women of child-bearing age in developing countries, are the main risk groups for HIV infection. Despite the achievements in the management of HIV infections, the virus persists in the latency organs of the host for entire life.

HIV is associated with the central nervous system (CNS) in two ways. First, without antiretroviral treatment, the progressing decline of CD4+ cells leads to the development of CNS opportunistic infections (cryptococcosis, tuberculosis, toxoplasmosis). Second, HIV enters the brain soon after the peripheral infection of circulating T cells and monocytes, and HIV is detectable in the cerebrospinal fluid (CSF) even without an apparent involvement of CNS in the very early stages of the infection. A consensus research definition of HIV-associated neurocognitive disorder includes manifestations of asymptomatic neurocognitive impairment, mild neurocognitive disorder and HIV-associated dementia (formerly AIDS associated dementia) (Antinori et al. 2007). HIV-associated dementia is a progressive disabling disorder characterised by a subcortical dementia that manifests with a loss of attention and concentration, notable motor slowing and various behavioural disorders and generally leads to death within a year (Navia et al. 1986). Compared to the general population, about a half of patients with HIV infection have lower cognitive performance levels, categorised as a mild neurocognitive disorder. The main difference between CNS infections and HIV-associated neurocognitive disorders is their response to antiretroviral therapy. While CNS opportunistic infections and the prevalence of HIV-associated dementia have significantly decreased in the era of effective antiretroviral therapies, still about a half of all treated patients with HIV have cognitive impairment.

HIV infection is diagnosed by detection of specific antibodies against HIV-1 or HIV-2 in serum by ELISA and confirmed by using immunoblotting.

15.1.2 Cerebrospinal Fluid

Detection of HIV in CSF HIV ribonucleic acid (RNA) has been found in CSF from patients regardless of CSF involvement, but the viral load in CSF is usually lower than in plasma (Ho et al. 2013). While initial studies suggested correlation between CSF HIV RNA (viral load) and the HIV-associated dementia (Brew et al. 1997), subsequent reports have shown that virus load correlated neither with the severity of the HIV-associated dementia nor abnormal quantitative neurological performance (Spudich et al. 2005).

CSF Inflammatory Parameters CSF pleocytosis, consisting mostly of lymphocytes and to a lesser extent of monocytes, is present early in the course of HIV infection even in neurologically asymptomatic subjects suggesting that it is directly linked to HIV infection itself, rather than an undiagnosed opportunistic infection or neurological complications (Ho et al. 2013). Longitudinal trials have indicated resolution of baseline pleocytosis in all patients after the beginning of the antiretroviral treatment. In untreated patients, CSF pleocytosis correlates with plasma and CSF HIV RNA levels and with levels of CSF and blood CD8+ cell activation (Spudich et al. 2005). Recent studies have demonstrated that even during treatment, an increase in CD8+ T cells, as well as a generalised increase in most other cell types present in normal CSF, is characteristic to HIV infection. The ratio of CD4+ to CD8+ T cells is in favour of CD8+ T cells, similarly to findings in the plasma (Ho et al. 2013). B and NK cells, which are extremely rare in normal CSF, are found in HIV-positive subjects even without CNS involvement. Their role and importance are still poorly investigated.

CSF Immunological and Other Markers While CSF biomarkers have been useful in defining the natural history of HIV infection and their responses to treatment, they have been found to be of a very limited clinical use for either patient management or clinical trials. The CSF biomarkers could be divided into viral (presented above), immune and neural markers. The immunological markers that have been studied include neopterin as a cardinal marker but also other soluble markers such as chemokines CCL2 (MCP-1, monocyte chemokine protein 1), CXCL10 (IP-10, interferon protein 10) and β2M (beta-2-microglobulin); a component of the MHC-I complex increased in CSF in HIV-associated dementia; and TNFα (tumour necrosis factor alpha), sCD14 (a soluble LPS ligand), sCD163 (a macrophage chemokine), sVCAM-1 (soluble vascular adhesion molecule 1), MMP-9 (matrix metallopeptidase 9) and TIMP-1 (tissue inhibitor of metalloproteinases 1). All these markers mostly indicate the presence of CNS inflammation during HIV infection rather being specific for HIV infection (Price et al. 2013).

Neopterin, a pteridine biomarker metabolite, is produced by cells of the monocyte–macrophage lineage and likely also by astrocytes within the CNS compartment and increases as systemic HIV infection progresses, with the highest levels observed in HIV-associated dementia and CNS opportunistic infections (Hagberg et al. 2010). The neopterin levels in patients receiving effective antiretroviral treatment are low but still greater than in HIV negative controls (Price et al. 2013).

A number of neural biomarkers have been explored, including neuronal injury neurofilament (NFL) and indicators of disturbed amyloid and tau metabolism t-tau (total tau) and p-tau (phosphorylated tau) proteins. While none of these neural biomarkers are specific for HIV neuropathology, they importantly indicate active CNS injury (Gisslen et al. 2009).

15.2 Neurosyphilis

15.2.1 Clinical Background

Syphilis is a systemic infectious disease caused by the spirochete *Treponema pallidum*. The incidence of syphilis decreased after the introduction of penicillin in the 1940s, but during the era of HIV infection, the incidence has increased again. In recent years, young men who have sex with men have accounted for an increasing proportion of syphilis, and co-infection with HIV has changed clinical and laboratory profiles, demonstrating higher antigen titres and more malignant course of neurosyphilis (CDC 2014; ECDC 2013; Chahine et al. 2011; Gitai et al. 2009; Poliseli et al. 2008).

CNS involvement can occur at any stage of syphilis. In asymptomatic cases, there are no neurological manifestations except CSF abnormalities. Symptomatic neurosyphilis can occur as an early meningeal form within 12 months after infection, or late or chronic forms as meningovascular syphilis that usually occur 5–10 years after the initial infection, or parenchymatous findings 15–25 years after the onset of the disease. The pathological basis of chronic neurosyphilis is persistence of spirochetes in affected tissues: walls of brain arteries, leptomeninges, brain parenchyma, dorsal roots or spinal cord (Miklossy 2012).

Neurosyphilis has various clinical manifestations, but they lack specificity and may mimic several other diseases. Meningovascular neurosyphilis with endarteritis leads to multiple ischaemic lesions, presenting with pareses, aphasia and seizures. Parenchymatous syphilis may manifest as (1) paretic neurosyphilis ('general paresis' or 'dementia paralytica') with neuropsychiatric features including behavioural and cognitive disorders, depression, confusion and hallucinations, sleep impairment, dysarthria, movement disorders and Argyll Robertson phenomenon (anisocoria) or (2) tabetic neurosyphilis (*tabes dorsalis*) characterised by sensory ataxia, sphincter disorders, peripheral neuropathy with pain and paraesthesias and cranial nerve lesions including facial nerve disorder, optic atrophy and Argyll Robertson pupils. Uveitis or other ocular manifestations or auditory signs may be associated with neurosyphilis, but gummas of CNS are very rare (Zhang et al. 2013; Ghanem 2010; Danielsen et al. 2004).

Parenteral penicillin G is the preferred treatment for all stages of syphilis. There are inconsistent data on the effectiveness of procaine penicillin/probenecid combination. If the CSF abnormalities are not resolved within 2 years, re-treatment is recommended (CDC 2010; Ghanem 2010; French et al. 2009).

15.2.2 Diagnosis of Neurosyphilis

T. pallidum is difficult to culture, and dark field examination and direct fluorescent antibody stains from ulcers are not highly sensitive. Historically, the Wassermann test has been used for laboratory testing.

For confirmation of syphilis, combination of reactive serological tests is used: there are two modern non-treponemal (or lipoidal/cardiolipin) serological tests, the venereal disease research laboratory (VDRL) and rapid plasma reagin test (RPR), and treponemal tests including *T. pallidum* haemagglutination assay (TPHA), microhaemagglutination for *T. pallidum* (MHA-TP), *T. pallidum* particle agglutination (TPPA), fluorescent treponemal antibody (FTA), fluorescent treponemal antibody absorption (FTA-abs) or treponemal enzyme immunoassay (EIA) test (Ghanem 2010; French et al. 2009). Sensitivity of *T. pallidum* PCR is moderate, while its specificity is very good: PCR may be helpful in detecting *T. pallidum*, but a negative result does not exclude the diagnosis of neurosyphilis (Gayet-Ageron et al. 2013; Kingston et al. 2008, 2011).

By the CDC surveillance case definitions, confirmed neurosyphilis is defined as any stage of syphilis that meets the laboratory criteria for neurosyphilis: a reactive serologic test for syphilis and a reactive non-treponemal test in CSF. Probable neurosyphilis is defined as syphilis of any stage with a negative non-treponemal test in the CSF, with elevated CSF protein or pleocytosis and clinical signs consistent with neurosyphilis, in the absence of other known causes for abnormalities (CDC 2014).

15.2.3 Cerebrospinal Fluid

Lumbar puncture for a CSF examination is mandatory in patients with serological evidence and clinical signs suggestive of neurosyphilis; it is the only way to diagnose asymptomatic neurosyphilis. In guidelines of the HIV era, a CSF examination is recommended in asymptomatic cases not responding with a fourfold decrease of serum RPR titres 6–12 months after therapy (CDC 2010; Sparling 2010; Choe et al. 2010; Marra et al. 2008).

Detection of *T. pallidum*   *T. pallidum* has been recovered from the CSF during secondary syphilis in 30 % of patients, mostly in those with abnormal CSF (Miklossy 2012). High numbers of *T. pallidum* has been detected in spinal dorsal roots, brain parenchyma and brain arteries. Demonstration of *T. pallidum* specific DNA in CSF is a strong indicator of active disease, but PCR is more efficient to confirm than to exclude the diagnosis: the sensitivity estimates of CSF PCR have been close to 50 % and the specificity 80–90 % (Gayet-Ageron et al. 2013; Marra et al. 2004). In some patients, *T. pallidum* DNA could be detected up to 3 years after adequate treatment (French et al. 2009).

CSF Inflammatory Parameters   In neurosyphilis, lymphocyte-predominant CSF pleocytosis with >5 mononuclear cells/µL as a standard cut-off, and elevated CSF proteins are characteristic but insensitive and non-specific findings; CSF may be normal in some patients. In the presence of HIV infection, pleocytosis greater than

20 is relatively typical for neurosyphilis (CDC 2014; Marra et al. 2004). If CSF pleocytosis was present initially, follow-up CSF examinations should be repeated every 6 months until the cell count is normal (CDC 2010; Marra et al. 2008). However, neurosyphilis may progress despite appropriate therapy and serological responses; thus a CSF examination should be considered in any treated patient with evidence of clinical progression (Zhou et al. 2012).

CSF Immunological Markers To establish a diagnosis of neurosyphilis, serological testing is used, combining non-specific (non-treponemal/lipoidal) and specific treponemal tests in CSF. A positive CSF non-treponemal test (VDRL/PRP) is considered a highly specific diagnostic marker for neurosyphilis, but its sensitivity is limited; it shows a positive result only in about half of symptomatic cases; thus a negative CSF non-treponemal test does not exclude neurosyphilis (Marra et al. 2012; Sparling 2010; Castro et al. 2008).

Treponemal-specific CSF tests are more sensitive than lipoidal tests, and a TPHA index >70 and a CSF TPHA titre >320 support the diagnosis. A negative test excludes neurosyphilis. However, it lacks specificity, and a positive reaction may not reflect neurosyphilis but can be caused by other conditions (Harding and Ghanem 2012; Ho and Marra 2012; French et al. 2009). The IgG index $\geq$0.7 is an indicator for intrathecal antibody production; data on detecting of *T. pallidum* specific IgG have been inconsistent (French et al. 2009; Kingston et al. 2008).

Diagnosis of neurosyphilis is more complicated in co-infection with HIV and opportunistic infections. Recent studies suggest that the concentration of CXCL13 in CSF has a potential to be used for the diagnosis of neurosyphilis in HIV-infected patients (Tsai et al. 2014; Marra et al. 2010). However, increased levels of CXCL13 have been described also in patients with Lyme neuroborreliosis, thus it is not a specific finding (Cerar et al. 2013).

15.3   Tuberculosis of the Central Nervous System

15.3.1 Clinical Background

Tuberculosis is an infectious disease declared by the WHO as a global public health emergency that caused 8.6 million new cases and 1.3 million deaths in the world in 2012, including 320,000 deaths among HIV-positive people (WHO 2013). In Europe, there were more than 70,000 cases reported in 2011, with a significant proportion of multidrug-resistant cases though overall incidence has slightly decreased (ECDC 2013).

Tuberculosis is caused by *Mycobacterium tuberculosis*, affecting multiple organs but the lungs most frequently. CNS involvement accounts about 1 % of cases of active tuberculosis but is highly predominant in children in endemic areas. CNS tuberculosis develops by haematogenous dissemination with a release of bacteria to subarachnoid space and manifests most commonly as tuberculous meningitis or tuberculomas but also as tuberculous abscess, cerebral miliary tuberculosis, arteritis or spinal cord lesions (Isabel and Rogelio 2014; Thwaites et al. 2009; Katti 2004).

Clinical presentations of tuberculous meningitis are non-specific. A prodromal period with mild fever, headache, vomiting and confusion is followed by variable manifestations due to of meningeal involvement, cranial nerve lesions or vasculitis causing ischaemic lesions with focal neurological findings. Tuberculomas without meningitis may manifest with seizures or focal neurological signs including pareses and cerebellar signs. Spinal tuberculosis presents with upper or lower motor neuron involvement (Daniele 2014; Gunawardhana et al. 2013; Christensen et al. 2011; Christie et al. 2008). Co-infection with HIV is associated with increased risk for other CNS infections and malignancies and leads to worse outcome (Chamie et al. 2014; Cecchini et al. 2009).

Treatment of CNS tuberculosis is suggested as a combination of isoniazid, pyrazinamide, rifampicin and ethambutol for 2 months followed by two drugs for 7–10 months, with adjunctive corticosteroid administration. For tuberculomas, chemotherapy is recommended before surgery, and ventricular shunting may be beneficial for hydrocephalus. All patients with tuberculosis should be tested for HIV and in case of co-infection, treated concomitantly with antiretroviral drugs additionally to anti-tuberculosis drugs that are used by the same principles as for patients without HIV (Chamie et al. 2014; Thwaites et al. 2004, 2009).

The mortality rate of tuberculous meningitis in case series has ranged from 7 to 41 % (Daniele 2014; Gunawardhana et al. 2013; Christensen et al. 2011; Hsu et al. 2010). A poor outcome is associated with older age, severity of disease, impaired consciousness, seizures, hydrocephalus, HIV co-infection and delayed anti-tuberculosis therapy (Achazi et al. 2011; Hsu et al. 2010; Cecchini et al. 2009). Drug-resistant tuberculosis is associated with more severe manifestations and higher mortality (Garg et al. 2013).

15.3.2 Diagnosis of Tuberculous Meningitis

Various diagnostic criteria for tuberculous meningitis have been used. The consensus case definition proposed by an expert panel in 2009 includes scoring for clinical, CSF and cerebral imaging criteria, evidence of tuberculosis elsewhere and exclusion of alternative diagnosis. A definite case of tuberculous meningitis is described as (A) clinical criteria plus acid-fast bacilli seen in the CSF; *M. tuberculosis* cultured in the CSF or a CSF positive nucleic acid amplification (NAA) test; or (B) acid-fast bacilli identified, with suggestive symptoms and CSF changes or visible meningitis in autopsy (Marais et al. 2010). Age, length of history, white blood cell count, clear CSF appearance with white cell count <1,000 cells/µl, lymphocytes proportion >30 % and protein >1 g/L and neurological focal findings have been shown as predictive for the diagnosis (Thwaites et al. 2002, 2009). Results of tuberculin skin testing in CNS tuberculosis are variable with a sensitivity of 17–32 % in adult and 30–77 % in children, but specificity may be reduced by BCG vaccination. Peripheral blood interferon-gamma release assays (IGRA) have higher specificity, but sensitivity varies. Magnetic resonance imaging (MRI) may reveal tuberculomas (Fig. 15.1), vascular lesions, hydrocephalus, basilar

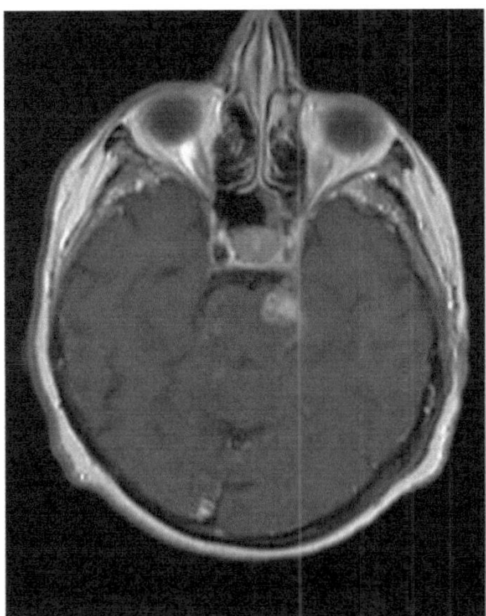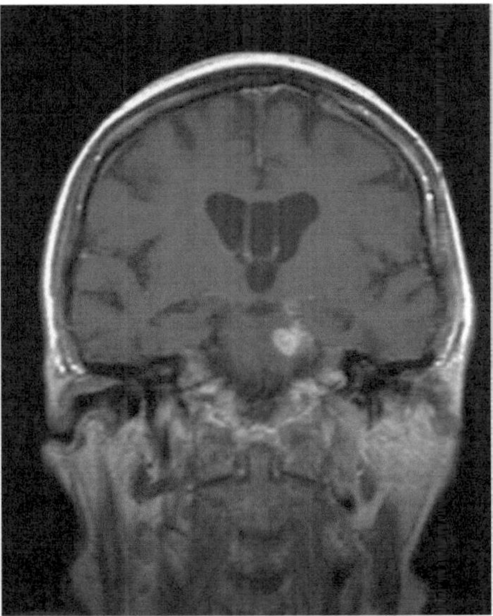

Fig. 15.1   MRI revealing a tuberculoma in the left pons area, in a patient with tuberculous meningitis, manifesting with paresis of n. abducens

arachnoiditis and spinal cord lesions, but the findings are non-specific (Marais et al. 2010; Thwaites et al. 2009).

15.3.3 Cerebrospinal Fluid

Detection of *M. tuberculosis*   The gold standard for diagnosis confirmation is demonstration of *M. tuberculosis* in the CSF by smear examination after Ziehl–Neelsen staining or culture. In CSF microscopy, acid-fast bacilli may be seen in up to 80 % of adult cases but only 15–20 % in children; large volumes (>6 ml) of CSF increase the diagnostic yield. Acid-fast bacilli are less frequently found in CSF with tuberculoma or spinal tuberculosis, compared to tuberculous meningitis (Marais et al. 2010; Thwaites et al. 2009).

Mycobacteria are slow-growing organisms; in conventional solid media (Lowenstein–Jensen), the growth can take up to 6–8 weeks. The BACTEC liquid media used in most microbiology labs has improved culture yields and enables detection of mycobacteria in average of 15 days. After anti-tuberculosis treatment is started, the sensitivity of smear or culture is lower. For susceptibility testing, direct culture methods are used, including liquid culture microscopic observation drug susceptibility (MODS), colorimetric redox indicator methods and the nitrate reductase assay (Thwaites et al. 2009; Garg et al. 2013).

Molecular-based PCR assay techniques including nucleic acid amplification tests (NAAT) are effective methods with high specificity but low sensitivity for rapid detection of mycobacterial DNA in CSF and other specimens. Molecular methods may be useful even in partially treated patients as mycobacterial DNA in CSF can be detected for 1 month after the initiation of the treatment (Solomons et al. 2014; Nhu et al. 2014; Garg et al. 2013). Quantitative RT-PCR for *M. tuberculosis* DNA and multiplex PCR using different primers have been introduced as possible useful methods for a rapid diagnosis (Takahashi et al. 2012; Kusum et al. 2011).

CSF Inflammatory Parameters For the diagnosis of CNS tuberculosis, examination of CSF is mandatory; the volume of CSF is important, and repeated lumbar punctures may be needed. Typical CSF findings included in the consensus diagnostic criteria set are: a clear appearance, pleocytosis 10–500 cells/µL with a lymphocytic predominance of >50 %, elevated protein >1 g/L and decreased glucose levels (<2.2 mmol/L; CSF/plasma ratio <50 %), but atypical findings have been demonstrated. Lower protein levels and white cell counts or non-inflammatory CSF are more frequent in patients with HIV co-infection (Marais et al. 2010; Chamie et al. 2014; Cecchini et al. 2009).

Adenosine deaminase (ADA) is an enzyme, considered as an indicator of immunity, and a potential diagnostic marker to improve the diagnosis of tuberculous meningitis. In some studies, increased ADA levels in the CSF have been demonstrated in tuberculous meningitis but not in bacterial or viral meningitis; however, the results are inconsistent (Agarwal et al. 2014; Tuon et al. 2010).

CSF Immunological Markers At present, there is insufficient evidence of CSF antibody or IGRA tests for diagnosis of active tuberculosis, but there are a few promising reports on possible innovative diagnostic markers (Song et al. 2014; Kim et al. 2010; Marais et al. 2010).

15.4 Chronic Neuroborreliosis

15.4.1 Clinical Background

Lyme borreliosis, or Lyme disease, is a tick-borne illness caused by a spirochete *Borrelia burgdorferi sensu lato* complex that can result in dermatological, neurological, cardiac and musculoskeletal disorders. Lyme neuroborreliosis develops usually within 2–6 weeks after the tick bite, most frequently as lymphocytic meningoradiculitis (Bannwarth syndrome) in Europe, meningitis in the United States and facial nerve palsy in children. The number of cases of neuroborreliosis has increased in recent years that may be partially explained by higher incidence but also by improved diagnostic methods (Aguero-Rosenfeld et al. 2005; Stanek et al. 2012).

Chronic or late Lyme neuroborreliosis occurs in less than 5 % of neuroborreliosis patients, lasting for more than 6 months after tick-transmitted infection. Chronic neuroborreliosis is defined as a continuous active disease process with CNS inflammation and is characterised by various manifestations like recurrent or progressive encephalomyelitis with pareses, movement disorders, seizures, gait and bladder disturbances or stroke-like syndrome caused by vasculitis, radiculopathy or peripheral neuropathy (Ljostad and Mygland 2013; Hansen et al. 2013; Mygland et al. 2010). Psychiatric features include cognitive impairment, psychosis with visual and auditory hallucinations and obsessive–compulsive disorders. Depressive state among patients with late Lyme disease is reported to be common, ranging in 20–66 %. Whether the chronic Lyme neuroborreliosis is caused by the persistence of spirochetes in the brain leading directly to tissue damage or it is a result of immunological changes in the absence of continuing infection is still debated. It is believed that the pathological processes in neurosyphilis and neuroborreliosis are similar as spirochetes are known to be neurotrophic (Miklossy 2012). For treatment of chronic neuroborreliosis, intravenous penicillin G and ceftriaxone are empirically effective, and theoretically doxycycline could be as effective, but there is not enough evidence from trials. Response to antibiotic treatment in chronic Lyme disease is usually slow and may be incomplete (Ljostad and Mygland 2013; Hansen et al. 2013; Mygland et al. 2010).

15.4.2 Diagnosis of Chronic Neuroborreliosis

The European guidelines define chronic neuroborreliosis by the following criteria: (1) clinical syndrome with neurologic manifestation, without other possible causes; (2) CSF pleocytosis; and (3) intrathecally produced anti-Borrelia antibodies, except for peripheral neuropathy with antibodies in serum (Stanek et al. 2011, 2012; Mygland et al. 2010). A diagnosis of chronic Lyme disease based on persistence of non-specific symptoms without objective clinical and laboratory findings, which has been reported in the United States but also in other countries, cannot be supported (Ljostad and Mygland 2013; Feder et al. 2007; Cameron et al. 2004). Imaging is not essential for the diagnosis, but in chronic neuroborreliosis, MRI may reveal meningeal enhancement due to chronic inflammation or ischaemic-like white matter lesions (Agarwal and Sze 2009; Aalto et al. 2007).

15.4.3 Cerebrospinal Fluid

Detection of *B. burgdorferi* in CSF Direct detection of the causing agent in later manifestation of Lyme borreliosis is limited. There is not enough evidence for microscope-based assays for use as a diagnostic tool, due to low sensitivity and specificity (Mygland et al. 2010). Recovery of *B. burgdorferi sensu lato* from CSF is complicated and can be done only in 10–17 % of untreated patients (Cerar et al. 2013; Aguero-Rosenfeld et al. 2005). Furthermore, by most conventional bacteriologic standards, borrelial cultures are poorly standardised, labour intensive, expensive and slow, requiring up to 12 weeks of incubation before being considered negative. Thus direct culture technique is hardly ever used in diagnosis of neuroborreliosis in clinical practice.

B. burgdorferi sensu lato DNA has been detected by PCR in CSF specimens, but it is of low diagnostic sensitivity, being positive in only 10–30 % cases with lower detection levels in longer duration of the disease that prevents implementation of this method in clinical practice (Aguero-Rosenfeld 2008; Wilske et al. 2007). The sensitivity of the PCR may depend also on the clinical presentations, CSF WBC count and whether antibiotic treatment is given or not. The spirochetes have been detected in the brain biopsy specimens and in autopsy samples (Miklossy 2012). PCR and CSF culture may be corroborative in the early stage of the disease when antibodies are absent or in immunosuppressed individuals, but otherwise not recommended for diagnosis (Mygland et al. 2010).

CSF Inflammatory Parameters Most patients with ongoing neuroborreliosis regardless of clinical symptoms have increased WBC, typically 10–1,000 cells/mm^3 (in 60 % in a range of 30 and 300 cells/mm^3), mainly lymphocytes and plasma cells, with an exception in cases with peripheral neuropathies. Further supporting findings include elevated CSF protein up to 1–3 g/L or even higher and oligoclonal IgG bands. Unlike in early Lyme neuroborreliosis, chronic patients may have low CSF glucose levels. In contrast to other meningitides of bacterial origin, the CSF lactate concentration is in normal ranges (Ljostad and Mygland 2013; Hansen et al. 2013; Djukic et al. 2012; Stanek et al. 2011).

CSF Immunological Markers: Detection of Antibodies Specific intrathecal production of IgM and IgG antibodies is one of the key features of neuroborreliosis (Ljostad and Mygland 2013; Stanek et al. 2012; Aguero-Rosenfeld 2008; Blanc et al. 2007). However, there are no uniformly accepted tests to measure *Borrelia* antibodies in CSF. Methods that have been used include capture immunoassays, CSF/serum antibodies determined by ELISA and Western immunoblots (Coyle et al. 1995, Wilske et al. 2007). Diagnostic yield of CSF antibodies could be improved when at least two antigens, flagella and one of the new antigens or two of the new antigens (decorin-binding protein A, BBK32, and outer surface protein C, and IR(6) peptide of borrelial VlsE protein) are used (Panelius et al. 2003). Positive intrathecal production of *Borrelia*-specific antibodies is indicated by an antibody index >1.3 (antibody index=CSF/serum *Borrelia* antibody concentration ratios: CSF/serum IgG concentration ratios, see also Chaps. 10 and 16); a pathological antibody index has a sensitivity of 80 % in early Lyme neuroborreliosis and nearly 100 % in longer duration (Wilske et al. 1986), Tumani et al. 1995). Intrathecal production can also be determined by testing CSF and serum at matching concentrations using immunoblotting. Of note anti-Borrelia antibodies may persist for years after the infection, and thus the specificity is low without other criteria of chronic neuroborreliosis (Djukic et al. 2012; Mygland et al. 2010; Wilske et al. 2007).

Detection of Chemokines and Cytokines in the CSF *Borreliae* that enter the CNS are recognised by monocytes, macrophages or dendritic cells, which produce proinflammatory cytokines and induce chemokines. Increased concentrations of interleukin 4 (IL-4), IL-5, IL-6, IL-8, IL-10, IL-12, IL-18 and gamma interferon (IFN-γ) have been found in the CSF samples of patients suffering from Lyme neuroborreliosis (Cerar et al. 2013). Various chemokines (CXCL8, CXCL10, CXCL11, CXCL12, CXCL13) are released as a result of inflammation and stimulate chemotaxis involved in the CNS (Moniuszko et al. 2014). Studies have suggested that measuring CXCL13 enables to distinguish neuroborreliosis from other inflammatory diseases of the CNS and to evaluate treatment response (Cerar et al. 2013; Senel et al. 2010). However, it is not specific as described also in other viral and spirochetal infections such as tick-borne encephalitis (TBE), neurosyphilis and CNS lymphoma (Moniuszko et al. 2014; Marra et al. 2010; Schmidt et al. 2011). The exact diagnostic cut-off values, however, are not established, and thus potential diagnostic usefulness of CXCL13 levels in CSF in chronic neuroborreliosis is still debatable (Ljostad and Mygland 2013; Bremell et al. 2013; Schmidt et al. 2011).

15.5 Tick-Borne Encephalitis (Chronic Form)

15.5.1 Clinical Background

Tick-borne encephalitis (TBE) is caused by the tick-borne encephalitis virus (TBEV), which is a single-stranded RNA virus that has European, Siberian and Far-Eastern subtypes. The course of the European subtype is mainly asymptomatic or if symptomatic then characterised by a biphasic course with development of meningitis, meningoencephalitis or myelitis which can be followed by a postencephalitic syndrome. The case fatality rate in the European subtype is low around 1–2 % (Holzmann 2003; Dumpis et al. 1999). In contrast, in the Far-Eastern subtype, the disease is mostly monophasic but causes more severe forms with neurological sequelae and the fatality rates of up to 30 %. The Siberian subtype characteristically induces a less severe acute period with a case fatality rate of 6–8 %, but there is a tendency to develop chronic TBE (Dumpis et al. 1999).

Acute forms of tick-borne encephalitis (TBE) are described in Chap. 14.a i. A chronic form of TBE mainly affects people <35 years and has been associated exclusively with the Siberian subtype of TBEV in Siberia and Far East. Hyperkinesias (54 %), epilepsia partialis continua, encephalopoliomyelitis and lateral amyotrophic sclerosis syndrome have been described (Mukhin et al. 2012; Poponnikova 2006; Gritsun et al. 2003a; Nadezhdina 2001). In the chronic form of TBE, a relapsing course following the acute TBE has been described or delayed development of the progressive disease after a long incubation period without the typical acute stage (Gritsun et al. 2003b; Frolova et al. 1987; Vasilenko and Grigor'eva 1987). Chronic TBE is very rare in Europe, with only two cases reported in Lithuania (Mickiene et al. 2002). Experimental studies have demonstrated the ability of TBEV Siberian subtype to persist and produce the chronic disease in animal models (Gritsun et al. 2003a; Frolova et al. 1987). The chronic form of TBE has been associated with mutations in the TBEV NS1 gene (Gritsun et al. 2003b) and immunological changes with defective T-cell response and imbalance in production of cytokines (Naslednikova et al. 2005).

The diagnostic criteria of chronic TBE are poorly defined, and there is no uniform consensus.

15.5.2 Cerebrospinal Fluid

Detection of TBEV in CSF TBEV is very rarely if ever isolated from CSF. The RT-PCR to detect TBE RNA in CSF has not been successful either

(Holzmann 2003). In a study in which TBE RNA was successfully detected in all blood samples, only 1 of 31 CSF samples tested positive during early viraemic period (Saksida et al. 2005). In fatal cases, the virus has been detected by RT-PCR in the brain tissue (Holzmann 2003). A strain of the Siberian subtype of TBEV was isolated postmortem from a patient who died of a progressive (2-year) form of TBE 10 years after being bitten by a tick, and another strain was detected in CSF of a 11-year-old girl with relapsing course of epilepsia partialis continua during 5 years (Gritsun et al. 2003a).

CSF Inflammatory Parameters Patients with TBE have shown CSF pleocytosis in the range of 12–1,100 cells with a predominance of segmented granulocytes (60–70 %) over lymphocytes (30–40 %) and a moderate impairment of the blood–CSF barrier (increased CSF–to–serum albumin ratio) (Holzmann 2003).

Detection of Antibodies in CSF The diagnosis of TBE is based on the demonstration of TBE-specific IgM and IgG antibodies in blood, which are usually detectable at the beginning of the second phase and increase to high titres. IgG antibodies persist over a lifetime and prevent reinfection. In CSF, intrathecally produced specific antibodies can only be found in 50 % of patients early after the disease onset, but within 10 days, they almost invariably become detectable (Holzmann 2003). However, there are limited data on antibodies in chronic TBE. In two patients in Siberia with progressive or relapsing course of chronic TBE, the TBEV Siberian serotype strains were isolated, but virus-specific antibodies were not detected that might show a possible defect of immune mechanisms, contributing to the persistence of the virus (Gritsun et al. 2003b).

15.6 Prion Diseases

15.6.1 Clinical Background

Prion diseases are rare fatal transmissible neurodegenerative disorders, characterised by the accumulation of protease-resistant prion protein (PrP), an isoform of a normal cellular protein. Aetiologically, human prion diseases can be divided into sporadic, inherited and acquired forms, with a diversity of clinical presentations (Araujo 2013; Wadsworth and Collinge 2007).

About 85 % of prion disease cases occur as sporadic Creutzfeldt–Jakob disease (CJD), with a yearly incidence rate of 1–2 cases per million of population. Clinically, it presents with rapidly progressive dementia, fast development of akinetic mutism, along with generalised myoclonus, ataxia, extrapyramidal and pyramidal signs and cortical blindness. Inherited cases that are classified as familial CJD, Gerstmann–Sträussler–Scheinker syndrome or fatal familial insomnia are associated with mutations in the human prion protein gene. Iatrogenic CJD may occur due to transmission through medical procedures. Variant CJD represents bovine-to-human transmission associated with the consumption of meat products that was described first in 1996 in the United Kingdom. Around 230 variant CJD cases have been reported, and global monitoring continues through the EuroCJD network. Kuru was endemic in Papua

New Guinea, transmitted by ritual cannibalism and manifested after a long incubation period with ataxia and dementia developing later (ECDC 2013; Araujo 2013;
Wadsworth and Collinge 2007).

Human prion diseases are ultimately fatal – death follows symptom onset within
2 years. The therapeutic approaches include polyanionic and polycyclic drugs to
prevent conversion of PrP and laminin receptor antagonists that have provided some
experimental promises. Active and passive immunisation against PrP in animals has
shown divergent effects and can trigger neurotoxic pathways (Panegyres and Armari
2013; Aguzzi et al. 2013).

15.6.2 Diagnosis of Creutzfeldt–Jakob Disease

Diagnostic criteria for CJD were formulated in 1979 and updated in 2009, including
clinical criteria and tests/investigations. For probable or possible sporadic CJD, two
clinical signs of the following four should be fulfilled: (1) dementia, (2) cerebellar
or visual signs, (3) pyramidal or extrapyramidal signs and (4) akinetic mutism.
Additionally, for a probable case, one of the following tests should be positive: (1)
periodic sharp wave complexes in EEG that are of high specificity and low sensitivity or (2) 14-3-3 protein in CSF that has a high sensitivity but modest specificity or
(3) high signal abnormalities in the caudate nucleus and putamen or at least two
cortical regions in MRI (Fig. 15.2). However, the accuracy of diagnostic criteria has
been assessed in a series of rapid progressive dementia and the level of the tau protein considered as a possible additional marker for the diagnosis (Felix-Morais et al.
2014; Tagliapietra et al. 2013; Zerr et al. 2009).

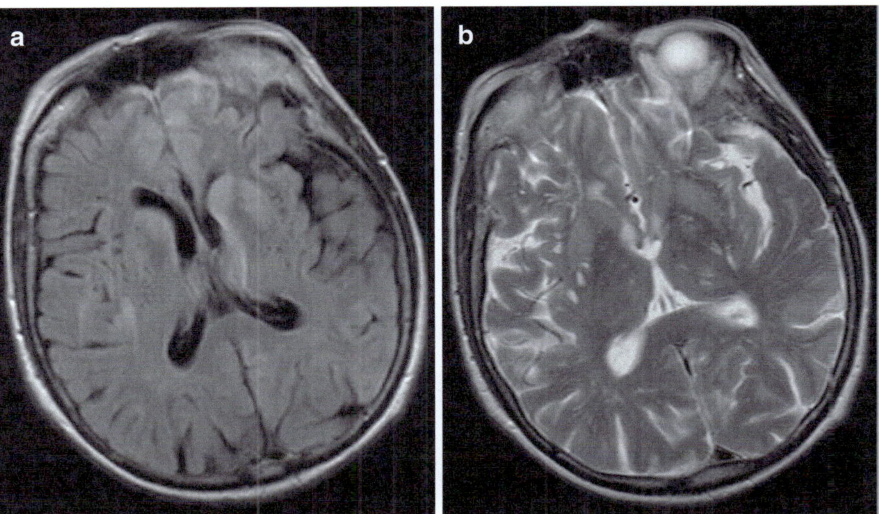

Fig. 15.2 MRI in sporadic CJD demonstrating bilateral hyperintensities in striatum and fronto-
medial cortex: (**a**) FLAIR; (**b**) T2

For variant CJD, the case definition for reporting communicable diseases has been approved in the Commission Implementing Decision of the European Council in 2012, combining preconditions of medical history, of at least four clinical criteria out of five (early psychiatric symptoms; painful sensory symptoms; ataxia; myoclonus or chorea or dystonia; dementia), epidemiological criteria and negative EEG findings without periodical complexes typical for sporadic CJD. The diagnostic criteria for a confirmed case are neuropathological findings: spongiform degeneration, neuronal loss, astrocytosis and PrP immunohistochemistry (EC 2012).

15.6.3 Cerebrospinal Fluid

Detection of Prions PrP cannot be detected in CSF by currently available methods. A promising novel method of real-time quaking-induced conversion has been developed for detection of PrP in the diluted CJD brain homogenate, but further studies are needed for more evidence (Atarashi et al. 2011).

CSF Inflammatory Parameters Typically there are no changes in inflammatory parameters in CSF in prion diseases, but a routine CSF examination may be of importance for differential diagnosis to exclude potentially treatable inflammatory conditions. A large study on standard CSF examination showed isolated mild increases of white cell count or total protein in a small proportion of patients with sporadic CJD. The presence of >20 cells/µL or 1 g/L of protein in CSF suggests an alternative diagnosis (Green et al. 2007).

CSF Immunological Markers In patients with rapidly progressive dementia and suspected sporadic CJD, it is recommended to examine CSF to detect 14-3-3 protein as a marker with a high sensitivity of 92 % and specificity of 80 % for CJD (Muayqil et al. 2012; Stoeck et al. 2012). However, the positive results have also been reported in other dementias and encephalopathies, infections and cerebrovascular diseases and metastases (Deisenhammer et al. 2009). Other brain-derived proteins have also been considered as diagnostic markers for CJD. In a Swedish study, the combination of t-tau levels and t-tau to p-tau ratios in CJD patients had a high specificity against important differential diagnoses (Skillback et al. 2014). However, CSF 14-3-3 protein had higher sensitivity than tau protein and S100b in the United Kingdom 10-year review (Chohan et al. 2010).

15.7 Progressive Multifocal Leucoencephalopathy

15.7.1 Clinical Background and Diagnosis

Progressive multifocal leucoencephalopathy (PML) is a potentially fatal CNS infection with progressive deterioration, caused by a polyoma virus (JC virus/John Cunningham virus). Polyoma viruses are double-stranded enveloped DNA viruses. Subclinical infection may occur in childhood, and about a half of an adult population with sclerosis multiplex have been tested as seropositive for JCV (Steiner and

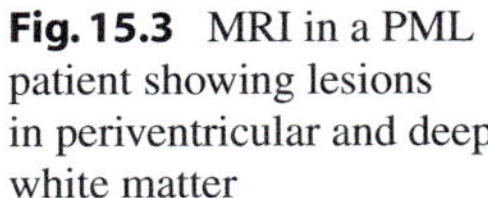

Fig. 15.3 MRI in a PML patient showing lesions in periventricular and deep white matter

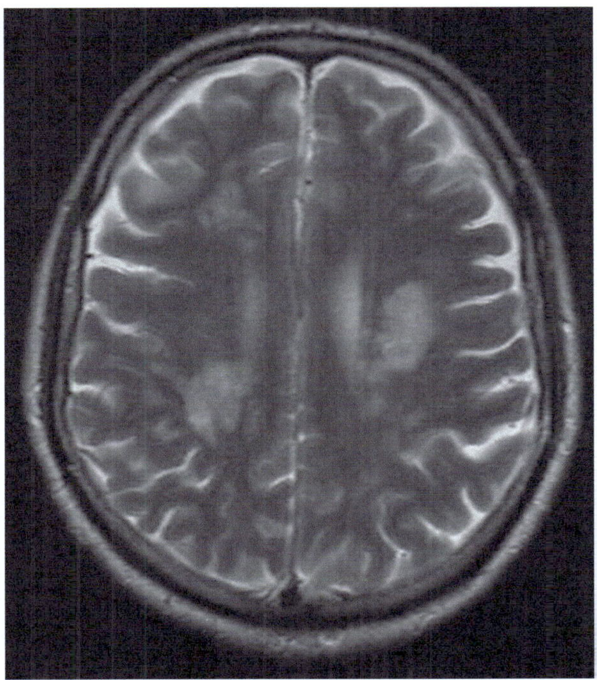

Berger 2012). PML occurs as an opportunistic infection in patients with monoclonal antibody immunosuppressive therapies, HIV infection or lymphoproliferative disorders. It has been reported in association with natalizumab treatment of multiple sclerosis, rituximab for lymphoproliferative and rheumatic disorders, efalizumab for psoriasis and brentuximab vedotin therapy (Carson et al. 2014; Mancuso et al. 2012; Mentzer et al. 2012; Carson et al. 2009). There is no antiviral therapy against the JCV, and the prognosis is poor. Highly active antiretroviral therapy has a beneficial impact to the prognosis of PML in HIV patients (Casado et al. 2014; Steiner and Berger 2012).

The proposed case definition is based on detection of JCV DNA in CSF or positive DNA and viral antigens with typical histopathology in the brain biopsy or autopsy tissue, in appropriate clinical settings and in brain MRI findings. Clinically, cognitive and behavioural disorders, pareses, ataxia, sensory loss, speech and visual disturbances and seizures have been described. PML damage is related to the brain demyelination, and MRI typically reveals lesions in subcortical and periventricular white matter (Fig. 15.3), cerebellum or peduncles, but also grey matter involvement can occur rarely. Typical histopathological findings include enlarged oligodendroglial nuclei, bizarre astrocytes and demyelination (Berger et al. 2013; Mentzer et al. 2012; Steiner and Berger 2012).

The 2-step enzyme-linked immunosorbent assay (ELISA) assay is used to detect the anti-JCV serostatus in patients with multiple sclerosis, as a tool for PML risk stratification, but not for confirmation of the diagnosis of PML (Gorelik et al. 2010).

15.7.2 Cerebrospinal Fluid

In a routine CSF examination, most PML patients demonstrate a normal cell count (usually less than 20 cells/µL) but mildly increased protein levels (Berger et al. 2013). The JCV DNA can be detected by PCR in a laboratory with specific expertise. However, positive PCR without typical clinical and radiological findings is not sufficient to provide evidence for the diagnosis, and a negative JCV PCR does not exclude PML. In HIV-infected patients who have developed PML-immune reconstitution inflammatory syndrome as a result of antiretroviral therapy, detection of JCV declines substantially. Repeated testing of CSF may be needed, but testing of blood or urine for JCV has no diagnostic value (Berger et al. 2013; Mentzer et al. 2012; Fong et al. 1995). A novel method for mutation scanning has been developed with the potential to serve as an additional diagnostic method when combined with routine RT-PCR testing (Nakamichi et al. 2014).

A CSF JCV antibody index has been suggested as a complementary tool for the diagnosis of natalizumab-associated PML in cases with low levels of JC virus DNA in CSF, but it needs additional evidence (Warnke et al. 2014).

15.8 Subacute Sclerosing Panencephalitis

15.8.1 Clinical Background and Diagnosis

Subacute sclerosing panencephalitis (SSPE) is a chronic encephalitis secondary to measles infection that causes demyelination damage of CNS. The measles virus (a single-stranded, negative-sense, enveloped RNA virus in the family of *Paramyxoviridae*) occurs predominantly in regions with low vaccination rates. The SSPE clinical manifestations occur on average 6 years after measles and include cognitive and behavioural disorders, myoclonic seizures, pareses, rigidity and akinetic mutism, rarely cerebellar signs and speech disorder and, in some patients, early visual symptoms with macular and retinal changes. SSPE is more prevalent in males, and the presentations usually occur in childhood, but adult cases have been described as well. The incidence of SSPE is decreasing as a result of measles vaccination (Colpak et al. 2012; Erturk et al. 2011; Gutierrez et al. 2010).

The diagnosis of SSPE is based on clinical manifestations, EEG findings with periodic complexes, demyelinating lesions in MRI and immunological evidence of intrathecal anti-measles antibody production. Clinically, measles have been demonstrated by a history in about half of SSPE patients (Gutierrez et al. 2010; Lakshmi et al. 1993).

There is no effective treatment for SSPE. Oral isoprinosine and intrathecal alpha-interferon may prolong survival but do not change the long-term outcome. The prognosis of SSPE is poor, with a lethal outcome in a majority of cases. The best method for prevention of SSPE is vaccination against measles (Gutierrez et al. 2010; Eroglu et al. 2008).

15.8.2 Cerebrospinal Fluid

In CSF examination the SSPE patients have a mild pleocytosis, normal or elevated protein and normal glucose CSF-to-serum ratio. Diagnosis of SSPE is confirmed by CSF anti-measles antibodies; ELISA for CSF antibodies has a sensitivity of 100 % and specificity of 93 % and a positive predictive value in appropriate clinical settings (Gutierrez et al. 2010; Lakshmi et al. 1993). IgG titre range in CSF has been demonstrated from 1:40 to 1:1,280 and the CSF-serum IgG ratio from 5:1 to 40:1 (Manayani et al. 2002). Results of studies on CSF cytokine levels show discrepancies between reports (Aydin et al. 2010).

15.9 Toxoplasmosis

15.9.1 Clinical Background

Toxoplasmosis is caused by the obligate intracellular protozoal parasite *Toxoplasma gondii*, transmitted by the oral or transplacental route. Common sources of human infection are consumption of undercooked lamb or pork meat that contains viable tissue cysts or direct ingestion of oocytes from contaminated soil, water, goat's milk or unwashed vegetables (Finsterer and Auer 2013). In immunocompetent adults, most *T. gondii* infections are subclinical, but severe clinical manifestations occur in immunocompromised patients (Patil et al. 2011). The prevalence rates of latent *Toxoplasma* infections in HIV-infected patients have been found to vary greatly from 3 to 97 % (Ammassari et al. 2000). Prior to the introduction of effective antiretroviral therapy, about half of seropositive patients had cerebral toxoplasmosis (Oksenhendler et al. 1994).

The involvement of cerebral grey or white matter in these patients results in encephalitis or a CNS mass lesion, which manifests clinically as headache, epilepsy, hemiparesis, psychosis, cognitive dysfunction or movement disorders. The basal ganglia, thalamus and corticomedullar junction are most frequently affected (Finsterer and Auer 2013). Neurotoxoplasmosis is diagnosed upon clinical, serological, CSF or imaging investigations. MRI findings include lesions with mass effect in cerebral cortex, subcortical white matter, basal ganglia, brain stem or cerebellum (Fig. 15.4).

15.9.2 Cerebrospinal Fluid

The combination of mononuclear pleocytosis, elevated protein count and normal glucose levels in CSF of immunocompromised patients is highly suggestive of toxoplasma encephalitis.

Detection of *T. gondii* in CSF A definite diagnosis of cerebral toxoplasmosis could be made by histologic demonstration of tachyzoites in brain biopsies taken

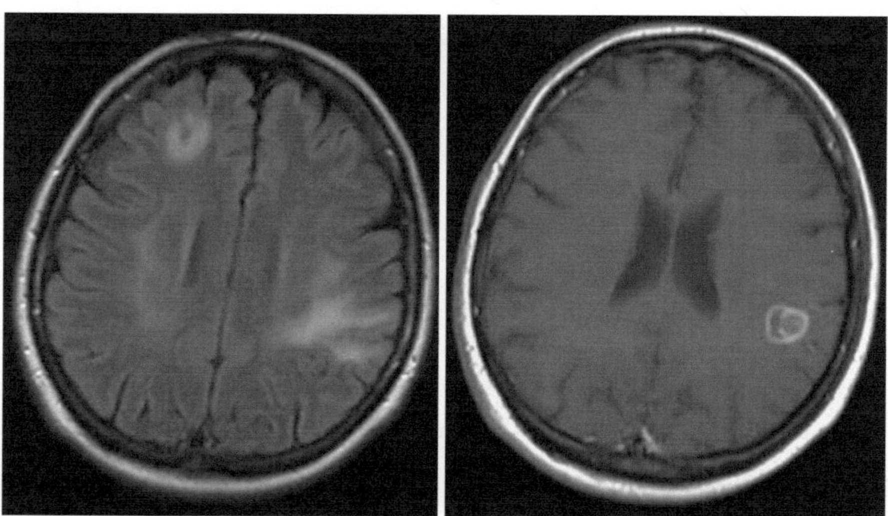

Fig. 15.4 MRI of a HIV patient with toxoplasmosis, revealing lesions in corticomedullar junction

from lesions. This procedure is hardly ever used in clinics due to the high rate of serious complications. Furthermore the sensitivity of tissue cultures that have been used in the past was lower than of PCR (Dupon et al. 1995). However, the PCR for *T. gondii* DNA in CSF has shown variable sensitivity values from 0 to 100 % that depend on various factors, including the site of a puncture: studies have shown that the sensitivity of samples taken by ventricular tap is higher than those taken by lumbar puncture (Adurthi et al. 2011; Contini 2008; Contini et al. 1998). Direct identification of *T gondii* tachyzoites in CSF of adult patients is apparently extremely rare. In all but one reported case, the organisms have been identified in the ventricular rather than lumbar specimen (Brogi and Cibas 2000; Palm et al. 2008).

Detection of Antibodies in CSF It is believed that more than 50 % of patients with cerebral toxoplasmosis present specific antibodies in the CSF due to permeability changes of the blood–CSF barrier allowing passive passage of antibodies from serum to the CSF (Dannemann et al. 1992). CSF serology appears to be remarkably sensitive for the diagnosis of cerebral toxoplasmosis (Adurthi et al. 2011) but has relatively low specificity in discriminating between recent, active and past dormant toxoplasma infection (Luft and Remington 1988). This could be overcome by measuring antibodies against excretory–secretory antigens which are the majority of the circulating antigens in sera in patients with acute toxoplasmosis. These antibodies measured in CSF by ELISA or immunoblotting appear to be good markers for cerebral toxoplasmosis also in patients with HIV infections (Meira et al. 2011).

15.10 Sleeping Sickness/African Trypanosomiasis

15.10.1 Clinical Background and Diagnosis

African trypanosomiasis is a parasitosis, caused by the protozoa *Trypanosoma brucei gambiense* (West African form) or *Trypanosoma brucei rhodesiense* (East African form), transmitted by tsetse flies. Incidence of African trypanosomiasis has decreased, but the WHO estimates a large population being at risk, and has classified this as a neglected tropical disease by 2020 (WHO 2014b; Truc et al. 2012). Sleeping sickness is endemic to Sub-Saharan Africa with the highest number of cases in Congo, but an increasing number of cases has been reported in non-endemic areas including Europe and North America, in travellers, military personnel and immigrants (Migchelsen et al. 2011).

There are two clinical stages of African trypanosomiasis – the first or haemolymphatic stage starts with fever, lymphadenopathy and chancres, followed by invasion of protozoa into CNS. The second or meningoencephalitic stage is characterised by severe headaches, disruption of the circadian rhythm with daytime somnolence and night time insomnia, cognitive and behavioural disorders, pareses and movement disorders. The disease eventually may progress to apallic syndrome, coma and death (Migchelsen et al. 2011; Brun et al. 2010).

For laboratory large-scale screening of the populations at risk, the card agglutination test for trypanosomiasis/*T. b. gambiense* (CATT) in serum is used, and the diagnosis is confirmed by microscopic verification of the parasite, followed by CSF examination for staging of the disease (WHO 2014b). Novel rapid serological tests have been introduced recently, but they need further evaluation of their diagnostic accuracy (Buscher et al. 2013). MRI may show diffuse white matter abnormalities, basal ganglia hyperintensities and ventricular enlargement, but neuroimaging is often not available in endemic areas (Brun et al. 2010; Kennedy 2008).

African trypanosomiasis is fatal if untreated, but current anti-trypanosomal therapies have limitations due to toxicity. Pentamidine or suramin are recommended for the first stage and melarsoprol and eflornithine for the neurological stage of sleeping sickness (WHO 2014b; Migchelsen et al. 2011; Kennedy 2008).

15.10.2 Cerebrospinal Fluid

Examination of CSF is essential for the diagnosis of human African trypanosomiasis with CNS involvement and also for selection of treatment and post-treatment follow-up. A pleocytosis >5 cells/µL is an indicator of CNS infection, but typically there are 100–300 cells/µL of lymphocytic origin. A slightly elevated cell count may persist for several months even after successful treatment. The microscopic detection of trypanosomes in CSF is diagnostic for the meningoencephalitis stage of the disease. Molecular amplification tests to detect trypanosomal DNA are sensitive; however, the accuracy of these tests as diagnostic tools has not been fully verified (Mugasa et al. 2012). Increased IgM concentrations in CSF are an early and specific diagnostic marker, and the intrathecal IgM response is higher than the IgG response, but detection of trypanosome specific antibodies is of low sensitivity (Brun et al. 2010; Lejon and Buscher 2005). Novel promising biomarkers including neopterin have been proposed for stage determination of human African trypanosomiasis but need further evidence (Tiberti et al. 2013; Burchmore 2012). CSF cytokines have not demonstrated sufficient sensitivity to be of clinical value for staging of the disease (MacLean et al. 2012).

15.11 Nipah Encephalitis

The Nipah virus along with the Hendra virus are the members of a newly identified genus of emerging paramyxoviruses, henipaviruses. Since their discovery in the 1990s, henipavirus outbreaks have been described mainly in Asian countries. The viruses have high economic and public health threat potential. When compared to other paramyxoviruses, henipaviruses appear to have unique characteristics. They are zoonotic viruses with a broader tropism and host range than most other paramyxoviruses and can cause severe acute encephalitis with unique features among viral encephalitides. Both henipaviruses are very likely to be transmitted to their amplifying or dead-end host (pigs, horses) by several species of fruit bats (Vigant and Lee 2011). The Nipah virus infects a wide range of mammalian species (pigs, dogs, goats and cats). It is extremely contagious among pigs and is readily transmitted to humans (Parashar et al. 2000). Moreover, direct transmission to humans and between humans has been reported (Chua 2012). Human may also become infected through consumption of raw fruit or date palm juice contaminated with the virus.

One of the most unusual features of Nipah infection is the propensity for patients to develop relapsing or late-onset encephalitis up to 53 months after acute infection (median 8 months); some patients may have a second relapse. Late-onset encephalitis, in patients who do not initially have neurological symptoms, occurs in about 3 % of cases. Eight percent of survivors of acute encephalitis have recurrent neurological disease (relapsed encephalitis). Patients with relapses are likely to have fever (46 %) and headache (42 %) and more likely to have seizures (50 %) and focal neurological signs (42 %) than those with acute encephalitis (Tan and Chua 2008). As in acute encephalitis, CSF is usually abnormal with mild lymphocytic pleocytosis. However, the absence of the virus in CSF suggests that the pathophysiology of acute and relapsed or late-onset encephalitis is different but needs further investigation. MRI findings usually involve damage of grey matter. As many as 35–75 % of symptomatic Nipah virus infections are fatal, and approximately 15 % of survivors have neurological sequelae (Sawatsky et al. 2007).

The diagnosis is made by detecting Nipah virus by RT-PCR or cell culture of CSF in the early stage or by detecting Nipah virus-specific IgM and IgG antibodies in serum by using ELISA in the later stages (www.cdc.gov. last accessed 21.09.2014). The CSF in Nipah virus encephalitis shows lymphocytic pleocytosis, elevated protein content and normal glucose concentration. MRI features consist of disseminated small (<7 mm) signal hyperintensities, best seen on FLAIR sequences, predominately involving white matter.

15.12 Mollaret Meningitis

Recurrent lymphocytic meningitis was first described in 1944 by Pierre Mollaret. The syndrome, also known as Mollaret meningitis, occurs very rarely and is characterised by recurrent attacks of sudden-onset aseptic meningitis that usually lasts for 2–7 days, with a complete recovery but unpredictable recurrences. In the first 24 h, large mononuclear cells with blunt pseudopods and bean-shaped, bilobed nuclei – termed 'Mollaret cells' – are typical in CSF but may be absent. Using electron microscopy (de Chadarevian and Becker 1980) proved that Mollaret endothelial cells were epithelioid-looking monocytes or macrophages.

With improving of diagnostic techniques, Mollaret meningitis has been associated with human herpes virus 2 since recurrent herpes encephalitis is clinically indistinguishable from cases of idiopathic Mollaret meningitis (Munoz-Sanz et al. 2013; Miller et al. 2013). It has been argued that the term 'Mollaret meningitis' should be restricted to idiopathic recurrent aseptic meningitis, whereas cases of recurrent meningitis known to be associated with herpes simplex virus or, rarely, other viruses should be referred to as 'recurrent viral meningitis' (Pearce 2008).

Conclusions

There is a number of diseases that can cause a chronic infection of CNS. Distinguishing rare patients with chronic CNS infections from those with more common syndromes of acute neuroinfections or other CNS diseases may be difficult, and when unrecognised, the delayed diagnosis and treatment may result in the most unfavourable outcome. Immunocompromised patients require special considerations for differential diagnosis. In summary, the diagnosis of chronic infections of CNS is a complex issue, often based on combination of variable clinical manifestations and different laboratory methods, including novel PCR methods and immunological assays.

References

Aalto A, Sjowall J, Davidsson L, Forsberg P, Smedby O (2007) Brain magnetic resonance imaging does not contribute to the diagnosis of chronic neuroborreliosis. Acta Radiol 48(7):755–762

Achazi K, Ruzek D, Donoso-Mantke O, Schlegel M, Ali HS, Wenk M et al (2011) Rodents as sentinels for the prevalence of tick-borne encephalitis virus. Vector Borne Zoonotic Dis 11(6):641–647

Adurthi S, Mahadevan A, Bantwal R, Satishchandra P, Ramprasad S, Sridhar H et al (2011) Diagnosis of cerebral toxoplasmosis. Ann Indian Acad Neurol 14(2):145–146

Agarwal R, Sze G (2009) Neuro-lyme disease: MR imaging findings. Radiology 253(1):167–173

Agarwal AK, Bansal S, Nand V (2014) A Hospital Based Study on Estimation of Adenosine Deaminase Activity (ADA) in Cerebrospinal Fluid (CSF) in Various Types of Meningitis. J Clin Diagn Res 8(2):73–76

Aguero-Rosenfeld ME (2008) Lyme disease: laboratory issues. Infect Dis Clin North Am 22(2):301–313, vii

Aguero-Rosenfeld ME, Wang G, Schwartz I, Wormser GP (2005) Diagnosis of lyme borreliosis. Clin Microbiol Rev 18(3):484–509

Aguzzi A, Nuvolone M, Zhu C (2013) The immunobiology of prion diseases. Nat Rev Immunol 13(12):888–902

Ammassari A, Cingolani A, Pezzotti P, De Luca DA, Murri R, Giancola ML et al (2000) AIDS-related focal brain lesions in the era of highly active antiretroviral therapy. Neurology 55(8):1194–1200

Antinori A, Arendt G, Becker JT, Brew BJ, Byrd DA, Cherner M et al (2007) Updated research nosology for HIV-associated neurocognitive disorders. Neurology 69(18):1789–1799

Araujo AQ (2013) Prionic diseases. Arq Neuropsiquiatr 71(9b):731–737

Atarashi R, Satoh K, Sano K, Fuse T, Yamaguchi N, Ishibashi D et al (2011) Ultrasensitive human prion detection in cerebrospinal fluid by real-time quaking-induced conversion. Nat Med 17(2):175–178

Aydin OF, Ichiyama T, Anlar B (2010) Serum and cerebrospinal fluid cytokine concentrations in subacute sclerosing panencephalitis. Brain Dev 32(6):463–466

Berger JR, Aksamit AJ, Clifford DB, Davis L, Koralnik IJ, Sejvar JJ et al (2013) PML diagnostic criteria: consensus statement from the AAN Neuroinfectious Disease Section. Neurology 80(15):1430–1438

Blanc F, Jaulhac B, Fleury M, de Seze J, de Martino SJ, Remy V et al (2007) Relevance of the antibody index to diagnose Lyme neuroborreliosis among seropositive patients. Neurology 69(10):953–958

Bremell D, Mattsson N, Edsbagge M, Blennow K, Andreasson U, Wikkelso C et al (2013) Cerebrospinal fluid CXCL13 in Lyme neuroborreliosis and asymptomatic HIV infection. BMC Neurol 13:2

Brew BJ, Pemberton L, Cunningham P, Law MG (1997) Levels of human immunodeficiency virus type 1 RNA in cerebrospinal fluid correlate with AIDS dementia stage. J Infect Dis 175(4): 963–966

Brogi E, Cibas ES (2000) Cytologic detection of Toxoplasma gondii tachyzoites in cerebrospinal fluid. Am J Clin Pathol 114(6):951–955

Brun R, Blum J, Chappuis F, Burri C (2010) Human African trypanosomiasis. Lancet 375(9709): 148–159

Burchmore R (2012) Parasites in the brain? The search for sleeping sickness biomarkers. Expert Rev Anti Infect Ther 10(11):1283–1286

Buscher P, Gilleman Q, Lejon V (2013) Rapid diagnostic test for sleeping sickness. N Engl J Med 368(11):1069–1070

Cameron D, Gaito A, Harris N, Bach G, Bellovin S, Bock K et al (2004) Evidence-based guidelines for the management of Lyme disease. Expert Rev Anti Infect Ther 2(1 Suppl):S1–S13

Carson KR, Evens AM, Richey EA, Habermann TM, Focosi D, Seymour JF et al (2009) Progressive multifocal leukoencephalopathy after rituximab therapy in HIV-negative patients: a report of 57 cases from the Research on Adverse Drug Events and Reports project. Blood 113(20): 4834–4840

Carson KR, Newsome SD, Kim EJ, Wagner-Johnston ND, von Geldern G, Moskowitz CH et al (2014) Progressive multifocal leukoencephalopathy associated with brentuximab vedotin therapy: a report of 5 cases from the Southern Network on Adverse Reactions (SONAR) project. Cancer 120:2464–2471

Casado JL, Corral I, Garcia J. Martinez-San Millan J, Navas E, Moreno A et al (2014) Continued declining incidence and improved survival of progressive multifocal leukoencephalopathy in HIV/AIDS patients in the current era. Eur J Clin Microbiol Infect Dis 33(2):179–187

Castro R, Prieto ES, da Luz Martins Pereira F (2008) Nontreponemal tests in the diagnosis of neurosyphilis: an evaluation of the Venereal Disease Research Laboratory (VDRL) and the Rapid Plasma Reagin (RPR) tests. J Clin Lab Anal 22(4):257–261

CDC (Centers for Disease Control) (2010) STD treatment guidelines 2010 [cited 02/05/2014]. Available from: http://www.cdc.gov/std/default.htm

CDC (Centers for Disease Control) (2014) National notifiable diseases surveillance system. Syphilis (Treponema pallidum), 2014 case definition [cited 5/18/2014]. Available from: http://wwwn.cdc.gov/nndss/script/casedef.aspx?condyrid=941&datepub=1/1/2014

Cecchini D, Ambrosioni J, Brezzo C, Corti M, Rybko A, Perez M et al (2009) Tuberculous meningitis in HIV-infected and non-infected patients: comparison of cerebrospinal fluid findings. Int J Tuberc Lung Dis 13(2):269–271

Cerar T, Ogrinc K, Lotric-Furlan S, Kobal J, Levicnik-Stezinar S, Strle F et al (2013) Diagnostic value of cytokines and chemokines in lyme neuroborreliosis. Clin Vaccine Immunol 20(10):1578–1584

Chahine LM, Khoriaty RN, Tomford WJ, Hussain MS (2011) The changing face of neurosyphilis. Int J Stroke 6(2):136–143

Chamie G, Marquez C, Luetkemeyer A (2014) HIV-associated central nervous system tuberculosis. Semin Neurol 34(1):103–115

Choe PG, Song JS, Song KH. Jeon JH, Park WB, Park KU et al (2010) Usefulness of routine lumbar puncture in non-HIV patients with latent syphilis of unknown duration. Sex Transm Infect 86(1):39–40

Chohan G, Pennington C, Mackenzie JM, Andrews M, Everington D, Will RG et al (2010) The role of cerebrospinal fluid 14-3-3 and other proteins in the diagnosis of sporadic Creutzfeldt-Jakob disease in the UK: a 10-year review. J Neurol Neurosurg Psychiatry 81(11):1243–1248

Christensen AS, Andersen AB, Thomsen VO, Andersen PH, Johansen IS (2011) Tuberculous meningitis in Denmark: a review of 50 cases. BMC Infect Dis 11:47

Christie LJ, Loeffler AM, Honarmand S, Flood JM, Baxter R, Jacobson S et al (2008) Diagnostic challenges of central nervous system tuberculosis. Emerg Infect Dis 14(9):1473–1475

Chua KB (2012) Introduction: Nipah virus – discovery and origin. Curr Top Microbiol Immunol 359:1–9

Colpak AI, Erdener SE, Ozgen B, Anlar B, Kansu T (2012) Neuro-ophthalmology of subacute sclerosing panencephalitis: two cases and a review of the literature. Curr Opin Ophthalmol 23(6):466–471

Contini C (2008) Clinical and diagnostic management of toxoplasmosis in the immunocompromised patient. Parassitologia 50(1–2):45–50

Contini C, Fainardi E, Cultrera R, Canipari R, Peyron F, Delia S et al (1998) Advanced laboratory techniques for diagnosing Toxoplasma gondii encephalitis in AIDS patients: significance of intrathecal production and comparison with PCR and ECL-western blotting. J Neuroimmunol 92(1–2):29–37

Coyle PK, Schutzer SE, Deng Z, Krupp LB, Belman AL, Benach JL et al (1995) Detection of Borrelia burgdorferi-specific antigen in antibody-negative cerebrospinal fluid in neurologic Lyme disease. Neurology 45(11):2010–2015

Daniele B (2014) Characteristics of central nervous system tuberculosis in a low-incidence country: a series of 20 cases and a review of the literature. Jpn J Infect Dis 67(1):50–53

Danielsen AG, Weismann K, Jorgensen BB, Heidenheim M, Fugleholm AM (2004) Incidence, clinical presentation and treatment of neurosyphilis in Denmark 1980–1997. Acta Derm Venereol 84(6):459–462

Dannemann B, McCutchan JA, Israelski D, Antoniskis D, Leport C, Luft B et al (1992) Treatment of toxoplasmic encephalitis in patients with AIDS. A randomized trial comparing pyrimethamine plus clindamycin to pyrimethamine plus sulfadiazine The California Collaborative Treatment Group. Ann Intern Med 116(1):33–43

de Chadarevian JP, Becker WJ (1980) Mollaret's recurrent aseptic meningitis: relationship to epidermoid cysts. Light microscopic and ultrastructural cytological studies of the cerebrospinal fluid. J Neuropathol Exp Neurol 39(6):661–669

Deisenhammer F, Egg R, Giovannoni G, Hemmer B, Petzold A, Sellebjerg F et al (2009) EFNS guidelines on disease-specific CSF investigations. Eur J Neurol 16(6):760–770

Djukic M, Schmidt-Samoa C, Lange P, Spreer A, Neubieser K, Eiffert H et al (2012) Cerebrospinal fluid findings in adults with acute Lyme neuroborreliosis. J Neurol 259(4):630–636

Dumpis U, Crook D, Oksi J (1999) Tick-borne encephalitis. Clin Infect Dis 28(4):882–890

Dupon M, Cazenave J, Pellegrin JL, Ragnaud JM, Cheyrou A, Fischer I et al (1995) Detection of Toxoplasma gondii by PCR and tissue culture in cerebrospinal fluid and blood of human immunodeficiency virus-seropositive patients. J Clin Microbiol 33(9):2421–2426

EC (The European Commission) (2012) Commission Implementing Decision of 8 August 2012 amending Decision 2002/253/EC laying down case definitions for reporting communicable diseases to the Community network under Decision No 2119/98/EC of the European Parliament and of the Council. Off J Eur Union 55:L262/1-59 2012

ECDC (European Centre for Disease Prevention and Control) (2013) Annual epidemiological report: reporting on 2011 surveillance data and 2013 epidemic intelligence data. ECDC, Stockholm

Eroglu E, Gokcil Z, Bek S, Ulas UH, Ozdag MF, Odabasi Z (2008) Long-term follow-up of patients with adult-onset subacute sclerosing panencephalitis. J Neurol Sci 275(1–2):113–116

Erturk O, Karsligil B, Cokar O, Yapici Z, Demirbilek V, Gurses C et al (2011) Challenges in diagnosing SSPE. Childs Nerv Syst 27(12):2041–2044

Feder HM Jr, Johnson BJ, O'Connell S, Shapiro ED, Steere AC, Wormser GP et al (2007) A critical appraisal of "chronic Lyme disease". N Engl J Med 357(14):1422–1430

Felix-Morais R, Andrade LC, Rebelo O (2014) Creutzfeldt-Jakob disease: typical imaging findings. BMJ Case Rep 2014. doi:10.1136/bcr-2014-203997

Finsterer J, Auer H (2013) Parasitoses of the human central nervous system. J Helminthol 87(3):257–270

Fong IW, Britton CB, Luinstra KE, Toma E, Mahony JB (1995) Diagnostic value of detecting JC virus DNA in cerebrospinal fluid of patients with progressive multifocal leukoencephalopathy. J Clin Microbiol 33(2):484–486

French P, Gomberg M, Janier M, Schmidt B, van Voorst VP, Young H (2009) IUSTI: 2008 European guidelines on the management of syphilis. Int J STD AIDS 20(5):300–309

Frolova TV, Frolova MP, Pogodona VV, Sobolev SG, Karmysheva V (1987) Pathogenesis of persistent and chronic forms of tick-borne encephalitis (experimental study). Zh Nevropatol Psikhiatr Im S S Korsakova 87(2):170–178

Garg RK, Jain A, Malhotra HS, Agrawal A, Garg R (2013) Drug-resistant tuberculous meningitis. Expert Rev Anti Infect Ther 11(6):605–621

Gayet-Ageron A, Lautenschlager S, Ninet B, Perneger TV, Combescure C (2013) Sensitivity, specificity and likelihood ratios of PCR in the diagnosis of syphilis: a systematic review and meta-analysis. Sex Transm Infect 89(3):251–256

Ghanem KG (2010) REVIEW: neurosyphilis: a historical perspective and review. CNS Neurosci Ther 16(5):e157–e168

Gisslen M, Krut J, Andreasson U, Blennow K, Cinque P, Brew BJ et al (2009) Amyloid and tau cerebrospinal fluid biomarkers in HIV infection. BMC Neurol 9:63

Gitai LL, Jalali PS, Takayanagui OM (2009) Neurosyphilis in the age of AIDS: clinical and laboratory features. Neurol Sci 30(6):465–470

Gorelik L, Lerner M, Bixler S, Crossman M, Schlain B, Simon K et al (2010) Anti-JC virus antibodies: implications for PML risk stratification. Ann Neurol 68(3):295–303

Green A, Sanchez-Juan P, Ladogana A, Cuadrado-Corrales N, Sanchez-Valle R, Mitrova E et al (2007) CSF analysis in patients with sporadic CJD and other transmissible spongiform encephalopathies. Eur J Neurol 14(2):121–124

Gritsun TS, Frolova TV, Zhankov AI, Armesto M, Turner SL, Frolova MP et al (2003a) Characterization of a siberian virus isolated from a patient with progressive chronic tick-borne encephalitis. J Virol 77(1):25–36

Gritsun TS, Lashkevich VA, Gould EA (2003b) Tick-borne encephalitis. Antiviral Res 57(1–2): 129–146

Gunawardhana SA, Somaratne SC, Fernando MA, Gunaratne PS (2013) Tuberculous meningitis in adults: a prospective study at a tertiary referral centre in Sri Lanka. Ceylon Med J 58(1):21–25

Gutierrez J, Issacson RS, Koppel BS (2010) Subacute sclerosing panencephalitis: an update Dev Med Child Neurol 52(10):901–907

Hagberg L, Cinque P, Gisslen M, Brew BJ, Spudich S, Bestetti A et al (2010) Cerebrospinal fluid neopterin: an informative biomarker of central nervous system immune activation in HIV-1 infection. AIDS Res Ther 7:15

Hansen K, Crone C, Kristoferitsch W (2013) Lyme neuroborreliosis. Handb Clin Neurol 115: 559–575

Harding AS, Ghanem KG (2012) The performance of cerebrospinal fluid treponemal-specific antibody tests in neurosyphilis: a systematic review. Sex Transm Dis 39(4):291–297

Ho EL, Marra CM (2012) Treponemal tests for neurosyphilis – less accurate than what we thought? Sex Transm Dis 39:298–299, United States

Ho EL, Ronquillo R, Altmeppen H, Spudich SS, Price RW, Sinclair E (2013) Cellular composition of cerebrospinal fluid in HIV-1 infected and uninfected subjects. PLoS One 8(6):e66188

Holzmann H (2003) Diagnosis of tick-borne encephalitis. Vaccine 21(Suppl 1):S36–S40

Hsu PC, Yang CC, Ye JJ, Huang PY, Chiang PC, Lee MH (2010) Prognostic factors of tuberculous meningitis in adults: a 6-year retrospective study at a tertiary hospital in northern Taiwan. J Microbiol Immunol Infect 43(2):111–118

Isabel BE, Rogelio HP (2014) Pathogenesis and immune response in tuberculous meningitis. Malays J Med Sci 21(1):4–10

Katti MK (2004) Pathogenesis, diagnosis, treatment, and outcome aspects of cerebral tuberculosis. Med Sci Monit 10(9):Ra215–Ra229

Kennedy PG (2008) The continuing problem of human African trypanosomiasis (sleeping sickness). Ann Neurol 64(2):116–126

Kim SH, Cho OH, Park SJ, Lee EM, Kim MN, Lee SO et al (2010) Rapid diagnosis of tuberculous meningitis by T cell-based assays on peripheral blood and cerebrospinal fluid mononuclear cells. Clin Infect Dis 50(10):1349–1358

Kingston M, French P, Goh B, Goold P, Higgins S, Sukthankar A et al (2008) UK National guidelines on the management of syphilis 2008. Int J STD AIDS 19(11):729–740

Kingston M, Goold P, Radcliffe K (2011) Amendment and correction to the 2008 UK national guideline on the management of syphilis. Int J STD AIDS 22:613–614, England

Kusum S, Aman S, Pallab R, Kumar SS, Manish M, Sudesh P et al (2011) Multiplex PCR for rapid diagnosis of tuberculous meningitis. J Neurol 258(10):1781–1787

Lakshmi V, Malathy Y, Rao RR (1993) Serodiagnosis of subacute sclerosing panencephalitis by enzyme linked immunosorbent assay. Indian J Pediatr 60(1):37–41

Lejon V, Buscher P (2005) Review Article: cerebrospinal fluid in human African trypanosomiasis: a key to diagnosis, therapeutic decision and post-treatment follow-up. Trop Med Int Health 10(5):395–403

Ljostad U, Mygland A (2013) Chronic Lyme; diagnostic and therapeutic challenges. Acta Neurol Scand Suppl 196:38–47

Luft BJ, Remington JS (1988) AIDS commentary. Toxoplasmic encephalitis. J Infect Dis 157(1):1–6

MacLean L, Reiber H, Kennedy PG, Sternberg JM (2012) Stage progression and neurological symptoms in Trypanosoma brucei rhodesiense sleeping sickness: role of the CNS inflammatory response. PLoS Negl Trop Dis 5(10):e1857

Manayani DJ, Abraham M, Gnanamuthu C, Solomon T, Alexander M, Sridharan G (2002) SSPE – the continuing challenge: a study based on serological evidence from a teritary care centre in India. Indian J Med Microbiol 20(1):16–18

Mancuso R, Saresella M, Hernis A, Marventano I, Ricci C, Agostini S et al (2012) JC virus detection and JC virus-specific immunity in natalizumab-treated multiple sclerosis patients. J Transl Med 10:248

Marais S, Thwaites G, Schoeman JF, Torok ME, Misra UK, Prasad K et al (2010) Tuberculous meningitis: a uniform case definition for use in clinical research. Lancet Infect Dis 10(11):803–812

Marra CM, Maxwell CL, Smith SL, Lukehart SA, Rompalo AM, Eaton M et al (2004) Cerebrospinal fluid abnormalities in patients with syphilis: association with clinical and laboratory features. J Infect Dis 189(3):369–376

Marra CM, Maxwell CL, Tantalo LC, Sahi SK, Lukehart SA (2008) Normalization of serum rapid plasma reagin titer predicts normalization of cerebrospinal fluid and clinical abnormalities after treatment of neurosyphilis. Clin Infect Dis 47(7):893–899

Marra CM, Tantalo LC, Sahi SK, Maxwell CL, Lukehart SA (2010) CXCL13 as a cerebrospinal fluid marker for neurosyphilis in HIV-infected patients with syphilis. Sex Transm Dis 37(5):283–287

Marra CM, Tantalo LC, Maxwell CL, Ho EL, Sahi SK, Jones T (2012) The rapid plasma reagin test cannot replace the venereal disease research laboratory test for neurosyphilis diagnosis. Sex Transm Dis 39(6):453–457

Meira CS, Vidal JE, Costa-Silva TA, Frazatti-Gallina N, Pereira-Chioccola VL (2011) Immunodiagnosis in cerebrospinal fluid of cerebral toxoplasmosis and HIV-infected patients using Toxoplasma gondii excreted/secreted antigens. Diagn Microbiol Infect Dis 71(3):279–285

Mentzer D, Prestel J, Adams O, Gold R, Hartung HP, Hengel H et al (2012) Case definition for progressive multifocal leukoencephalopathy following treatment with monoclonal antibodies. J Neurol Neurosurg Psychiatry 83(9):927–933

Mickiene A, Laiskonis A, Gunther G, Vene S, Lundkvist A, Lindquist L (2002) Tickborne encephalitis in an area of high endemicity in lithuania: disease severity and long-term prognosis. Clin Infect Dis 35(6):650–658

Migchelsen SJ, Buscher P, Hoepelman AI, Schallig HD, Adams ER (2011) Human African trypanosomiasis: a review of non-endemic cases in the past 20 years. Int J Infect Dis 15(8): e517–e524

Miklossy J (2012) Chronic or late lyme neuroborreliosis: analysis of evidence compared to chronic or late neurosyphilis. Open Neurol J 6:146–157

Miller S, Mateen FJ, Aksamit AJ Jr (2013) Herpes simplex virus 2 meningitis: a retrospective cohort study. J Neurovirol 19(2):166–171

Moniuszko A, Czupryna P, Pancewicz S, Rutkowski K, Zajkowska O, Swierzbinska R et al (2014) Evaluation of CXCL8, CXCL10, CXCL11, CXCL12 and CXCL13 in serum and cerebrospinal fluid of patients with neuroborreliosis. Immunol Lett 157(1–2):45–50

Muayqil T, Gronseth G, Camicioli R (2012) Evidence-based guideline: diagnostic accuracy of CSF 14-3-3 protein in sporadic Creutzfeldt-Jakob disease: report of the guideline development subcommittee of the American Academy of Neurology. Neurology 79(14):1499–1506

Mugasa CM, Adams ER, Boer KR, Dyserinck HC, Buscher P, Schallig HD et al (2012) Diagnostic accuracy of molecular amplification tests for human African trypanosomiasis – systematic review. PLoS Negl Trop Dis 6(1):e1438

Mukhin KY, Mameniskiene R, Mironov MB, Kvaskova NE, Bobylova MY, Petrukhin AS et al (2012) Epilepsia partialis continua in tick-borne Russian spring-summer encephalitis. Acta Neurol Scand 125(5):345–352

Munoz-Sanz A, Rodriguez-Vidigal FF, Nogales-Munoz N, Vera-Tome A (2013) Herpes simplex type-2 recurrent meningitis: Mollaret or not Mollaret? Enferm Infecc Microbiol Clin 31(4): 271–272

Mygland A, Ljostad U, Fingerle V, Rupprecht T, Schmutzhard E, Steiner I (2010) EFNS guidelines on the diagnosis and management of European Lyme neuroborreliosis. Eur J Neurol 17(1): 8–16, e1–4

Nadezhdina MV (2001) Clinical pathogenic peculiarities of chronic Russian tick-born encephalitis. Zh Nevrol Psikhiatr Im S S Korsakova 101(4):10–15

Nakamichi K, Tajima S, Lim CK, Saijc M (2014) High-resolution melting analysis for mutation scanning in the non-coding control region of JC polyomavirus from patients with progressive multifocal leukoencephalopathy. Arch Virol 159(7):1687–1696

Naslednikova IO, Ryazantseva NV, Novitskii VV, Lepekhin AV, Antoshina MA, Belokon VV et al (2005) Chronic tick-borne encephalitis virus antigenemia: possible pathogenesis pathways. Bull Exp Biol Med 139(4):451–454

Navia BA, Jordan BD, Price RW (1986) The AIDS dementia complex: I. Clinical features. Ann Neurol 19(6):517–524

Nhu NT, Heemskerk D, DA T d, Chau TT, Mai NT, Nghia HD et al (2014) Evaluation of GeneXpert MTB/RIF for diagnosis of tuberculous meningitis. J Clin Microbiol 52(1):226–33

Oksenhendler E, Charreau I, Tournerie C, Azihary M, Carbon C, Aboulker JP (1994) Toxoplasma gondii infection in advanced HIV infection. AIDS 8(4):483–487

Palm C, Tumani H, Pietzker T, Bengel D (2008) Diagnosis of cerebral toxoplasmosis by detection of *Toxoplasma gondii* tachyzoites in cerebrospinal fluid. J Neurol 255(6):939–941

Panegyres PK, Armari E (2013) Therapies for human prion diseases. Am J Neurodegener Dis 2(3):176–186

Panelius J, Lahdenne P, Saxén H, Carlsson SA, Heikkilä T, Peltomaa M et al (2003) Diagnosis of Lyme neuroborreliosis with antibodies to recombinant proteins DbpA, BBK32, and OspC, and VlsE IR6 peptide. J Neurol 250(11):1318–1327

Parashar UD, Sunn LM, Ong F, Mounts AW, Arif MT, Ksiazek TG et al (2000) Case–control study of risk factors for human infection with a new zoonotic paramyxovirus, Nipah virus, during a 1998–1999 outbreak of severe encephalitis in Malaysia. J Infect Dis 181(5):1755–1759

Patil HV, Patil VC, Rajmane V, Raje V (2011) Successful treatment of cerebral toxoplasmosis with cotrimoxazole. Indian J Sex Transm Dis 32(1):44–46

Pearce JM (2008) Mollaret's meningitis. Eur Neurol 60(6):316–317

Poliseli R, Vidal JE, Penalva De Oliveira AC, Hernandez AV (2008) Neurosyphilis in HIV-infected patients: clinical manifestations, serum venereal disease research laboratory titers, and associated factors to symptomatic neurosyphilis. Sex Transm Dis 35(5):425–9

Poponnikova TV (2006) Specific clinical and epidemiological features of tick-borne encephalitis in Western Siberia. Int J Med Microbiol 296(Suppl 40):59–62

Price RW, Peterson J, Fuchs D, Angel TE, Zetterberg H, Hagberg L et al (2013) Approach to cerebrospinal fluid (CSF) biomarker discovery and evaluation in HIV infection. J Neuroimmune Pharmacol 8(5):1147–1158

Saksida A, Duh D, Lotric-Furlan S, Strle F, Petrovec M, Avsic-Zupanc T (2005) The importance of tick-borne encephalitis virus RNA detection for early differential diagnosis of tick-borne encephalitis. J Clin Virol 33(4):331–335

Sawatsky B, Grolla A, Kuzenko N, Weingartl H, Czub M (2007) Inhibition of henipavirus infection by Nipah virus attachment glycoprotein occurs without cell-surface downregulation of ephrin-B2 or ephrin-B3. J Gen Virol 88(Pt 2):582–591

Schmidt C, Plate A, Angele B, Pfister HW, Wick M, Koedel U et al (2011) A prospective study on the role of CXCL13 in Lyme neuroborreliosis. Neurology 76(12):1051–1058

Senel M, Rupprecht TA, Tumani H, Pfister HW, Ludolph AC, Brettschneider J (2010) The chemokine CXCL13 in acute neuroborreliosis. J Neurol Neurosurg Psychiatry 81(8):929–933

Skillback T, Rosen C, Asztely F, Mattsson N, Blennow K, Zetterberg H (2014) Diagnostic performance of cerebrospinal fluid total tau and phosphorylated tau in Creutzfeldt-Jakob disease: results from the Swedish Mortality Registry. JAMA Neurol 71(4):476–483

Solomons RS, van Elsland SL, Visser DH, Hoek KG, Marais BJ, Schoeman JF et al (2014) Commercial nucleic acid amplification tests in tuberculous meningitis – a meta-analysis. Diagn Microbiol Infect Dis 78(4):398–403

Song F, Sun X, Wang X, Nai Y, Liu Z (2014) Early diagnosis of tuberculous meningitis by an indirect ELISA protocol based on the detection of the antigen ESAT-6 in cerebrospinal fluid. Ir J Med Sci 183(1):85–88

Sparling PF (2010) Diagnosis of neurosyphilis: new tools. Sex Transm Dis 37(5):288–289

Spudich SS, Nilsson AC, Lollo ND, Liegler TJ, Petropoulos CJ, Deeks SG et al (2005) Cerebrospinal fluid HIV infection and pleocytosis: relation to systemic infection and antiretroviral treatment. BMC Infect Dis 5:98

Stanek G, Fingerle V, Hunfeld KP, Jaulhac B, Kaiser R, Krause A et al (2011) Lyme borreliosis: clinical case definitions for diagnosis and management in Europe. Clin Microbiol Infect 17(1):69–79

Stanek G, Wormser GP, Gray J, Strle F (2012) Lyme borreliosis. Lancet 379(9814):461–473

Steiner I, Berger JR (2012) Update on progressive multifocal leukoencephalopathy. Curr Neurol Neurosci Rep 12(6):680–686

Stoeck K, Sanchez-Juan P, Gawinecka J, Green A, Ladogana A, Pocchiari M et al (2012) Cerebrospinal fluid biomarker supported diagnosis of Creutzfeldt-Jakob disease and rapid dementias: a longitudinal multicentre study over 10 years. Brain 135(Pt 10):3051–3061

Tagliapietra M, Zanusso G, Fiorini M, Bonetto N, Zarantonello G, Zambon A et al (2013) Accuracy of diagnostic criteria for sporadic creutzfeldt-jakob disease among rapidly progressive dementia. J Alzheimers Dis 34(1):231–238

Takahashi T, Tamura M, Takasu T (2012) The PCR-based diagnosis of central nervous system tuberculosis: up to date. Tuberc Res Treat 2012:831292

Tan CT, Chua KB (2008) Nipah virus encephalitis. Curr Infect Dis Rep 10(4):315–320

Thwaites GE, Chau TT, Stepniewska K, Phu NH, Chuong LV, Sinh DX et al (2002) Diagnosis of adult tuberculous meningitis by use of clinical and laboratory features. Lancet 360(9342): 1287–1292

Thwaites GE, Nguyen DB, Nguyen HD, Hoang TQ, Do TT, Nguyen TC et al (2004) Dexamethasone for the treatment of tuberculous meningitis in adolescents and adults. N Engl J Med 351(17): 1741–1751

Thwaites G, Fisher M, Hemingway C, Scott G, Solomon T, Innes J (2009) British Infection Society guidelines for the diagnosis and treatment of tuberculosis of the central nervous system in adults and children. J Infect 59(3):167–187

Tiberti N, Lejon V, Hainard A, Courtioux B, Robin X, Turck N et al (2013) Neopterin is a cerebrospinal fluid marker for treatment outcome evaluation in patients affected by Trypanosoma brucei gambiense sleeping sickness. PLoS Negl Trop Dis 7(2):e2088

Truc P, Lando A, Penchenier L, Vatunga G, Josenando T (2012) Human African trypanosomiasis in Angola: clinical observations, treatment, and use of PCR for stage determination of early stage of the disease. Trans R Soc Trop Med Hyg 106(1):10–14

Tsai HC, Ye SY, Lee SS, Wann SR, Chen YS (2014) Expression of CXCL2 in the serum and cerebrospinal fluid of patients with HIV and syphilis or neurosyphilis. Inflammation 37(3):950–955

Tumani H, Nölker G, Reiber H (1995) Relevance of cerebrospinal fluid variables for early diagnosis of neuroborreliosis. Neurology 45(9):1663–1670

Tuon FF, Higashino HR, Lopes MI, Litvoc MN, Atomiya AN, Antonangelo L et al (2010) Adenosine deaminase and tuberculous meningitis – a systematic review with meta-analysis. Scand J Infect Dis 42(3):198–207

UNAIDS. (The Joint United Nations Programme on HIV/AIDS). 2013 global fact sheet. UNAIDS communications 2013 [5/18/2014]. Available from: http://www.unaids.org/en/media/unaids/contentassets/documents/epidemiology/2013/gr2013/20130923_FactSheet_Global_en.pdf

Vasilenko FI, Grigor'eva IG (1987) Early and late acute recurrences of tick-borne encephalitis. Zh Nevropatol Psikhiatr Im S S Korsakova 87(2):178–181

Vigant F, Lee B (2011) Hendra and nipah infection: pathology, models and potential therapies. Infect Disord Drug Targets 11(3):315–336

Wadsworth JD, Collinge J (2007) Update on human prion disease. Biochim Biophys Acta 1772(6):598–609

Warnke C, von Geldern G, Markwerth P, Dehmel T, Hoepner R, Gold R et al (2014) Cerebrospinal fluid JC virus antibody index for diagnosis of natalizumab-associated progressive multifocal leukoencephalopathy. Ann Neurol 76(6):792–801

WHO (World Health Organization) (2013) Global tuberculosis report

WHO (World Health Organization) (2014a) World Health Statistics [5/18/2014]. Available from: http://apps.who.int/iris/bitstream/10665/112738/1/9789240692671_eng.pdf?ua=1

WHO (World Health Organization) (2014b) Trypanosomiasis, human African (sleeping sickness). World Health Organization Fact Sheet No 259; [02/05/2014]. Available from: http://www.who.int/mediacentre/factsheets/fs259/en/

Wilske B, Fingerle V, Schulte-Spechtel U (2007) Microbiological and serological diagnosis of Lyme borreliosis. FEMS Immunol Med Microbiol 49(1):13–21

Zerr I, Kallenberg K, Summers DM, Romero C, Taratuto A, Heinemann U et al (2009) Updated clinical diagnostic criteria for sporadic Creutzfeldt-Jakob disease. Brain 132(Pt 10):2659–2668

Zhang HL, Lin LR, Liu GL, Zeng YL, Wu JY, Zheng WH et al (2013) Clinical spectrum of neurosyphilis among HIV-negative patients in the modern era. Dermatology 226(2):148–156

Zhou P, Gu X, Lu H, Guan Z, Qian Y (2012) Re-evaluation of serological criteria for early syphilis treatment efficacy: progression to neurosyphilis despite therapy. Sex Transm Infect 88(5): 342–345

Autoimmune Encephalitis

Agnes van Sonderen and Maarten J. Titulaer

Contents

A. van Sonderen
Department of Neurology, Erasmus Medical Center,
Rotterdam, The Netherlands

Department of Neurology,
Haga Hospital,
The Hague, The Netherlands
e-mail: A.vanSonderen@hagaziekenhuis.nl

M.J. Titulaer (⊠)
Department of Neurology,
Erasmus Medical Center,
Rotterdam, The Netherlands
e-mail: M.Titulaer@erasmusmc.nl

© Springer International Publishing Switzerland 2015
F. Deisenhammer et al. (eds.), *Cerebrospinal Fluid in Clinical Neurology*,
DOI 10.1007/978-3-319-01225-4_16

Abstract

This chapter gives an overview of the syndromes associated with antibodies directed to membrane-bound or synaptic proteins. In contrast to the classical syndromes, disease occurs in younger patients as well; patients are also seen by non-neurologists like psychiatrists and pediatricians, and patients tend to have a more favorable response to immunotherapy. The focus in this chapter is on the clinical characteristics which distinguishes these disorders and on the relevance of cerebrospinal fluid (CSF) analysis. Comparison of sensitivity and specificity for serum and CSF is extensively discussed. N-methyl-D-aspartate receptor (NMDAR) encephalitis is relatively common and discussed first. Alpha-amino-3-hydroxy-5-methyl-4-isoxazolepropionic acid receptor (AMPAR) encephalitis and encephalitis associated with antibodies to the metabotropic glutamate receptors mGluR1 and mGluR5 are rare and will be reviewed briefly. Subsequently, syndromes associated with antibodies to the glycine receptor, VGKC complex, and dipeptidyl-peptidase-like protein-6 (DPP6) are described. Encephalitis with antibodies directed to the γ-aminobutyric acid (GABA) receptor type B and type A are reviewed last.

16.1   Introduction

The first reports of the association between limbic encephalitis and tumors date back to the 1960s (Corsellis et al. 1968). In the following decades, several paraneoplastic syndromes were described. The first antigens were detected in the 1980s–1990s. In these classical paraneoplastic syndromes, the antibodies are directed to intracellular antigens, like Hu and Yo (Anderson et al. 1988; Szabo et al. 1991). In the year 2007, the discovery of N-methyl-D-aspartate receptor (NMDAR) antibodies was a major breakthrough recognizing cell surface proteins as antigens in encephalitis (Dalmau et al. 2007). Several other cell surface antigens and their clinical syndrome have been reported more recently. In contrast to the classical syndromes, disease occurs in younger patients as well; patients are also seen by non-neurologists like psychiatrists and pediatricians, and patients tend to have a more favorable response to immunotherapy. Only a minority of these patients have an associated tumor, although the incidence of cancer differs per antigen.

This chapter gives an overview of the syndromes associated with antibodies directed to membrane-bound or synaptic proteins. Focus is on the clinical characteristics which distinguishes these disorders and on the relevance of cerebrospinal fluid (CSF) analysis. Antibodies directed to the ionotropic glutamate receptors are described first. N-methyl-D-aspartate receptor (NMDAR) encephalitis is relatively common. Alpha-amino-3-hydroxy-5-methyl-4-isoxazolepropionic acid receptor (AMPAR) encephalitis and encephalitis associated with antibodies to the metabotropic glutamate receptors mGluR1 and mGluR5 are rare and will be reviewed briefly. Subsequently, syndromes associated with antibodies to the glycine receptor, VGKC complex, and dipeptidyl-peptidase-like protein-6 (DPP6) are described. Encephalitis with antibodies directed to the γ-aminobutyric acid (GABA) receptor type B and type A are reviewed at the end of this chapter. Classical paraneoplastic syndromes are described elsewhere (Chap. 21) in this book.

16.2 *N*-methyl-D-aspartate Receptor (NDMAR)

16.2.1 Introduction

In 2005, the clinical picture of acute psychiatric symptoms, memory deficit, seizures, decreased level of consciousness, and central hypoventilation was described in four young women. All four had ovarian teratoma and CSF abnormalities with a distinct pattern of reactivity to the cytoplasmic membrane of hippocampal neurons (Vitaliani et al. 2005). A study of eight additional patients has led to the identification of a subunit of the *N*-methyl-D-aspartate receptor (NMDAR) as the target antigen of disease in the year 2007 (Dalmau et al. 2007). Since then, this antibody-mediated encephalitis has been reported in hundreds of patients with and without teratoma, mostly young women. Generally, patients do well on tumor removal and immunotherapy.

16.2.2 Pathophysiology

The NMDAR consists of two NR1 and two NR2 subunits. One specific epitope of the amino terminal domain of the NR1 subunit, around the N368/G369 amino acids, is the target antigen in all patients. Binding of antibodies results in prolongation of the opening time of the receptor (Gleichman et al. 2012). This hyperfunction might induce excessive calcium influx, resulting in damage to the receptor, although the exact mechanism is yet undetermined. In neuronal cultures, patients' antibodies are shown to induce capping and internalization of the NMDAR. The amount of NMDAR clusters in the postsynaptic dendrites decreases. Overall these two contradictory effects result in NMDAR-mediated synaptic hypofunctioning. The reversibility of this process has been shown in vitro (Dalmau et al. 2008; Hughes et al. 2010; Mikasova et al. 2012).

The crucial amino terminal domain of the NR1 subunit is found in NMDARs across the brain. However, immunohistochemistry shows staining of the hippocampus and to a lesser degree staining of cortical regions, whereas the cerebellum is spared. This is in accordance with the lack of clinical cerebellar symptoms seen in most patients. There is no structural difference in NR1 subunits underlying this cerebellar sparing and the reason for selective immune reactivity in the brain is currently unknown (Gleichman et al. 2012).

The trigger for the immune reaction in patients with a teratoma seems to be the expression of NMDARs by neurons in the tumor (Tuzun et al. 2009). The trigger for antibody production in patients without a teratoma is unknown. Over 10 cases of anti-NMDAR encephalitis occurring within 6 weeks after herpes simplex virus-1 encephalitis are reported, suggesting that NMDAR antibody production was triggered by the viral infection (Armangue et al. 2012, 2013; Leypoldt et al. 2013; Hacohen et al. 2014; Titulaer and Dalmau 2014; Mohammad et al. 2014).

Antibody production is thought to start systemically. Activated B cells cross the blood–brain barrier, resulting in intrathecal synthesis of antibodies

(Moscato et al. 2012; Martinez-Hernandez et al. 2011). Although complement reactivity is seen in teratoma, complement-mediated neural toxicity does not seem to play a pathogenic role in the brain (Martinez-Hernandez et al. 2011).

Animal models in which NMDAR function is decreased either pharmacologically or genetically show symptoms comparable to patients with anti-NMDAR encephalitis, such as behavioral abnormalities and breathing problems (Dalmau et al. 2011). Injection of patient CSF in mice caused reversible memory and behavioral deficits due to antibody-mediated decrease of hippocampal NMDAR (Planaguma et al. 2014).

16.2.3 Epidemiology

The exact incidence is unknown, but anti-NMDAR encephalitis is thought to be the most common antibody-mediated encephalitis on account of the considerably high number of patients included in recent studies (Dalmau et al. 2011; Titulaer et al. 2013a). In a prospective analysis of infectious and noninfectious encephalitis in the United Kingdom, 4 % of the patients were diagnosed with anti-NMDAR encephalitis (Granerod et al. 2010). Incidence of anti-NMDAR encephalitis was also analyzed in a retrospective study of intensive care patients diagnosed with encephalitis of unknown origin. Five hundred five patients age 18–35 years were screened for encephalitis with psychiatric symptoms, seizures, CSF inflammation, and exclusion of viral and bacterial etiology. Seven patients fulfilled these criteria, of whom six retrospectively tested positive for anti-NMDAR antibodies (Pruss et al. 2010).

Eighty percent of the patients with anti-NMDAR encephalitis are female. In an observational study of 577 patients, age of onset ranged from 8 months to 85 years, but the vast majority of the patients were 18–45 years of age. Only 5 % of the patients were over 45 years. In this group of late-onset anti-NMDAR encephalitis, almost half of the patients were male, similar to the male to female ratio in patients under the age of 12 (Titulaer et al. 2013a, b).

In this observational study, 38 % of the patients had a tumor, of which 94 % were ovarian teratoma. Tumors were less frequently diagnosed in girls under 12 years of age, in women over 45 years of age, and in men (Titulaer et al. 2013a, b).

16.2.4 Clinical Features

Just over half of the adult patients have prodromal symptoms such as headache, fever, nausea, vomiting, diarrhea, or upper respiratory tract symptoms, suggesting a nonspecific infection (Titulaer et al. 2013a). In the following days to weeks, patients develop psychiatric symptoms, most commonly hallucinations, anxiety, and behavioral problems. Many patients are initially analyzed in a psychiatric clinic (Dalmau et al. 2008), although after four weeks less than 1 % of the patients still have psychiatric symptoms only (Kayser et al. 2013). Short-term memory deficit, confusion, insomnia, and language deterioration are common features early in the course of the disease (Dalmau et al. 2011; Irani et al. 2010a). Most patients show abnormal movements, such as orofacial dyskinesias and chorea. Level of consciousness decreases and autonomic instability and hypoventilation may occur, requiring admission to the intensive care unit in 75 % of the patients. Generalized or complex partial seizures are seen in about 70 % of the patients, both in early and late disease stages.

Onset of disease is somewhat different in patients under 18 years of age. Prodromal symptoms are seen less often (Armangue et al. 2012; Florance et al. 2009). In children under 12 years of age, seizures and movement disorders are the presenting symptom in half the patients, which is less common in adolescents or adults (Titulaer et al. 2013a). Eighty-four to eighty-nine percent of the children develop stereotyped movements within the first month (Titulaer et al. 2013a; Florance et al. 2009). Overall, the clinical picture in children becomes similar to adults within 4 weeks (Titulaer et al. 2013a). Late-onset anti-NMDAR encephalitis is related to behavioral, cognitive, or memory problems, milder disease, less often requiring admission to the intensive care unit (Titulaer et al. 2013b).

Recovery from anti-NMDAR encephalitis occurs in the reverse order of symptom presentation. Autonomic functions and respiration improve after which patients awake from their coma. Psychiatric symptoms may temporarily reoccur. Social behavior and language function return with further recovery. Recovery may take well over 18 months (Titulaer et al. 2013a).

16.2.5 Diagnosis

Routine CSF analysis shows slight abnormalities in most patients. Lymphocytic pleocytosis is seen in early course of the disease but then disappears, whereas CSF-specific oligoclonal bands may become apparent a few weeks after disease onset (Irani et al. 2010a). CSF protein can be mildly elevated (Dalmau et al. 2011). IgG antibodies directed to the NR1 subunit of the NMDAR can be detected in both serum and CSF and can be detected using several tests: immunohisto-chemistry (IHC) of rat brain, cell-based assay (CBA) using HEK293 cells, or cultures of rat hippocampal neurons. The latter is useful in research but has no additional value to IHC and is therefore infrequently used in clinical practice. The accuracy of serum and CSF examination was analyzed side by side in an observational cohort study of 250 patients. In CSF, the sensitivity of both IHC and CBA was 100 % (CI 98.5–100 %). In serum, only 85.6 % (CI 80.7–89.4) of the samples was tested positive for both ICH and CBA, with 7 % negative in either one of the tests and 7 % negative in both. These findings show that serum examination is insufficient to exclude anti-NMDAR encephalitis. Specificity was 100 % (CI 96.3–100 %) for both serum and CSF (Gresa-Arribas et al. 2013), although another study mentioned a false-positive rate of 3 % in serum (Viaccoz et al. 2014). In addition, NMDAR antibodies directed to the NR1 subunit have been mentioned in isolated cases of Creutzfeldt-Jakob disease and dementia, all only in serum (Mackay et al. 2012).

Serial dilution of serum or CSF in IHC can be used to measure antibody titer. In our opinion, CBA is less suitable as transfection can differ within and between slides, making serial dilutions more variable. Higher titers, either serum and/or CSF, are seen in patients with an underlying tumor and in patients with poorer outcome, but these predictions are not useful in individual patients. CSF titers correlate better with clinical course in relapses than serum titers (Gresa-Arribas et al. 2013).

Initial cerebral magnetic resonance imaging (MRI) shows abnormalities in about a third of the patients, mostly nonspecific hyperintensities on T_2/FLAIR sequences in several brain regions (Dalmau et al. 2008; Titulaer et al. 2013a). Cerebral PET may show abnormal glucose metabolism in the brain, with temporal and frontal hypermetabolism and occipital hypometabolism, which is reversible upon recovery (Leypoldt et al. 2012).

EEG usually shows diffuse background slowing. One fourth of the patients have electrographic seizures (Titulaer et al. 2013a). A unique EEG pattern characterized by rhythmic delta activity with superimposed bursts of beta activity was seen in 7 out of 23 patients (Schmitt et al. 2012). It has been described in a pediatric patient as well (Armangue et al. 2012). This pattern of "extreme delta brushes" was named after the delta brush EEG pattern known in premature infants.

16.2.6 Treatment

Trials concerning treatment of anti-NMDAR encephalitis have not been performed. However, the favorable effect of immunotherapy has been reported since the description of the "treatment-responsive paraneoplastic encephalitis" which was shown to be related to the NMDAR, and data have been analyzed for a large cohort of (>500) patients (Titulaer et al. 2013a). Early treatment is related to better outcome. First-line immunotherapy usually consists of any combination of steroids, intravenous immunoglobulin, and plasma exchange. In patients with teratoma, first-line treatment includes tumor removal. In an observational study, half of the patients improved in the 4 weeks following initiation of first-line immunotherapy or tumor removal (Titulaer et al. 2013a).

If the effect of first-line treatment is insufficient, second-line immunotherapy such as rituximab or cyclophosphamide should be started. This has been shown to be an independent factor associated with better outcome in patients with first-line treatment failure, although this was not analyzed as part of an RCT. After first-line treatment failure, 78 % of the patients who received second-line treatment had a favorable outcome, compared to 55 % in patients not receiving second-line therapy (Titulaer et al. 2013a). No preference of rituximab, cyclophosphamide, or combination could be found in this study, but the study was not designed for this purpose. Choice of drug is dependent on patient-specific features and the treating physician's experiences. In children, there is slight preference of rituximab as there is more experience with that drug (expert opinion) (Fig. 16.1).

No trials addressed to symptomatic treatment have been performed. Based on expert opinion, psychiatric symptoms and dyskinesias can be controlled

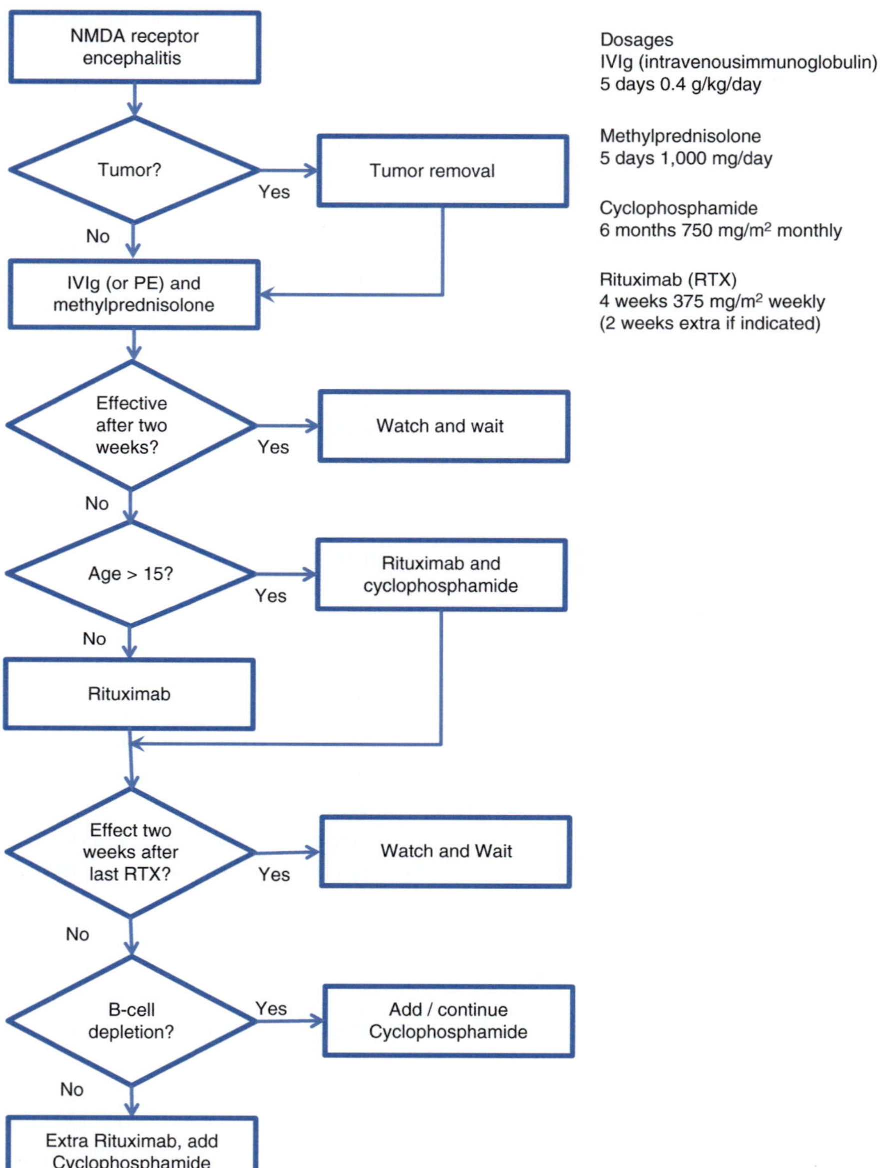

Fig. 16.1 Treatment scheme for anti-NMDAR encephalitis. Can also be useful for other autoimmune encephalitis (expert opinion). *PE* plasma exchange

with benzodiazepines, clonidine, or dexmedetomidine. The latter two might reduce autonomic instability as well (Kayser et al. 2013; Babbitt et al. 2014). The use of haloperidol should be carefully considered due to the antidopaminergic effect associated with severe exacerbation of motor symptoms.

Seizures are treated with common antiepileptic drugs, but refractory seizures and status epilepticus are not uncommon, resulting in the need for long-lasting pharmacological coma.

16.2.7 Prognosis and Follow-Up

Of 501 patients in an observational cohort study, the vast majority was treated with first-line therapy. Overall, at 24 months follow-up, 81 % had a favorable outcome, defined as a modified Rankin scale (mRS) of 0–2. Good outcome was associated with milder disease in the first month, no need for admission to the intensive care unit, and early initiation of treatment. Mortality at 24 months was estimated on 7 % (Titulaer et al. 2013a).

Although late-onset anti-NMDAR encephalitis is related to milder disease, outcome in older patients is poorer (60 % good outcome at 24 months). This might be due to longer delay to diagnosis and treatment (Titulaer et al. 2013b).

Even in patients who appear to be fully recovered, slight residual deficits are common. In order to analyze long-term cognitive outcome, neuropsychological assessment was performed in nine patients who had returned to their homes and/or professional life. Time of testing from disease onset was differing largely (median 43 months). Although most patients did not report persistent problems, cognitive deficit on neuropsychological assessment was observed in eight out of nine patients, mainly concerning impairment of executive function and memory (Finke et al. 2012).

Anti-NMDAR encephalitis can relapse months to years after recovery from the first episode. Relapses tend to be less severe than the initial disease episode (Titulaer et al. 2013a). Relapses can present with psychiatric symptoms only (Kayser et al. 2013). Relapse risk was initially identified to be 24–30 % in retrospective analyses (Irani et al. 2010a; Gabilondo et al. 2011). This is possibly an overestimation due to a diagnostic bias. More patients with milder disease or only one disease episode might be unrecognized in the early years. Relapse rate has dropped to 12 % within 2 years in an observational cohort study (Titulaer et al. 2013a). This can be a true decrease in relapse rate, due to better therapy, but relapse rate will eventually become somewhat higher with longer follow-up. About 35 % of the patients have more than one relapse (Titulaer et al. 2013a; Gabilondo et al. 2011). The risk of relapses is lower in patients with a tumor and seems to decrease with more aggressive immunotherapy (Titulaer et al. 2013a).

After recovery, NMDAR antibodies can still be detected in serum and CSF in most patients.

Measurement of CSF titer at recovery might be useful to compare with titer when clinical symptoms reoccur as a re-increase in titer may indicate a relapse. Immediate diagnosis of a relapse will advance treatment (Gresa-Arribas et al. 2013).

There is no need for scheduled antibody measurements during follow-up.

16.2.8 CSF in Clinical Practice

- CSF analysis can be helpful in cases with a diagnostic dilemma. In a patient with atypical clinical picture but anti-NMDAR antibodies in serum, CSF can either confirm or refute the diagnosis. In a patient with classical clinical picture but no antibodies in serum, CSF can still confirm the diagnosis or support refusal.
- Higher serum and/or CSF antibody titers are seen in patients with an underlying tumor and in patients with poorer outcome. However, titers are of limited significance in the analysis of the individual patient.
- CSF titers tend to remain higher for a prolonged period after treatment in patients with poor outcome. Titers are insufficient to be leading clinical decisions of alternative treatments.
- If a patient deteriorates after recovery, a re-increase of CSF titer may indicate a relapse.

16.3 Alpha-Amino-3-Hydroxy-5-Methyl-4-Isoxazolepropionic Acid Receptor (AMPAR)

16.3.1 Introduction

In 2009, 43 patients with limbic encephalitis of unknown origin were investigated in order to identify the antigen. Among these, antibodies of ten patients showed a similar pattern of reactivity to neuropil of brain and cerebellum. Further tests showed that the alpha-amino-3-hydroxy-5-methyl-4-isoxazolepropionic acid receptor (AMPAR) was the target antigen in these patients. Until now, this series of 10 patients is the major source of information concerning anti-AMPA receptor encephalitis (Lai et al. 2009).

16.3.2 Pathophysiology

The AMPAR is an ionotropic glutamate receptor concentrated at synapses, mediating most of the fast excitatory neurotransmission in the brain (Shepherd and Huganir 2007). The receptors are composed of various combinations of four subunit proteins, GluR1-4 (Lai et al. 2009; Shepherd and Huganir 2007; Granger et al. 2011). Expression of subunits is developmentally regulated and is brain region specific. Most receptors consist of two different subunits, mainly GluR1-2 or GluR2-3 (Shepherd and Huganir 2007). In anti-AMPAR encephalitis, antibodies are shown to react to cell surface GluR1 and GluR2 subunits. Antibody reaction leads to a decrease in the number of receptors at synapses and a decrease of receptors along dendrites. Removal of antibodies from neuronal cultures has shown to restore receptor number and localization of AMPAR clusters (Lai et al. 2009).

16.3.3 Epidemiology

The patients investigated to isolate the antigen were nine women and one man. Age ranged from 38 to 87 years; median age was 60 years. A series of four female patients age 51–71 has been reported as well (Graus et al. 2010). These data suggest that the disease predominantly occurs in older women. Seven out of ten patients had a tumor. In four patients tumor was diagnosed concurrent with the first episode of encephalitis, in two patients concurrent with a relapse, and in one patient 6 months after limbic encephalitis. Tumors were thymic carcinoma, thymoma, non-SCLC, SCLC, and breast cancer. Four tumors were tested on GluR1 and GluR2 proteins and all showed to be positive (Lai et al. 2009).

16.3.4 Clinical Features

Eleven of fourteen reported patients had presented with classical limbic encephalitis, showing confusion, disorientation, and memory loss evolving within 8 weeks. One patient presented with a 4-month history of symptoms suggesting a rapidly progressive dementia and two patients had atypical acute psychosis. Four out of ten patients had seizures (Lai et al. 2009; Graus et al. 2010).

16.3.5 Diagnosis

Most patients have CSF lymphocytic pleocytosis (Lai et al. 2009). Antibodies to the AMPAR can be detected with both immunohistochemical staining of neuropil or cell-based assay, using either serum or CSF. However, one patient was tested negative in serum although CSF was positive (Graus et al. 2010). Brain MRI shows increased FLAIR signal in medial temporal lobes (Lai et al. 2009). Rapid brain atrophy evolving within 5 days was seen on serial MRIs in a pregnant 30-year-old woman with anti-AMPAR encephalitis (Wei et al. 2013; Hutchinson et al. 2003).

16.3.6 Treatment

In the series of ten patients, nine were treated with immunotherapy and tumor treatment when appropriate. Immunotherapy usually consisted of combinations of plasma exchange, corticosteroids, and/or intravenous immunoglobulin. Azathioprine and cyclophosphamide were both used in one patient (Lai et al. 2009).

16.3.7 Prognosis and Follow-Up

All nine treated patients showed major improvement after first episode of limbic encephalitis. Three patients had fully recovered without relapse. One patient had mild persistent depression, apathy, and reduced verbal fluency at 3 months. Five patients had one to three relapses. Relapses occurred up to 101 months after the initial disease episode. Recovery from relapses can be incomplete, with persistent memory loss and behavior problems. One patient died shortly after prolonged status epilepticus at second relapse (Lai et al. 2009).

16.3.8 CSF in Clinical Practice

- Antibodies directed to the AMPAR can be detected in serum and/or CSF using immunohistochemistry or cell-based assay.
- Limited data suggest that CSF analysis might be more sensitive than serum analysis.

16.4 Metabotropic Glutamate Receptors (mGluR)

16.4.1 Introduction

The NMDA receptor and AMPA receptor are ionotropic glutamate receptors, as mentioned earlier. In contrast, there are several metabotropic subtypes of glutamate receptors (mGluR). These receptors indirectly activate ion channels through a signaling cascade involving G proteins. Antibodies directed to the mGluR5 and mGluR1 subtype have been reported in patients with encephalitis. The mGluR5 and mGluR1 receptors are very similar in their amino acid sequences, but antibodies to these receptors do not cross react. The brain distributions differ between the receptors, just as the clinical picture described in disease (van Coevorden-Hameete et al. 2014; Lancaster et al. 2011a).

16.4.2 mGluR5

In 1982, Ian Carr wrote a moving personal paper about the subacute loss of memory and psychosis in his 15-year-old daughter Jane, who subsequently appeared to have Hodgkin's lymphoma (Carr 1982). He called this paraneoplastic disease the Ophelia syndrome, after the character in Shakespeare's Hamlet. More recently three patients with a comparable clinical picture in Hodgkin lymphoma were reported. In these patients mGluR5 was detected as the target antigen of the antibodies (Lancaster et al. 2011a; Mat et al. 2013; Sillevis et al. 2000). Antibodies were detected in serum in two patients (CSF not available) and in CSF in the third patient (serum not available). All three patients received tumor treatment, either chemotherapy or radiotherapy. Only one patient had immunotherapy with intravenous methylprednisolone. All patients had a favorable outcome of both oncological and neurological disease, similar to Carr's daughter.

16.4.3 mGluR1

Subacute cerebellar ataxia has been associated with antibodies to mGluR1 in serum and CSF in five patients. The first two patients had had Hodgkin's disease 2 and 9 years earlier and were in remission (Sillevis et al. 2000). A third had an adenocarcinoma of the prostate and two patients had no tumor (Lancaster et al. 2011a; Iorio et al. 2013; Marignier et al. 2010). The pathogenic role of mGluR1 antibodies has been demonstrated by the induction of cerebellar symptoms in mice after passive transfer of patient's antibodies (Sillevis et al. 2000). Biopsy specimen of lymph node of one patient with mGluR1 antibodies and Hodgkin's disease failed to show mGluR1 RNA. In contrast, immunohistochemistry analysis showed mGluR1 expression in the adenocarcinoma of the patient with prostate cancer (Sillevis et al. 2000; Iorio et al. 2013). Neurological outcome in the five reported patients is variable, ranging from complete recovery to no improvement, despite immunotherapy.

16.5 Glycine Receptor (GlyR)

16.5.1 Introduction

Antibodies to the glycine receptor (GlyR) were initially detected in a patient with progressive encephalomyelitis with rigidity and myoclonus (PERM) in 2008 (Hutchinson et al. 2008). In the following years, antibodies were seen in several patients with the clinical spectrum of both stiff person syndrome (SPS) and PERM (Alexopoulos et al. 2013; McKeon et al. 2013).

16.5.2 Pathophysiology

GlyRs are chloride channels facilitating inhibitory neurotransmission in the brain and spinal cord. GlyRs are expressed on the cell surface membrane and are composed of two GlyRα subunits, with four variants, GlyRα1–4, and three GlyRβ subunits. GlyR antibodies are thought to be directed to the GlyRα1 subunit (van Coevorden-Hameete et al. 2014). Receptor dysfunction results in loss of inhibitory neurotransmission in the brainstem and spinal cord, leading to abnormal discharges of motor neurons and widespread muscular rigidity (Bourke et al. 2013; De Blauwe et al. 2013).

16.5.3 Epidemiology

SPS and PERM are part of a clinical spectrum of antibody-mediated disease in both children and adults (Clardy et al. 2013). Several antibodies have been associated with these syndromes. Antibodies directed to the intracellular protein glutamic acid decarboxylase (GAD65) are detected in 60–80 % of the patients with SPS, but the pathogenic role of these antibodies remains controversial (De Blauwe et al. 2013). Anti-amphiphysin antibodies have been detected in some patients, associated with breast cancer. Passive transfer of patients' immunoglobulin to rats has been reported to induce stiffness and spasms, suggesting some pathogenic role of these antibodies (Geis et al. 2010; Sommer et al. 2005), even though these antibodies act to intracellular antigens. Anti-GlyR antibodies are detected in only 9–15 % of the patients with SPS but are probably much more common in PERM. Several arguments support the pathogenic role of anti-GlyR antibodies in these disorders. Mutations in the GlyRα gene are identified in hereditary hyperekplexia. Pharmacological disturbance of the GlyR causes muscle cramps. The favorable effect of immunotherapy is also supporting the pathogenicity of antibodies, especially antibodies directed to extracellular proteins such as GlyR (Hutchinson et al. 2008; van Coevorden-Hameete et al. 2014).

Whether anti-GlyR antibody production is a paraneoplastic phenomenon is unknown. SPS and PERM with anti-GlyR antibodies have been reported in patients with thymoma, small cell lung cancer, breast cancer, and chronic lymphocytic leukemia but in a considerable amount of patients without a tumor as well (Kyskan et al. 2013; Derksen et al. 2013).

Anti-GlyR antibodies have been detected in 3–6 % of the patients with epilepsy of unknown cause (Brenner et al. 2013; Ekizoglu et al. 2014).

16.5.4 Clinical Features

Patients with SPS show lower extremity and lumbar stiffness and spasms. PERM has been described as a severe variant of SPS with whole-body stiffness, myoclonic jerks, autonomic features, and brainstem signs, usually ocular motility disorders. Patients may experience hyperekplexia and bulbar signs such as trismus and laryngospasm (Hutchinson et al. 2008; Alexopoulos et al. 2013; Iizuka et al. 2012; Vincent et al. 2011).

16.5.5 Diagnosis

Standard CSF examination in PERM is usually normal or shows mild lymphocytosis.

Anti-GlyR antibodies can be detected in both serum and CSF using cell-based assay. Immunohistochemistry of the brain shows no staining.

MRI of the brain and spinal cord is unremarkable. Electromyography findings can be characteristic for hyperekplexia, showing involuntary continuous motor unit activity.

16.5.6 Treatment

Successful treatment of SPS and PERM has been described in case reports. Immunotherapy with either steroids, intravenous immunoglobulin, or plasmapheresis might be beneficial. Azathioprine and rituximab have been used with success as well (Bourke et al. 2013; Clardy et al. 2013; Kyskan et al. 2013; Damasio et al. 2013). Stiffness and spasms can be symptomatically treated with clonazepam, diazepam, baclofen, phenytoin, or gabapentin (Bourke et al. 2013; Kyskan et al. 2013; Mas et al. 2011).

16.5.7 Prognosis and Follow-Up

After initial improvement on immunotherapy, PERM patients tend to relapse. Three reported patients responded well on immunotherapy during relapse, although one of them had sustained disabilities (Hutchinson et al. 2008; Kyskan et al. 2013; Damasio et al. 2013).

16.5.8 CSF in Clinical Practice

- Anti-GlyR antibodies can be detected in both serum and CSF using cell-based assay.
- The pathogenic role of anti-GAD65 antibodies in the clinical spectrum of stiff person syndromes is controversial. Some patients have both anti-GAD65 antibodies and anti-GlyR antibodies.

16.6 Voltage-Gated Potassium Channel Complex (VGKC Complex): LGI1 and Caspr2

16.6.1 Introduction

Antibodies to the voltage-gated potassium channel (VGKC) were initially detected in patients with acquired neuromyotonia, a peripheral nerve disorder characterized by muscle cramps, impaired relaxation, and stiffness (Shillito et al. 1995). A pathogenic role of anti-VGKC antibodies was subsequently suspected in Morvan's syndrome, showing neuromyotonia accompanied by autonomic and cognitive symptoms and insomnia (Barber et al. 2000). The similarity of the central nervous system symptoms of Morvan's syndrome with symptoms seen in limbic encephalitis has led to the analysis and identification of anti-VGKC antibodies in two patients with limbic encephalitis in 2001 (Buckley et al. 2001). Antibodies were eventually thought to be directed to the Kv1.1, 1.2, and 1.6 subunits of the VGKC receptor (Kleopa et al. 2006). However, the exact role of VGKC antibodies remained controversial as no laboratory succeeded in showing staining with serum in VGKC-transfected cells. In the year 2010, this reconsideration led two laboratories to identify simultaneously that these antibodies are not directed to the subunits of the VGKC itself but to the VGKC-associated proteins leucine-rich glioma-inactivated protein 1 (LGI1) and contactin-associated protein 2 (Caspr2) (Irani et al. 2010b; Lai et al. 2010). Anti-LGI1 antibodies are mainly associated with CNS disorders such as limbic encephalitis and epilepsy. Caspr2 antibodies are predominantly associated with peripheral nerve hyperexcitability and the combination of CNS and PNS symptoms in Morvan's syndrome but have been described with (limbic) encephalitis as well.

A significant part of the patients testing positive in the VGKC-radioimmunoassay (VGKC-RIA) do not have anti-LGI1 or anti-Caspr2 antibodies. This is an emerging heterogeneous group of patients. The clinical significance of a positive VGKC-RIA in these patients is currently unknown, which poses a threat for both under- and overdiagnosis as well as under- and overtreatment.

The use of several cutoff values for positive VGKC-RIA titers and the tendency to perform grouped analysis of all VGKC-RIA-positive patients, even after the discovery of the LGI1 and Caspr2 subtypes, are a significant limitation in reviewing clinical symptoms and response to treatment.

16.6.2 Pathophysiology

LGI1 is a secreted glycoprotein, in contrast to the previously described membrane-bound proteins. LGI1 binds to the cell membrane via a disintegrin and metallo-protease domain-containing protein (ADAM). LGI1 connects presynaptic ADAM23 to postsynaptic ADAM22, thereby influences synaptic transmission (van Coevorden-Hameete et al. 2014; Fukata et al. 2010). This LGI1 transsynaptic fine-tuning is thought to have an antiepileptic effect (Fukata et al. 2010). Antibodies are thought to react to LGI1 co-expressed with ADAM22 or ADAM23 (Fukata et al. 2010; Shin et al. 2013; Ohkawa et al. 2013). No in vivo studies have been performed to establish a pathogenic role of LGI1 antibodies in limbic encephalitis. However, genetic disruption of LGI1 is known to cause an epileptic syndrome and, as seizures are a hallmark symptom in anti-LGI encephalitis, makes its pathogenic role more likely.

Caspr2 is a membrane protein in the juxtaparanodes in myelinated axons in both the peripheral and central nervous system (Irani et al. 2010b; Lancaster et al. 2011b). Caspr2 stabilizes Kv1.1 and 1.2 channels. The role of Caspr2 antibodies has not been studied in vivo. Caspr2 antibodies reactivity might disrupt this colocalization of Kv1.1 and 1.2, diminishing repolarization and thereby causing hyperexcitability. Mutation in the Caspr2 coding gene, CNTNAP2, is known to cause childhood-onset refractory epilepsy with mental retardation (van Coevorden-Hameete et al. 2014).

16.6.3 Epidemiology

The exact incidence of VGKC-complex encephalitis and its subtypes is unknown. Pooling of study results is impeded by the differences between countries in test technics and its interpretation.

The VGKC-RIA is requested for several indications. High titers are most commonly seen in limbic encephalitis. In a cohort of 125 patients with antibody-mediated encephalitis, 11.2 % had anti-LGI antibodies and only 0.8 % showed anti-Caspr2 antibodies (Shin et al. 2013). In two cohorts of VGKC-RIA-positive patients with limbic encephalitis, LGI antibodies were detected in respectively 49/64 (77 %) and 9/10 (90 %) patients (Irani et al. 2010b; Butler et al. 2014). Median age at onset of anti-LGI antibody-mediated limbic encephalitis is 60 years (range 30–80) and there is a male predominance (Lai et al. 2010; Shin et al. 2013). Tumors are uncommon (Irani et al. 2010b).

Anti-Caspr2 antibodies are rarely seen in limbic encephalitis and are more often associated with peripheral nervous system disorders, such as neuromyotonia, or in Morvan's syndrome, showing both PNS and CNS features. Tumors, most frequently thymoma, are seen in the minority of anti-Caspr2 antibody-positive patients, mainly in those with Morvan's syndrome (Irani et al. 2010b).

Positive VGKC-RIA is seen in unexplained adult-onset epilepsy in 4–6 % of the patients (Lilleker et al. 2013; Majoie et al. 2006). In one cohort of six VGKC-RIA-positive patients with unexplained epilepsy, only one patient showed anti-LGI1 and one other patient had anti-Caspr2 antibodies (Lilleker et al. 2013). Another cohort of 18 epilepsy patients with positive VGKC-RIA showed positive CBA for LGI1 in 14 patients and Caspr2 in 1 patient, but the clinical picture of this cohort is different. Most patients had cognitive symptoms as well, suggesting limbic encephalitis (Quek et al. 2012).

Patients with a positive test result by VGKC-RIA who do not show anti-LGI1 or anti-Caspr2 antibodies might react to a VGKC-complex protein yet to be identified. This mainly applies to patients with a clear clinical syndrome such as limbic encephalitis or Morvan's syndrome. The clinical relevance of antibodies is highly controversial in patients with an atypical or peripheral nervous system syndrome showing positive VGKC-RIA without LGI1 or Caspr2 antibodies.

A positive VGKC-RIA is unfrequently seen in children, although several cases of movement disorders, insomnia, peripheral nervous system disorders, seizures, and limbic encephalitis have been reported. Unfortunately, reactivity to LGI1 and Caspr2 in these patients is unknown (Dhamija et al. 2011).

16.6.4 Clinical Features

Patients with anti-LGI1 encephalitis show the typical features of limbic encephalitis such as seizures, memory deficit, confusion, and behavioral problems. A minority of the patients show autonomic dysfunction (Irani et al. 2010b; Shin et al. 2013). Hyponatremia is common (~60 %). Typical for anti-LGI1 encephalitis is the occurrence of faciobrachial dystonic seizures (FBDS). These brief involuntary abnormal movements are unilateral, involving the arm, usually ipsilateral face, and less commonly the trunk or a leg. A minority of the patients produce vocalizations at the start of the FBDS, and loss of consciousness is uncommon. FBDS occur very frequent, up to 100 times per day (Andrade et al. 2011; Irani et al. 2011). The etiology of FBDS was analyzed in three patients. Longer events showed generalized flattened EEG pattern just before the onset of movement, confirming that these events are tonic seizures (Andrade et al. 2011; Irani et al. 2011). In the majority of the patients, FBDS precede the onset of limbic encephalitis. Patients usually have other seizure types and cognitive symptoms within a few weeks. Early recognition of FBDS as a prodromal feature of anti-LGI encephalitis might enable early treatment.

Patients with anti-Caspr2 antibodies may have limbic encephalitis. More common, these antibodies are seen in Morvan's syndrome, a combination of central and peripheral nervous system symptoms, showing muscle weakness, cramps, autonomic features, and insomnia. Anti-Caspr2 antibodies are also associated with neuromyotonia, a peripheral nerve hyperexcitability syndrome.

16.6.5 Diagnosis

Standard CSF examination is usually unremarkable, although mild pleocytosis or mildly elevated protein can be seen. Serum hyponatremia is common in anti-LGI1 encephalitis (Lai et al. 2010; Shin et al. 2013).

A commercial 125-I-α-dedrotoxin RIA is available to test reactivity to the Kv1.1, 1.2, and 1.6 subunits of the VGKC. Values and cutoff values vary among laboratories. Usually titer >100 pM or >400 pM is interpreted as positive. The test is only applicable on serum and is not able to discriminate between LGI1, Caspr2, or "double negatives."

Immunocytochemistry and immunohistochemistry can be used to further analyze both serum and CSF. LGI1 tests are complicated by the fact that LGI1 is a secreted protein. LGI1-encoded cell-based assay improves when human embryonic kidney cells are co-transfected with receptors ADAM22 or ADAM23. Immunochemistry on rat hippocampal neuronal cultures are used to detect the specific reactivity pattern to LGI1 or Caspr2 (Lai et al. 2010). No studies to compare serum and CSF sensitivity have been performed.

MRI shows increased signal of the medial temporal lobe on T2 or FLAIR sequences, indicating limbic encephalitis in about 60 % of anti-LGI1 encephalitis patients (Irani et al. 2010b; Shin et al. 2013). PET scan may show hypermetabolism in the medial temporal lobe or basal ganglia (Shin et al. 2013).

Little is known of the frequency of EEG abnormalities in anti-LGI1 encephalitis. In a series 10/14 patients showed abnormalities, with 8 patients showing epileptic discharges and two others showing focal rhythmic slowing (Shin et al. 2013). Continuous video-EEG monitoring in three patients showed electrodecremental events preceding FBDS (Andrade et al. 2011), but this has not been reported with standard EEG examination.

16.6.6 Treatment

Therapeutic strategy is mainly based on experience with other groups of antibody-mediated encephalitis such as NMDAR encephalitis. First-line therapy consists of high-dose corticosteroids, IVIg, and/or plasma exchange. Second-line therapy with cyclophosphamide, rituximab, or mycophenolate mofetil has been used.

Response to immunotherapy is fairly good. A systemic review of 60 VGKC-RIA-positive patients with limbic encephalitis reported significant improvement in 83 %, minimal improvement in 10 %, no change in 5 %, and worsening in 2 % of the patients after immunotherapy. However, LGI1/Caspr2 subtyping was not reported (Radja and Cavanna 2013).

Favorable response to immunotherapy is seen in most patients with anti-LGI1 encephalitis (Irani et al. 2010b; Shin et al. 2013). Immunotherapy seems to be beneficial in Caspr2-related syndromes as well (Lancaster et al. 2011b).

Symptomatic treatment of FBDS with antiepileptic drugs has little effect (Irani et al. 2011).

16.6.7 Prognosis and Follow-Up

A neuropsychological test battery has been used to analyze cognitive deficit before and after immunotherapy in patients with limbic encephalitis and positive VGKC-RIA. Unfortunately, only 10 of 34 patients were tested for LGI1 and Caspr2 antibodies, of which 9 showed anti-LGI1 antibodies. Overall, improvement of cognitive function is seen in most patients (Butler et al. 2014; Frisch et al. 2013). However, residual cognitive impairment is seen, mainly concerning verbal memory. These long-lasting cognitive deficits can seriously impact quality of life. Higher antibody titer at presentation predicted more residual deficit (Butler et al. 2014).

The relapse rate of anti-LGI1 encephalitis seems to be low. In a series 2/14 patients had a relapse; both patients were treated initially with corticosteroids only (Shin et al. 2013).

The value of antibody titer monitoring during follow-up is yet unknown.

16.6.8 CSF in Clinical Practice

- Radioimmunoassay (RIA) is used to detect reactivity to the VGKC complex. However, patients' antibodies are not directed to the VGKC itself but to associated proteins, such as LGI1 and Caspr2, which cannot be detected on RIA. RIA can only be performed on serum.
- Anti-LGI1 and anti-Caspr2 antibodies can be detected in both serum and CSF using cell-based assay or immunohistochemistry.
- The clinical relevance of a positive VGKC-RIA in absence of antibodies directed to LGI1 or Caspr2 is still unknown.

16.7 Dipeptidyl-Peptidase-Like Protein-6 (DPP6)

16.7.1 Introduction

Antibodies to the dipeptidyl-peptidase-like protein-6 (DPP6 or DPPX) were identified in four patients with rapidly progressive encephalopathy in the year 2012. In 2014, DPP6 antibodies were detected in three patients with PERM, not showing antibodies against GAD65, glycine, or amphiphysin (Balint et al. 2014).

16.7.2 Pathophysiology

DPP6 is a cell surface auxiliary subunit of the Kv4.2 potassium channel, most prominent in hippocampal neurons. Immunohistochemical analysis of the small bowel demonstrated antibody reactivity to DPP6 in myenteric plexus as well, explaining diarrhea in a part of the patients (van Coevorden-Hameete et al. 2014; Boronat et al. 2013).

16.7.3 Clinical Features

The four patients with rapidly progressive encephalopathy had severe disease, characterized by agitation, delusions, hallucinations, myoclonic jerks, and seizures, requiring long-lasting hospital admission. Interestingly, three of these patients had severe prodromal diarrhea (Boronat et al. 2013).

Two patients were male and two were female, age ranging from 45 to 76 years.

The three patients with clinical syndrome of PERM had insidious, progressive trunk stiffness, hyperekplexia, and marked cerebellar ataxia. One of these patients had prodromal diarrhea; another suffered from excessive obstipation, resolving on steroids (Balint et al. 2014).

No tumors were reported (Balint et al. 2014; Boronat et al. 2013).

16.7.4 Diagnosis

CSF showed pleocytosis and intrathecal IgG production. Anti-DPP6 antibodies were detected in both serum and CSF (Balint et al. 2014; Boronat et al. 2013).

16.7.5 Therapy and Prognosis

All seven anti-DPP6-positive patients showed at least partial improvement on either first-line or second-line immunotherapy. Relapses were frequently seen, mostly after tapering of immunotherapy (Balint et al. 2014; Boronat et al. 2013).

16.8 γ-Aminobutyric Acid-B Receptor (GABA$_B$)

16.8.1 Introduction

The γ-aminobutyric acid-B (GABA$_B$) receptor was identified as target antigen in limbic encephalitis in 2010. Serum and CSF of 15 patients with limbic encephalitis showed a pattern of reactivity with the neuropil of rat brain reminiscent of AMPAR and Caspr2, but different from the pattern known from antibodies to the NMDAR, and LGI1. Further analysis using confocal microscopy, immunoprecipitation, and mass spectrometry has led to the identification of the $GABA_B$ receptor as the auto-antigen (Lancaster et al. 2010).

16.8.2 Pathophysiology

$GABA_B$ receptors are G-protein-coupled receptors composed of a $GABA_{B1}$ and a $GABA_{B2}$ subunit. The highest level of receptors is found in the hippocampus, thalamus, and cerebellum. $GABA_B$ receptors have an inhibitory function both presynaptic and postsynaptic. Pharmacological and genetic disruption of the inhibitory $GABA_B$ in rodents results in a clinical picture similar to limbic encephalitis, with seizures, memory deficits, and anxiety (Lancaster et al. 2010).

16.8.3 Epidemiology

Anti-$GABA_B$ receptor antibodies are detected in about 0.2 % of the patients with auto-immune or paraneoplastic encephalitis (Hoftberger et al. 2013; Jeffery et al. 2013). In a cohort of 19 patients with limbic encephalitis without a tumor or classical onconeural antibodies, two patients (14 %) had anti-$GABA_B$ antibodies (Boronat et al. 2011). There is a male predominance (Hoftberger et al. 2013; Boronat et al. 2011).

Over half of the patients have a tumor, mainly SCLC. These patients tend to be older with a median age of 67.5 years in one series, compared to a median age of 39 years in non-tumor patients (Hoftberger et al. 2013). Other tumors reported in patients with anti-$GABA_B$ receptor antibodies are neuroendocrine lung tumor, malignant melanoma, and esophagus carcinoma (Lancaster et al. 2010; Jarius et al. 2013; Mundiyanapurath et al. 2013). Limbic encephalitis usually precedes the diagnosis of a tumor.

16.8.4 Clinical Features

Seizures, often refractory, are prominent in anti-$GABA_B$ patients. The majority of the patients have memory deficit and confusion as well, meeting the criteria for limbic encephalitis (Lancaster et al. 2010; Hoftberger et al. 2013; Jeffery et al. 2013). Cases of cerebellar ataxia, brainstem encephalitis, and opsoclonus myoclonus have been reported (Hoftberger et al. 2013; Jarius et al. 2013; Mundiyanapurath et al. 2013).

16.8.5 Diagnosis

Antibodies in serum or CSF can be detected using immunohistochemistry, live neurons, or cell-based assay. A study about the accuracy of serum and CSF testing has not been performed, but paired analysis in 12 patients detected antibodies in CSF in all samples and in serum in only 8 samples. This suggests that CSF analysis might be more reliable than serum (Hoftberger et al. 2013). Some patients may have $GABA_B$ antibodies in addition to GAD65 antibodies (Boronat et al. 2011).

16.8.6 Treatment and Prognosis

The majority of the patients respond well to immunotherapy, combined with oncologic therapy when appropriate (Lancaster et al. 2010; Hoftberger et al. 2013; Jeffery et al. 2013). In paraneoplastic cases, survival depends on the tumor (Hoftberger et al. 2013).

16.8.7 CSF in Clinical Practice

- Anti-$GABA_B$ receptor antibodies can be detected in either serum of CSF, using immunohistochemistry, live neurons, or cell-based assay.
- CSF is probably more sensitive than serum.

16.9 γ-Aminobutyric Acid-A Receptor (GABA$_A$)

16.9.1 Introduction

In 2014, two patients with encephalitis and refractory seizures showed an immunohistochemistry pattern similar to $GABA_B$ receptor antibodies, but CBA for $GABA_B$ was negative. In these two patients, and in four others, antibodies to the $GABA_A$ receptor were detected (Petit-Pedrol et al. 2014).

16.9.2 Pathophysiology

Antibodies react to subunits of the $GABA_A$ receptor: $\alpha 1$, $\beta 3$, or both. Neuronal cultures exposed to patient's antibodies showed a reduction of synaptic $GABA_A$ receptors. This might cause loss of inhibition, thereby inducing status epilepticus. Lengthy seizures are thought to reduce $GABA_A$ receptors further, resulting in a pathogenic reinforcement. This hypothesis can explain the refractory nature of seizures in $GABA_A$ receptor encephalitis and suggests a beneficial role of early treatment.

Mutations in genes encoding $GABA_A$ receptor subunits are known to be associated with epilepsy, supporting a pathogenic role of antibodies in encephalitis. The autoimmune mechanism for $GABA_A$ receptor encephalitis is supported by the co-occurrence of other antibodies in most patients; 3/6 had thyroid peroxidase antibodies, 1/6 had GAD65 antibodies, and 2/6 patients had $GABA_B$ antibodies (Petit-Pedrol et al. 2014).

16.9.3 Epidemiology

Five of the six patients were male. Three were children and three were adults, age ranging from 3 to 63 years. Patients did not have a tumor.

Another 12 patients with low-titer antibodies were reported, but the clinical relevance of antibodies in these patients remains unclear for now (Petit-Pedrol et al. 2014).

16.9.4 Clinical Features

All six patients had developed a rapidly progressive encephalopathy resulting in refractory seizure. Five patients had status epilepticus. One patient developed a progressive hemiparesis before seizures (Petit-Pedrol et al. 2014).

16.9.5 Diagnosis

CSF pleocytosis was seen in 4/6 patients, elevated protein in 4/6 patients, and oligoclonal bands in 2/6. One patient had unremarkable CSF.

All patients had abnormal brain MRI. T2 and FLAIR sequences showed multifocal or diffuse cortical involvement without contrast enhancement (Petit-Pedrol et al. 2014).

16.9.6 Prognosis and Follow-Up

Five patients had immunotherapy. Three of them showed partial or complete recovery. One untreated patient had substantial recovery, although antiepileptic drugs needed to be continued (Petit-Pedrol et al. 2014).

16.10 Conclusion and Future Directions

Encephalitis associated with antibodies directed to cell surface proteins are new, exciting disease entities (Table 16.1). In a short period, a dozen antigens have been discovered and new discoveries are to be expected in upcoming years. These discoveries have high impact in clinical practice. The number of patients diagnosed with antibody-mediated encephalitis or comparable neurological syndromes is rising rapidly. Response to therapy is generally fairly good, in contrast to patients with classical paraneoplastic syndromes. The therapeutic options underline the need for immediate diagnosis, which is especially challenging in patients not primarily seen by neurologists, like children or patients mainly showing psychiatric symptoms.

The increasing amount of patient samples tested for multiple indications and multiple antibodies raise concerns for sensitivity and specificity. Both serum and CSF can be used in diagnosing patients. However, false-positive NMDAR

Table 16.1 Overview of characteristics of antigen in antibody-mediated autoimmune encephalitis

Antigen	No. of patients reported	Epidemiology	Clinical features	Tumor association	CSF characteristics	Antibody detection
NMDA receptor	>700	All ages, most 12–45 years; female predominance; 37 % children	Prodromal symptoms, psychiatric symptoms, memory deficit, confusion, orofacial dyskinesias, seizures	35–40 % (94 % ovarian teratoma); tumor association age dependent	Pleocytosis common in early disease, oligoclonal bands >10 days	CSF more sensitive than serum[a]
AMPA receptor	~23	Median age 60 years, range 38–87 years	Limbic encephalitis	7/10 tumor (thymic carcinoma, thymoma, non-SCLC, SCLC)	Common lymphocytic pleocytosis	CSF or serum[a]
mGluR1	~5		Subacute cerebellar ataxia	3/5 tumor (Hodgkin lymphoma, prostate adenocarcinoma)		CSF or serum[a]
mGluR5	~4		Subacute memory loss and psychosis (Ophelia syndrome)	Hodgkin lymphoma		CSF or serum[a]
Glycine receptor	>20	Children and adults	Stiff person syndrome, PERM	Unknown (thymoma, SCLC, breast cancer, leukemia are reported)	Normal or mild pleocytosis	CSF or serum[a]
LGI1	>100	Median age 60 years; male predominance	Limbic encephalitis, faciobrachial dystonic seizures, hyponatremia	Uncommon: ~5 %	Normal or mild pleocytosis	CSF or serum (VGKC test in serum only)[a]
Caspr2	>50	Common age ~60 years Male predominance	Morvan's syndrome Neuromyotonia Limbic encephalitis	10–15 % (thymoma)	Normal or mild pleocytosis	CSF or serum (VGKC test in serum only)[a]

DPPX	~7	Age 45–76	Rapidly progressive encephalopathy, PERM	No tumor reported	Pleocytosis and intrathecal IgG production	CSF or serum[a]
GABA-B	>60	With tumor: median age 67.5 years. Without tumor: median age 39 years	Limbic encephalitis with prominent refractory seizures	50–60 % (SCLC)	Common lymphocytic pleocytosis	CSF probably more sensitive than serum[a]
GABA-A	6	3 children and 3 adults, age 3–63 years. 5/6 male	Rapidly progressive encephalopathy with (refractory) seizures	No tumor	Common pleocytosis and elevated protein	CSF or serum[a]

[a]If disease pattern is not completely specific, CSF confirmation or additional serum testing (immunohistochemistry or live neuron testing) is necessary. *CSF* cerebrospinal fluid, *PERM* progressive encephalomyelitis with rigidity and myoclonus, *SCLC* small cell lung cancer, *VGKC* voltage-gated potassium channel

antibodies and VGKC-complex tests have been identified in those tested in serum only, while this has not been described for CSF. Additionally, CSF analysis is more sensitive than serum in anti-NMDAR encephalitis and probably also for $GABA_B$ and AMPAR encephalitis. Serial measurements of antibody titer have limited value so far.

Anti-NMDAR encephalitis is most prevalent and most extensively analyzed. Although studied retrospectively, the need for immunotherapy in these patients is beyond doubt.

Immunotherapy is usually given to patients with other antibodies as well, with beneficial response reported in small series and case reports. The indication for immunotherapy is less clear in cases where the pathogenesis of disease is still unclear, such as patients with positive VGKC-RIA without proven antibodies. Further research addressing these issues is necessary.

References

Alexopoulos H, Akrivou S, Dalakas MC (2013) Glycine receptor antibodies in stiff-person syndrome and other GAD-positive CNS disorders. Neurology 81(22):1962–1964

Anderson NE, Rosenblum MK, Posner JB (1988) Paraneoplastic cerebellar degeneration: clinical-immunological correlations. Ann Neurol 24(4):559–567

Andrade DM, Tai P, Dalmau J, Wennberg R (2011) Tonic seizures: a diagnostic clue of anti-LGI1 encephalitis? Neurology 76(15):1355–1357

Armangue T, Titulaer MJ, Malaga I, Bataller L, Gabilondo I, Graus F et al (2012) Pediatric anti-N-methyl-D-aspartate receptor encephalitis-clinical analysis and novel findings in a series of 20 patients. J Pediatr 162:850–856.e2

Armangue T, Leypoldt F, Malaga I, Raspall-Chaure M, Marti I, Nichter C et al (2013) Herpes simplex virus encephalitis is a trigger of brain autoimmunity. Ann Neurol 75(2):317–323

Babbitt CJ, Levine GK, Lake J (2014) Use of dexmedetomidine as adjunctive therapy for anti-NMDA receptor encephalitis. J Pediatr Intensive Care (in press)

Balint B, Jarius S, Nagel S, Haberkorn U, Probst C, Blocker IM et al (2014) Progressive encephalomyelitis with rigidity and myoclonus: a new variant with DPPX antibodies. Neurology 82(17):1521–1528

Barber PA, Anderson NE, Vincent A (2000) Morvan's syndrome associated with voltage-gated K+ channel antibodies. Neurology 54(3):771–772

Boronat A, Sabater L, Saiz A, Dalmau J, Graus F (2011) GABA(B) receptor antibodies in limbic encephalitis and anti-GAD-associated neurologic disorders. Neurology 76(9):795–800

Boronat A, Gelfand JM, Gresa-Arribas N, Jeong HY, Walsh M, Roberts K et al (2013) Encephalitis and antibodies to dipeptidyl-peptidase-like protein-6, a subunit of Kv4.2 potassium channels. Ann Neurol 73(1):120–128

Bourke D, Roxburgh R, Vincent A, Cleland J, Jeffery O, Dugan N et al (2013) Hypoventilation in glycine-receptor antibody related progressive encephalomyelitis, rigidity and myoclonus. J Clin Neurosci 21(5):876–878

Brenner T, Sills GJ, Hart Y, Howell S, Waters P, Brodie MJ et al (2013) Prevalence of neurologic autoantibodies in cohorts of patients with new and established epilepsy. Epilepsia 54(6):1028–1035

Buckley C, Oger J, Clover L, Tuzun E, Carpenter K, Jackson M et al (2001) Potassium channel antibodies in two patients with reversible limbic encephalitis. Ann Neurol 50(1):73–78

Butler CR, Miller TD, Kaur MS, Baker IW, Boothroyd GD, Illman NA et al (2014) Persistent anterograde amnesia following limbic encephalitis associated with antibodies to the voltage-gated potassium channel complex. J Neurol Neurosurg Psychiatry 85(4):387–391

Carr I (1982) The Ophelia syndrome: memory loss in Hodgkin's disease. Lancet 1(8276):844–845

Clardy SL, Lennon VA, Dalmau J, Pittock SJ, Jones HR Jr, Renaud DL et al (2013) Childhood onset of stiff-man syndrome. JAMA Neurol 70(12):1531–1536

Corsellis JA, Goldberg GJ, Norton AR (1968) "Limbic encephalitis" and its association with carcinoma. Brain 91(3):481–496

Dalmau J, Tuzun E, Wu HY, Masjuan J, Rossi JE, Voloschin A et al (2007) Paraneoplastic anti-N-methyl-D-aspartate receptor encephalitis associated with ovarian teratoma. Ann Neurol 61(1):25–36

Dalmau J, Gleichman AJ, Hughes EG, Rossi JE, Peng X, Lai M et al (2008) Anti-NMDA-receptor encephalitis: case series and analysis of the effects of antibodies. Lancet Neurol 7(12): 1091–1098

Dalmau J, Lancaster E, Martinez-Hernandez E, Rosenfeld MR, Balice-Gordon R (2011) Clinical experience and laboratory investigations in patients with anti-NMDAR encephalitis. Lancet Neurol 10(1):63–74

Damasio J, Leite MI, Coutinho E, Waters P, Woodhall M, Santos MA et al (2013) Progressive encephalomyelitis with rigidity and myoclonus: the first pediatric case with glycine receptor antibodies. JAMA Neurol 70(4):498–501

De Blauwe SN, Santens P, Vanopdenbosch LJ (2013) Anti-glycine receptor antibody mediated progressive encephalomyelitis with rigidity and myoclonus associated with breast cancer. Case Rep Neurol Med 2013, 589154

Derksen A, Stettner M, Stocker W, Seitz RJ (2013) Antiglycine receptor-related stiff limb syndrome in a patient with chronic lymphocytic leukaemia. BMJ Case Rep 2013 [Epub ahead of print] doi: 10.1136/bcr-2013-008667

Dhamija R, Renaud DL, Pittock SJ, McKeon A, Lachance DH, Nickels KC et al (2011) Neuronal voltage-gated potassium channel complex autoimmunity in children. Pediatr Neurol 44(4): 275–281

Ekizoglu E, Tuzun E, Woodhall M, Lang B, Jacobson L, Icoz S et al (2014) Investigation of neuronal autoantibodies in two different focal epilepsy syndromes. Epilepsia 55(3): 414–422

Finke C, Kopp UA, Pruss H, Dalmau J, Wandinger KP, Ploner CJ (2012) Cognitive deficits following anti-NMDA receptor encephalitis. J Neurol Neurosurg Psychiatry 83(2):195–198

Florance NR, Davis RL, Lam C, Szperka C, Zhou L, Ahmad S et al (2009) Anti-N-methyl-D-aspartate receptor (NMDAR) encephalitis in children and adolescents. Ann Neurol 66(1): 11–18

Frisch C, Malter MP, Elger CE, Helmstaedter C (2013) Neuropsychological course of voltage-gated potassium channel and glutamic acid decarboxylase antibody related limbic encephalitis. Eur J Neurol 20(9):1297–1304

Fukata Y, Lovero KL, Iwanaga T, Watanabe A, Yokoi N, Tabuchi K et al (2010) Disruption of LGI1-linked synaptic complex causes abnormal synaptic transmission and epilepsy. Proc Natl Acad Sci U S A 107(8):3799–3804

Gabilondo I, Saiz A, Galan L, Gonzalez V, Jadraque R, Sabater L et al (2011) Analysis of relapses in anti-NMDAR encephalitis. Neurology 77(10):996–999

Geis C, Weishaupt A, Hallermann S, Grunewald B, Wessig C, Wultsch T et al (2010) Stiff person syndrome-associated autoantibodies to amphiphysin mediate reduced GABAergic inhibition. Brain 133(11):3166–3180

Gleichman AJ, Spruce LA, Dalmau J, Seeholzer SH, Lynch DR (2012) Anti-NMDA receptor encephalitis antibody binding is dependent on amino acid identity of a small region within the GluN1 amino terminal domain. J Neurosci 32(32):11082–11094

Granerod J, Ambrose HE, Davies NW, Clewley JP, Walsh AL, Morgan D et al (2010) Causes of encephalitis and differences in their clinical presentations in England: a multicentre, population-based prospective study. Lancet Infect Dis 10(12):835–844

Granger AJ, Gray JA, Lu W, Nicoll RA (2011) Genetic analysis of neuronal ionotropic glutamate receptor subunits. J Physiol 589(Pt 17):4095–4101

Graus F, Boronat A, Xifro X, Boix M, Svigelj V, Garcia A et al (2010) The expanding clinical profile of anti-AMPA receptor encephalitis. Neurology 74(10):857–859

Gresa-Arribas N, Titulaer MJ, Torrents A, Aguilar E, McCracken L, Leypoldt F et al (2013) Antibody titres at diagnosis and during follow-up of anti-NMDA receptor encephalitis: a retrospective study. Lancet Neurol 13:167–177

Hacohen Y, Deiva K, Pettingill P, Waters P, Siddiqui A, Chretien P et al (2014) N-methyl-D-aspartate receptor antibodies in post-herpes simplex virus encephalitis neurological relapse. Mov Disord 29(1):90–96

Hoftberger R, Titulaer MJ, Sabater L, Dome B, Rozsas A, Hegedus B et al (2013) Encephalitis and GABAB receptor antibodies: novel findings in a new case series of 20 patients. Neurology 81(17):1500–1506

Hughes EG, Peng X, Gleichman AJ, Lai M, Zhou L, Tsou R et al (2010) Cellular and synaptic mechanisms of anti-NMDA receptor encephalitis. J Neurosci 30(17):5866–5875

Hutchinson M, Waters P, McHugh J, Gorman G, O'Riordan S, Connolly S et al (2008) Progressive encephalomyelitis, rigidity, and myoclonus: a novel glycine receptor antibody. Neurology 71(16):1291–1292

Iizuka T, Leite MI, Lang B, Waters P, Urano Y, Miyakawa S et al (2012) Glycine receptor antibodies are detected in progressive encephalomyelitis with rigidity and myoclonus (PERM) but not in saccadic oscillations. J Neurol 259(8):1566–1573

Iorio R, Damato V, Mirabella M, Vita MG, Hulsenboom E, Plantone D et al (2013) Cerebellar degeneration associated with mGluR1 autoantibodies as a paraneoplastic manifestation of prostate adenocarcinoma. J Neuroimmunol 263(1–2):155–158

Irani SR, Bera K, Waters P, Zuliani L, Maxwell S, Zandi MS et al (2010a) N-methyl-D-aspartate antibody encephalitis: temporal progression of clinical and paraclinical observations in a predominantly non-paraneoplastic disorder of both sexes. Brain 133(Pt 6):1655–1667

Irani SR, Alexander S, Waters P, Kleopa KA, Pettingill P, Zuliani L et al (2010b) Antibodies to Kv1 potassium channel-complex proteins leucine-rich, glioma inactivated 1 protein and contactin-associated protein-2 in limbic encephalitis, Morvan's syndrome and acquired neuromyotonia. Brain 133(9):2734–2748

Irani SR, Michell AW, Lang B, Pettingill P, Waters P, Johnson MR et al (2011) Faciobrachial dystonic seizures precede Lgi1 antibody limbic encephalitis. Ann Neurol 69(5):892–900

Jarius S, Steinmeyer F, Knobel A, Streitberger K, Hotter B, Horn S et al (2013) GABAB receptor antibodies in paraneoplastic cerebellar ataxia. J Neuroimmunol 256(1–2):94–96

Jeffery OJ, Lennon VA, Pittock SJ, Gregory JK, Britton JW, McKeon A (2013) GABAB receptor autoantibody frequency in service serologic evaluation. Neurology 81(10):882–887

Kayser MS, Titulaer MJ, Gresa-Arribas N, Dalmau J (2013) Frequency and characteristics of isolated psychiatric episodes in anti-NMDA receptor encephalitis. JAMA Neurol 70(9):1133–1139, Ref Type: Journal (Full)

Kleopa KA, Elman LB, Lang B, Vincent A, Scherer SS (2006) Neuromyotonia and limbic encephalitis sera target mature Shaker-type K+channels: subunit specificity correlates with clinical manifestations. Brain 129(Pt 6):1570–1584

Kyskan R, Chapman K, Mattman A, Sin D (2013) Antiglycine receptor antibody and encephalomyelitis with rigidity and myoclonus (PERM) related to small cell lung cancer. BMJ Case Rep 2013 [Epub ahead of print] doi: 10.1136/bcr-2013-010027

Lai M, Hughes EG, Peng X, Zhou L, Gleichman AJ, Shu H et al (2009) AMPA receptor antibodies in limbic encephalitis alter synaptic receptor location. Ann Neurol 65(4):424–434

Lai M, Huijbers MG, Lancaster E, Graus F, Bataller L, Balice-Gordon R et al (2010) Investigation of LGI1 as the antigen in limbic encephalitis previously attributed to potassium channels: a case series. Lancet Neurol 9(8):776–785

Lancaster E, Lai M, Peng X, Hughes E, Constantinescu R, Raizer J et al (2010) Antibodies to the GABA(B) receptor in limbic encephalitis with seizures: case series and characterisation of the antigen. Lancet Neurol 9(1):67–76

Lancaster E, Martinez-Hernandez E, Titulaer MJ, Boulos M, Weaver S, Antoine JC et al (2011a) Antibodies to metabotropic glutamate receptor 5 in the Ophelia syndrome. Neurology 77(18):1698–1701

Lancaster E, Huijbers MG, Bar V, Boronat A, Wong A, Martinez-Hernandez E et al (2011b) Investigations of caspr2, an autoantigen of encephalitis and neuromyotonia. Ann Neurol 69(2):303–311

Leypoldt F, Buchert R, Kleiter I, Marienhagen J, Gelderblom M, Magnus T et al (2012) Fluorodeoxyglucose positron emission tomography in anti-N-methyl-D-aspartate receptor encephalitis: distinct pattern of disease. J Neurol Neurosurg Psychiatry 83(7):681–686

Leypoldt F, Titulaer MJ, Aguilar E, Walther J, Bonstrup M, Havemeister S et al (2013) Herpes simplex virus-1 encephalitis can trigger anti-NMDA receptor encephalitis: case report. Neurology 81(18):1637–1639

Lilleker JB, Jones MS, Mohanraj R (2013) VGKC complex antibodies in epilepsy: diagnostic yield and therapeutic implications. Seizure 22(9):776–779

Mackay G, Ahmad K, Stone J, Sudlow C, Summers D, Knight R et al (2012) NMDA receptor autoantibodies in sporadic Creutzfeldt-Jakob disease. J Neurol 259(9):1979–1981

Majoie HJ, de Baets M, Renier W, Lang B, Vincent A (2006) Antibodies to voltage-gated potassium and calcium channels in epilepsy. Epilepsy Res 71(2–3):135–141

Marignier R, Chenevier F, Rogemond V, Sillevis SP, Renoux C, Cavillon G et al (2010) Metabotropic glutamate receptor type 1 autoantibody-associated cerebellitis: a primary autoimmune disease? Arch Neurol 67(5):627–630

Martinez-Hernandez E, Horvath J, Shiloh-Malawsky Y, Sangha N, Martinez-Lage M, Dalmau J (2011) Analysis of complement and plasma cells in the brain of patients with anti-NMDAR encephalitis. Neurology 77(6):589–593

Mas N, Saiz A, Leite MI, Waters P, Baron M, Castano D et al (2011) Antiglycine-receptor encephalomyelitis with rigidity. J Neurol Neurosurg Psychiatry 82(12):1399–1401

Mat A, Adler H, Merwick A, Chadwick G, Gullo G, Dalmau JO et al (2013) Ophelia syndrome with metabotropic glutamate receptor 5 antibodies in CSF. Neurology 80(14):1349–1350

McKeon A, Martinez-Hernandez E, Lancaster E, Matsumoto JY, Harvey RJ, McEvoy KM et al (2013) Glycine receptor autoimmune spectrum with stiff-man syndrome phenotype. JAMA Neurol 70(1):44–50

Mikasova L, De RP, Bouchet D, Georges F, Rogemond V, Didelot A et al (2012) Disrupted surface cross-talk between NMDA and Ephrin-B2 receptors in anti-NMDA encephalitis. Brain 135(Pt 5):1606–1621

Mohammad SS, Sinclair K, Pillai S, Merheb V, Aumann TD, Gill D et al (2014) Herpes simplex encephalitis relapse with chorea is associated with autoantibodies to N-methyl-D-aspartate receptor or dopamine-2 receptor. Mov Disord 29(1):117–122

Moscato E, Peng XY, Parsons T, Dalmau J, Balice-Gordon R (2012) Acute mechanisms underlying antibody effects in anti-NMDA receptor encephalitis. J Neuroimmunol 253(1–2):145

Mundiyanapurath S, Jarius S, Probst C, Stocker W, Wildemann B, Bosel J (2013) GABA-B-receptor antibodies in paraneoplastic brainstem encephalitis. J Neuroimmunol 259(1–2):88–91

Ohkawa T, Fukata Y, Yamasaki M, Miyazaki T, Yokoi N, Takashima H et al (2013) Autoantibodies to epilepsy-related LGI1 in limbic encephalitis neutralize LGI1-ADAM22 interaction and reduce synaptic AMPA receptors. J Neurosci 33(46):18161–18174

Petit-Pedrol M, Armangue T, Peng X, Bataller L, Cellucci T, Davis R et al (2014) Encephalitis with refractory seizures, status epilepticus, and antibodies to the GABAA receptor: a case series, characterisation of the antigen, and analysis of the effects of antibodies. Lancet Neurol 13(3):276–286

Planaguma J, Leypoldt F, Mannara F, Gutierrez-Cuesta J, Martin-Garcia E, Aguilar E et al (2014) Human N-methyl-D-aspartate receptor antibodies alter memory and behaviour in mice. Brain (in press)

Pruss H, Dalmau J, Harms L, Holtje M, Ahnert-Hilger G, Borowski K et al (2010) Retrospective analysis of NMDA receptor antibodies in encephalitis of unknown origin. Neurology 75(19):1735–1739

Quek AM, Britton JW, McKeon A, So E, Lennon VA, Shin C et al (2012) Autoimmune epilepsy: clinical characteristics and response to immunotherapy. Arch Neurol 69(5):582–593

Radja GK, Cavanna AE (2013) Treatment of VGKC complex antibody-associated limbic encephalitis: a systematic review. J Neuropsychiatry Clin Neurosci 25(4):264–271

Schmitt SE, Pargeon K, Frechette ES, Hirsch LJ, Dalmau J, Friedman D (2012) Extreme delta brush: a unique EEG pattern in adults with anti-NMDA receptor encephalitis. Neurology 79(11):1094–1100

Shepherd JD, Huganir RL (2007) The cell biology of synaptic plasticity: AMPA receptor trafficking. Annu Rev Cell Dev Biol 23:613–643

Shillito P, Molenaar PC, Vincent A, Leys K, Zheng W, van den Berg RJ et al (1995) Acquired neuromyotonia: evidence for autoantibodies directed against K+channels of peripheral nerves. Ann Neurol 38(5):714–722

Shin YW, Lee ST, Shin JW, Moon J, Lim JA, Byun JI et al (2013) VGKC-complex/LGI1-antibody encephalitis: clinical manifestations and response to immunotherapy. J Neuroimmunol 265(1–2):75–81

Sillevis SP, Kinoshita A, de Leeuw B, Moll W, Coesmans M, Jaarsma D et al (2000) Paraneoplastic cerebellar ataxia due to autoantibodies against a glutamate receptor. N Engl J Med 342(1): 21–27

Sommer C, Weishaupt A, Brinkhoff J, Biko L, Wessig C, Gold R et al (2005) Paraneoplastic stiff-person syndrome: passive transfer to rats by means of IgG antibodies to amphiphysin. Lancet 365(9468):1406–1411

Szabo A, Dalmau J, Manley G, Rosenfeld M, Wong E, Henson J et al (1991) HuD, a paraneoplastic encephalomyelitis antigen, contains RNA-binding domains and is homologous to Elav and Sex-lethal. Cell 67(2):325–333

Titulaer MJ, Dalmau J (2014) Antibodies to NMDA and other synaptic receptors in choreoathetosis and relapsing symptoms post-Herpes Virus Encephalitis. Mov Dis 29(1):3–6

Titulaer MJ, McCracken L, Gabilondo I, Armangue T, Glaser C, Iizuka T et al (2013a) Treatment and prognostic factors for long-term outcome in patients with anti-NMDA receptor encephalitis: an observational cohort study. Lancet Neurol 12:157–165

Titulaer MJ, McCracken L, Gabilondo I, Iizuka T, Kawachi I, Bataller L et al (2013b) Late-onset anti-NMDA receptor encephalitis. Neurology 81(12):1058–1063

Tuzun E, Zhou L, Baehring JM, Bannykh S, Rosenfeld MR, Dalmau J (2009) Evidence for antibody-mediated pathogenesis in anti-NMDAR encephalitis associated with ovarian teratoma. Acta Neuropathol 118(6):737–743

van Coevorden-Hameete MH, de Graaff GE, Titulaer MJ, Hoogenraad CC, Sillevis Smitt PA (2014) Molecular and cellular mechanisms underlying anti-neuronal antibody mediated disorders of the central nervous system. Autoimmun Rev 13(3):299–312

Viaccoz A, Desestret V, Ducray F, Picard G, Cavillon G, Rogemond V et al (2014) Clinical specificities of adult male patients with NMDA receptor antibodies encephalitis. Neurology 82(7):556–563

Vincent A, Bien CG, Irani SR, Waters P (2011) Autoantibodies associated with diseases of the CNS: new developments and future challenges. Lancet Neurol 10(8):759–772

Vitaliani R, Mason W, Ances B, Zwerdling T, Jiang Z, Dalmau J (2005) Paraneoplastic encephalitis, psychiatric symptoms, and hypoventilation in ovarian teratoma. Ann Neurol 58(4):594–604

Wei YC, Liu CH, Lin JJ, Lin KJ, Huang KL, Lee TH et al (2013) Rapid progression and brain atrophy in anti-AMPA receptor encephalitis. J Neuroimmunol 261(1–2):129–133

Chronic Noninfectious Inflammatory CNS Diseases   17

Irina Elovaara, Sanna Hagman, and Aki Hietaharju

Contents

I. Elovaara, MD, PhD (✉)
Department of Neurology and Rehabilitation,
Tampere University Hospital,
Tampere, Finland

Neuroimmunology Unit,
Medical School, University of Tampere
Tampere, Finland
e-mail: irina.elovaara@uta.fi

S. Hagman, PhD
Neuroimmunology Unit,
Medical School, University of Tampere
Tampere, Finland

A. Hietaharju, MD, PhD
Department of Neurology and Rehabilitation,
Tampere University Hospital,
Tampere, Finland

© Springer International Publishing Switzerland 2015
F. Deisenhammer et al. (eds.), *Cerebrospinal Fluid in Clinical Neurology*,
DOI 10.1007/978-3-319-01225-4_17

Abstract

In clinical practice the differentiation between inflammatory diseases of the central nervous system (CNS) as well as chronic and subacute CNS diseases may be challenging due to similarities in the symptomatology and overlapping changes on magnetic resonance imaging (MRI). However, the distinction between these diseases is important due to major differences in the treatment strategies. Since cerebrospinal fluid (CSF) is in direct contact with the brain and spinal tissue, the analysis of CSF composition provides additional information needed in differential diagnostics. Changes in the composition of the CSF occur in primary autoimmune diseases of the CNS but also in nearly all infection-induced inflammation and neurological manifestations of systemic autoimmune diseases such as systemic lupus erythematosus (SLE), primary Sjögren's syndrome (PSS), and mixed connective tissue disease (MCTD). Inflammatory lesions in the brain in primary angiitis of the CNS and in systemic vasculitides such as granulomatosis with polyangitis, Behcet's disease, and polyarteritis nodosa may also mimic MS. This chapter reviews the CSF findings in CNS diseases including multiple sclerosis and other inflammatory demyelinating diseases as well as in major chronic and subacute CNS manifestations associated with systemic autoimmune diseases.

17.1 Multiple Sclerosis and Other Inflammatory Demyelinating CNS Diseases

MS is the most common disabling autoimmune disease of the CNS in young adults that has a major socioeconomic impact. Immunopathogenesis of MS is complex, and pathology is characterized by inflammation, demyelination, axonal loss, and gliosis (Boppana et al. 2011; Lassmann 2013). The cause of MS is still unknown, but its pathogenesis is mediated by activated autoreactive CD4+ T-helper 1 (Th1) and Th17 cells, CD8+ cells, natural killer cells, and B cells that all contribute to neural damage (Comabella and Khoury 2012). In the majority of patients, MS presents as relapsing–remitting subtype (RRMS) that later on progresses into secondary progressive course (SPMS). Whether or not the relapsing and progressive phases of MS differ qualitatively is unknown. Currently several licensed immunomodulatory disease-modifying therapies are available stressing the importance of early diagnosis allowing initiating of appropriate therapy. The diagnosis of MS is based on a detailed clinical evaluation including a systematic history and neurological examination that are facilitated by supportive laboratory and magnetic resonance imaging (MRI) investigations that all provide the evidence of dissemination in space (DIS) and dissemination in time (DIT) needed for a diagnosis of MS (Polman et al. 2011). Other MS-resembling inflammatory or infectious conditions need to be excluded. Among such diseases are acute disseminated encephalomyelitis (ADEM), neuromyelitis optica (NMO, Devic's disease), transverse myelitis, neurosarcoidosis, systemic lupus erythematosus (SLE), primary Sjögren's syndrome (SS), isolated central nervous system vasculitis, human T-lymphocyte virus-1-associated myelopathy, and Behcet's disease.

The value of *CSF* in the diagnosis of MS is well known (Link and Tibbling 1977; Andersson et al. 1994; Freedman et al. 2005). Demonstration of oligoclonal immunoglobulin G (IgG) bands (OCBs) in the CSF (>1 band) or elevated IgG index (>0.7) indicating intrathecal IgG synthesis is widely used in the diagnosis of MS. IgG index has lower diagnostic sensitivity and has been shown to be increased in 50–75 % of MS patients, while OCBs are detected in 90–100 % of MS patients (Link and Huang 2006; Freedman et al. 2005; Stangel et al. 2013). Many studies have reported stability of OCBs, once established, throughout lifetime of MS (Petzold 2013). Additionally, OCBs can be used to predict conversion of clinically isolated syndrome (CIS) to MS (Senel et al. 2014). Their presence is not specific for MS as they may also be found in CNS infections and other autoimmune and paraneoplastic disorders (Petzold 2013). These disorders can usually be differentiated from MS on clinical and paraclinical grounds, which makes the finding of CSF OCBs relatively specific in a patient presenting with symptoms consistent with MS (Deisenhammer et al. 2006). The presence of low-grade mononuclear pleocytosis, typically less than 25×10^6 cells/l together with slightly elevated protein concentration (less than 1 g/l), is also typical of MS. Recently, also the measurement of CSF immunoglobulin kappa free light chain (KFLC) in MS has been shown to be almost equal to OCBs in regard to diagnostic sensitivity and specificity in patients with early MS (Senel et al. 2014). Analysis of KFLC is performed by nephelometric test, which is a more straightforward and easier methodology to standardize between the laboratories (Presslauer et al. 2014). In addition to IgG OCBs, 40 % of MS patients present IgM OCBs (Villar et al. 2010).

During the recent years, a large number of studies have been performed with the purpose to identify new clinically useful biomarkers specific for MS (Comabella and Montalban 2014). Several candidate biomarkers such as adhesion molecules, cytokines and cytokine receptors, chemokines such as CXCL13 and chemokine receptors, antibodies, apoptosis-related molecules, several proteases, oxidative stress-related free radicals, and adipocytokines have been suggested as diagnostic markers, but only minority of them have been validated and taken in the clinical use. In recent clinical studies, neurofilament (NF) protein, myelin basic protein (MBP), matrix metalloproteinase (MMP)-9, chemokine CXCL13, osteopontin (OPN), and nitric oxide metabolites have been used as surrogate end points of neuronal damage and disease activity in chronic progressive MS (Romme Christensen et al. 2014). Other candidate biomarkers are listed in Table 17.1. Neurofilament protein has been reported to be increased in the CSF of patients with MS during relapse, related to radiological activity and neurological disability. It is also reported to have prognostic value for conversion from CIS to MS (Teunissen and Khalil 2012). CXCL13, a B-cell-attracting chemokine, is also reported to be increased in patients with MS reflecting more active disease course. Elevated level of CXCL13 is also associated to an increased risk of conversion from CIS to MS (Khademi et al. 2011). Recently fetuin-A was linked to inflammatory disease activity and early conversion from CIS to RRMS (Harris et al. 2013).

Table 17.1 CSF markers in multiple sclerosis

Cerebrospinal fluid biomarkers	Origin	Target cells
Immune activation		
CXCL13	FDC	B cells, TFH cells
CXCL16	APC	T cells, NKT cells
CXCL10	Astrocytes, endothelial cells, fibroblast	Th1 cells, CD8+ cells, NK cells, endothelial cells, neurons, microglia, oligodendrocytes
Leptin	Adipocytes	Monocytes, macrophages, NK cells, T cells
Osteopontin	Macrophages, DC, T cells	Leukocytes
BAFF	Astrocytes, monocytes	B cells
Fetuin-A	Demyelinated lesions	Neuronal cells
KFLC	B cells	–
Blood–brain barrier damage		
MMP-2	Immune cells, endothelial cells	–
MMP-9	Immune cells, endothelial cells	–
sICAM	Endothelial cells	Immune cells
sP-selectin	Endothelial cells	Immune cells
sE-selectin	Endothelial cells	Immune cells
Demyelination		
Anti-MOG	B cells	Oligodendrocytes
Anti-MBP	B cells	Oligodendrocytes
Axonal/neuronal damage and gliosis		
Anti-neurofilament	B cells	Neurons
Neurofilament	Neurons	–
14-3-3	Neuron	–
Tau	Neurons	–
Oxidative stress and cytotoxicity		
NO metabolites	Macrophages, astrocytes	Neurons, oligodendrocytes
NO	Macrophages, astrocytes	Neurons, oligodendrocytes
NOS	Macrophages, astrocytes	–
Remyelination/neural repair		
BDNF	Astrocytes, neurons, T cells, B cells, monocytes	Oligodendrocytes
NCAM	Neurons	Neurons
CTNF	Oligodendrocytes, microglia cells, astrocytes, neurons	Neurons

Table 17.1 (continued)

Cerebrospinal fluid biomarkers	Origin	Target cells
HGF	Microglia, astrocytes, neurons, OPG	Neurons, oligodendrocytes, astrocytes, microglia cells, DC, monocytes, T cells

FDC follicular dendritic cells, *TFH* follicular B helper T cells, *APC* antigen-presenting cells, *NK* natural killer cells, *NKT* natural killer T cells, *Th* T-helper cells, *DC* dendritic cells, *BAFF* B-cell-activating factor, *KFLC* immunoglobulin kappa free light chain, *MMP* matrix metalloproteinase, *ICAM* intracellular adhesion molecule, *MOG* myelin oligodendrocyte glycoprotein, *MBP* myelin basic protein, *NO* nitric oxide, *NOS* nitric oxide synthase, *BDNF* brain-derived neurotrophic factor, *NCAM* neuronal cell adhesion molecule, *CNTF* ciliary neurotrophic factor, *HGF* hepatocyte growth factor, *OPG* oligodendroglial progenitor cells

17.1.1 Acute Disseminated Encephalomyelitis (ADEM)

Acute disseminated encephalomyelitis (ADEM) is an inflammatory disorder of the CNS that is generally monophasic and self-limiting (Tselis and Lisak 1998). It is characterized by an acute or subacute encephalopathy with or without myelopathy related to diffuse demyelination of white matter and variable neurological symptoms and signs (Bennetto and Scolding 2004). ADEM is a relatively rare disease that occurs more frequently in young persons than in adults (Schwarz et al. 2001). The mean incidence varies from 0.07/100,000 persons to 0.4/100,000 persons per year (Leake et al. 2004; Krupp et al. 2007). The distinction of ADEM from MS is an important issue and may be difficult in spite of relatively clear differences in clinical picture, MR images, and CSF findings. Typically ADEM manifests after viral infection or vaccination. A prodromal phase with fever, malaise, headache, nausea, and vomiting may be observed shortly before the development of meningeal signs and drowsiness. The clinical course is rapidly progressive, developing maximum deficits within 4–5 days (Tenembaum et al. 2002). The diagnosis is based on the presence of subacute or acute illness characterized by febrile disease, frequent changes in consciousness, multifocal neurological deficits coupled with CSF, and imaging abnormalities. Although typically ADEM is a monophasic condition new episodes of neurological manifestations may occur, causing difficulties in the differentiation from MS.

CSF findings are abnormal and unspecific. There is often low-grade mononuclear pleocytosis (less than 100×10^6/l cells) with mild elevation of protein concentration. Increased intrathecal synthesis of IgG detected by isoelectric focusing (OCBs) is infrequent (0–29 %) (Tselis and Lisak 1998; Dale et al. 2001; Pohl et al. 2004). CSF viral, fungal, and bacterial cultures together with viral polymerase chain reaction assay and serological tests for suspected etiological agent should also be performed. Recently the presence of antibodies to myelin oligodendrocyte glycoprotein (MOG) in sera of children with ADEM was shown to be associated with widespread bilateral lesions in MRI and better prognosis in comparison to children without such antibodies (Baumann et al. 2014). However, in CSF such marker has not been reported.

17.1.2 Neuromyelitis Optica (NMO, Devic's Disease)

Neuromyelitis optica (NMO, Devic's disease) is defined as a severely disabling chronic autoimmune disorder of the CNS associated with the presence of aquaporin-4 antibodies in a subset (60–80 %) of patients (aquaporin-4 antibody positive NO) (Jarius et al. 2011). Less than 10 % of NMO patients have been reported to have seronegative NMO (Kitley et al. 2014). Until discovery of these antibodies in 2005 (Lennon et al. 2005), NMO was defined clinically by the presence of inflammatory myelitis and optic neuritis without symptomatic disease outside of these regions (Wingerchuk et al. 1999). Currently due to high specificity of antibodies (termed NMO-IgG or AQP4-Ab), the clinical phenotype of NMO has been broadened to include disease forms with monophasic or recurrent longitudinally extensive transverse myelitis (LETM) or less frequently bilateral or recurrent optic neuritis or brain disease together designated NMO spectrum disorders (NMOSD) (Wingerchuk et al. 2007; Jurynczyk et al. 2014). NMO is a chronic disease that typically manifests with new episodes causing difficulties in the differentiation from MS.

In patients with NMO, CSF usually shows $\geq 50 \times 10^6$ white cells/l, but their absence does not exclude the diagnosis of NMO (Jurynczyk et al. 2014). Their CSF may contain neutrophils (typically $\geq 5 \times 10^6$ cells/l) and eosinophils. Neutrophils are detected in 44 % and eosinophils in 10 % of patients (Jarius et al. 2011). In MS these cells are normally absent, while lymphocytes and macrophages predominate in CSF (Jurynczyk et al. 2014). In contrast to MS, increased CSF/serum albumin ratio indicating disturbance of blood–brain barrier (BBB) is detected in half of NMO patients (Jarius et al. 2011). OCBs are found only in 10–25 % of patients with NMO but in 95 % of patients with MS (Jurynczyk et al. 2014). The presence of OCB in CSF was associated mainly to relapses in NMO (Jarius et al. 2011). Occasionally, the intrathecal production of IgM antibodies was also observed. Lactate levels in CSF were reported to be elevated in ca. one-third of the patients, and therefore lactate was suggested as a marker of disease activity in NMO (Jarius et al. 2011).

17.1.3 Idiopathic Transverse Myelitis

Idiopathic transverse myelitis is an acute or subacute monofocal disease of the spinal cord resulting in motor, sensory, and autonomic dysfunction and requiring evidence of inflammation within the spinal cord by MRI and/or CSF studies (Transverse Myelitis Consortium Working Group 2002). Transverse myelitis is a relatively rare condition, with 1–4/1,000,000 new cases per year (Berman et al. 1981). Neurological dysfunction in acute myelitis reaches a maximum no later than 4 weeks after onset. Myelitis may be associated with potential risk of developing MS (Ghezzi et al. 2001). The disease affects individuals of all ages but mainly pediatric age groups, adolescents, and subjects between 30 and 39 years (Transverse myelitis consortium working group 2002; Kerr et al. 2005; Altrocchi 1963; Christensen et al. 1990; Jeffery et al. 1993). In contrast to most autoimmune CNS diseases, there is no sex preference in transverse myelitis. The clinical features of transverse myelitis depend on the location of the lesion which may be cervical, thoracic, or lumbar. Inflammation of the spinal cord can be detected by contrast enhancement MRI or by the analysis of the CSF (the consensus of the Transverse Myelitis Consortium 98 Working Group 2002).

Abnormalities of CSF in transverse myelitis include pleocytosis (white blood cell count >5 cells $\times 10^6$/l) or an elevated immunoglobulin G (IgG) index or presence of OCBs. If MRI and CSF analyses are not consistent with inflammation at disease onset, the lumbar puncture and MR imaging should be repeated within a week to reliably detect or exclude abnormal findings. Approximately 10 % of patients with idiopathic transverse myelitis have been reported to convert to MS after a median follow-up of ca. 3 years (Calvo et al. 2013). The likelihood of conversion of idiopathic transverse myelitis to MS increases in cases with increased IgG index and/or OCBs and brain lesions in MRI (Ghezzi et al. 2001).

17.2 Systemic Inflammatory and Autoimmune Disorders

17.2.1 Neurosarcoidosis (NS)

Neurosarcoidosis (NS) occurs in 5–15 % of patients with systemic sarcoidosis and may affect the brain, spinal cord, meninges, cranial nerves, and peripheral nervous system (Oksanen 1986; Wengert et al. 2013). Sarcoidosis is a systemic disease histologically characterized by noncaseating epithelioid granulomas, most often localized in the lungs and mediastinal lymph nodes (Zajicek et al. 1999). Neurological symptoms are the primary manifestation of the disease in ca. two-thirds of cases of NS (Zajicek et al. 1999; Ferriby et al. 2001). Thus most patients with NS only develop systemic symptoms after presenting with neurological signs of the disease. The clinical course may be acute, subacute, or chronic with insidious onset. The diagnosis of NS is based on demonstration of variable combination of neurological deficits, CNS imaging and CSF abnormalities, histological findings consistent with sarcoidosis, a positive Kveim–Siltzbach test, and positive results for at least two of the following tests: gallium scan, serum angiotensin-converting enzyme (ACE) level, and chest radiology including high-resolution computed tomography of the chest and bronchoalveolar lavage fluid analysis (Zajicek et al. 1999; Marangoni et al. 2006). The most typical MRI abnormalities include diffuse leptomeningeal enhancement in the brain and/or spinal cord and parenchymal hyperintense lesions with contrast enhancement (Wengert et al. 2013). In spite of this complexity, histological evidence of systemic disease together with compatible alterations in the CNS is sufficient for diagnosis in most cases (Marangoni et al. 2006). Other etiologies have to be ruled out.

CSF in patients with neurosarcoidosis may show several abnormalities: elevated leukocyte counts ($\geq 50 \times 10^6$/l cells), increased protein concentration (≥ 2 g/l), elevated level of lactate, and decreased level of glucose (Wengert et al. 2013). Intrathecal synthesis of IgG, IgA, and IgG has been detected in ca. one-fifth to one-third of the cases. Such CSF abnormalities were most pronounced in patients with active disease and correlated with changes on MRI.

Angiotensin-converting enzyme activity in sarcoidosis is regarded both as a diagnostic feature and as an index of disease activity that is elevated in the serum of patients with sarcoidosis (Parrish et al. 1982). Increase of its activity in the CSF has been reported in half of the patients with NS (Oksanen et al. 1985). Increased activity of this enzyme is thought to parallel macrophage and epithelioid cell activity. Also increase of the levels of lysozyme and beta-2 microglobulin, a low-molecular-weight protein associated with the histocompatibility antigens, has been reported in both the CSF and serum of majority of patients with NS (Oksanen et al. 1986). Notably, both CSF lysozyme and beta-2 microglobulin correlated to CSF leukocytes but not to CSF albumin suggesting that these markers were secreted from cells within the CNS. Elevations of CSF lysozyme and beta-2 microglobulin reveal disease activity in the CNS, and therefore both analyses are useful in monitoring disease activity in this illness.

17.2.2 Systemic Lupus Erythematosus (SLE)

Systemic lupus erythematosus (SLE) is a chronic, relapsing–remitting autoimmune disease of unknown etiology with a broad spectrum of clinical and immunologic manifestations affecting multiple organ systems. Neuropsychiatric SLE (NPSLE) encompasses central, peripheral, and autonomic nervous system as well as psychiatric manifestations observed in SLE patients. These features are classified using the American College of Rheumatology case definitions for 19 neuropsychiatric syndromes, which are listed in Table 17.2 (American College of Rheumatology 1999). The prevalence of NPSLE is highly variable, ranging from 21 to 95 % (Hanly 2014). However, only one-third of neuropsychiatric events can be directly attributed to SLE (Hanly 2014). These events can also be a consequence of complications of the disease or its treatment or totally unrelated to SLE.

Cornerstones of NPSLE diagnosis are (1) serum autoantibody profiling, (2) CSF examination, (3) neuroimaging (mainly MRI) in evaluation of brain structural abnormalities, (4) electrophysiological assessment (EEG to exclude underlying seizure disorder), and (5) neuropsychological assessment (Hanly 2014). The most important autoantibodies are antineuronal, antiribosomal P, and antiphospholipid antibodies (aPL). Antiribosomal P antibodies are mainly associated with SLE psychosis and aPL with stroke and seizure disorders.

In practice, the examination of CSF is primarily done to exclude CNS infections as a secondary cause of neuropsychiatric events and rarely in differential diagnosis of MS. In general, mild CSF abnormalities are common (40–50 %) but not specific to NPSLE (Bertsias et al. 2010). CSF findings include lymphocytic pleocytosis and OCBs, which may be detected in 25–80 % of cases (Ernerudh et al. 1983; Winfield et al. 1983; McLean et al. 1995; Reske et al. 2005). Unlike in MS, OCBs are not stable: they may disappear after treatment with corticosteroids (McLean et al. 1995).

Table 17.2 Neuropsychiatric syndromes in SLE (American College of Rheumatology 1999)

Central nervous system
Aseptic meningitis
Cerebrovascular disease
Demyelinating syndrome
Headache
Movement disorder
Myelopathy
Seizure disorders
Acute confusional state
Anxiety disorder
Cognitive dysfunction
Mood disorder
Psychosis
Peripheral nervous system
Acute inflammatory demyelinating polyneuropathy
Autonomic neuropathy
Mononeuropathy
Myasthenia gravis
Cranial neuropathy
Plexopathy
Polyneuropathy

Anti-NR2 antibodies are directed against the NR2 subtype of N-methyl-D-aspartate (NMDA) receptors, which are important in memory and learning functions. A Japanese study of 80 SLE patients found a strong association between CSF anti-NR2 antibodies and neuropsychiatric events (Yoshio et al. 2006). In another study, antiNR2 antibodies were detected in CSF of 44 and 82 % of patients with focal and diffuse NPSLE, respectively (Arinuma et al. 2008). These antibodies are also associated with hippocampal atrophy (Lauvsnes et al. 2014).

17.2.3 Primary Sjögren's Syndrome (PSS)

Primary Sjögren's syndrome (PSS) is a relatively common autoimmune disease affecting approximately 3–4 % of adults (Thomas et al. 1998). It is characterized by chronic inflammation of exocrine glands, specifically the salivary and lacrimal glands, often leading to the dryness of the mouth and eyes. The diagnosis of PSS is based on (1) ocular and oral symptoms; (2) autoantibody testing; (3) objective measures of dry eyes by Schirmer's test and Rose Bengal testing; (4) objective evidence of salivary gland involvement by unstimulated whole salivary flow, parotid sialography, or salivary scintigraphy; and (5) demonstration of focal lymphocytic infiltration in lip minor salivary gland biopsy (Vitali et al. 2002). The nuclear autoantibodies associated with but not specific for PSS are anti-SSA (formerly known as anti-Ro) and anti-SSB (anti-La). Their occurrence in patients with PSS is 33–74 % and 23–52 %, respectively (Bournia and Vlachoyiannopoulos 2012).

At least one-third of PSS patients develop extraglandular manifestations, which may be pulmonary, gastrointestinal, rheumatological, or neurological (Vitali et al. 2002). Due to the diverse criteria formerly used in the definition of PSS and selection bias in study populations, the prevalence of neurological manifestations has varied between 10 and 60 % (Chai and Logigian 2010). Unlike in SLE, CNS involvement in PSS is much less common than peripheral nervous system (PNS) involvement. According to a large Spanish cohort study of 1,010 PSS patients, 11 % had peripheral neuropathy and only 2 % CNS involvement (Ramos-Casals et al. 2008).

PNS and CNS manifestations of PSS are listed in Table 17.3. Even though NMO and PSS-associated myelitis share many clinical features, NMOSD is not currently considered as a neurological manifestation of PSS. It is more likely that these two conditions coexist in the same autoimmune milieu (Berkowitz and Samuels 2014; Carvalho et al. 2014).

The first reports on diverse CNS manifestations of SS, including the description of MS-mimicking brain lesions, were based on data from a tertiary referral center (Alexander et al. 1986; Alexander and Alexander 1983; Alexander 1993; Malinow et al. 1985). In some of these patients, CSF analysis showed lymphocytic pleocytosis with evidence of plasma cells, elevated protein content, and reduced glucose. IgG index was found to be increased in up to 50 % of patients, and OCBs were detected in nearly 90 % of CSF samples. Compared to patients with MS, patients with PSS-associated CNS manifestations had fewer OCBs (1–2 bands in patients with PSS and 2–10 bands in patients with MS).

In a Swedish study of 17 PSS patients, evidence of intrathecal IgG synthesis was found in 6 of 8 patients with clinical nervous system involvement but also in 5 of 9

Table 17.3 Neurological manifestations of primary Sjögren's syndrome

Peripheral nervous system
Sensorimotor polyneuropathy
Polyradiculopathy
Chronic inflammatory demyelinating polyneuropathy (CIDP)
Selective nerve root inflammation
Sensory ganglionopathy (sensory ataxic neuropathy)
Small fiber neuropathy
Multiple mononeuropathy
Autonomic neuropathy
Cranial neuropathies (most common are trigeminal neuropathy and optic neuritis)
Central nervous system
Aseptic meningitis
Encephalopathy
Seizures
Transverse myelitis
Brainstem and cerebellar symptoms
Cognitive dysfunction

patients without neurological manifestations (Vrethem et al. 1990). Based on data from a hospital specializing in inflammatory diseases, focal or multifocal CNS disorder was diagnosed in 56 of 86 consecutive PSS patients (68 %). In CSF analysis, 30 % of the CNS subgroup had OCBs (Delalande et al. 2004). CSF of eight patients with PSS-associated myelitis was examined and only one had OCBs (one band) (Kim et al. 2009). Like in SLE, recent studies have indicated the association between CSF anti-NR2 antibodies and memory dysfunction in patients with PSS (Lauvsnes et al. 2013).

17.2.4 Behcet's Disease

Behcet's disease is a chronic systemic relapsing inflammatory disease involving the small blood vessels. It is characterized by combination of oral and/or genital ulcerations, papulopustular skin lesions, erythema nodosum, ophthalmologic lesions (uveitis, retinal vasculitis), and arthritis (Pohl and Benseller 2013). Less frequently, subcutaneous thrombophlebitis and gastrointestinal lesions may also occur. The disease is more frequent and severe in patients from the eastern Mediterranean and Asia (Akmar-Demir et al. 1999). Neurologic manifestations may occur in up to 50 % of patients and present as aseptic meningitis, encephalitis, myelitis, thrombosis, or arteritis. Neurological manifestations commonly develop within 6 years after the onset of systemic features (Pohl and Benseller 2013). Patients with Behcet's disease and neurological injury are associated with a poorer prognosis (Cikes et al. 2008). The differential diagnosis between neurological Behcet's disease and MS may be difficult especially if neurological manifestations develop before the systemic appearance fulfilling diagnostic criteria for BD.

CSF may be abnormal in 70–80 % of patients with neurological Behcet's disease. Abnormalities include increase in protein levels and pleocytosis up to 400 cells/l (initially neutrophilic, later lymphocytic). OCBs are typically absent, but in a subset of patients, they may be present in the CSF (Serdaroglu et al. 1998).

17.2.5 Primary Cerebral Vasculitis

Primary cerebral vasculitis may occur as primary angiitis of the central nervous system (PACNS) or as CNS manifestation in the setting of systemic vasculitis. PACNS is a rare inflammatory disease typically affecting middle-aged patients. It involves small- and medium-sized leptomeningeal and intracranial vessels and has focal and segmental distribution. PACNS has to be distinguished from secondary CNS vasculitis that is an inflammation of cerebral blood vessels, which may occur in the context of an underlying systemic inflammatory disease, a malignancy, or an infection, as well as a number of other diseases. The most frequent symptoms of PACNS and cerebral vasculitis are headache, focal neurologic deficits, confusion, seizures, and neuropsychological deficits (Berlit and Kraemer 2013). Diagnostic workup includes history and general medical examination especially focusing on the skin, lungs, kidney, and other signs of systemic disease, laboratory and CSF studies, MRI, angiography, and brain biopsy (Berlit and Kraemer 2013; Kinsella et al. 2009). Differential diagnosis is of key importance to exclude other more frequent diseases.

Laboratory analyses should include determination of acute phase proteins like erythrocyte sedimentation rate, C-reactive protein, immunoglobulin G levels, complement C3 levels, von Willebrand factor antigen, lupus anticoagulant, antinuclear antibodies, double-stranded DNA antibodies, rheumatoid factor, anticytoplasmic antibodies (cANCA, pANCA), anticardiolipin antibodies, antithrombin III, fibrinogen, plasminogen, homocysteine, factor V, Leiden gene mutation, and MTHFR gene mutation. Cerebrospinal fluid analysis includes determination of opening pressure, cell count, protein, glucose, lactate, OCBs and IgG index, cytology, serology, and CSF polymerase chain reaction which is required to exclude infections. Normal inflammatory markers and CSF analysis do not rule out the diagnosis of cerebral vasculitis.

References

Akmar-Demir G, Serdaroglu P, Tasci B et al (1999) Clinical patterns of neurological involvement in Behcet's disease: evaluation of 200 patients. Brain 122:2171–2182

Alexander EL (1993) Neurologic disease in Sjogren's syndrome: mononuclear inflammatory vasculopathy affecting central/ peripheral nervous system and muscle. A clinical review and update of immunopathogenesis. Rheum Dis Clin North Am 19:869–908

Alexander EL, Alexander GE (1983) Aseptic meningoencephalitis in primary Sjogren's syndrome. Neurology 33:593–598

Alexander EL, Malinow K, Lejewski JE, Jerdan MS, Provost TT, Alexander GE (1986) Primary Sjogren's syndrome with central nervous system disease mimicking multiple sclerosis. Ann Intern Med 104:323–330

Altrocchi PH (1963) Acute transverse myelopathy. Arch Neurol 9:111–119

Andersson M, Alvarez-Cermeno J, Bernardi G et al (1994) Cerebrospinal fluid in the diagnosis of multiple sclerosis: a consensus report. J Neurol Neurosurg Psychiatry 57:897–902

Arinuma Y, Yanagida T, Hirohata S (2008) Association of cerebrospinal fluid anti-NR2 glutamate receptor antibodies with diffuse neuropsychiatric systemic lupus erythematosus. Arthritis Rheum 58:1130–1135

Baumann M, Sahin K, Lechner C, Hennes EM, Schanda K et al (2014) Clinical and neuroradiological differences of paediatric acute disseminating encephalomyelitis with and without antibodies to myelin oligodendrocyte glycoprotein. J Neurol Neurosurg Psychiatry pii:jnnp-2014-308346. doi:10.1136/jnnp-2014-308346. [Epub ahead of print]

Bennetto L, Scolding N (2004) Inflammatory/post-infectious encephalomyelitis. J Neurol Neurosurg Psychiatry 75:2–8

Berkowitz AL, Samuels MA (2014) The neurology of Sjögren's syndrome and the rheumatology of peripheral neuropathy and myelitis. Pract Neurol 14:14–22

Berlit P, Kraemer M (2013) Cerebral vasculitis in adults: what are the steps in order to establish the diagnosis? Red flags and pitfalls. Clin Exp Immunol 175:419–424

Berman M, Feldman S, Alter M, Zilber N, Kahana E (1981) Acute transverse myelitis: incidence and etiologic considerations. Neurology 31:966–971

Bertsias GK, Ioannidis JPA, Aringer M et al (2010) EULAR recommendations for the management of systemic lupus erythematosus with neuropsychiatric manifestations: report of a task force of the EULAR standing committee for clinical affairs. Ann Rheum Dis 69:2074–2082

Boppana S, Huang H, Ito K, Dhib-Jalbut S (2011) Immunologic aspects of multiple sclerosis. Mt Sinai J Med 78(2):207–220

Bournia VK, Vlachoyiannopoulos PG (2012) Subgroups of Sjögren syndrome patients according to serological profiles. J Autoimmun 39:15–26

Calvo AC, Martinez AMM, Alentorn-Palau A et al (2013) Idiopathic acute transverse myelitis: outcome and conversion to multiple sclerosis in a large series. BMC Neurol 13:135

Carvalho DC, Tironi TS, Freitas DS, Kleinpaul R, Talim NC, Lana-Peixoto MA (2014) Sjögren syndrome and neuromyelitis optica spectrum disorder co-exist in a common autoimmune milieu. Arq Neuropsiquiatr 72:619–624

Chai J, Logigian EL (2010) Neurological manifestations of primary Sjögren's syndrome. Curr Opin Neurol 23:509–513

Christensen PB, Wermuth L, Hinge HH, Bømers K (1990) Clinical course and long-term prognosis of acute transverse myelopathy. Acta Neurol Scand 81:431–435

Cikes N, Bosnik D, Sentic M (2008) Non-MS autoimmune demyelination. Clin Neurol Neurosurg 110:905–912

Comabella M, Khoury SJ (2012) Immunopathogenesis of multiple sclerosis. Clin Immunol 142(1):2–8

Comabella M, Montalban X (2014) Body fluid biomarkers in multiple sclerosis. Lancet Neurol 13(1):113–126

Dale RC, Church AJ, Cardoso F et al (2001) Post streptococcal acute disseminated encephalomyelitis with basal ganglia involvement and autoreactive antibasal ganglia antibodies. Ann Neurol 50:588–595

Deisenhammer F, Bartos A, Egg R et al (2006) Guidelines on routine cerebrospinal fluid analysis. Report from an EFNS task force. Eur J Neurol 13:913–922

Delalande S, de Seze J, Fauchais AL et al (2004) Neurologic manifestations in primary Sjögren syndrome: a study of 82 patients. Medicine (Baltimore) 83(5):280–291

Ernerudh J, Olsson T, Lindstrom F, Skogh T (1983) Cerebrospinal fluid immunoglobulin abnormalities in systemic lupus erythematosus. J Neurol Neurosurg Psychiatry 48:807–813

Ferriby D, de Seze J, Stojkovic T et al (2011) Long-term follow-up of neurosarcoidosis. Neurology 11;57(5):927–929

Freedman MS, Thompson EJ, Deisenhammer F (2005) Recommended standard of cerebrospinal fluid analysis in the diagnosis of multiple sclerosis: a consensus statement. Arch Neurol 62:865–870

Ghezzi A, Baldini SM, Zaffaroni M (2001) Differential diagnosis of acute myelopathies. Neurol Sci 22:S60–S64

Hanly JG (2014) Diagnosis and management of neuropsychiatric SLE. Nat Rev Rheumatol 10:338–347

Harris VK, Donelan N, Yan QJ, Clark K, Touray A, Rammal M, Sadiq SA (2013) Cerebrospinal fluid fetuin-A is a biomarker of active multiple sclerosis. Mult Scler 19(11):1462–1472

Jarius S, Paul F, Franciotta D, Ruprecht K et al (2011) Cerebrospinal fluid findings in aquaporin-4 antibody positive neuromyelitis optica: results from 211 lumbar punctures. J Neurol Sci 306(1–2):82–90

Jeffery DR, Mandler RN, Davis LE (1993) Transverse myelitis. Retrospective analysis of 33 cases, with differentiation of cases associated with multiple sclerosis and parainfectious events. Arch Neurol 50:532–535

Jurynczyk M, Craner M, Palace M (2014) Overlapping CNS inflammatory diseases: differentiating features of NMO and MS. J Neurol Neurosurg Psychiatry doi:10.1136/jnnp-2014-303984

Kerr D, Chrishnan C, Piddock F (2005) Acute transverse myelitis. In: Singer H, Kossof EH, Hartman AL, Crawford TO (eds) Treatment of pediatric neurologic disorders. Taylor & Francis, Boca Raton, pp 445–451

Khademi M, Kockum I, Andersson ML, Iacobaeus E, Brundin L, Sellebjerg F, Hillert J, Piehl F, Olsson T (2011) Cerebrospinal fluid CXCL13 in multiple sclerosis: a suggestive prognostic marker for the disease course. Mult Scler 17(3):335–343

Kim SM, Waters P, Vincent A et al (2009) Sjögren's syndrome myelopathy: spinal cord involvement in Sjögren's syndrome might be a manifestation of neuromyelitis optica. Mult Scler 15:1062–1068

Kinsella JA, O'Brien WO, Mullins GM, Brewer J, Whyte S (2009) Primary angiitis of the central nervous system with diffuse cerebral mass effect and giant cells. J Clin Neurosci 17:674–676

Kitley J, Waters P, Woodhall M, Leite MI, Murchison A, George J, Küker W, Chandratre S, Vincent A, Palace J (2014) Neuromyelitis optica spectrum disorders with aquaporin-4 and myelin-oligodendrocyte glycoprotein antibodies: a comparative study. JAMA Neurol 71(3):276–283

Krupp LB, Banwell B, Tenembaum S, International Paediatric MS Study Group (2007) Consensus definitions proposed for pediatric multiple sclerosis and related disorders. Neurology 68(Suppl 2):S7–S12

Lassmann H (2013) Pathology and disease mechanisms in different stages of multiple sclerosis. J Neurol Sci 15;333(1-2):1–4. Review

Lauvsnes MB, Maroni SS, Appenzeller S et al (2013) Memory dysfunction in primary Sjögren's syndrome is associated with anti-NR2 antibodies. Arthritis Rheum 65:3209–3217

Lauvsnes MB, Beyer MK, Kvalöy JT et al (2014) Hippocampal atrophy is associated with cerebrospinal fluid anti-NR2 antibodies in patients with systemic lupus erythematosus and primary Sjögren's syndrome. Arthritis Rheumatol 66:3387–3394

Leake JA, Albani S, Kao AS et al (2004) Acute disseminated encephalomyelitis in childhood: epidemiologic, clinical and laboratory features. Pediatr Infect Dis J 23:756–764

Lennon VA, Kryzer TJ, Pittock SJ, Verkman AS et al (2005) IgG marker of optic-spinal multiple sclerosis binds to the aquaporin-4 water channel. J Exp Med 202:473–477

Link H, Huang YM (2006) Oligoclonal bands in multiple sclerosis cerebrospinal fluid: an update on methodology and clinical usefulness. J Neuroimmunol 180(1–2):17–28

Link H, Tibbling G (1977) Principles of albumin and IgG analyses in neurological disorders. III. Evaluation of IgG synthesis within the central nervous system in multiple sclerosis. Scand J Clin Lab Invest 37:397–401

Malinow KL, Molina R, Gordon B, Selnes OA, Provost TT, Alexander EL (1985) Neuropsychiatric dysfunction in primary Sjogren's syndrome. Ann Intern Med 103:344–350

Marangoni S, Argentiero V, Tavolato B (2006) Neurosarcoidosis: clinical description of 7 cases with a proposal for a new diagnostic strategy. J Neurol 253:488–495

McLean BN, Miller D, Thompson EJ (1995) Oligoclonal banding of IgG in CSF, blood–brain barrier function, and MRI findings in patients with sarcoidosis, systemic lupus erythematosus, and Behcet's disease involving the nervous system. J Neurol Neurosurg Psychiatry 58:548–554

Oksanen V (1986) Neurosarcoidosis: clinical presentation and course in 50 patients. Acta Neurol Scand 73(3):283–290

Oksanen V, Fyhrquist F, Grönhagen-Riska C, Somer H (1985) CSF angiotensin-converting enzyme in neurosarcoidosis. Lancet 1(8436):1050–1051

Oksanen V, Grönhagen-Riska C, Tikanoja S, Somer H, Fyhrquist F (1986) Cerebrospinal fluid lysozyme and beta 2-microglobulin in neurosarcoidosis. J Neurol Sci 73(1):79–87

Parrish RW, Williams JD, Davies BH (1982) Serum beta-2-microglobulin and angiotensin converting enzyme activity in sarcoidosis. Thorax 37(12):936–940

Petzold A (2013) Intrathecal oligoclonal IgG synthesis in multiple sclerosis. J Neuroimmunol 262(1–2):1–10

Pohl D, Benseller S (2013) Systemic inflammatory and autoimmune disorders. Handb Clin Neurol 112:1243–1252

Pohl D, Rostasy K, Reiber H, Hanefeld F (2004) CSF characteristics in early-onset multiple sclerosis. Neurology 63:1966–1967

Polman CH, Reingold SC, Banwell B et al (2011) Diagnostic criteria for multiple sclerosis: 2010 revisions to the McDonald criteria. Ann Neurol 69:292–302

Presslauer S, Milosavljevic D, Huebl W, Parigger S, Schneider-Koch G, Bruecke T (2014) Kappa free light chains: diagnostic and prognostic relevance in MS and CIS. PLoS One 9(2):e89945

Ramos-Casals M, Solans R, Rosas J et al (2008) Primary Sjögren syndrome in Spain: clinical and immunologic expression in 1010 patients. Medicine (Baltimore) 87:210–219

Reske D, Petereit H-F, Heiss W-D (2005) Difficulties in the differentiation of chronic inflammatory diseases of the central nervous system – value of cerebrospinal fluid analysis and immunological abnormalities in the diagnosis. Acta Neurol Scand 112:207–213

Romme Christensen J, Ratzer R, Bornsen L, Lyksborg M, Garde E, Dyrby TB, Siebner HR, Sorensen PS, Sellebjerg F (2014) Natalizumab in progressive MS: results of an open-label, phase 2A, proof-of-concept trial. Neurology 82(17):1499–1507

Schwarz S, Mohr A, Knauth M, Wildemann B, Storch-Hagenlocher B (2001) Acute disseminated encephalomyelitis. A follow-up study of 40 adult patients. Neurology 56:1313–1318

Senel M, Tumani H, Lauda F, Presslauer S, Mojib-Yezdani R, Otto M, Brettschneider J (2014) Cerebrospinal fluid immunoglobulin kappa light chain in clinically isolated syndrome and multiple sclerosis. PLoS One 9(4):e88680

Serdaroglu P et al (1998) Behcet's disease and the nervous system. J Neurol 245:197–205

Stangel M, Fredrikson S, Meinl E, Petzold A, Stuve O, Tumani H (2013) The utility of cerebrospinal fluid analysis in patients with multiple sclerosis. Nat Rev Neurol 9(5):267–276

Tenembaum S, Chamoles N, Fejerman N (2002) Acute disseminated encephalomyelitis: a long-term follow-up study of 84 pediatric patients. Neurology 59:1224–1232

Teunissen CE, Khalil M (2012) Neurofilaments as biomarkers in multiple sclerosis. Mult Scler 18(5):552–556

The American College of Rheumatology nomenclature and case definitions for neuropsychiatric lupus syndromes (1999) Arthritis Rheum 42:599–608

Thomas E, Hay EM, Hajeer A, Silman AJ (1998) Sjögren's syndrome: a community based study of prevalence and impact. Br J Rheumatol 37:1069–1076

Transverse Myelitis Consortium Working Group (2002) Proposed diagnostic criteria and nosology of acute transverse myelitis. Neurology 59:499–505

Tselis AC, Lisak RP (1998) Acute disseminated encephalomyelitis. In: Antel J, Birnbaum G, Hartung H-P (eds) Clinical neuroimmunology. Blackwell Sciences, Malden

Villar LM, Espiño M, Cavanillas ML, Roldán E, Urcelay E, de la Concha EG, Sádaba MC, Arroyo R, González-Porqué P, Álvarez-Cermeño JC (2010) Immunological mechanisms that associate with oligoclonal IgM band synthesis in multiple sclerosis. Clin Immunol 137(1):51–59

Vitali C, Bombardieri S, Jonsson R et al (2002) Classification criteria for Sjögren's syndrome: a revised version of the European criteria proposed by the American-European Consensus Group. Ann Rheum Dis 61:554–558

Vrethem M, Ernerudh J, Lindstrom F, Skogh T (1990) Immunoglobulins within the central nervous system in primary Sjogren's syndrome. J Neurol Sci 100:186–192

Wengert O, Rothenfusser-Korber E, Vollrath B, Bohner B et al (2013) Neurosarcoidosis: correlation of cerebrospinal fluid findings with diffuse leptomeningeal gadolinium enhancement on MRI and clinical disease activity. J Neurol Sci 335:124–130

Winfield JB, Shaw M, Silverman LM, Eisenberg RA, Wilson HA III, Koffler D (1983) Intrathecal IgG synthesis and blood–brain barrier impairment in patients with systemic lupus erythematosus and central nervous system dysfunction. Am J Med 74:837–844

Wingerchuk DM, Hogancamp WF, O'Brien PC, Weinshenker BG (1999) The clinical course of neuromyelitis optica (Devic's syndrome). Neurology 53(5):1107–1114

Wingerchuk DM, Lennon VA, Lucchinetti CF, Pittock SJ, Weinshenker BG (2007) The spectrum of neuromyelitis optica. Lancet Neurol 6(9):805–815

Yoshio T, Onda K, Nara H, Minota S (2006) Association of IgG anti-NR2 glutamate receptor antibodies in cerebrospinal fluid with neuropsychiatric systemic lupus erythematosus. Arthritis Rheum 54:675–678

Zajicek JP, Scolding NJ, Foster O, Rovaris M, Evanson J, Moseley IF, Scadding JW, Thompson EJ, Chamoun V, Miller DH, McDonald WI, Mitchell D (1999) Central nervous system sarcoidosis–diagnosis and management. QJM 92(2):103–117

CSF Findings in Guillain-Barré Syndrome: Demyelinating and Axonal Acute Inflammatory Polyneuropathies

18

Zsolt Illes and Morten Blaabjerg

Contents

Abstract

The clinical picture of Guillain-Barré syndrome (GBS) is heterogeneous and involves the classical demyelinating type of inflammatory polyradiculoneuropathy (AIDP), the more rapid and usually less benign motor or motor-sensory axonal forms (AMAN, AMSAN), and the anti-GQ1b spectrum of Miller Fisher syndrome (MFS) characterized by the triad of external ophthalmoparesis, ataxia,

Z. Illes (✉)
Department of Neurology,
Odense University Hospital,
Sdr. Boulevard 29, Odense 5000, Denmark

Institute of Clinical Research, University of Southern Denmark,
Odense, Denmark
e-mail: zsolt.illes@rsyd.dk

M. Blaabjerg
Department of Neurology,
Odense University Hospital,
Sdr. Boulevard 29, Odense 5000, Denmark

© Springer International Publishing Switzerland 2015
F. Deisenhammer et al. (eds.), *Cerebrospinal Fluid in Clinical Neurology*,
DOI 10.1007/978-3-319-01225-4_18

and areflexia and the Bickerstaff brainstem encephalitis (BBE). In addition, GBS-like disease has been described in other medical conditions, e.g., associated with acquired immunodeficiencies, transplantations, lymphomas, and biological treatments. Albuminocytological dissociation, the classical alteration of the CSF in GBS, was already described in the original paper by Guillain, Barré, and Strohl. Since then, a number of studies have examined molecular changes of the CSF using different methodologies. Considering the presumably autoimmune pathogenesis, antibodies, complement components, cytokine, and chemokine patterns have been explored. Molecules considered being neuroprotective or reflecting axonal damage have been compared among different subtypes of GBS. Analysis of the proteome in GBS has been also performed and revealed several potential biomarkers. Although most of these studies indicate alteration of the CSF and support the immunopathogenesis of GBS, albuminocytological dissociation described 100 years ago remains the only consistent CSF biomarker supporting the diagnosis of GBS after the second week of disease onset.

Abbreviations

AIDP	Acute inflammatory demyelinating polyneuropathy
AMAN	Acute motor axonal neuropathy
AMSAN	Acute motor-sensory axonal neuropathy
ART	Antiretroviral therapy
BBE	Bickerstaff brainstem encephalitis
CIDP	Chronic inflammatory demyelinating polyneuropathy
CMV	Cytomegalovirus
EBV	Epstein-Barr virus
ENG	Electroneurography
GALT	Galactose-1-phosphate uridylyltransferase
GBS	Guillain-Barré syndrome
GVHD	Graft-versus-host disease
HHV-6	Human herpesvirus 6
HIV	Human immunodeficiency virus
HSP	Heat shock protein
HSV	Herpes simplex virus
ICAM-1	Intercellular adhesion molecule 1
IRIS	Immune reconstitution inflammatory syndrome
MFS	Miller Fisher syndrome
NfH	Neurofilament heavy chain
NRTI	Nucleoside reverse transcriptase inhibitors
NSE	Neuron-specific enolase
PCB	Acute pharyngo-cervico-brachial palsy
PGDS	Prostaglandin D2 synthetase
SCT	Stem cell transplantation
VCAM-1	Vascular cell adhesion molecule 1
VEGF	Vascular endothelial growth factor
VZV	Varicella-zoster virus

The classical Guillain-Barré syndrome (GBS) is an acute, inflammatory polyradiculoneuropathy characterized by ascending symmetric motor weakness in the majority of cases (Kuwabara et al. 2013; Rinaldi 2013; Yuki and Hartung 2012). The original conception of GBS as an acute demyelinating polyneuropathy has changed considerably. In 1951 Bickerstaff and Cloake described the brainstem encephalitis, which later became part of the anti-GQ1b disease spectrum together with the Miller Fisher syndrome (MFS, described in 1956) characterized by ataxia and external ocular palsy (Bickerstaff and Cloake 1951; Ito et al. 2008; Chavada and Willison 2012; Shahrizaila and Yuki 2013). Axonal forms of GBS were described from 1990 first in Asia (acute motor axonal neuropathy, AMAN and acute motor-sensory axonal neuropathy, AMSAN) (Kuwabara et al. 2013). Thereafter, the most common and classic type of demyelinating GBS has been termed acute inflammatory demyelinating polyradiculoneuropathy (AIDP) (Fig. 18.1).

Based on well-designed epidemiological studies, the annual incidence of GBS is 1–2 cases/100,000. Meta-analysis indicated a higher incidence in men and in

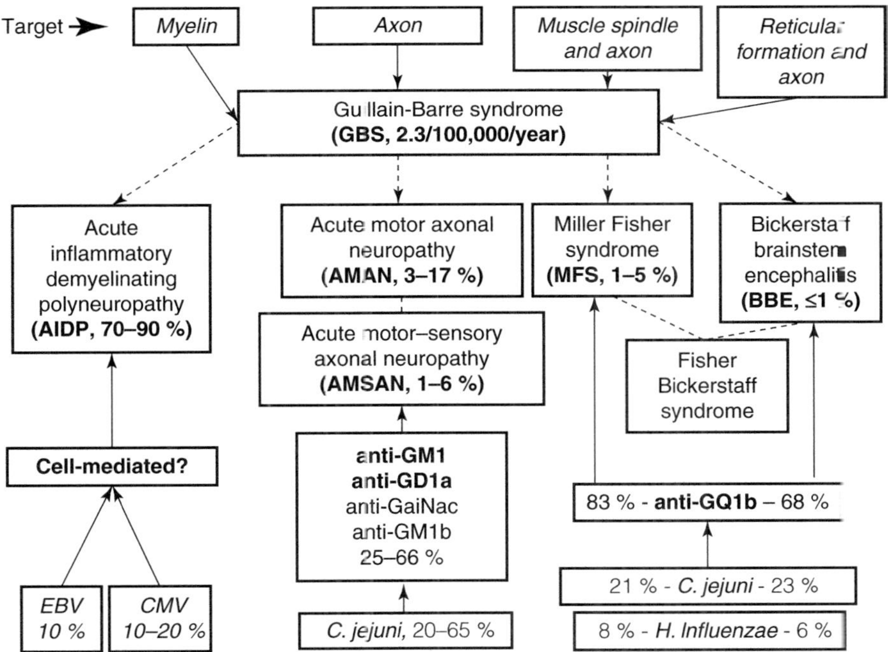

Fig. 18.1 Major syndromes of acute demyelinating polyneuropathies. The figure indicates the heterogeneous pathology and clinical picture of GBS. Demyelination is responsible for the most common form of AIDP, while axonal lesion and involvement of the muscle spindles and reticular formation may be responsible for the rarer forms of AMAN, AMSAN, MFS, and BBE. Antibody responses may differentially contribute and characterize the different subtypes of GBS, most typically by anti-GM1 antibodies in AMAN and AMSAN and by anti-GQ1b antibodies in MFS and BBE. Bacterial infection in the axonal forms and viral infection in AIDP may precede the disease. *GBS* Guillain-Barré syndrome, *AIDP* acute inflammatory demyelinating polyneuropathy, *AMAN* acute motor axonal neuropathy, *AMSAN* acute motor-sensory axonal neuropathy, *MFS* Miller Fisher syndrome, *BBE* Bickerstaff brainstem encephalitis, *EBV* Epstein-Barr virus, *CMV* cytomegalovirus

elderlies. In Europe and North America, about 70–90 % of the cases are AIDP; 3–17 %, AMAN; and 1–6 %, AMSAN. There are no epidemiological studies regarding BBE and MFS; about 1–5 % of the GBS cases are estimated to be MFS, and BBE is even rarer. AMAN, MFS, and BBE are characterized by a preceding infection in a large number of cases, which is most commonly caused by *C. jejuni*. Cytomegalovirus (CMV) and Epstein-Barr virus (EBV) infection can be also associated with GBS (Kuwabara et al. 2013; Rinaldi 2013; Yuki and Hartung 2012).

The pathogenesis of GBS is unclear and most likely heterogeneous: some data suggest the importance of T cell responses in AIDP. Molecular mimicry involving antibodies reacting with axonal gangliosides might be important in the axonal forms. Although genetic association has been suggested, a recent meta-analysis of 1,600 patients and 2,150 controls was unable to confirm most of the previously suggested associations (Kuwabara et al. 2013; Rinaldi 2013; Yuki and Hartung 2012; Chavada and Willison 2012; Hadden et al. 2001; Rajabally and Uncini 2012).

18.1 Acute Inflammatory Demyelinating Polyneuropathy (AIDP)

The progressive phase of the disease is less than 4 weeks long and usually starts with ascending distal paresthesia of the lower extremities. Symmetric motor weakness is always present in the plateau phase, and deep reflexes are lost in 90 % of the cases. Involvement of the cranial nerves, especially bilateral peripheral facial nerve palsy, can be characteristic of AIDP. Autonomic symptoms and respiratory failure are the major concerns of life-threatening complications. Electroneurography (ENG) indicates distal and proximal multifocal demyelination: the motor nerve conduction is decreased, the distal motor latency and F wave latency are long, and temporal dispersion and conduction blocks can be present (Kuwabara et al. 2013; Rinaldi 2013; Yuki and Hartung 2012; Chavada and Willison 2012; Hadden et al. 2001; Rajabally and Uncini 2012; Uncini and Kuwabara 2012; Verma et al. 2013).

CSF Alterations in AIDP (Table 18.1) The albuminocytologic dissociation defined as high CSF protein but normal cell count is a key feature of GBS and was described by Guillain, Barré, and Strohl in 1916. However, total protein levels may be initially normal in around half of the patients. Nevertheless, when lumbar puncture is performed during the second week of GBS, around 80 % of patients or more have increased total CSF protein levels (Van der Meché et al. 2001), and 6 days after symptom onset, >84 % have elevated CSF/serum albumin ratio consistent with blood–CSF barrier dysfunction (Brettschneider et al. 2005).

The CSF white cell count is usually below 50 cells/μl, and in a case series of 134 patients, only 15 patients (11 %) had more than 3 cells/μl (Van der Meché et al. 2001). One study with a limited number of patients showed an increased number of CD123+ dendritic cells in the CSF (Press et al. 2005).

Several different antibodies have been found in the CSF of patients with GBS, and a matched pattern of oligoclonal bands may be seen in up to 65 % of patients (Krüger et al. 1981; Segurado et al. 1986). A key feature of GBS is myelin

Table 18.1 Alteration of CSF in Guillain-Barré syndrome

	Change	References
Protein	Elevated (>80 % second week)	Van der Meché et al. (2001)
	Elevated CSF/serum albumin ratio	Brettschneider et al. (2005)
Cells	<50 cells; 89 % have 3 cells or less	Van der Meché et al. (2001)
Cell type	Increased number of CD123[+] dendritic cells	Press et al. (2005)
Oligoclonal bands	Matched pattern in 65 %	Krüger et al. (1981)
		Segurado et al. (1986)
Antibodies	IgG-MBP (56.2 %) and IgM-MBP (53 %)	Marchiori et al. (1990)
	Cerebrosides IgG (38.5 %) and IgM (23 %)	
	Cardiolipin IgG (50 %)	
	GM1 IgG and IgM (48 %)	Simone et al. (1993)
	GD1a, GD1b, GM2 IgG and IgM	Matà et al. (2006)
	GM3, AGM1, GD1a, GD1b IgM or IgG	
	HSP27, HSP60, HSP70, and HSP90	Yonekura et al. (2004)
	$\alpha\beta$-crystallin	Wanschitz et al. (2008)
Complement	C3a, C5a	Hartung et al. (1987)
	C4d	Koguchi et al. (1995)
	Fluid phase complement complex C5b-9	Sanders et al. (1986)
Enzymes	Cystatin C (decreased), cathepsin B (increased)	Nagai et al. (2000)
	Prostaglandin D2 synthetase (increased in AIDP)*	Huang et al. (2009)
Cyto- and chemokines	CXCL10 (IP-10) (elevated)	Kieseier et al. (2002)
	MCP-1 (elevated)	Press et al. (2003)
	CX3CL1 (elevated)	Kastenbauer et al. (2003)
	CCL2, CCL7, CCL27 CXCL9 CXCL10, CXCL12 (elevated)	Sainaghi et al. (2010)
	IL-18 (elevated)	Jander and Stoll (2001)
	IL-17 (acute phase), IL-22 and IL-37 (elevated)	Li et al. 2012; 2013
	IL-8 and IL-1ra (higher in GBS than CIDP)	Sainaghi et al. (2010)
	Osteopontin (elevated acute phase)	Han et al. (2014)
	Tumor necrosis factor α mRNA (elevated)	Petzold et al. (1998)
	sTNF-R p60 (elevated)	
Cell adhesion	ICAM-1, VCAM-1 (elevated)	Sainaghi et al. (2010)
Growth factors	VEGF (elevated)	Sainaghi et al. (2010)
Axonal markers	Neurofilament heavy chain (elevated)	Merkies et al. (2002)
		Petzold et al. (2006, 2009)
		Dujmovic et al. (2013)
	Tau (elevated)	Süssmuth et al. (2001)
	Neuron-specific enolase (elevated)	Vermuyten et al. (1990)
	S100B	Mokuno et al. (1994)
	Protein 14-3-3[a]	Satoh et al. (1999)

(continued)

Table 18.1 (continued)

	Change	References
Protein components (proteome analysis)	*Upregulated:* apolipoprotein A-IV, PRO2044, serine/threonine kinase 10, alpha-1-antitrypsin, SNC73, alpha II spectrin, IgG kappa chain, cathepsin D preprotein, haptoglobin, Orosomucoid, apolipoprotein A-IV Vitamin D-binding protein, beta-2 glycoprotein I (ApoH), complement component C3 isoform alpha-1-antitrypsin, and neurofilaments	Lehmensiek et al. (2007) Chang et al. (2007) D'Aguanno et al. (2010) Yang et al. (2009) Jin et al. (2007)
	Downregulated; fibrinogen, transferrin, caldesmon, GALT, human heat shock protein 70, transthyretin, amyloidosis patient HL-heart-peptide 127aa, prostaglandin D2 synthase, apolipoprotein E, albumin and five of its fragments, cystatin C, apolipoprotein E and heat shock protein 70	

[a]Changes only found in some studies

disruption; IgG and IgM antibodies against myelin basic protein (MBP) have been found in the CSF of 56.2 and 53 % of patients, respectively (Marchiori et al. 1990). These antibodies could, however, not distinguish GBS from other inflammatory diseases such as MS and are therefore not suitable as biomarkers (Marchiori et al. 1990). IgG and IgM antibodies against cerebrosides (38.5 and 23 %, respectively) and IgG antibodies against cardiolipin (50 %) were also found (Marchiori et al. 1990). One of the major targets of antibodies detected in the CSF is gangliosides (Marchiori et al. 1990). These include anti-GM1 IgG and IgM in 48 % of GBS cases (Simone et al. 1993); GM1, GD1a, GD1b, and GM2 IgG/IgM (Mata et al. 2006); and GM1, GM2, GM3, AGM1, GD1a, and GD1b IgM or IgG (Brettschneider et al. 2009). Antibodies reacting with heat shock proteins (HSP) have also been found. These include HSP27, HSP60, HSP70, and HSP90 (Yonekura et al. 2004). Antibodies (IgG) targeting another stress protein, αβ-crystallin (αBC), was found to be elevated in the CSF. When using a cutoff of αBC-IgG index >0.8, the specificity was 85 % and the sensitivity was 76 % for GBS (Wanschitz et al. 2008).

Evidence also points to an activation of the complement system in GBS. Elevated levels of complement fragments C3a, C5a (Hartung et al. 1987), and C4d (Koguchi et al. 1995) and the fluid phase complement complex C5b-9 (Sanders et al. 1986) in the CSF have been described. The membrane attack complex C5b-9 was associated with a more severe disease course, being higher in patients dependent on respiratory support (Sanders et al. 1986).

Not surprisingly, levels of cytokines and chemokines are also altered in CSF of patients with GBS. Thus, studies have found increased levels of CXCL10 (IP-10) (Kieseier et al. 2002), MCP-1 (Press et al. 2003), and CX3CL1 (fractalkine) (Kastenbauer et al. 2003). Elevated concentrations of IL-18 (Jander and Stoll 2001), IL-17, IL-22 (Li et al. 2012, 2013), and IL-37 (Li et al. 2013) have been detected. Concentrations of IL-17 and IL-37 correlated with functional disability

(Li et al. 2013). A recent study found increased IL-17 levels in the acute but not in the stable phase of both AMAN and AIDP (Han et al. 2014). The same study found an increased CSF osteopontin level in the CSF of both AIDP and AMAN patients (Han et al. 2014). Tumor necrosis factor (TNF)-α mRNA and its soluble 60 kDa receptor (sTNF-R p60) were also upregulated in the CSF (Petzold et al. 1998). Using a multiplex bead-based ELISA assay investigating 32 inflammatory mediators, increased levels of CCL2, CCL7, CCL27, CXCL9, CXCL10, CXCL12, ICAM-1, VCAM-1, and VEGF were detected similar to CIDP (Sainaghi et al. 2010). Moreover, concentrations of IL-8 and IL-1ra were higher in GBS compared to CIDP or controls (Sainaghi et al. 2010).

Levels of the proteolytic enzyme cystatin C were decreased, whereas cathepsin B concentration was increased in the CSF of patients with GBS, similar to CIDP (Nagai et al. 2000). The concentration of another abundant brain protein, prostaglandin D2 synthetase (PGDS), was elevated in the CSF of patients with AIDP compared to controls despite of a decreased intrathecal synthesis, in contrast to Miller Fisher syndrome or CIDP (Huang et al. 2009). However, data regarding PGDS are conflicting, since it was found to be downregulated in a recent proteome analysis (Chang et al. 2007).

Markers of axonal damage have also been investigated. The level of heavy chain subunit of neurofilament (NfH) was 12.5-fold higher in the CSF of patients with electrophysiological evidence of axonal involvement, and high NfH concentration seemed to be associated with worse outcome (Merkies et al. 2002; Petzold et al. 2006, 2009; Dujmovic et al. 2013). Other axonal proteins, such as tau, have not been found to be elevated in GBS, when compared to controls (Süssmutt Süssmuth et al. 2001). However, a small study has suggested that CSF levels might be higher in patients with worse outcome (Jin et al. 2006).

Other neuronal and glial markers investigated include neuron-specific enolase (NSE), which was higher in the CSF of patients with GBS compared to controls, and S100B (Vermuyten et al. 1990; Mokuno et al. 1994). Both have been described to correlate with the number of months to recovery (Mokuno et al. 1994). A more recent multicenter study, however, found that only NfH but not tau, GFAP, or S100B correlated with outcome (Petzold et al. 2009).

One study also reported detectable level of protein 14-3-3 in 29 of 38 patients with GBS (Bersano et al. 2006), in contrast to others (Satoh et al. 1999); this controversy may be explained by methodological differences.

Several recent studies have focused on potential biomarkers by analyzing the CSF proteome in GBS. Almost all studies have found an upregulation of haptoglobin and a downregulation of transthyretin, besides other potentially interesting molecular alterations. These include upregulation of apolipoprotein A-IV, PRO2044, serine/threonine kinase 10, alpha-1-antitrypsin, SNC73, alpha II spectrin, IgG kappa chain, and cathepsin D preprotein (Lehmensiek et al. 2007) orosomucoid and apolipoprotein A-IV (Chang et al. 2007); vitamin D-binding protein, beta-2 glycoprotein I (ApoH), and a complement component C3 isoform (D'Aguanno et al. 2010); and alpha-1-antitrypsin, apolipoprotein A-IV, and neurofilaments (Yang et al. 2009).

Downregulation was reported for fibrinogen (Jin et al. 2007); transferrin, caldesmon, galactose-1-phosphate uridylyltransferase (GALT), human heat shock protein 70, amyloidosis patient HL-heart-peptide 127aa (Lehmensiek et al. 2007); prostaglandin D2 synthase (Chang et al. 2007); apolipoprotein E, albumin, and five of its fragments (D'Aguanno et al. 2010); and cystatin C, apolipoprotein E, and heat shock protein 70 (Yang et al. 2009).

18.2 Miller Fisher Syndrome (MFS) and Bickerstaff Brainstem Encephalitis (BBE)

In 1951, Bickerstaff and Cloake described the first cases characterized by external ophthalmoparesis, ataxia, and alteration of consciousness; the syndrome was preceded by infection, and symptoms improved spontaneously (Bickerstaff and Cloake 1951). Bickerstaff described additional cases in 1957. One year earlier, in 1956, Miller Fisher published a similar syndrome with areflexia, ocular nerve palsies, ataxia, and spontaneous improvement. Both authors discussed the similarities to GBS. In 1992, the presence of anti-GQ1b antibodies was discovered in MFS (Chiba et al. 1992), and similar antibodies have later been found in BBE. In 2008, an analysis of 581 cases (53 BBE and 466 MFS) was published, which indicated the clinical and serological overlap of the two diseases (Ito et al. 2008). In MFS, ataxia, ophthalmoparesis, and areflexia are characteristic symptoms without major motor weakness. In BBE, alteration of consciousness is characteristic, deep reflexes can be increased, and Babinski reflex is present in about 10 % of the cases. Ptosis, mydriasis, facial nerve palsy, and peripheral sensory symptoms can be present in both diseases. The spectrum may contain additional rare variants: anti-GQ1b-seropositive acute isolated ophthalmoparesis (n. III and n. VI), acute ataxic neuropathy without ophthalmoparesis, and acute pharyngo-cervico-brachial palsy (PCB). MFS and BBE are most probably caused by antibodies cross-reacting with axonal GQ1b antigens in the paranodal region and at the neuromuscular junction. GQ1b is highly expressed in cranial nerves and Ia afferents of the muscle spindles, which may explain ataxia. Involvement of the brainstem reticular formation may be responsible for the alteration of consciousness in BBE, but experimental evidences are lacking. Both MFS and BBE are preceded by *C. jejuni* (21–23 %) and *H. influenzae* (6–8 %) infection, similar to AMAN and AMSAN (Fig. 18.1). In a small number of patients, an overlap syndrome of AMAN, MFS, and BBE may occur characterized by coexistence of anti-GM1, anti-GD1a, and anti-GQ1b antibodies. Despite the alarming symptoms, more than half of the patients completely recover within 6 months; the presence of anti-GQ1b antibodies suggests good prognosis with high sensitivity and specificity (Ito et al. 2008; Odaka et al. 2001; Shahrizaila and Yuki 2013; Chavada and Willison 2012; Yuki et al. 2004).

CSF Alterations in MFS and BBE In the original publication, Bickerstaff and Cloake speculated about a similar etiology of BBE and GBS due to the albuminocytological dissociation (Bickerstaff and Cloake 1951).

Reviewing CSF alterations in 375 cases of MFS and 44 cases of BBE indicated albuminocytological dissociation in 37 and 25 %, respectively, during the first week of illness. Pleocytosis was more characteristic for BBE (32 %, 0–668 cells/µl) and occurred only in 4 % (0–105 cells/µl) of patients with MFS. In the second week, albuminocytological dissociation became more frequent in MFS and occurred in 76 % of patients in contrast to 46 % in BBE. There was no change in the frequency of pleocytosis, which remained 5 % in MFS and 31 % in BBE. These data may indicate a more severe breakdown of the blood-CSF barrier in BBE, but examination of the CSF cannot discriminate between BBE and MFS (Ito et al. 2008).

Analyzing the anti-GQ1b syndrome, 58 % of patients had albuminocytological dissemination: it was the highest among patients with BBE/GBS (75 %) and occurred in 66 % of patients with MFS, in 43 % of those with MFS/GBS, and in 42 % of those with BBE (Odaka et al. 2001). Comparing CSF protein concentrations between MFS and GBS, protein content was higher in GBS in the first week (25 % vs 44 %) but increased continuously during the first 3 weeks in both diseases (84 % vs. 75 %) up to 1.5 g/l. CSF albuminocytological dissociation was present in 59 % of patients with MFS and in 62 % of those with GBS. One-third of patients with MFS had anti-GQ1b antibody in the sera but no albuminocytological dissociation in the CSF; in contrast, only 7 % presented albuminocytological dissociation without anti-GQ1b antibodies, indicating the higher sensitivity of antibody testing in MFS. In GBS, the frequency of albuminocytological dissociation was higher than the presence of anti-ganglioside antibodies (anti-GM1, anti-GD1a, and anti-GQ1b) without albuminocytological dissociation. These findings suggest that during the first 3 weeks, testing of such antibodies is inferior to the examination of the CSF for supporting a diagnosis of GBS, whereas anti-GQ1b antibody testing is superior to a CSF examination for the diagnosis of MFS. This is, however, true only in the first week of MFS (anti-GQ1b 48 % vs. albuminocytological dissociation only 4 %): after the second week, there is no difference in the frequency of anti-GQ1b antibodies and albuminocytological dissociation in MFS (Nishimoto et al. 2004).

Recurrent MFS is a rare condition, altogether 28 cases are described. It is slightly more common in men (16 vs. 12 cases) with an average age at onset of 34 years and an average age at the last episode of 47 years. Cerebrospinal fluid in 41 such episodes displayed elevated protein in 52 % of the cases (0.2–2.1 g/l). Pleocytosis was present only in two cases. Repeated CSF examination in two cases indicated a slight increase in the protein content (Heckmann and Dütsch 2012).

Some special biomarkers have been also examined in the CSF of patients with MFS, mostly validating previous data obtained in GBS. Proteomic analysis of the CSF indicated several proteins to be up- and downregulated in patients with GBS: cathepsin D preprotein, haptoglobin, cystatin C, and prostaglandin D_2 synthase were validated by Western blot or ELISA (Chang et al. 2007; Jin et al. 2007; Lehmensiek et al. 2007; Yang et al. 2009). Transthyretin, considered to be neuroprotective in traumatic brain injury and Alzheimer disease (Zou et al. 1998; Long et al. 2003; Merched et al. 1998; Stein et al. 2004), was consistently downregulated; therefore, it was later examined by ELISA in the CSF of patients with neurological diseases including GBS and MFS (Chiang et al. 2009). The mean protein content

(1.08 and 1.23 g/l) was elevated in both diseases, while the albumin level, the albumin ratio, the transthyretin concentration, and the ratio of transthyretin/total protein were elevated only in GBS. The authors discussed that such elevation in GBS in contrast to downregulation in other studies might be explained by methodological differences, measuring the target protein relative to the total protein content in the previous studies; the elevated transthyretin concentration may be caused by barrier dysfunction. In the four patients with MFS, transthyretin concentration in the CSF was not different compared to controls or GBS. Another downregulated protein, prostaglandin D_2 synthase (PGDS), the most abundant brain-synthetized protein in the CSF catalyzing the synthesis of the proinflammatory prostaglandin D_2 (PGD_2), was also investigated in 18 patients with AIDP and nine patients with MFS by using Western blot (Huang et al. 2009). In contrast to AIDP, where concentration of PGDS was increased in the CSF despite of a presumably decreased intrathecal synthesis, neither the concentration nor the PGDS/albumin ratio was different from controls.

In a single case, cytokines and chemokines were measured in the serum and CSF in the acute and recovery phase of MFS. Concentration and CSF/serum ratio of two chemokines, MCP-1 and IL-8, were elevated in the acute phase and decreased after IVIG treatment (Sato et al. 2009). MCP-1 has been suggested to be involved in the infiltration of spinal nerve roots by macrophages in GBS (Press et al. 2003). IL-8, a chemoattractant for neutrophils and monocytes, has not been implicated in MFS or GBS earlier.

CSF hypocretin-1 levels were reported to be reduced in MFS similar to GBS and CIDP (Nishino et al. 2003).

18.3 Acute Motor and Acute Motor-Sensory Axonal Neuropathy (AMAN and AMSAN)

The first cases of GBS without demyelination were described in 1986. Thereafter, two Japanese cases were published in 1990, which were characterized by preceding infection with *C jejuni* and by association with anti-GM1 antibodies. The disease was termed AMAN in 1993 (Kuwabara and Yuki 2013; Rinaldi 2013). Based on experimental data, pathogenetic antibodies generated against the lipo-oligosaccharides of *C. jejuni* (mainly anti-GM1 and anti-GD1a) cross-react with the motor axolemma (Chavada and Willison 2012; Yuki et al. 2004). This results in the disappearance of the sodium channels at the Ranvier nodules and complement-mediated disruption of the paranodal myelin. The antibodies can also interfere with the function of the sodium channels, which may be responsible for the reversible conduction failure. In contrast to Asia, AMAN is rare in Europe and North America and is responsible for about 3–17 % of cases (Fig. 18.1). Characteristically, the progression of the disease is faster compared to AIDP: the ascending, symmetric peripheral motor weakness peaks within 5–9 days. Cranial nerve palsies and autonomic dysfunction are less frequent. Rapid atrophy of the muscles may evolve, and the prognosis is usually poorer (Kuwabara et al. 2013; Rinaldi 2013; Yuki and Hartung 2012).

AMSAN is less frequent than AMAN and was first described in the 1980s. In contrast to AMAN, sensory symptoms are also observed. This form of GBS has the worse prognosis. Both diseases are usually associated with anti-GM1, anti-GM1b, and anti-GD1b antibodies (Kuwabara et al. 2013; Rinaldi 2013; Yuki and Hartung 2012).

CSF Alterations in AMAN and AMSAN Considering that the primary target in AIDP and AMAN differs, the glial marker S100B, the exoskeletal marker phosphorylated neurofilament heavy protein (pNfH), and the cytoskeletal protein tau were examined in the CSF of patients with AIDP and AMAN (Wang et al. 2013). The albumin ratio (CSF/serum) was increased in both AIDP and AMAN compared to OND controls, but was not different between AMAN and AIDP. The IgG index (IgG in CSF/IgG in serum divided by albumin in CSF/albumin in serum) was also elevated in both diseases; however, it was significantly higher in AMAN compared to AIDP. Concentrations of S100B, tau, and pNfH were elevated in the serum and CSF of patients with both GBS and AMAN. CSF levels of tau and pNfH correlated with the clinical severity of AMAN and predicted poor prognosis.

18.4 Rare Acute Neuropathies

Acute autonomic neuropathy (pandysautonomia) is a rare condition characterized by dysfunction of the sympathetic or parasympathetic nervous system with spontaneous improvement. Hodgkin disease, HIV, iatrogenic immunosuppression (e.g., peripheral stem cell transplantation, bone marrow transplantation, organ transplantation), and autoimmune diseases may be occasionally associated with GBS-like disease. GBS has been also described during biological treatments with monoclonal antibodies: anti-CD20 (rituximab), anti-TNF-α (infliximab, etanercept, adalimumab), and bortezomib used in treating multiple myeloma. Treatment of hepatitis C virus infection with pegylated interferon-alfa-2a can be also complicated with GBS.

CSF Alterations Both AIDP and CIDP are more frequent in HIV-1 seropositive patients. AIDP occurs mostly at seroconversion or in the early stage of infection, when patients are otherwise asymptomatic (Verma 2000; Gabbai et al. 2013). In the pre-ART area, its frequency was estimated to be about one-third of HIV-related neuropathies (Verma and Bradley 2000). The clinical features are similar to conventional AIDP: motor deficit predominates and sensory symptoms are relatively minor. The CSF protein is usually elevated, and lymphocytic pleocytosis of 10–50 cells/µl may raise suspicion of a "complicated" AIDP (Snider et al. 1983). However, a review series of 10 patients showed that 7 had cell counts of less than 10/µl, indicating that pleocytosis may be less common and may be related with frequent recurrent episodes (Brannagan and Zhou 2003). Miller Fisher syndrome and the axonal variants of GBS are rare in patients with HIV; a few cases are published. GBS-like syndromes, including MFS can be rarely associated with lactic acidosis attributed to NRTI-induced mitochondrial toxicity (Shah et al. 2003; Wooltorton 2002). MFS with anti-GQ1b antibodies may occur also at the late stage and improves after IVIG treatment (Hiraga et al. 2007; Sillevis Smitt and Portegies

1990; Arranz Caso et al. 1997; Shah et al. 2003). Only a few cases with AMAN are known in both the early and late phases after seroconversion: it usually occurs without confirmed *C. jejuni* infection, and anti-GM1 IgG/IgM antibodies may be absent. CSF may be normal or may indicate mononuclear pleocytosis with elevated protein, oligoclonal bands, and increased IgG index (Wagner and Bromberg 2007; Jadhav et al. 2014; Millogo et al. 2004; Goldstein et al. 1993). Progressive radiculopathy in the advanced stages of HIV immunodeficiency should raise the suspicion of CMV-related disease. Cauda equina syndrome develops over a few days or weeks with asymmetric motor deficit followed by saddle anesthesia and progressive leg weakness. CSF analysis indicates polymorphonuclear pleocytosis, low glucose level, elevated protein content, and presence of the viral genome by PCR. Other etiologies include tuberculosis, coinfection with HTLV-1, lymphoma, syphilis, *Cryptococcus* infection, and IRIS (Eidelberg et al. 1986; Verma 2001; Gabbai et al. 2013). Mononeuropathy multiplex or simplex is characterized by motor, sensory, or mixed somatic/cranial neuropathy and generally occurs in early HIV-1 infection, sometimes later (Wulff et al. 2000; Bradley and Verma 1996; Snider et al. 1983). It is usually dysimmune or vasculitic of origin, and the course is self-limiting (Wulff et al. 2000; Bradley and Verma 1996). CSF analysis reveals mild mononuclear pleocytosis and elevated protein. Superimposed infection (herpes zoster, CMV, syphilis), lymphomatous infiltration, or necrotizing vasculitis should be also considered (Gabbai et al. 2013).

A rare condition of acute erythromelalgia associated with acute neuropathy has been described in a few patients (Dabby et al. 2006; Pfund et al. 2009). CSF examination was only presented in 1 out of 4 cases with small fiber neuropathy and revealed no pathology (Dabby et al. 2006).

Complications of the peripheral nervous system occur in approximately 0.1–2 % of lymphoma patients, 5 % of patients with non-Hodgkin lymphoma (NHL), and least commonly in Hodgkin's disease (Hughes et al. 1994; Nobile-Orazio 2013). Infiltration of the nerve roots or nerves mostly occurs in NHL, while immunological disorders such as GBS are usually associated with Hodgkin's disease (Kelly and Karcher 2005). Depending on the etiology, CSF may show lymphoma cells (infiltration of roots) and mononuclear pleocytosis (e.g., paraneoplastic) or can be acellular; protein content may be elevated or normal.

Bone marrow, peripheral stem cell, and solid organ transplantation can be also associated with GBS (Openshaw 1997; Delios et al. 2012; Karam et al. 2014; El-Sabrout et al. 2001). Two recent studies reviewed immune-mediated peripheral nervous system diseases after stem cell transplantation (SCT) (Delios et al. 2012; Karam et al. 2014). The pathogenesis may involve paraneoplasia, GVHD, de novo autoimmune disease, and viral infection; almost all cases of GBS in the setting of solid organ transplantation are associated with CMV infection at or before the onset of GBS (El-Sabrout et al. 2001). The overall frequency of immune-mediated neuropathies was 0.36 %; the frequency of GBS was 0.12–0.2 % in these series. No CIDP was observed in one of these large studies reviewing data of 3,305 patients, who underwent SCT: four patients had acute polyradiculoneuropathies, seven patients had radiculoplexus neuropathy, and one patient had multiple mononeuropathy (Karam et al. 2014). CSF was examined in six cases in this cohort: the median level of protein was 0.56 g/l in 3 GBS cases and 0.78 g/l in three cases with radiculoplexus neuropathy; cell count ranged from 0 to 12 cells/µl and 1–42 cell/µl, respectively. In the other study involving 1,484 patients, acute inflammatory neuropathy developed in 3 patients. CSF examination indicated 1–9 cells/µl and protein concentration of 1.44–3 g/l; PCR analysis for CMV, VZV, EBV, HSV, and HHV-6 was negative (Delios et al. 2012).

All existing forms of acute demyelinating neuropathies have been reported to occur in patients treated with TNF-α antagonists, especially with infliximab: AIDP, MFS, acute axonal neuropathy, and optic neuropathy; CSF may be normal (Shin et al. 2006; Tracey et al. 2008; Faivre et al. 2010; Chan and Castellanos 2010). Peripheral neuropathy can also be a rare side effect of interferon-alpha treatment: sensory neuropathy, autonomic neuropathy, Bell's palsy, CIDP, and rarely AIDP have all been described; increased protein concentration may be found in the CSF (Lahbabi et al. 2012; Irioka et al. 2001).

Conclusion

A number of studies investigated the molecular composition of the CSF in different types of GBS, mainly in AIDP. These data support the immunopathogenesis of GBS and also indicate that biomarkers of axonal damage may be associated with worse outcome. Analysis of the CSF proteome in different types of GBS may provide an additional opportunity of biomarker discovery, but validation of data in large international cohorts is needed.

References

Arranz Caso JA, Martinez R, Cabrera F, Tejeiro J (1997) Miller Fisher syndrome in a patient with HIV infection. AIDS 11:550–551

Bersano A, Fiorini M, Allaria S, Zanusso G, Fasoli E, Gelati M, Monaco H, Squintani G, Monaco S, Nobile-Orazio E (2006) Detection of CSF 14-3-3 protein in Guillain-Barré syndrome. Neurology 67:2211–2216

Bickerstaff ER, Cloake PC (1951) Mesencephalitis and rhombencephalitis. Br Med J 2:77–81

Bradley WG, Verma A (1996) Painful vasculitic neuropathy in HIV-1 infection: relief of pain with prednisone therapy. Neurology 47:1446–1451

Brannagan TH 3rd, Zhou Y (2003) HIV-associated Guillain-Barré syndrome. J Neurol Sci 208:39–42

Brettschneider J, Claus A, Kassubek J, Tumani H (2005) Isolated blood-cerebrospinal fluid barrier dysfunction: prevalence and associated diseases. J Neurol 252:1067–1073

Brettschneider J, Petzold A, Süssmuth S, Tumani H (2009) Cerebrospinal fluid biomarkers in Guillain-Barré syndrome–where do we stand? J Neurol 256:3–12

Chan JW, Castellanos A (2010) Infliximab and anterior optic neuropathy: case report and review of the literature. Graefes Arch Clin Exp Ophthalmol 248:283–287

Chang KH, Lyu RK, Tseng MY, Ro LS, Wu YR, Chang HS, Hsu WC, Kuo HC, Huang CC, Chu CC, Hsieh SY, Chen CM (2007) Elevated haptoglobin level of cerebrospinal fluid in Guillain-Barré syndrome revealed by proteomics analysis. Proteomics Clin Appl 1:467–475

Chavada G, Willison HJ (2012) Autoantibodies in immune-mediated neuropathies. Curr Opin Neurol 25:550–555

Chiang HL, Lyu RK, Tseng MY, Chang KH, Chang HS, Hsu WC, Kuo HC, Chu CC, Wu YR, Ro LS, Huang CC, Chen CM (2009) Analyses of transthyretin concentration in the cerebrospinal fluid of patients with Guillain-Barré syndrome and other neurological disorders. Clin Chim Acta 405:143–147

Chiba A, Kusunoki S, Shimizu T, Kanazawa I (1992) Serum IgG antibody to ganglioside GQ1b is a possible marker of Miller Fisher syndrome. Ann Neurol 31:677–9

Dabby R, Gilad R, Sadeh M, Lampl Y, Watemberg N (2006) Acute steroid responsive small-fiber sensory neuropathy: a new entity? J Peripher Nerv Syst 11:47–52

D'Aguanno S, Franciotta D, Lupisella S, Barassi A, Pieragostino D, Lugaresi A, Centonze D, D'Eril GM, Bernardini S, Federici G, Urbani A (2010) Protein profiling of Guillain-Barrè syndrome cerebrospinal fluid by two-dimensional electrophoresis and mass spectrometry. Neurosci Lett 485:49–54

Delios AM, Rosenblum M, Jakubowski AA, DeAngelis LM (2012) Central and peripheral nervous system immune mediated demyelinating disease after allogeneic hemopoietic stem cell transplantation for hematologic disease. J Neurooncol 110:251–256

Dujmovic I, Lunn MP, Reilly MM, Petzold A (2013) Serial cerebrospinal fluid neurofilament heavy chain levels in severe Guillain-Barré syndrome. Muscle Nerve 48:132–134

Eidelberg D, Sotrel A, Vogel H, Walker P, Kleefield J, Crumpacker CS 3rd (1986) Progressive polyradiculopathy in acquired immune deficiency syndrome. Neurology 36:912–916

El-Sabrout RA, Radovancevic B, Ankoma-Sey V, Van Buren CT (2001) Guillain-Barré syndrome after solid organ transplantation. Transplantation 71:1311–1316

Faivre A, Franques J, De Paula AM, Gutierrez M, Bret S, Aubert S, Attarian S, Pouget J (2010) Acute motor and sensory axonal neuropathy and concomitant encephalopathy during tumor necrosis factor-alpha antagonist therapy. J Neurol Sci 291:103–106

Gabbai AA, Castelo A, Oliveira AS (2013) HIV peripheral neuropathy. Handb Clin Neurol 115:515–529

Goldstein JM, Azizi SA, Booss J, Vollmer TL (1993) Human immunodeficiency virus-associated motor axonal polyradiculoneuropathy. Arch Neurol 50:1316–1319

Guillain G, Barré JA, Strohl A (1916) Sur un syndrome de radiculonevrite avec hyperalbuminose du liquid cephalo-rachidien sans reaction cellulaire. Remarques sur les caracteres cliniques et graphiques des reflexes tendineaux. Bull Soc Med Hop Paris 40:1462–1470

Hadden RDM, Karch H, Hartung HP, Zielasek J, Weissbrich B, Schubert J, Weishaupt A, Cornblath DR, Swan AV, Hughes RA, Toyka KV, Plasma Exchange/Sandoglobulin Guillain-Barré Syndrome Trial Group (2001) Preceding infections, immune factors and outcome in Guillain-Barré syndrome. Neurology 56:758–765

Han RK, Cheng YF, Zhou SS, Guo H, He RD, Chi LJ, Zhang LM (2014) Increased circulating Th17 cell populations and elevated CSF osteopontin and IL-17 concentrations in patients with Guillain-Barré syndrome. J Clin Immunol 34:94–103

Hartung HP, Schwenke C, Bitter-Suermann D, Toyka KV (1987) Guillain-Barré syndrome: activated complement components C3a and C5a in CSF. Neurology 37:1006–1009

Heckmann JG, Dütsch M (2012) Recurrent Miller Fisher syndrome: clinical and laboratory features. Eur J Neurol 19:944–954

Hiraga A, Kuwabara S, Nakamura A, Yuki N, Hattori T, Matsunaga T (2007) Fisher/Guillain-Barré overlap syndrome in advanced AIDS. J Neurol Sci 258:148–150

Huang YC, Lyu RK, Tseng MY, Chang HS, Hsu WC, Kuo HC, Chu CC, Wu YR, Ro LS, Huang CC, Chen CM (2009) Decreased intrathecal synthesis of prostaglandin D2 synthase in the cerebrospinal fluid of patients with acute inflammatory demyelinating polyneuropathy. J Neuroimmunol 206:100–105

Hughes RA, Britton T, Richards M (1994) Effects of lymphoma on the peripheral nervous system. J R Soc Med 87:526–530

Irioka T, Yamada M, Yamawaki M, Saito Y, Mizusawa H, Yamada M, Miura H (2001) Acute autonomic and sensory neuropathy after interferon alpha-2b therapy for chronic hepatitis C. J Neurol Neurosurg Psychiatry 70:408–410

Ito M, Kuwabara S, Odaka M. Misawa S, Koga M, Hirata K, Yuki N (2008) Bickerstaff's brainstem encephalitis and Fisher syndrome form a continuous spectrum: clinical analysis of 581 cases. J Neurol 255:674–682

Jadhav S, Agrawal M, Rathi S (2014) Acute motor axonal neuropathy in HIV infection. Indian J Pediatr 81:193

Jander S, Stoll G (2001) Interleukin-18 is induced in acute inflammatory demyelinating polyneuropathy. J Neuroimmunol 114:253–258

Jin K, Takeda A, Shiga Y, Sato S, Ohnuma A, Nomura H, Arai H, Kusunoki S, Ikeda M, Itoyama Y (2006) CSF tau protein: a new prognostic marker for Guillain-Barré syndrome. Neurology 67:1470–1472

Jin T, Hu LS, Chang M, Wu J, Winblad B, Zhu J (2007) Proteomic identification of potential protein markers in cerebrospinal fluid of GBS patients. Eur J Neurol 14:563–568

Karam C, Mauermann ML, Johnston PB, Lahoria R, Engelstad JK, Dyck PJ (2014) Immune-mediated neuropathies following stem cell transplantation. J Neurol Neurosurg Psychiatry 85:638–642

Kastenbauer S, Koedel U, Wick M, Kieseier BC, Hartung HP, Pfister HW (2003) CSF and serum levels of soluble fractalkine (CX3CL1) in inflammatory diseases of the nervous system. J Neuroimmunol 137:210–217

Kelly JJ, Karcher DS (2005) Lymphoma and peripheral neuropathy: a clinical review. Muscle Nerve 31:301–313

Kieseier BC, Tani M, Mahad D, Oka N, Ho T, Woodroofe N, Griffin JW, Toyka KV, Ransohoff RM, Hartung HP (2002) Chemokines and chemokine receptors in inflammatory demyelinating neuropathies: a central role for IP-10. Brain 125:823–834

Koguchi Y, Yamada T, Kuwabara S, Nakajima M, Hirayama K (1995) Increased CSF C4d in demyelinating neuropathy indicates the radicular involvement. Acta Neurol Scand 91:58–61

Krüger H, Englert D, Pflughaupt KW (1981) Demonstration of oligoclonal immunoglobulin G in Guillain-Barré syndrome and lymphocytic meningoradiculitis by isoelectric focusing. J Neurol 226:15–24

Kuwabara S, Yuki N (2013) Axonal Guillain-Barré syndrome: concepts and controversies. Lancet Neurol 12:1180–1188

Lahbabi M, Ghissassi M, Belahcen F, Ibrahimi SA, Aqodad N (2012) Acute inflammatory demyelinating polyneuropathy after treatment with pegylated interferon alfa-2a in a patient with chronic hepatitis C virus infection: a case report. J Med Case Reports 6:278

Lehmensiek V, Süssmuth SD, Brettschneider J, Tauscher G, Felk S, Gillardon F, Tumani H (2007) Proteome analysis of cerebrospinal fluid in Guillain-Barré syndrome (GBS). J Neuroimmunol 185:190–194

Li S, Yu M, Li H, Zhang H, Jiang Y (2012) IL-17 and IL-22 in cerebrospinal fluid and plasma are elevated in Guillain-Barré syndrome. Mediators Inflamm. doi:10.1155/2012/260473

Li C, Zhao P, Sun X, Che Y, Jiang Y (2013) Elevated levels of cerebrospinal fluid and plasma interleukin-37 in patients with Guillain-Barré syndrome. Mediators Inflamm. doi:10.1155/2013/639712

Long Y, Zou L, Liu H, Lu H, Yuan X, Robertson CS, Yang K (2003) Altered expression of randomly selected genes in mouse hippocampus after traumatic brain injury. J Neurosci Res 71:710–720

Marchiori PE, Dos Reis M, Quevedo ME, Callegaro D, Hirata MT, Scaff M, De Oliveira RM (1990) Cerebrospinal fluid and serum antiphospholipid antibodies in multiple sclerosis Guillain-Barré syndrome and systemic lupus erythematosus. Arq Neuropsiquiatr 48:465–468

Matà S, Galli E, Amantini A, Pinto F, Sorbi S, Lolli F (2006) Anti-ganglioside antibodies and elevated CSF IgG levels in Guillain-Barré syndrome. Eur J Neurol 13:153–160

Merched A, Serot JM, Visvikis S, Aguillon D, Faure G, Siest G (1998) Apolipoprotein E, transthyretin and actin in the CSF of Alzheimer's patients: relation with the senile plaques and cytoskeleton biochemistry. FEBS Lett 425:225–228

Merkies IS, Schmitz PI, van der Meché FG, Samijn JP, van Doorn PA, Inflammatory Neuropathy Cause and Treatment (INCAT) group (2002) Quality of life complements traditional outcome measures in immune-mediated polyneuropathies. Neurology 59:84–91

Millogo A, Sawadogo A, Lankoandé D, Sawadogo AB (2004) Guillain-Barré syndrome in HIV-infected patients at Bobo-Dioulasso Hospital (Burkina Faso). [Article in French]. Rev Neurol (Paris) 160:559–562

Mokuno K, Kiyosawa K, Sugimura K, Yasuda T, Riku S, Murayama T, Yanagi T, Takahashi A, Kato K (1994) Prognostic value of cerebrospinal fluid neuron-specific enolase and S-100b protein in Guillain-Barré syndrome. Acta Neurol Scand 89:27–30

Nagai A, Murakawa Y, Terashima M, Shimode K, Umegae N, Takeuchi H, Kobayashi S (2000) Cystatin C and cathepsin B in CSF from patients with inflammatory neurologic diseases. Neurology 55:1828–1832

Nishimoto Y, Odaka M, Hirata K, Yuki N (2004) Usefulness of anti-GQ1b IgG antibody testing in Fisher syndrome compared with cerebrospinal fluid examination. J Neuroimmunol 148: 200–205

Nishino S, Kanbayashi T, Fujiki N, Uchino M, Ripley B, Watanabe M, Lammers GJ, Ishiguro H, Shoji S, Nishida Y, Overeem S, Toyoshima I, Yoshida Y, Shimizu T, Taheri S, Mignot E (2003) CSF hypocretin levels in Guillain-Barré syndrome and other inflammatory neuropathies. Neurology 61:823–825

Nobile-Orazio E (2013) Neuropathy and monoclonal gammopathy. Handb Clin Neurol 115: 443–459

Odaka M, Yuki N, Hirata K (2001) Anti-GQ1b IgG antibody syndrome: clinical and immunological range. J Neurol Neurosurg Psychiatry 70:50–55

Openshaw H (1997) Peripheral neuropathy after bone marrow transplantation. Biol Blood Marrow Transplant 3:202–209

Petzold T, Sindern E, Ossege-Pohle L, Malin JP (1998) The soluble 60-kDa tumour necrosis factor receptor: no difference found between patients with relapsing-remitting multiple sclerosis and controls: increasing levels are associated with the recovery from Guillain-Barré syndrome. J Neurol 245:803–808

Petzold A, Hinds N, Murray NM, Hirsch NP, Grant D, Keir G, Thompson EJ, Reilly MM (2006) CSF neurofilament levels: a potential prognostic marker in Guillain-Barré syndrome. Neurology 67:1071–1073

Petzold A, Brettschneider J, Jin K, Keir G, Murray NM, Hirsch NP, Itoyama Y, Reilly MM, Takeda A, Tumani H (2009) CSF protein biomarkers for proximal axonal damage improve prognostic accuracy in the acute phase of Guillain-Barré syndrome. Muscle Nerve 40:42–49

Pfund Z, Stankovics J, Decsi T, Illes Z (2009) Childhood steroid-responsive acute erythromelalgia with axonal neuropathy of large myelinated fibers: a dysimmune neuropathy? Neuromuscul Disord 19:49–52

Press R, Pashenkov M, Jin JP, Link H (2003) Aberrated levels of cerebrospinal fluid chemokines in Guillain-Barré syndrome and chronic inflammatory demyelinating polyradiculoneuropathy. J Clin Immunol 23:259–267

Press R, Nennesmo I, Kouwenhoven M, Huang YM, Link H, Pashenkov M (2005) Dendritic cells in the cerebrospinal fluid and peripheral nerves in Guillain-Barré syndrome and chronic inflammatory demyelinating polyradiculoneuropathy. J Neuroimmunol 159:165–176

Rajabally YA, Uncini A (2012) Outcome and its predictors in Guillain-Barre syndrome. J Neurol Neurosurg Psychiatry 83:711–718

Rinaldi S (2013) Update on Guillain-Barré syndrome. J Peripher Nerv Syst 18:99–112

Sainaghi PP, Collimedaglia L, Alciato F, Leone MA, Naldi P, Molinari R, Monaco F, Avanzi GC (2010) The expression pattern of inflammatory mediators in cerebrospinal fluid differentiates Guillain-Barré syndrome from chronic inflammatory demyelinating polyneuropathy. Cytokine 51:138–143

Sanders ME, Koski CL, Robbins D, Shin ML, Frank MM, Joiner KA (1986) Activated terminal complement in cerebrospinal fluid in Guillain-Barré syndrome and multiple sclerosis. J Immunol 136:4456–4459

Sato S, Suzuki K, Nagao R, Kashiwagi Y, Kawashima H, Tsuyuki K, Hoshika A (2009) Detection of MCP-1 and IL-8 in the serum and cerebrospinal fluid of a child with Miller Fisher syndrome. J Clin Neurosci 16:1698–1699

Satoh J, Kurohara K, Yukitake M, Kuroda Y (1999) The 14-3-3 protein detectable in the cerebro-spinal fluid of patients with prion-unrelated neurological diseases is expressed constitutively in neurons and glial cells in culture. Eur Neurol 41:216–225

Segurado OG, Krüger H, Mertens HG (1986) Clinical significance of serum and CSF findings in the Guillain-Barré syndrome and related disorders. J Neurol 233:202–208

Shah SS, Rodriguez T, McGowan JP (2003) Miller Fisher variant of Guillain-Barré syndrome associated with lactic acidosis and stavudine therapy. Clin Infect Dis 36:e131–e133

Shahrizaila N, Yuki N (2013) Bickerstaff brainstem encephalitis and Fisher syndrome: anti-GQ1b antibody syndrome. J Neurol Neurosurg Psychiatry 84:576–583

Shin IS, Baer AN, Kwon HJ, Papadopoulos EJ, Siegel JN (2006) Guillain-Barré and Miller Fisher syndromes occurring with tumor necrosis factor alpha antagonist therapy. Arthritis Rheum 54:1429–1434

Sillevis Smitt PA, Portegies P (1990) Fisher's syndrome associated with human immunodeficiency virus infection. Clin Neurol Neurosurg 92:353–355

Simone IL, Annunziata P, Maimone D, Liguori M, Leante R, Livrea P (1993) Serum and CSF anti-GM1 antibodies in patients with Guillain-Barré syndrome and chronic inflammatory demyelinating polyneuropathy. J Neurol Sci 114:49–55

Snider WD, Simpson DM, Nielsen S, Gold JW, Metroka CE, Posner JB (1983) Neurological complications of acquired immune deficiency syndrome: analysis of 50 patients. Ann Neurol 14:403–418

Stein TD, Anders NJ, DeCarli C, Chan SL, Mattson MP, Johnson JA (2004) Neutralization of transthyretin reverses the neuroprotective effects of secreted amyloid precursor protein (APP) in APPSW mice resulting in tau phosphorylation and loss of hippocampal neurons: support for the amyloid hypothesis. J Neurosci 24:7707–7717

Süssmuth SD, Reiber H, Tumani H (2001) Tau protein in cerebrospinal fluid (CSF): a blood-CSF barrier related evaluation in patients with various neurological diseases. Neurosc Lett 300:95–98

Tracey D, Klareskog L, Sasso EH, Salfeld JG, Tak PP (2008) Tumor necrosis factor antagonist mechanisms of action: a comprehensive review. Pharmacol Ther 117:244–279

Uncini A, Kuwabara S (2012) Electrodiagnostic criteria for Guillain-Barrè syndrome: a critical revision and the need for an update. Clin Neurophysiol 123:1487–1495

Van der Meché FG, Van Doorn PA, Meulstee J, Jennekens FG, GBS-consensus group of the Dutch Neuromuscular Research Support Centre (2001) Diagnostic and classification criteria for the Guillain-Barré syndrome. Eur Neurol 45:133–139

Verma A (2001) Epidemiology and clinical features of HIV-1 associated neuropathies. J Peripher Nerv Syst 6:8–13

Verma A, Bradley WG (2000) HIV-1-Associated Neuropathies. CNS Spectr 5:66–72

Verma R, Chaudhari TS, Raut TP, Garg RK (2013) Clinico-electrophysiological profile and predictors of functional outcome in Guillain-Barre syndrome (GBS). J Neurol Sci 335:105–11

Vermuyten K, Lowenthal A, Karcher D (1990) Detection of neuron specific enolase concentrations in cerebrospinal fluid from patients with neurological disorders by means of a sensitive enzyme immunoassay. Clin Chim Acta 187:69–78

Wagner JC, Bromberg MB (2007) HIV infection presenting with motor axonal variant of Guillain-Barré Syndrome. J Clin Neuromuscul Dis 9:303–305

Wang XK, Zhang HL, Meng FH, Chang M, Wang YZ, Jin T, Mix E, Zhu J (2013) Elevated levels of S100B, tau and pNFH in cerebrospinal fluid are correlated with subtypes of Guillain-Barré syndrome. Neurol Sci 34:655–661

Wanschitz J, Ehling R, Löscher WN, Künz B, Deisenhammer F, Kuhle J, Budka H, Reindl M, Berger T (2008) Intrathecal anti-alphaB-crystallin IgG antibody responses: potential inflammatory markers in Guillain-Barré syndrome. J Neurol 255:917–924

Wooltorton E (2002) HIV drug stavudine (Zerit, d4T) and symptoms mimicking Guillain-Barré syndrome. CMAJ 166:1067

Wulff EA, Wang AK, Simpson DM (2000) HIV-associated peripheral neuropathy: epidemiology, pathophysiology and treatment. Drugs 59:1251–1260

Yang Y, Liu S, Qin Z, Cui Y, Qin Y, Bai S (2009) Alteration of cystatin C levels in cerebrospinal fluid of patients with Guillain-Barré Syndrome by a proteomical approach. Mol Biol Rep 36:677–682

Yonekura K, Yokota S, Tanaka S, Kubota H, Fujii N, Matsumoto H, Chiba S (2004) Prevalence of anti-heat shock protein antibodies in cerebrospinal fluids of patients with Guillain-Barré syndrome. J Neuroimmunol 156:204–209

Yuki N, Hartung HP (2012) Guillain-Barré syndrome. N Engl J Med 366:2294–2304

Yuki N, Susuki K, Koga M, Nishimoto Y, Odaka M, Hirata K, Taguchi K, Miyatake T, Furukawa K, Kobata T, Yamada M (2004) Carbohydrate mimicry between human ganglioside GM1 and Campylobacter jejuni lipooligosaccharide causes Guillain-Barré syndrome. Proc Natl Acad Sci U S A 101:11404–11409

Zou L, Burmeister LA, Styren SD, Kochanek PM, DeKosky ST (1998) Up-regulation of type 2 iodothyronine deiodinase mRNA in reactive astrocytes following traumatic brain injury in the rat. J Neurochem 71:887–890

Alterations of the Cerebrospinal Fluid in Chronic Inflammatory Diseases of the Peripheral Nervous System

19

Zsolt Illes and Morten Blaabjerg

Contents

Abstract

Chronic inflammatory neuropathies comprise a heterogeneous group of diseases mainly characterized by a demyelinating pathology. The most common disease, CIDP (chronic inflammatory demyelinating polyneuropathy),

Z. Illes (✉)
Department of Neurology,
Odense University Hospital,
Sdr. Boulevard 29, Odense 5000, Denmark

Institute of Clinical Research,
University of Southern Denmark, Odense, Denmark
e-mail: zsolt.illes@rsyd.dk

M. Blaabjerg
Department of Neurology,
Odense University Hospital,
Sdr. Boulevard 29, Odense 5000, Denmark

© Springer International Publishing Switzerland 2015
F. Deisenhammer et al. (eds.), *Cerebrospinal Fluid in Clinical Neurology*,
DOI 10.1007/978-3-319-01225-4_19

can be further categorized based on the clinical symptoms and associated diseases. Three other syndromes have been well defined. Similar to CIDP, distal acquired demyelinating sensory polyneuropathy (DADS) evolves with symmetrical symptoms. In contrast, multifocal motor neuropathy (MMN) and multifocal acquired demyelinating sensory and motor neuropathy (MADSAM, Lewis-Sumner syndrome) are asymmetric polyneuropathies. In this chapter, we discuss CSF alterations in these four main syndromes of demyelinating chronic inflammatory neuropathies, the chronic neuropathies associated with M proteins, and the vasculitic neuropathies. Although we touch some of the hematological malignancies associated with paraproteinemic polyneuropathies, paraneoplastic neurological diseases of the PNS are described in a separate chapter. Altogether, increased protein in the CSF is a supportive factor of CIDP, especially when electrophysiological criteria are not definite. A number of specific markers have been also investigated in the CSF of patients with chronic inflammatory neuropathies, but their role in differentiating the different syndromes, supporting diagnosis of MMN, or predicting the clinical course and treatment responses is inconclusive.

Abbreviations

ANCA	Anti-neutrophil cytoplasmic antibody
CRP	C-reactive protein
EFNS	European Federation of Neurological Societies
ESR	Erythrocyte sedimentation rate
FGF	Fibroblast growth factor
G-CSF	Granulocyte colony-stimulating factor
GM-CSF	Granulocyte macrophage colony-stimulating factor
HBV	Hepatitis B virus
HCV	Hepatitis C virus
ICAM-1	Intercellular adhesion molecule 1
IFN	Interferon
IL	Interleukin
LIF	Leukemia inhibitory factor
M-CSF	Macrophage colony-stimulating factor
MIF	Macrophage migration inhibitory factor
MPA	Microscopic polyangiitis
PAN	Polyarteritis nodosa
PDGFbb	Platelet-derived growth factor-BB
SCGF-β	Stem cell growth factor beta
Th	T helper
TNF	Tumor necrosis factor
TRAIL	Tumor necrosis factor-related apoptosis-inducing ligand
VCAM-1	Vascular cell adhesion molecule 1
VEGF	Vascular endothelial growth factor

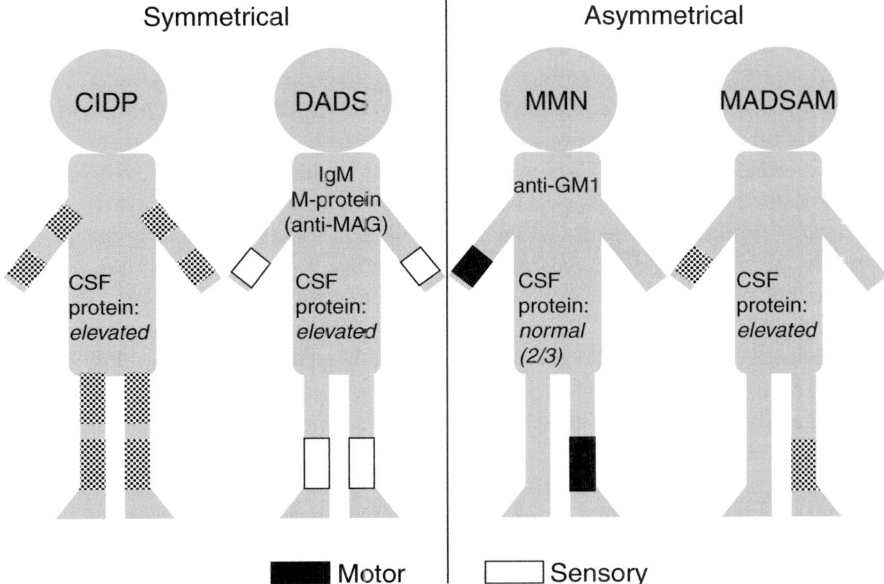

Fig. 19.1 Major syndromes of chronic demyelinating polyneuropathies

A common feature of chronic inflammatory neuropathies is the mainly demyelinating pathology, except for the vasculitic neuropathies, and a chronic progressive course. The major syndrome of chronic demyelinating polyneuropathies is chronic inflammatory demyelinating polyneuropathy (CIDP) characterized by symmetric, proximal, and distal symptoms (Barohn et al. 1989; Bouchard et al. 1999; Saic and Krarup 2013). EFNS (European Federation of Neurological Societies) guidelines also define CIDP associated with other diseases and atypical CIDP with focal, pure motor or pure sensory symptoms (Joint Task Force of the EFNS and the PNS 2010c). One of the atypical CIDP syndromes depicted by EFNS guidelines is characterized by mainly distal sensory symptoms, therefore called distal acquired demyelinating sensory polyneuropathy (DADS). It responds less to steroids than typical CIDP and is frequently associated with an IgM M protein reactive with myelin-associated glycoprotein (MAG) (Larue et al. 2011; Ramchandren and Lewis 2012; Nobile-Orazio 2013). Another atypical CIDP syndrome appears with asymmetric, multifocal motor and sensory symptoms (MADSAM, Lewis-Sumner syndrome) (Katz et al. 2000; Rajabally and Chavada 2009). An additional major asymmetric multifocal demyelinating polyneuropathy syndrome with pure motor symptoms has been also described: multifocal motor neuropathy (MMN), frequently associated with an antibody response similar to DADS (Fig. 19.1). The antibodies in MMN target gangliosides of the peripheral nerve (anti-GM1) similar to the acute demyelinating polyneuropathy AMAN/AMSAN, nevertheless without preceding infection with *C. jejuni* (Cats et al. 2010a; Joint Task Force of the EFNS and the PNS 2010a, b, c; Muley and Parry 2012; Vlam et al. 2013).

19.1 Chronic Inflammatory Demyelinating Polyneuropathy (CIDP)

CIDP is a rare disease: its prevalence is 0.5–1/100,000 in childhood and 1–2/100,000 in adult populations. CIDP responds well to corticosteroid and immunosuppressive treatments (Gorson et al. 1997; Laughlin et al. 2009; Hughes and Mehndiratta 2012; Mahdi-Rogers et al. 2013; Stübgen 2013).

A core criterion for the diagnosis is the subacute onset progressing for at least 8 weeks; in about 16 % of patients, the onset may be acute, but the progression extends over 8 weeks, or at least 3 relapses occur (Barohn et al. 1989; Joint Task Force of the EFNS and the PNS 2010c). Motor symptoms are usually symmetric and prominent, affect the lower extremities more than the upper extremities, and are present both distally and proximally. The rare pure motor and sensory variants are defined as atypical CIDP by the EFNS guidelines (Joint Task Force of the EFNS and the PNS 2010c).

The diagnosis of definite CIDP requires electrophysiological examination, which indicates primary demyelination of at least two peripheral nerves (Joint Task Force of the EFNS and the PNS 2010c). In case of axonal degeneration or demyelinating electrophysiological feature only in one nerve, supportive criteria are required. Such supportive data can be obtained by the examination of the CSF, MRI examination of the plexus and roots, or pathological examination of peripheral nerves (Bosboom et al. 2001; Joint Task Force of the EFNS and the PNS 2010c).

CSF Alterations in CIDP As described by the supportive criteria of CIDP (Joint Task Force of the EFNS and the PNS 2010c), the most prominent finding in CSF is the albuminocytologic dissociation: elevated protein levels with less than 10 cells per µl (Barohn et al. 1989) (Table 19.1). In some series, protein content of more than 0.45 g/l was mandatory for the diagnosis (Notermans et al. 1993; Saperstein et al. 2001). Others described subpopulations of patients with normal protein content (up to 14 %) but all with normal cell counts (Bouchard et al. 1999; Said and Krarup 2013). In these patients, the diagnosis is supported by demyelinating features revealed by electrophysiological and/or pathological examination. Among patients with sensory chronic demyelinating neuropathy, the frequency of CSF with normal protein content has been described as high as 44 % (Said and Krarup 2013). In patients with concurrent HIV infection, pleocytosis with up to 50 cells is widely accepted (on CIDP 2001).

Elevated CSF albumin levels in CIDP are likely caused by damage of the blood-CSF barrier permitting serum proteins to enter the CSF. One study looked at changes in protein levels and CSF index of proteins other than albumin using an ELISA approach (Table 19.1). They found higher levels of fibrinogen in CSF but not in plasma (low CSF index), as well as high levels of haptoglobin and normal CSF prealbumin index when comparing CIDP to controls (Zhang et al. 2012). Similarly, a proteome analysis of CSF from CIDP compared to controls also found upregulation of two haptoglobin isoforms as well as 8 other proteins (two transferrin isoforms, alpha-1 acid glycoprotein 1 precursor, apolipoprotein A IV, transthyretin,

Table 19.1 Alteration of CSF in CIDP

	Change	References
Protein	Elevated (>90 %), usually >0.45 g/l	Barohn et al. (1989)
		Notermans et al. (1993)
		Saperstein et al. (2001)
Protein components	Transferrin isoforms, alpha-1 acid glycoprotein 1 precursor, apolipoprotein A IV, transthyretin[a], retinol binding protein, and proapolipoprotein isoforms (upregulated); integrin beta 8 (downregulated)	Tumani et al. (2009)
Cells	<10 cells; up to 50 cells in cocurrent HIV	AAN Ad Hoc Subcommittee on CIDP (2001)
Cell type	Th1 elevated; Th17 elevated in active CIDP	Mei et al. (2005)
		Chi et al. (2010)
Enzymes	Cystatin C (decreased), cathepsin B (increased)	Nagai et al. (2000)
Cytokines and chemokines	CXCL10 (IP10) (elevated)	Kieseier et al. (2002)
		Mahad et al. (2002)
		Press et al. (2003)
		Sainaghi et al. (2010)
	CCL2, CCL3, CCL7, CCL19, CCL27, CXCL9[a]. CXCL12 (elevated)	Sainaghi et al. (2010)
		Mahad et al. (2002)
		Press et al. (2003)
	IL-6[a], IL-8, and IL-17 (elevated); IL-4, IL-5, and IL-7 (decreased)	Mei et al. (2005)
Cell adhesion	ICAM-1, VCAM-1 (elevated)	Sainaghi et al. (2010)
Growth factors	VEGF (elevated)	Sainaghi et al. (2010)

[a]Changes only found in some studies

retinol binding protein, and two isoforms of proapolipoprotein). In this study, one protein (integrin beta 8) was downregulated (Tumani et al. 2009). Another study that focused only on transthyretin using ELISA, however, found no difference between CIDP and controls (Chiang et al. 2009).

Several studies investigated immune cells, cytokine, and chemokine profiles of CSF obtained from CIDP patients (Table 19.1). One pioneering study found an increase in the chemokine receptor CXCR3 on infiltrating T cells in sural biopsies from inflammatory neuropathy (Kieseier et al. 2002). In accordance, they also found high expression of the CXCR3 ligand IP10 (now named CXCL10) in CSF from CIDP patients when compared to controls. There was however no significant increase in the expression of another main CXCR3 ligand Mig (now named CXCL9).

The increase in CXCL10 was later confirmed in other studies (Mahad et al. 2002; Press et al. 2003). These studies also found increased concentrations of other important chemoattractants such as MIP1-α (now named CCL3) (Mahad et al. 2002) and

MIP-3β (now named CCL19) (Press et al. 2003). In contrast to the initial study, Mahad and colleagues also found increased expression of the CXCL10 ligand CXCL9 in CSF from CIDP patients compared to controls.

By using an ELISA-based approach, no detectable levels of interleukin (IL)-1α, IL-1β, IL-2, IL-6, IL-10, interferon (IFN)-γ, tumor necrosis factor (TNF), and macrophage colony-stimulating factor (M-CSF) were found in the CSF (Sivieri et al. 1997). Others detected increased IL-6, IL-8, and IL-17 and decreased IL-4, IL-5, and IL-7 levels in CSF using a more sensitive bead assay. IL-17 and IL-8 correlated strongly with CSF protein levels, and this type 1 cytokine upregulation and type 2 downregulation coincided with an increase in IFN-γ-producing CD4$^+$ T cells, suggesting a T helper 1 (Th1) shift in CIDP (Mei et al. 2005). Accordingly, another study found increased Th1 cells in the CSF of active and remitting CIDP patients, whereas Th17 cell number was increased only in active patients (Chi et al. 2010). A recent multiplex bead-based ELISA assay investigating 32 inflammatory mediators also found an increased level of CXCL10 besides CCL2, CCL7, CCL27, CXCL9, CXCL12, ICAM-1, and VCAM-1 VEGF, when compared to control samples. No differences were found in the concentration of IL-6, IL-9, IL-15, IL-18, CCL4, CXCL1, LIF, MIF, PDGFbb, IFN-γ, IL-2ra, IL-12(p40), IL-16, SCGF-β, TRAIL, FGF, G-CSF, GM-CSF, and M-CSF. IL-17, IL-4, and IL-5 were not investigated (Sainaghi et al. 2010).

19.2 Multifocal Motor Neuropathy (MMN)

MMN has been considered as a separate chronic demyelinating polyneuropathy since 1988 (Parry and Clarke 1988). It is a rare disease with an incidence of 1–3/100,000 (Muley and Parry 2012). The disease is characterized by slowly progressive multifocal muscle weakness, which starts distally (Figure 19.1). Weakness of the finger extensors is considered typical. Sensory symptoms are absent except mild vibration sense abnormalities distally. Muscle atrophy and cramps appear in about half of the patients. The characteristic electrophysiological feature is conduction block of the peripheral nerves. MRI may indicate edema, T2 hyperintense signal, and thickening of the brachial plexus. The disease is progressive in about 80 % of the cases; stepwise worsening can be observed in about one-tenth of the patients, and relapses are exceptional (Nobile-Orazio et al. 2005; van Schaik et al. 2011; Muley and Parry 2012).

The pathological picture is similar to CIDP and indicates inflammatory demyelination, but the primary pathology is unclear. Antibody-mediated complement activation at the nodal axolemma has been considered similar to acute motor axonal neuropathy (AMAN) (Vlam et al. 2013). In about 30–80 % of patients, monoclonal or polyclonal IgM can be identified in the sera, which is reactive with the ganglioside GM1 (Pestronk et al. 1990; van Schaik et al. 1995; Willison et al. 2001; Cats et al. 2010b). The pathogenicity of the anti-GM1 antibodies is unclear, but they can activate complement in vitro (Uncini et al. 1993; Parry 1994; Harvey et al. 1995; Roberts et al. 1995; Yuki et al. 2011). The presence of anti-GM1 antibody is not specific, since it can be also identified in around 20 % of cases with lower motor neuron syndromes (Nobile-Orazio et al. 1990), but the titer is approximate tenfold higher in MMN (Muley and Parry 2012). EFNS guidelines consider the presence of anti-GM1 antibodies as a supportive factor of diagnosis. It may be especially important in cases with atypical clinical picture or mononeuropathy or in the absence of conduction block by electroneurography (ENG) (Joint Task Force of the EFNS and the PNS 2010a; van Schaik et al. 2011).

Four randomized, double-blind placebo-controlled studies showed the effectiveness of intravenous immunoglobulin (IVIG) in MMN, which supports the pathogenic role of autoantibodies (Azulay et al. 1994; Van den Berg et al. 1995; Federico et al. 2000; Léger et al. 2001; van Schaik et al. 2005; Parry and Clarke 1988). Remission can be achieved and maintained in about one-fifth of the patients. Seventy percent of the patients require long-term treatment with IVIG, and half of these need combination with another immunosuppressant (Meucci et al. 1997). The prognosis of the disease is relatively good (Cats et al. 2010a; van Schaik et al. 2011; Muley and Parry 2012).

CSF Alterations in MMN The EFNS guidelines define definite, probable and possible MMN (Joint Task Force of the EFNS and the PNS 2010a; van Schaik et al. 2011). In all these scenarios, obligatory clinical symptoms are required, and symptoms characteristic of motor neuron disease or CIDP are exclusive. Electrophysiological criteria of conduction block in motor but not sensory fibers are also required for definite diagnosis. In case of possible conduction block in only one nerve, at least two out of four supportive criteria have to be also fulfilled. One of the supportive factors is the elevation of protein in the CSF (<1 g/l), increased concentration of anti-GM1 antibodies in serum, increased T2 signal of the brachial plexus or any nerve on MRI, and clinical response to treatment with IVIG (Joint Task Force of the EFNS and the PNS 2010a; van Schaik et al. 2011).

Analysis of CSF in 32 patients found elevated protein concentrations in 41 %. The median value was 0.42 g/l, but the range was abnormal (0.21–0.97 g/l). Patients with elevated protein in the CSF did not differ clinically or electrophysiologically from those with normal CSF protein levels (Taylor et al. 2000). Other studies also found slightly increased protein levels (usually up to 0.8 g/l) in the CSF in about one-third of patients (Taylor et al. 1996; van den Berg-Vos et al. 2000; Nobile-Orazio 2001). CSF is normal in about two-thirds of the patients, including absence of oligoclonal bands. Such normal findings may help in distinguishing MMN from CIDP, in which protein level in the CSF is usually markedly increased (Nobile-Orazio et al. 2005).

19.3 MADSAM (Lewis-Sumner Syndrome, Asymmetric CIDP) (Multifocal Acquired Demyelinating Sensory and Motor Neuropathy)

The disease was described in 1982 (Lewis et al. 1982). Similarly to MMN and in contrast to CIDP and DADS, MADSAM is an asymmetric neuropathy, which usually starts in the upper extremity (Fig. 19.1) (Saperstein et al. 1999; Verschueren et al. 2005)

However, there are definite sensory symptoms, and ENG also proves the conduction abnormalities of sensory fibers. The EFNS guidelines describe MADSAM as atypical, asymmetric CIDP (Joint Task Force of the EFNS and the PNS 2010c). Corticosteroids may be effective in 65 % of patients according to a recent report reviewing 26 patients (Verschueren et al. 2005), but deterioration has been also described similar to MMN (Van den Berg-Vos et al. 2000; Rajabally and Chavada 2009). Efficacy of IVIG varies between 50 and 100 % (Saperstein et al. 1999; Van den Berg-Vos et al. 2000; Verschueren et al. 2005). Steroids appeared less effective than IVIG in other series (25 % vs 80 %) (Rajabally and Chavada 2009).

CSF Alterations in MADSAM A recent report reviewed 128 cases of asymmetric CIDP or MADSAM, including the CSF characteristics, and also compared cases with pure upper limb involvement at onset (90 cases) to cases with lower limb or mixed upper and lower limb onset (38 cases) (Rajabally and Chavada 2009). Moderate CSF protein elevation was seen in 42 % of patients with initially pure upper limb form; the mean protein level in 41 documented cases was 0.59 g/l. CSF protein was more frequently elevated in cases with asymmetric lower limb or simultaneous upper and lower limb onset (69 %), with a mean level of 0.62 g/l. The authors also concluded that the CSF protein level does not appear to help distinguish between upper limb-onset MADSAM and MMN, since in both conditions CSF protein concentrations are expected to be normal or only mildly elevated (Viala et al. 2004; Nobile-Orazio, et al. 2005; Rajabally and Chavada 2009). Earlier reports suggested increased CSF protein concentrations in 82 % of patients with MADSAM in contrast to 9 % of patients with MMN (Saperstein et al. 1999). In addition, comparing CSF protein levels between 12 patients with MADSAM and 11 patients with MMN, concentrations above 0.5 g/l were more common in MADSAM (50 %) than in MMN (18 %) (Verschueren et al. 2005).

19.4 Paraproteinemic Neuropathies: DADS and Neuropathies Associated with M Protein

The common feature of these diseases is the presence of an M protein (monoclonal gammopathy) in the serum (Fig. 19.1).

Monoclonal gammopathy is more common in the elderly: above 70 years of age, it is present in about 3 % of the population and rising to 10 % above 80 years of age (Crawford et al. 1987). In the majority of cases, the presence of a paraprotein is not associated with hematological diseases and is called MGUS (monoclonal gammopathy of unknown significance). Up to one-third of patients with MGUS have neuropathy, which is significantly more frequent in cases of IgM compared to IgG or IgA paraprotein (Osby et al. 1982; Nobile-Orazio et al. 1992; Vrethem et al. 1993). One study found that 10 % of polyneuropathy cases with undetermined etiology were associated with an M protein, and the frequency was equal to that of CIDP, alcoholic neuropathies, and other toxic neuropathies (Kelly et al. 1981). Moreover, others have found M protein in 8 of 29 patients diagnosed with CIDP or DADS

(Mygland and Monstad 2001). The frequency of neuropathy in hematological malignancies with paraproteinemia varies: 85–100 % in osteosclerotic multiple myeloma, 3–4 % in multiple myeloma, 2–8 % in lymphoma, and 5–50 % in Waldenström macroglobulinemia (Miralles et al. 1992; Nobile-Orazio et al. 1992; Latov 1995). Neuropathy associated with M protein is present in 17 % of cases with systemic amyloidosis (Kyle and Gertz 1995).

In cases of plasmacytoma (multiple myeloma) and POEMS (Crow-Fukase syndrome), the M protein is usually of the IgG or IgA classes; in Waldenström macroglobulinemia, chronic lymphocytic leukemia (CLL), and lymphoma, it is mainly an IgM antibody. The M protein belongs to the IgM class only in about 10–20 % of the cases; its prevalence in the population above 50 years of age is about 20/100,000. However, the proportion of paraprotein in patients with neuropathy is the highest for the IgM class (50 %) and less for IgG (35 %) and IgA (15 %); indeed, the proportion of IgM paraprotein without neuropathy is only 15 %, while it is 75 % for IgG paraprotein (Ramchandren and Lewis 2012). In neuropathies associated with IgM paraprotein, the M protein targets MAG in about 50–60 % of the cases (Nobile-Orazio 2013), and a characteristic symmetrical distal neuropathy (DADS, see below) may be present. The anti-MAG IgM paraprotein is associated with MGUS in about 80 % of the cases, but with malignant hematological disease (mainly Waldenström macroglobulinemia) only in 20 % of cases (Ramchandren and Lewis 2012; Nobile-Orazio 2013, 2014). In about 2 % of patients with neuropathy and IgM paraprotein, the M protein targets gangliosides containing disialosyl groups, and the characteristic clinical picture with prominent ataxia and recurrent ophthalmoplegia is present (CANOMAD) (Willison et al. 1996; Nobile-Orazio et al. 2008).

Neuropathies associated with M proteins have two major clinical significances: First, they should be considered in the differential diagnosis of CIDP. Second, the only clinical signs of MGUS might be the peripheral neuropathy, so the necessity of treatment is driven not by hematological but by neurological symptoms (Joint Task Force of the EFNS and the PNS 2010b).

19.4.1 DADS and Anti-MAG IgM Neuropathy

The disease (distal acquired demyelinating symmetric polyneuropathy, DADS) was described in 2000 (Katz et al. 2000). In about one-third of DADS patients, anti-MAG IgM cannot be identified in the sera. This group is designated as DADS-I (idiopathic DADS) and is differentiated from DADS-M where an IgM kappa light chain M protein is usually found (Ramchandren and Lewis 2012; Nobile-Orazio 2013, 2014). The EFNS guidelines classify DADS-I as atypical CIDP, while the presence of anti-MAG is an exclusion criterion (van Schaik et al. 2011).

The neurological syndrome is distal paresthesia, dysesthesia, and hypesthesia of the lower extremities and sensory ataxia (Fig. 19.1). Muscle weakness is not present at onset. Most of the patients are 60–70-year-old males. The course is usually slowly progressive, and about 25 % of the patients become disabled after 10 years. In spite of the relatively mild neurological symptoms, the ENG may indicate severe electrophysiological changes, prolonged distal motor latency, and decreased motor and sensory nerve conduction velocity.

The pathological role of the anti-MAG antibodies is not clear. Immunohistochemistry indicates IgM and complement colocalization, deposited according to the segmental demyelination in the peripheral nerves, and the presence of anti-MAG IgM antibodies in asymptomatic patients is predictive of neuropathy. Although transfer of immunoglobulins from patients induces experimental demyelination, removal of antibodies by plasma exchange or IVIG and immunosuppression/immunomodulation do not result in major improvement.

CSF Alterations in DADS In a case series of nine patients with DADS-I (no anti-MAG), the cell count was normal, but the protein concentration was elevated in the CSF in two-thirds of the patients. Half of these patients had protein levels between 1 and 1.6 g/l (Larue et al. 2011). A recent review considered examination of the CSF unnecessary in DADS, since it usually shows increased protein concentration (0.8–1 g/l) with normal cells and thus does not permit differentiation from CIDP (Nobile-Orazio 2013).

19.4.2 CANOMAD and Anti-ganglioside IgM Antibodies

IgM antibodies against gangliosides may cause sensory ataxic neuropathy associated with ophthalmoparesis in about 2 % of cases with IgM M proteins (Nobile-Orazio et al. 2008; Willison et al. 2001). The disease is designated as CANOMAD due to the chronic sensory ataxic neuropathy (CAN), the recurrent ophthalmoparesis (O), the M protein with cold-agglutinin activity (M), and the anti-disialosyl antibodies (AD): anti-GQ1b, anti-GD1b, anti-GD2, anti-GD3, and anti-GT1b (Willison et al. 1996). The symptoms can appear in relapses and may improve after treatment with IVIG. Similar sensory ataxic neuropathy can be associated with anti-sulfatide and anti-chondroitin sulfate antibodies in less than 2 % of cases with IgM M proteins (Nobile-Orazio 2013).

CSF Alterations in CANOMAD In a case series of 16 patients, concentrations of CSF protein were elevated in 68 %; protein levels were mildly increased in the majority of these cases (0.5–1 g/l in 82 %). Mild lymphocytic pleocytosis (7–16 cell/μl) was observed in 3 cases, two of whom had elevated protein levels as well. Oligoclonal bands were absent and glucose levels were normal (Willison et al. 2001).

In the majority of CANOMAD cases with Waldenström macroglobulinemia, CSF lymphocytosis has been described (McKelvie et al. 2013; Viala et al. 2012; Abad et al. 1999; Massengo et al. 2003; Sutter et al. 2007).

19.4.3 Neuropathies with IgG and IgA Paraproteins

Neuropathies associated with IgG and IgA MGUS are less frequent (3–4 %) compared to IgM MGUS (15 %) but may respond better to immunotherapies.

Hematological malignancies, i.e., multiple myeloma and POEMS (Crow-Fukase syndrome), should be always considered and excluded. About half of neuropathies associated with IgG MGUS are characterized by clinical and electrophysiological features of CIDP and respond similarly to immunotherapies. In the other half, the neuropathy is mainly sensory and axonal (CIAP, chronic idiopathic axonal polyneuropathy), and the treatment response is poor. IgA MGUS is rarely associated with neuropathy and can be demyelinating or axonal.

Chronic progressive sensorimotor polyneuropathy is a characteristic feature of Crow-Fukase syndrome (POEMS) characterized by organomegaly, endocrinopathy, lymphadenopathy, ascites, edema, M protein, and skin changes. Besides the distal weakness, sensory symptoms are prominent; sensory ataxia can be present. ENG and nerve biopsy indicates demyelination with axonal loss.

CSF Alterations in POEMS (Crow-Fukase) Syndrome Elevated cerebrospinal fluid protein levels were independently associated with papilledema in Crow-Fukase syndrome (Cui et al. 2014). High level of soluble IL-6 receptor in the CSF was also found in one case, which fluctuated in parallel with the clinical course and decreased after plasmapheresis (Atsumi et al. 1995).

19.5 Vasculitic Neuropathies

Neuropathy develops in about 40–80 % of cases with vasculitis. Neuropathy associated with systemic vasculitis is more common than isolated vasculitis localized to the PNS; however, nonsystemic vasculitic neuropathy is the most commonly encountered form with similar frequency to polyarteritis nodosa (PAN) and microscopic polyangiitis (MPA)-associated neuropathies (Collins and Periquet 2008). In systemic vasculitis, systemic signs may help diagnosis: loss of weight, leukocytosis, elevated C-reactive protein (CRP) and erythrocyte sedimentation rate (ESR), fever, purpura, muscle pain, arthralgia, and night sweats. However, neuropathy can be the only sign. Nevertheless, weight loss occurs in 35 % and fever in 15 % of patients with nonsystemic PNS vasculitis; most patients have elevated ESR, and 20–40 % have anemia, leukocytosis, and thrombocytosis (Collins 2003). In addition, 37 % of patients with isolated vasculitic neuropathy developed systemic manifestations during long-term follow-up (Said 1995).

The classical presenting syndrome (50 %) is multiple mononeuropathies in the fifth to eight decade (Davies et al. 1996; Dyck et al. 1987). ENG indicates asymmetric, multifocal, sensory, and motor axonal lesions in different nerves. Examination of the ANCA status is mandatory, since it can help to establish the diagnosis of the ANCA-associated vasculitis: Wegener granulomatosis, MPA, and Churg-Strauss syndrome. Nerve biopsy (n. suralis, n. peroneus superficialis) is needed to establish the diagnosis if localized vasculitis is suspected (Collins et al. 2010); its sensitivity is around 60 % (Dyck et al. 1987; Collins et al. 2000; Bennett et al. 2008). Secondary systemic vasculitis associated with connective tissue disorders, infections, mixed cryoglobulinemia, tumors, sarcoidosis, drugs, and toxins should be also considered (Collins 2012; Gwathmey et al. 2014; Vrancken and Said 2013).

The most common causes of vasculitic neuropathy are systemic vasculitis affecting the small and medium vessels: the three ANCA-associated vasculitis (MPA, Wegener granulomatosis, Churg-Strauss syndrome), PAN (hepatitis B virus), rheumatoid vasculitis, and cryoglobulinemic vasculitis (hepatitis C virus) (Collins 2012; Gwathmey et al. 2014; Vrancken and Said 2013; Vaglio et al. 2013). Neuropathy develops in about 11–13 % of patients with chronic HCV infection. The neuropathy in HCV-associated cryoglobulinemia is usually slowly progressive and distal with predominance of sensory symptoms and axonal loss. Neuropathic pain is present in half of the cases and small fiber neuropathy in 25 %. Symmetric polyneuropathy and asymmetric multiple mononeuropathy may be equally present and even overlap.

CSF Alterations in Vasculitic Neuropathies Guidelines of the Peripheral Nerve Society include CSF analysis for clinically probable nonsystemic vasculitis with nerve/muscle biopsy evidence of probable or possible vasculitis neuropathy: CSF pleocytosis and CSF protein concentrations >1.1 g/l are exclusion criteria (Collins et al. 2010).

In a clinical cohort of 19 patients with nonsystemic vasculitic neuropathy, mild pleocytosis was noted in one patient (5 %), and the CSF protein concentration was elevated in 26 % of the patients with a mean concentration of 0.47 ± 0.22 g/l and maximum concentration of 1.06 g/l (Collins et al. 2003).

By analyzing cytokine levels in the CSF of 8 patients with undefined vasculitic neuropathies, proinflammatory IL-6 and IL-8 and anti-inflammatory IL-10 levels were elevated (Mei et al. 2005). The authors concluded that increase of both IL-6 and IL-10 may exacerbate symptoms: IL-6 may contribute to vasculitis-related ischemia of the peripheral nerves, while IL-10 enhances autoantibody production. There was no increase of intracellular IFN-γ/IL-4 ratio in CSF cells in contrast to CIDP; thus, a contribution of Th1 cells may be less important. IFN-γ-producing cell percentages were distributed over a wide range in contrast to CIDP, indicating the heterogeneous nature of vasculitic neuropathies.

CSF was also analyzed in 61 patients with diabetic cervical or lumbosacral radiculoplexus neuropathy sharing many features with microvasculitis, including ischemic injury (Massie et al. 2012). Protein concentrations were abnormal in 90–100 %, respectively, while the cell count was mostly normal (≥ 90 %). IgG synthesis was elevated in 14 % of cases with cervical diabetic radiculoplexus neuropathy, but oligoclonal bands were not detected. These data indicate that the pathological process extends to the root levels in most of these patients.

CSF examination of patients with neuropathy associated with Churg-Strauss syndrome disclosed no abnormalities in a study investigating 28 patients, except one case (Hattori et al. 1999).

Conclusion

Studies investigating CSF alterations in chronic diseases of the peripheral nervous system are limited. This may be related to the fact that changes are expected only if parts of the PNS in close vicinity to the CSF compartment are affected or CNS alterations are associated.

In the routine clinical practice, examination of the CSF can help in establishing the diagnosis of CIDP and can support differentiation between MMN and CIDP in the majority of the cases.

References

Abad S, Zagdanski AM, Brechignac S et al (1999) Neurolymphomatosis in Waldenström's macroglobulinaemia. Br J Haematol 106:100–103

Atsumi T, Kato K, Kurosawa S, Abe M, Fujisaku A (1995) A case of Crow-Fukase syndrome with elevated soluble interleukin-6 receptor in cerebrospinal fluid. Response to double-filtration plasmapheresis and corticosteroids. Acta Haematol 94:90–94

Azulay JP, Blin O, Pouget J et al (1994) Intravenous immunoglobulin treatment in patients with motor neuron syndromes associated with anti-GM1 antibodies: a double-blind, placebo-controlled study. Neurology 44:429–32

Barohn RJ, Kissel JT, Warmolts JR et al (1989) Chronic inflammatory demyelinating polyradiculoneuropathy. Clinical characteristics, course, and recommendations for diagnostic criteria. Arch Neurol 46:878–884

Bennett DL, Groves M, Blake J et al (2008) The use of nerve and muscle biopsy in the diagnosis of vasculitis: a 5 year retrospective study. J Neurol Neurosurg Psychiatry 79:1376–1381

Bosboom WM, van den Berg LH, Franssen H et al (2001) Diagnostic value of sural nerve demyelination in chronic inflammatory demyelinating polyneuropathy. Brain 124:2427–2438

Bouchard C, Lacroix C, Planté V et al (1999) Clinicopathologic findings and prognosis of chronic inflammatory demyelinating polyneuropathy. Neurology 52:498–503

Cats EA, van der Pol WL, Piepers S et al (2010a) Correlates of outcome and response to IVIg in 88 patients with multifocal motor neuropathy. Neurology 75:818–825

Cats EA, Jacobs BC, Yuki N et al (2010b) Multifocal motor neuropathy: association of anti-GM1 IgM antibodies with clinical features. Neurology 75:1961–1967

Chi LJ, Xu WH, Zhang ZW et al (2010) Distribution of Th17 cells and Th1 cells in peripheral blood and cerebrospinal fluid in chronic inflammatory demyelinating polyradiculoneuropathy. J Peripher Nerv Syst 15:345–356

Chiang HL, Lyu RK, Tseng MY et al (2009) Analyses of transthyretin concentration in the cerebrospinal fluid of patients with Guillain-Barré syndrome and other neurological disorders. Clin Chim Acta 405:143–147. doi:10.1016/j.cca.2009.04.022, Epub 2009 May 3

Collins MP (2012) The vasculitic neuropathies: an update. Curr Opin Neurol 25:573–585

Collins MP, Periquet MI, Mendell et al (2003) Nonsystemic vasculitic neuropathy: insights from a clinical cohort. Neurology 61:623–30

Collins MP, Periquet MI (2008) Isolated vasculitis of the peripheral nervous system. Clin Exp Rheumatol 26(3 Suppl 49):S118–S130

Collins MP, Mendell JR, Periquet MI et al (2000) Superficial peroneal nerve/peroneus brevis muscle biopsy in vasculitic neuropathy. Neurology 55:636–643

Collins MP, Dyck PJ, Gronseth GS et al Peripheral Nerve Society (2010) Peripheral Nerve Society Guideline on the classification, diagnosis, investigation, and immunosuppressive therapy of non-systemic vasculitic neuropathy: executive summary. J Peripher Nerv Syst 15:176–184

Crawford J, Eye MK, Cohen HJ (1987) Evaluation of monoclonal gammopathies in the 'well' elderly. Am J Med 82:39–45

Cui R, Yu S, Huang X, Zhang J, Tian C, Pu C (2014) Papilloedema is an independent prognostic factor for POEMS syndrome. J Neurol 261:60–65

Davies L, Spies JM, Pollard JD, McLeod JG (1996) Vasculitis confined to peripheral nerves. Brain 119:1441–1448

Dyck PJ, Benstead TJ, Conn DL et al (1987) Nonsystemic vasculitic neuropathy. Brain 110:843–853

Federico P, Zochodne DW, Hahn AF et al (2000) Multifocal motor neuropathy improved by IVIG randomized double-blind, placebo-controlled study. Neurology 55:1256–1262

Gorson KC, Allam G, Ropper AH (1997) Chronic inflammatory demyelinating polyneuropathy: clinical features and response to treatment in 67 consecutive patients with and without a monoclonal gammopathy. Neurology 48:321–328

Gwathmey KG, Burns TM, Collins MP, Dyck PJ (2014) Vasculitic neuropathies. Lancet Neurol 13:67–82

Harvey GK, Toyka KV, Zielasek J et al (1995) Failure of anti-GM1 IgG or IgM to induce conduction block following intraneural transfer. Muscle Nerve 18:388–394

Hattori N, Ichimura M, Nagamatsu M et al (1999) Clinicopathological features of Churg-Strauss syndrome-associated neuropathy. Brain 122:427–39

Hughes RA, Mehndiratta MM (2012) Corticosteroids for chronic inflammatory demyelinating polyradiculoneuropathy. Cochrane Database Syst Rev (8):CD002062. doi:10.1002/14651858. CD002062.pub2

Joint Task Force of the EFNS and the PNS (2010a) European Federation of Neurological Societies/ Peripheral Nerve Society guideline on management of multifocal motor neuropathy. Report of a joint task force of the European Federation of Neurological Societies and the Peripheral Nerve Society – first revision. J Peripher Nerv Syst 15:295–301

Joint Task Force of the EFNS and the PNS (2010b) European Federation of Neurological Societies/Peripheral Nerve Society Guideline on management of paraproteinaemic demyelinating neuropathies. Report of a Joint Task Force of the European Federation of Neurological Societies and the Peripheral Nerve Societ–irst revision. J Peripher Nerv Syst 15:185–195

Joint Task Force of the EFNS and the PNS (2010c) EFNS/PNS CIDP guidelines. European Federation of Neurological Societies/Peripheral Nerve Society Guideline on management of chronic inflammatory demyelinating polyradiculoneuropathy: Report of a joint task force of the European Federation of Neurological Societies and the Peripheral Nerve Society – First Revision. J Peripher Nerv Syst 15:1–9

Katz JS, Saperstein DS, Gronseth G et al (2000) Distal acquired demyelinating symmetric neuropathy. Neurology 54:615–620

Kelly JJ Jr, Kyle RA, O'Brien PC, Dyck PJ (1981) Prevalence of monoclonal protein in peripheral neuropathy. Neurology 31:1480–1483

Kieseier BC, Tani M, Mahad D et al (2002) Chemokines and chemokine receptors in inflammatory demyelinating neuropathies: a central role for IP-10. Brain 125:823–834

Kyle RA, Gertz MA (1995) Primary systemic amyloidosis: clinical and laboratory features in 474 cases. Semin Hematol 32:45–59

Larue S, Bombelli F, Viala K et al (2011) Non-anti-MAG DADS neuropathy as a variant of CIDP: clinical, electrophysiological, laboratory features and response to treatment in 10 cases. Eur J Neurol 18:899–905

Latov N (1995) Pathogenesis and therapy of neuropathies associated with monoclonal gammopathies. Ann Neurol 37(Suppl 1):S32–S42

Laughlin RS, Dyck PJ, Melton LJ 3rd et al (2009) Incidence and prevalence of CIDP and the association of diabetes mellitus. Neurology 73:39–45

Léger JM, Chassande B, Musset L et al (2001) Intravenous immunoglobulin therapy in multifocal motor neuropathy: a double- blind, placebo controlled study. Brain 124:145–153

Lewis RA, Sumner AJ, Brown MJ, Asbury AK (1982) Multifocal demyelinating neuropathy with persistent conduction block. Neurology 32:958–964

Mahad DJ, Howell SJ, Woodroofe MN (2002) Expression of chemokines in cerebrospinal fluid and serum of patients with chronic inflammatory demyelinating polyneuropathy. J Neurol Neurosurg Psychiatry 73:320–323

Mahdi-Rogers M, van Doorn PA, Hughes RA (2013) Immunomodulatory treatment other than corticosteroids, immunoglobulin and plasma exchange for chronic inflammatory demyelinating polyradiculoneuropathy. Cochrane Database Syst Rev (6):CD003280. doi:10.1002/14651858. CD003280.pub4

Massengo S, Riffaud L, Morandi X, Bernard M, Verin M (2003) Nervous system lymphoid infiltration in Waldenström's macroglobulinemia. A case report. J Neurooncol 62:353–358

Massie R, Mauermann ML, Staff NP et al (2012) Diabetic cervical radiculoplexus neuropathy: a distinct syndrome expanding the spectrum of diabetic radiculoplexus neuropathies. Brain 135:3074–88

McKelvie PA, Gates PC, Day T (2013) Canomad: report of a case with a 40-year history and autopsy. Is this a sensory ganglionopathy with neuromuscular junction blockade? Muscle Nerve 48:599–603

Mei FJ, Ishizu T, Murai H et al (2005) Th1 shift in CIDP versus Th2 shift in vasculitic neuropathy in CSF. J Neurol Sci 228:75–85

Meucci N, Cappellari A, Barbieri S et al (1997) Long term effect of intravenous immunoglobulins and oral cyclophosphamide in multifocal motor neuropathy. J Neurol Neurosurg Psychiatry 63:765–769

Miralles GD, O'Fallon JR, Talley NJ (1992) Plasma-cell dyscrasia with polyneuropathy. The spectrum of POEMS syndrome. N Engl J Med 327:1919–1923

Muley SA, Parry GJ (2012) Multifocal motor neuropathy. J Clin Neurosci 19:1201–1209

Mygland A, Monstad P (2001) Chronic polyneuropathies in Vest-Agder, Norway. Eur J Neurol 8:157–165

Nagai A, Murakawa Y, Terashima M et al (2000) Cystatin C and cathepsin B in CSF from patients with inflammatory neurologic diseases. Neurology 55:1828–32

Nobile-Orazio E (2001) Multifocal motor neuropathy. J Neuroimmunol 115:4–18

Nobile-Orazio E (2013) Neuropathy and monoclonal gammopathy. Handb Clin Neurol 115: 443–459

Nobile-Orazio E, Carpo M, Legname G et al (1990) Anti-GM1 IgM antibodies in motor neuron disease and neuropathy. Neurology 40:1747–1750

Nobile-Orazio E, Barbieri S, Baldini L, Marmiroli P, Carpo M, Premoselli S, Manfredini E, Scarlato G (1992) Peripheral neuropathy in monoclonal gammopathy of undetermined significance: prevalence and immunopathogenetic studies. Acta Neurol Scand 85:383–390

Nobile-Orazio E, Cappellari A, Priori A (2005) Multifocal motor neuropathy: current concepts and controversies. Muscle Nerve 31:663–680

Nobile-Orazio E, Gallia F, Terenghi F, Allaria S, Giannotta C, Carpo M (2008) How useful are anti-neural IgM antibodies in the diagnosis of chronic immune-mediated neuropathies? J Neurol Sci 266:156–163

Nobile-Orazio E (2014) Chronic inflammatory demyelinating polyradiculoneuropathy and variants: where we are and where we should go.J Peripher Nerv Syst 19:2–13

Notermans NC, Wokke JH, Franssen H et al (1993) Chronic idiopathic polyneuropathy presenting in middle or old age: a clinical and electrophysiological study of 75 patients. J Neurol Neurosurg Psychiatry 56:1066–1071

Osby E, Noring L, Hast R, Kjellin KG, Knutsson E, Sidén A (1982) Benign monoclonal gammopathy and peripheral neuropathy. Br J Haematol 51:531–539

Parry GJ (1994) Antiganglioside antibodies do not necessarily play a role in multifocal motor neuropathy. Muscle Nerve 17:97–99

Parry GJ, Clarke S (1988) Multifocal acquired demyelinating neuropathy masquerading as motor neuron disease. Muscle Nerve 11:103–7

Pestronk A, Chaudhry V, Feldman EL et al (1990) Lower motor neuron syndromes defined by patterns of weakness, nerve conduction abnormalities, and high titers of antiglycolipid antibodies. Ann Neurol 27:316–26

Press R, Pashenkov M, Jin JP et al (2003) Aberrated levels of cerebrospinal fluid chemokines in Guillain-Barré syndrome and chronic inflammatory demyelinating polyradiculoneuropathy. J Clin Immunol 23:259–267

Rajabally YA, Chavada G (2009) Lewis-Sumner syndrome of pure upper-limb onset: diagnostic, prognostic, and therapeutic features. Muscle Nerve 39:206–220

Ramchandren S, Lewis RA (2012) An update on monoclonal gammopathy and neuropathy. Curr Neurol Neurosci Rep 12:102–110

Roberts M, Willison HJ, Vincent A et al (1995) Multifocal motor neuropathy human sera block distal motor nerve conduction in mice. Ann Neurol 38:111–8

Said G (1995) Vasculitic neuropathy. Ballieres Clin Neurol 4:489–503

Said G, Krarup C (2013) Chronic inflammatory demyelinative polyneuropathy. Handb Clin Neurol 115:403–413

Sainaghi PP, Collimedaglia L, Alciato F et al (2010) The expression pattern of inflammatory mediators in cerebrospinal fluid differentiates Guillain-Barré syndrome from chronic inflammatory demyelinating polyneuropathy. Cytokine 51:138–143

Saperstein DS, Amato AA, Wolfe GI et al (1999) Multifocal acquired demyelinating sensory and motor neuropathy: the Lewis-Sumner syndrome. Muscle Nerve 22:560–566

Saperstein DS, Katz JS, Amato AA, Barohn RJ (2001) Clinical spectrum of chronic acquired demyelinating polyneuropathies. Muscle Nerve 24:311–24

Sivieri S, Ferrarini AM, Lolli F et al (1997) Cytokine pattern in the cerebrospinal fluid from patients with GBS and CIDP. J Neurol Sci 147:93–95

Stübgen JP (2013) A review of the use of biological agents for chronic inflammatory demyelinating polyradiculoneuropathy. J Neurol Sci 326:1–9

Sutter R, Arber C, Tichelli A et al (2007) Cranial and peripheral neuropathy due to leptomeningeal infiltration in a patient with Waldenstrom's macroglobulinemia. J Neurol 254:1122–3

Taylor BV, Gross L, Windebank AJ (1996) The sensitivity and specificity of anti-GM1 antibody testing. Neurology 47:951–955

Taylor BV, Wright RA, Harper CM, Dyck PJ (2000) Natural history of 46 patients with multifocal motor neuropathy with conduction block. Muscle Nerve 23:900–908

Tumani H, Pfeifle M, Lehmensiek V et al (2009) Candidate biomarkers of chronic inflammatory demyelinating polyneuropathy (CIDP): proteome analysis of cerebrospinal fluid. J Neuroimmunol 214:109–112

Uncini A, Santoro M, Corbo M et al (1993) Conduction abnormalities induced by sera of patients with multifocal motor neuropathy and anti-GM1 antibodies. Muscle Nerve 16:610–615

Vaglio A, Buzio C, Zwerina J (2013) Eosinophilic granulomatosis with polyangiitis (Churg-Strauss): state of the art. Allergy 68:261–273

Van den Berg LH, Kerkhoff H, Oey PL et al (1995) Treatment of multifocal motor neuropathy with high dose intravenous gammaglobulin: a double-blind, placebo-controlled study. J Neurol Neurosurg Psychiatry 59:28–52

Van den Berg-Vos RM, Van den Berg LH, Franssen H et al (2000) Multifocal inflammatory demyelinating neuropathy: a distinct clinical entity? Neurology 54:26–32

van Schaik IN, Bossuyt PMM, Brand A, Vermeulen M (1995) The diagnostic value of GM1 antibodies in motor neuron disorders and neuropathies: a meta-analysis. Neurology 45:1570–1577

van Schaik IN, Van den Berg LH, de Haan R, Vermeulen M (2005) Intravenous immunoglobulin for multifocal motor neuropathy. Cochrane Database Syst Rev (2):CD004429

van Schaik IN, Léger J-M, Nobile-Orazio E et al (2011) Multifocal motor neuropathy. In: Gilhus NE, Barnes MP, Brainin M (eds) European handbook of neurological management, vol 1, 2nd edn. Blackwell Publishing LTD, Chichester, pp 343–350

Verschueren A, Azulay JP, Attarian S et al (2005) Lewis-Sumner syndrome and multifocal motor neuropathy. Muscle Nerve 31:88–94

Viala K, Renié L, Maisonobe T, Béhin A et al (2004) Follow-up study and response to treatment in 23 patients with Lewis-Sumner syndrome. Brain 127:2010–2017

Viala K, Stojkovic T, Doncker AV et al (2012) Heterogeneous spectrum of neuropathies in Waldenström's macroglobulinemia: a diagnostic strategy to optimize their management. J Peripher Nerv Syst 17:90–101

Vlam L, van den Berg LH, Cats EA et al (2013) Immune pathogenesis and treatment of multifocal motor neuropathy. J Clin Immunol 33(Suppl 1):S38–S42

Vrancken AF, Said G (2013) Vasculitic neuropathy. Handb Clin Neurol 115:463–483

Vrethem M, Cruz M, Wen-Xin H et al (1993) Clinical, neurophysiological and immunological evidence of polyneuropathy in patients with monoclonal gammopathies. J Neuro Sci 114:193–199

Willison HJ, Yuki N (2002) Peripheral neuropathies and antiglycolipid antibodies. Brain 125: 2591–2625

Willison HJ, O'Hanlon GM, Paterson G et al (1996) A somatically mutated human antiganglioside IgM antibody that induces experimental neuropathy in mice is encoded by the variable region heavy chain gene, V1-18. J Clin Invest 97:1155–1164

Willison HJ, O'Leary CP, Veitch J et al (2001) The clinical and laboratory features of chronic sensory ataxic demyelinating neuropathy with anti-disialosyl IgM antibodies. Brain 124:1968–1977

Yuki N, Watanabe H, Nakajima T et al (2011) IVIG blocks complement deposition mediated by anti-GM1 antibodies in multifocal motor neuropathy. J Neurol Neurosurg Psychiatry 82:87–91

Zhang HL, Zhang XM, Mao XJ et al (2012) Altered cerebrospinal fluid index of prealbumin, fibrinogen, and haptoglobin in patients with Guillain-Barré syndrome and chronic inflammatory demyelinating polyneuropathy. Acta Neurol Scand 125:129–135

Alzheimer's Disease and Other Neurodegenerative Disorders

Christoffer Rosén, Henrik Zetterberg, and Kaj Blennow

Contents

C. Rosén (✉) • K. Blennow
Clinical Neurochemistry Laboratory, Department of Psychiatry and Neurochemistry,
Institute of Neuroscience and Physiology,
The Sahlgrenska Academy at the University of Gothenburg,
Mölndal, Sweden
e-mail: christoffer.rosen@neuro.gu.se

H. Zetterberg
Clinical Neurochemistry Laboratory, Department of Psychiatry and Neurochemistry,
Institute of Neuroscience and Physiology,
The Sahlgrenska Academy at the University of Gothenburg,
Mölndal, Sweden

UCL Institute of Neurology, Department of Molecular Neuroscience,
Queen Square, London WC1N 3BG, UK

© Springer International Publishing Switzerland 2015
F. Deisenhammer et al. (eds.), *Cerebrospinal Fluid in Clinical Neurology*,
DOI 10.1007/978-3-319-01225-4_20

Abstract

Traditionally, patients suffering from Alzheimer's disease (AD) have been diagnosed according to clinical criteria, and a diagnosis has only been made in the dementia stage of the disease. Definite diagnosis required autopsy to confirm the neuropathological findings associated with AD, namely, extracellular depositions of amyloid β (Aβ) protein and intraneuronal neurofibrillary tangles consisting of hyperphosphorylated tau (P-tau) protein, together with gross cortical atrophy caused by neuronal degeneration and loss. These findings are reflected in the cerebrospinal fluid (CSF) of patients with AD. Numerous studies have shown that AD patients have lower levels of Aβ42 and higher levels of P-tau and total tau (T-tau) in CSF than cognitively healthy controls. In the new diagnostic criteria for AD, these CSF biomarkers are included as in vivo evidence of AD neuropathology together with positron emission tomography (PET) measurements of global cortical amyloid load. Further, AD is now divided into several disease stages, namely, preclinical AD and mild cognitive impairment and dementia due to AD. In this chapter, we review CSF biomarker characteristics for the various disease stages for AD and how to use them in the differentiation against other common neurodegenerative disorders. New candidate CSF biomarkers for AD are also presented, as well as a discussion on the standardization of biomarkers and their application in clinical trials.

20.1   Introduction

20.1.1 How It All Began

More than a century has passed since Doctor Alois Alzheimer in 1906 was the first to present a case of the disease that later would be named after him: Alzheimer's disease (AD). The patient was a woman that he had followed over time who displayed progressive memory disturbances and cognitive symptoms, and finally dementia. Upon her death at an age of 51 years, he performed an autopsy and noticed specific findings in her brain, namely, "miliary bodies" (plaques) and "dense bundles of fibrils" (tangles), which now are considered the main neuropathological characteristics of AD (Alzheimer 1987). Except for elucidating that disturbances in the cholinergic neuronal systems are a characteristic of AD, this was what was known on AD pathogenesis during the forthcoming 80 years. However, subsequent research efforts have given detailed knowledge on the molecular pathogenesis linked to these initial discoveries.

20.1.2 Amyloid Plaques

That the plaques mainly consisted of the 4 kDa β-amyloid (Aβ) peptide was discovered in 1985 (Masters et al. 1985). It is now known that the major isoforms of Aβ in the plaques are Aβ4-42, Aβ1-42, and Aβ1-40 (Portelius et al. 2010). Plaques also contain deformed neurites and are often surrounded by microglia and sometimes astrocytes (Perl 2010).

Aβ originates from the amyloid precursor protein (APP) and is released after enzymatic action of β- and γ-secretase. Mutations in the gene for APP, as well as in the genes for presenilin 1 and 2, which are components of the γ-secretase, lead to altered levels of Aβ and are seen in the rare familial variant of AD (FAD) (Mullan et al. 1992; van Duijn et al. 1991; Chartier-Harlin et al. 1991; Selkoe 2001). This, together with the findings of cerebral Aβ plaque pathology in patients with Down syndrome, who have one extra of the APP containing chromosome 21 (trisomy 21), led to the hypothesis that Aβ is a driving force in the disease process (Hardy and Higgins 1992; Hardy 2009). This hypothesis, called the "amyloid cascade hypothesis," states that increased levels of Aβ serve as a key initiating event in the disease process that ultimately results in neuronal degeneration and dementia.

20.1.3 Neurofibrillary Tangles

The neurofibrillary tangles are composed of abnormally phosphorylated tau protein (Grundke-Iqbal et al. 1986). Tau is an axonal protein that in its unphosphorylated state provides stabilizing functions for the microtubules (Goedert et al. 1989). When phosphorylated, however, this ability is disrupted, which leads to tau aggregation, impaired axonal transport, and eventually death of the neuron (Spires-Jones et al. 2009). Loss of neurons is a third feature of AD and can be seen at the gross anatomical levels—patients with AD have a significant thinning of the cerebral cortex compared to healthy controls (Ahn et al. 2011).

20.1.4 Diagnosis

The gold standard for the diagnosis of AD has since long been to perform an autopsy after the patient has deceased. The pathological hallmarks of plaques and tangles must be present to a certain extent to confer a pathological diagnosis. In 1984, clinical criteria for probable AD were published by a working group established by the National Institute of Neurological and Communicative disorders and Stroke and the Alzheimer's Disease and Related Disorders Association (McKhann et al. 1984). By these criteria, a diagnosis of AD could only be made when the patient was demented, and the diagnosis was mainly made by excluding other causes of dementia. Revision of these guidelines was made by the National Institute on Aging (NIA) in 2011 (Jack et al. 2011). Now, cerebrospinal fluid (CSF) and imaging biomarkers (magnetic resonance imaging measurements of hippocampal atrophy and positron emission tomography [PET] measurements of amyloid load and cortical glucose metabolism) were implemented for providing in vivo evidence of AD neuropathology. Also, the whole spectrum of the disease was acknowledged, from cognitively healthy individuals to patients experiencing some cognitive deficits (i.e., mild cognitive impairment [MCI]), and ultimately patients with full-blown dementia. According to these NIA 2011 guidelines, a diagnosis of AD could be made irrespective of disease stage, and criteria for preclinical AD, mild cognitive impairment (MCI) due to AD, and dementia due to AD were given (Sperling et al. 2011a; Albert et al. 2011).

20.1.5 Roles of CSF Biomarkers for AD

Biomarkers are variables (physiological, biochemical, anatomical) that can be measured in vivo and that indicate specific features of disease-related pathological changes (Jack et al. 2010). CSF has been the most successful source for finding fluid biomarkers for AD pathology. Since it surrounds the brain, it is close to the pathologies of interest, which may explain the success rate. As mentioned above, biomarkers are becoming increasingly important in the diagnosis of AD. However, there are also other potential roles.

As of today, the only treatments available for AD are symptomatic, and studies have shown significant but limited effects (Raina et al. 2008). Hence, disease-modifying drugs are needed. Over the past 20 years, there have been a large number of drug candidates, mainly focusing on the amyloid cascade hypothesis, but all have failed in late-stage clinical trials (Karran et al. 2011). This has raised critical voices about this hypothesis, especially since it has not been proven with certainty in late onset AD, which is the most common form. However, drug studies have mainly targeted patients in later stages of AD. Since disease-modifying drugs probably will be most effective in the earlier stages of the disease, before plaque and tangle load and neurodegeneration become too severe, it is possible that the recent drug failures partly may depend on including too severely affected patients (Garcia-Alloza et al. 2009; Das et al. 2001; Levites et al. 2006; Sperling et al. 2011b). A need to find patients early in the disease process, maybe even at a presymptomatic stage, has arisen. Here, CSF biomarkers may have an important role in providing early evidence of ongoing AD pathology. Even though the longitudinal trajectories of the AD biomarkers need to be further elucidated, it is known that biomarker abnormalities can be found before patients experience their first symptoms, reflecting the long asymptomatic phase of the disease (Jack et al. 2010). Further, biomarkers can provide indirect evidence that disease-modifying drugs really affect the central disease process and hallmark neuropathology, which is central together with a beneficial effect on cognition (Siemers 2009). Together, this has created a need for biomarkers corresponding to core element of the disease process for use in diagnostics and to

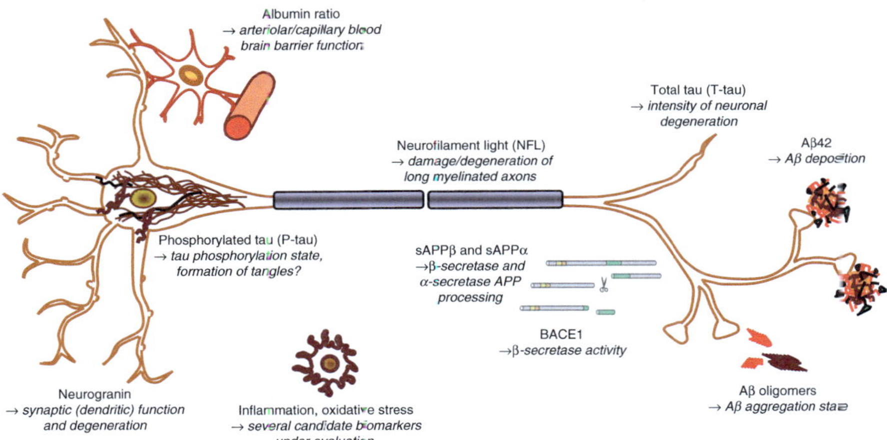

Fig. 20.1 Cartoon of CSF biomarkers and their relation to physiological and pathogenic processes. *Aβ* amyloid β, *BACE1* β-site APP cleaving enzyme 1, *sAPP* soluble amyloid precursor protein

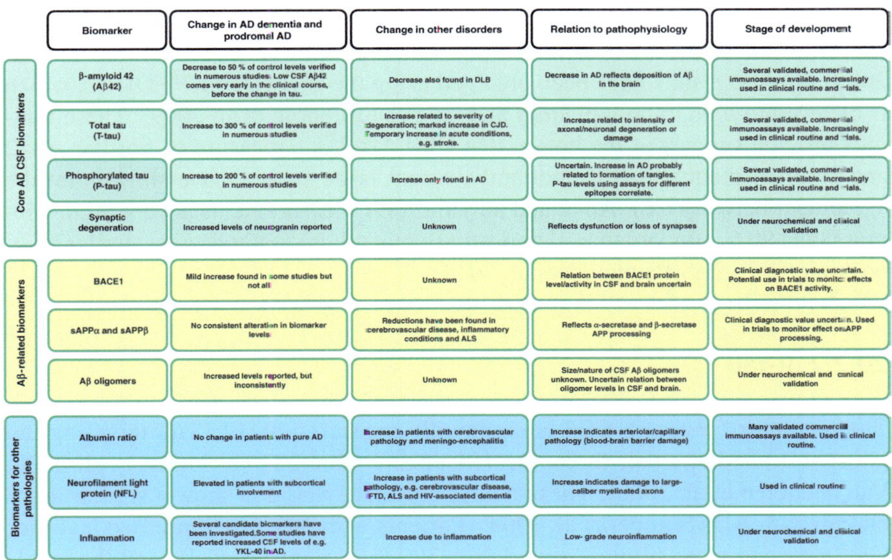

	Biomarker	Change in AD dementia and prodromal AD	Change in other disorders	Relation to pathophysiology	Stage of development
Core AD CSF biomarkers	β-amyloid 42 (Aβ42)	Decrease to 50 % of control levels verified in numerous studies. Low CSF Aβ42 comes very early in the clinical course, before the change in tau.	Decrease also found in DLB	Decrease in AD reflects deposition of Aβ in the brain	Several validated, commercial immunoassays available. Increasingly used in clinical routine and trials.
	Total tau (T-tau)	Increase to 300 % of control levels verified in numerous studies	Increase related to severity of degeneration; marked increase in CJD. Temporary increase in acute conditions, e.g. stroke.	Increase related to intensity of axonal/neuronal degeneration or damage	Several validated, commercial immunoassays available. Increasingly used in clinical routine and trials.
	Phosphorylated tau (P-tau)	Increase to 200 % of control levels verified in numerous studies	Increase only found in AD	Uncertain. Increase in AD probably related to formation of tangles. P-tau levels using assays for different epitopes correlate.	Several validated, commercial immunoassays available. Increasingly used in clinical routine and trials.
	Synaptic degeneration	Increased levels of neurogranin reported	Unknown	Reflects dysfunction or loss of synapses	Under neurochemical and clinical validation
Aβ-related biomarkers	BACE1	Mild increase found in some studies but not all	Unknown	Relation between BACE1 protein level/activity in CSF and brain uncertain	Clinical diagnostic value uncertain. Potential use in trials to monitor effects on BACE1 activity.
	sAPPα and sAPPβ	No consistent alteration in biomarker levels	Reductions have been found in cerebrovascular disease, inflammatory conditions and ALS	Reflects α-secretase and β-secretase APP processing	Clinical diagnostic value uncertain. Used in trials to monitor effect on APP processing.
	Aβ oligomers	Increased levels reported, but inconsistently	Unknown	Size/nature of CSF Aβ oligomers unknown. Uncertain relation between oligomer levels in CSF and brain.	Under neurochemical and clinical validation
Biomarkers for other pathologies	Albumin ratio	No change in patients with pure AD	Increase in patients with cerebrovascular pathology and meningo-encephalitis	Increase indicates arteriolar/capillary pathology (blood-brain barrier damage)	Many validated commercial immunoassays available. Used in clinical routine.
	Neurofilament light protein (NFL)	Elevated in patients with subcortical involvement	Increase in patients with subcortical pathology, e.g. cerebrovascular disease, FTD, ALS and HIV-associated dementia	Increase indicates damage to large-caliber myelinated axons	Used in clinical routine
	Inflammation	Several candidate biomarkers have been investigated. Some studies have reported increased CSF levels of e.g. YKL-40 in AD.	Increase due to inflammation	Low- grade neuroinflammation	Under neurochemical and clinical validation

Fig. 20.2 Table of CSF biomarkers reviewed in this chapter. *AD* Alzheimer's disease, *ALS* amyotrophic lateral sclerosis, *BACE1* β-site APP cleaving enzyme 1, *CJD* Creutzfeldt-Jakob disease, *CSF* cerebrospinal fluid, *DLB* dementia with Lewy bodies, *FTD* frontotemporal dementia, *HIV* human immunodeficiency virus, *sAPP* soluble amyloid precursor protein

monitor biochemical actions of upcoming drugs. In this chapter, we review the literature of biomarkers related to AD and highlight their diagnostic capability as well as their relation to AD pathology. Figures 20.1 and 20.2 show a summary of the biomarkers reviewed in this chapter.

20.2 Core CSF AD Biomarkers

The CSF biomarkers for AD that have been most successful reflect the core cerebral pathologies of the disease.

20.2.1 Aβ42

Aβ is produced during normal cell metabolism and is secreted into the CSF (Seubert et al. 1992). The finding that Aβ42 is the most common isoform of Aβ in senile plaques led to development of assays for its quantification (Jarrett et al. 1993). The levels of CSF Aβ1-42 (Aβ42) are approximately 50 % lower in AD patients compared to controls, which has been shown with several different enzyme-linked immunosorbent assay (ELISA) methods (Sunderland et al. 2003; Blennow 2004). The most prevalent explanation for the reduced Aβ42 in CSF is that the sequestration into plaques in the brain leaves less available for diffusion into the CSF. Cerebral plaque load at autopsy correlates inversely with Aβ42 levels in lumbar CSF *antemortem* and ventricular CSF *postmortem* (Tapiola et al. 2009; Strozyk et al. 2003). Studies using PET for in vivo amyloid imaging have also found an inverse relationship between amyloid brain load and CSF Aβ42 (Fagan et al. 2006; Forsberg et al. 2008; Tolboom et al. 2009; Grimmer et al. 2009). Similar results have been obtained using the PET ligand [18F]FDDNP, which is believed to bind to both plaques and tangles (Tolboom et al. 2009). These findings provide support of the notion that CSF Aβ42 is a measure of fibrillar Aβ42 and cerebral plaque load. Importantly, recent large studies have shown that the agreement between CSF Aβ42 and amyloid PET measurements is very high, with more than 90 % concordance, demonstrating that these methods give similar diagnostic information (Palmqvist et al. 2014).

20.2.2 P-tau

The amount of P-tau in CSF is commonly measured by ELISAs targeting tau phosphorylated at either threonine 181 or threonine 231 (Kohnken et al. 2000; Vanmechelen et al. 2000). These assays correlate well and show a similar association with AD (Hampel et al. 2004). Patients with AD have increased levels of CSF P-tau, in most studies around 200–300 % of control levels, and the levels in CSF have been shown to correlate with cerebral tangle pathology at autopsy (Blennow 2004; Tapiola et al. 2009; Buerger et al. 2006). In a study where cortical biopsies were taken from living patients with normal pressure hydrocephalus, a correlation between the amount of hyperphosphorylated tau in the biopsies and P-tau levels in CSF was found (Seppala et al. 2012). This supports the hypothesis that CSF P-tau reflects cerebral tangle pathology and the phosphorylation state of tau.

20.2.3 T-tau

CSF total tau corresponds to the intensity of neuronal and axonal damage and degeneration, which has been demonstrated in several studies. Levels increase after cardiac arrest, stroke, and brain trauma and are associated with amount of damaged tissue as well as clinical outcome (Hesse et al. 2001; Ost et al. 2006; Zetterberg et al. 2006; Rosen et al. 2014). In patients with Creutzfeldt-Jakob disease (CJD), a rapid rate of neurodegeneration is present, which is reflected in CSF by very high levels of T-tau (Otto et al. 1997). There are several isoforms and phosphorylation sites of the tau protein (Portelius et al. 2008). The ELISA assay most frequently used is capable of detecting all isoforms independent of phosphorylation state (Blennow et al. 1995). Studies have consistently shown that patients with AD have increased levels with about 300 % compared with normal controls (Sunderland et al. 2003; Blennow 2004). Also, it has been shown that levels of CSF T-tau *ante-mortem* correlate with the load of tangle pathology at autopsy, which indicates that release of tau from tangle-bearing neurons may contribute to levels of T-tau. In line with this, binding of the PET ligand ^{18}FDDNP has been shown to correlate with CSF T-tau levels (Tolboom et al. 2009).

20.3 Core Biomarkers in Various Stages of AD

20.3.1 Preclinical AD

Studies on preclinical AD have either been cross sectional, including patients with FAD, or longitudinal, with healthy elderly cohorts followed over time. The cross-sectional studies have calculated expected age of disease onset, which they relate biomarker levels to. One study showed that mutation carriers had elevated levels of CSF T-tau 15 years before expected symptom onset and reduced levels of CSF Aβ42 10 years before expected symptom onset (Bateman et al. 2012). Another study showed increased CSF Aβ42 in mutation carriers 20 years before estimated MCI onset (Reiman et al. 2012). Other studies that included cognitively normal mutation carriers closer to expected onset of AD have found increased levels of P-tau or T-tau, reduced Aβ42, and reduced Aβ42: Aβ40 ratio in CSF in these individuals compared with controls (Ringman et al. 2012; Moonis et al. 2005; Ringman et al. 2008).

The longitudinal studies have included cognitively healthy individuals, from which baseline biomarker levels have been related to future decrease in cognitive function or development of MCI or AD. CSF levels of Aβ42 alone or in combination with T-tau or P-tau have been associated with impending cognitive impairment (Gustafson et al. 2007; Fagan et al. 2007; Stomrud et al. 2007). Increased rates of brain atrophy have been found in cognitively normal individuals with low levels of CSF Aβ42 (Schott et al. 2010; Fagan et al. 2009; Fjell et al. 2010). Increased ratio of T-tau:Aβ42 or low levels of CSF Aβ42 have been found to predict conversion to

MCI in cognitively normal individuals or AD in nondemented elderly individuals, respectively (Li et al. 2007; Skoog et al. 2003). One study found that the predictive ability of CSF $A\beta42$ for the development of MCI or AD in individuals with subjective complaints was superior to that of P-tau or T-tau (van Harten et al. 2012). However, long-term prospective CSF studies on cognitively normal individuals followed for 10–20 years until development of AD are missing. Also, the longitudinal studies are in fact cross sectional with respect to biomarker measurements, since baseline biomarker data has been correlated with longitudinal clinical outcome. True longitudinal studies with repeated biomarker measurements to determine the longitudinal biomarker trajectories are needed.

20.3.2 MCI Due to AD

Patients with MCI have a risk for AD over a 4.5-year period that is roughly tripled compared to cognitively normal controls (Bennett et al. 2002). The yearly progression rate from MCI to AD is around 10–15 % (Petersen 2004). Hence, long follow-up periods are required so that late converters are caught. Also, it is important to remember the heterogeneous nature of MCI, since affected individuals may progress to other dementias than AD, including vascular dementia (VaD), frontotemporal dementia (FTD), and dementia with Lewy bodies (DLB), or remain relatively stable in cognition (Petersen 2003). Patients with impending AD can be accurately distinguished from stable MCI patients by the CSF biomarker profile of low levels of $A\beta42$ in combination with high levels of P-tau and T-tau (Blennow and Hampel 2003). Different combinations of these biomarkers have been used in several studies to successfully predict AD in MCI patients (Hansson et al. 2006; Buchhave et al. 2012; Hertze et al. 2010; Visser et al. 2009; Shaw et al. 2009; Mattsson et al. 2009; Johansson et al. 2011a). CSF T-tau and P-tau levels have been associated with brain atrophy in early stage MCI/AD (Fagan et al. 2009). Also, the levels of these two biomarkers were higher in MCI patients with a more rapid progression to AD, indication that they may be related to disease progress (Buchhave et al. 2012).

20.3.3 AD with Dementia

The combination of $A\beta42$, P-tau, and T-tau can accurately distinguish AD patients from controls, with sensitivity and specificity over 80 % (Blennow 2004; Blennow and Hampel 2003). P-tau is the most AD specific of the biomarkers and may therefore be valuable when differentiating against other dementias (Hampel et al. 2010). Increased levels of P-tau have been found in patients with AD compared with patients suffering from FTD and VaD, DLB, and Parkinson disease with dementia (Hampel et al. 2004; Hall et al. 2012a). However, a large study on patients with AD as well as DLB, FTD, and VaD showed that an AD biomarker profile was present in a substantial part of the non-AD patients (Schoonenboom et al. 2012).

Potential reasons for this overlap may be misdiagnosis or the presence of mixed dementias. Future autopsy studies will hopefully shed light on this issue. The presence of mixed pathologies increases with age, but the applicability of the core AD CSF biomarkers has been assessed in AD patients in different ages (Mattsson et al. 2012a). It was found that the accuracy decreased with age, but the combination of the biomarkers gave sufficiently strong results for the biomarkers to be used in old patients. Some studies have evaluated the longitudinal alterations of the core biomarkers in AD patients. Levels of Aβ42 and P-tau remain largely unaltered over time, while data concerning T-tau is more inconclusive (Blennow et al. 2007; Zetterberg et al. 2007; Mattsson et al. 2012b; Buchhave et al. 2009; Le Bastard et al. 2013). Some studies have found an increase of T-tau over time, while others have found stable levels. However, high levels of P-tau and T-tau have been associated with a more rapid disease progression (Samgard et al. 2010; Wallin et al. 2010; van Rossum et al. 2012).

20.3.4 Autopsy-Verified AD

The diagnostic performance of CSF AD biomarkers has been evaluated by performing subsequent autopsy of patients after death. They can with high sensitivity and specificity discriminate AD from cognitively normal elderly as well as patients with other dementias, such as FTD, DLB, and VaD (Sunderland et al. 2003; Shaw et al. 2009; Clark et al. 2003; Bian et al. 2008; Koopman et al. 2009). CSF biomarkers provide similar or better diagnostic accuracy compared with only using clinical criteria for diagnosis.

20.4 Aβ-Related Biomarkers

20.4.1 BACE1

The activity of BACE1 has been assessed in AD patients, but the results have not been consistent. Smaller studies have found increased BACE1 activity in CSF from AD patients (Holsinger et al. 2004; Holsinger et al. 2006; Verheijen et al. 2006). One study found that the activity was increased in patients with MCI and dementia due to AD compared with controls (Zetterberg et al. 2008). Another study found elevated levels in MCI patients, but not in AD patients (Mulder et al. 2010; Zhong et al. 2007). Finally, three studies found no differences between AD patients and controls (Mulder et al. 2010; Zhong et al. 2007; Rosén et al. 2012; Perneczky et al. 2014). However, in one of these studies, AD patients were stratified according to disease severity, which revealed that patients with moderate–severe dementia had lower levels of BACE1 activity than patients with mild dementia (Rosén et al. 2012). Although there is no clear-cut role for BACE1 activity in the diagnosis of AD, it may be useful in clinical trials on BACE1-inhibitors to monitor target engagement of the drug.

20.4.2 sAPPα/sAPPβ

The soluble ectodomain of APP (sAPP) is released when the protein is cut by α- or β-secretase. The levels of sAPPα and sAPPβ correlate very well in CSF in both AD patients and controls (Zetterberg et al. 2008). A large number of studies have not shown any differences in levels when comparing AD patients with controls (Hertze et al. 2010; Johansson et al. 2011a; Zetterberg et al. 2008; Perneczky et al. 2014; Rosen et al. 2012; Olsson et al. 2003). Some studies report elevated levels of sAPPβ in MCI patients compared to controls or in MCI patients with impending AD (Olsson et al. 2003; Perneczky et al. 2011). The latter differences were not seen in another study (Hertze et al. 2010). Studies using the core CSF AD biomarkers to characterize patients have found elevated levels of sAPPα and sAPPβ in patients with MCI or dementia that had a biomarker profile indicative of AD pathology, but with large overlaps between diagnostic groups (Lewczuk et al. 2010, 2012; Gabelle et al. 2010). The diagnostic value of sAPP levels appears low, but they may be utilized in clinical trials for studying effects on the APP metabolism, where a dose-dependent decrease in CSF sAPPβ indicates target engagement in clinical trials on BACE1 inhibitors (May et al. 2011).

20.4.3 Aβ Oligomers

The association between brain amyloid burden and neuronal loss is poor (Gomez-Isla et al. 1997). However, it has been shown that soluble oligomers of Aβ are capable of inhibiting long-term potentiation in vivo and cause abnormal tau phosphorylation and neuritic dystrophy (Walsh et al. 2002; Zempel et al. 2010; Jin et al. 2011; De Felice et al. 2008). Hence, many studies report attempts to measure the CSF levels of Aβ oligomers in patients with AD. This has proven to be difficult and studies have shown that the CSF levels of Aβ oligomers are very low, probably less than 1 % of total Aβ levels, which make reliable quantification challenging. Elevated oligomer levels have been found in the brains and CSF of AD patients (Bruggink et al. 2013; Shankar et al. 2008; Gao et al. 2010; Fukumoto et al. 2010; Georganopoulou et al. 2005; Pitschke et al. 1998). Increased levels were also reported in cognitively normal subjects with a CSF biomarker profile that indicated AD neuropathology (Handoko et al. 2013). Other studies have not been able to find altered levels of Aβ oligomers in CSF from AD patients (Bruggink and Jongbloed 2012; Santos et al. 2012; Yang et al. 2013). Apart from the difficulties of measuring minute amounts of Aβ oligomers in CSF samples, it is also possible that different assays measure different variants of Aβ oligomers, which might explain the divergent results. The studies provide little characterization of what the various assays are measuring.

20.5 Biomarkers for Other Pathologies

20.5.1 Blood-Brain Barrier Disturbances

The major biomarker for the integrity of the blood-brain barrier is the ratio between albumin measured in CSF and blood. This albumin ratio is typically normal in AD patients but tends to be elevated in patients with cerebral small vessel disease (Blennow et al. 1990; Wallin et al. 1999). An increased ratio may also be found in Lyme disease (neuroborreliosis), together with findings such as monocytosis and signs of immunoglobulin production in the CSF (Tumani et al. 1995). New potential biomarkers of the blood-brain barrier that need further verification include secretory Ca2+-dependent phospholipase A2 activity and antithrombin III (Chalbot et al. 2010; Zetterberg et al. 2009).

20.5.2 Neurofilament Light (NFL) Protein

NFL is mainly present in large-caliber myelinated axons, and increased levels are seen in conditions with subcortical axonal degeneration, such as cerebral small vessel disease, FTD, and human immunodeficiency virus (HIV)-associated dementia (Rosengren et al. 1999; Agren-Wilsson et al. 2007; Wallin and Sjogren 2001; de Jong et al. 2007; Landqvist Waldo et al. 2013; Gisslen et al. 2007). It may thus be of value in the differential diagnostics of AD. The simultaneous finding of elevated T-tau and NFL levels in CSF indicates mixed forms of AD and cerebrovascular disease, which appears to be very common in unselected patients undergoing evaluation because of a suspected neurodegenerative disease (Skillback et al. 2013).

20.5.3 Inflammatory, Glial, and Oxidative Stress Biomarkers

Neuroinflammation is a nonspecific feature of AD, and microglial cells can be found around senile plaques. In the 1990s and early 2000s, several studies reporting alterations in different inflammatory markers in CSF of AD patients (e.g., α1-antichymotrypsin, isoprostane, the interleukins, tumor necrosis factor α, interferon-gamma, complement C1q, and transforming growth factor β) were published (Craig-Schapiro et al. 2009; Zetterberg et al. 2004). The results have though been very inconsistent. A meta-analysis of cytokines in AD in 2010 showed great diversity in the study results (Swardfager et al. 2010). Reasons for discrepancies could include methodological differences (e.g., in the procedures for CSF collection and processing, assay differences, and criteria used for subject ascertainment), prevalence of comorbidities in the studied cohorts, and methods of diagnosis.

A recently described mutation in the microglia-controlling triggering receptor expressed on myeloid cells-2 (*TREM2*) gene was associated with an increased risk of AD. This has increased the interest of the role of microglia in the development of AD. Microglia are the macrophages of the brain. The enzyme chitotriosidase is secreted by activated macrophages and its levels of which are increased in the lysosomal storage disorder Gaucher disease (Renkema et al. 1998; Hollak et al. 1994). Studies on AD patients have revealed increased levels in CSF, although with overlaps with control groups (Mattsson et al. 2011a; Watabe-Rudolph et al. 2012; Rosén et al. 2014). A glycoprotein that has great homology with chitotriosidase but lacks its enzymatic activity is YKL-40 (Hakala et al. 1993). It is present in both microglial cells and astrocytes, and increased levels have been found in AD patients compared with controls (Rosén et al. 2014; Craig-Schapiro et al. 2010; Perrin et al. 2011; Olsson et al. 2013). One study did not find altered levels in AD patients compared with controls (Mattsson et al. 2011a).

A degree of oxidative stress is present in brains of AD patients and contributes to neuronal damage. Free radicals can cause lipid peroxidation, a feature that may be studied using biomarkers. A compound named isoprostane is produced by free radical-dependent peroxidation of arachidonic acid (Morrow and Roberts 1997). A certain subset, called F2-isoprostane, has been found in increased levels in CSF from AD patients (Montine et al. 1999; Pratico et al. 2000; Montine et al. 2001; Montine et al. 2007). Elevated levels are also reported among MCI patients with impending AD as well as asymptomatic patients with FAD-causing mutations (Ringman et al. 2008; Brys and Pirraglia 2007).

20.5.4 Synaptic Biomarkers

Loss of synapses correlates with decrease in neurocognitive function in AD patients (Terry et al. 1991). Biomarkers that reflect this pathology would therefore be desirable. Synaptic proteins such as synaptotagmin, growth-associated protein (GAP-43), synaptosomal-associated protein (SNAP-25), rab3a, and neurogranin have been identified in human CSF, and elevated CSF levels of neurogranin have been reported in both MCI and AD (Davidsson et al. 1999; Thorsell et al. 2010). More research is needed to determine the biomarker potential of synaptic proteins in the CSF.

20.6 Standardization of Biomarkers

The core CSF AD biomarkers have a high diagnostic accuracy for AD, especially in monocenter studies (Andreasen et al. 2001; Tabaraud et al. 2012; Johansson et al. 2011b). However, there is a large variability in measurements between centers and laboratories (Mattsson et al. 2011b). Standardization of pre-analytical and analytical factors is therefore needed before the biomarkers can be implemented in clinical practice. The Alzheimer's Association has launched a Quality Control Program for CSF biomarkers with the aim of monitoring longitudinal variations and measurements between laboratories (Mattsson et al. 2011b). There are also several other ongoing initiatives, such as the Global Biomarker Standardization Consortium, the CSF-Proteins Working Group of International Federation of Clinical Chemistry and Laboratory Medicine, and the BIOMARKAPD project of the EU Joint Programme in Neurodegenerative Disease Research, that strive towards biomarker standardization (Carrillo et al. 2013). An important step in these standardization efforts is the development of mass spectrometry–based techniques for matrix-independent absolute quantification of $A\beta42$ in CSF. The first fully validated candidate reference measurement procedure for CSF $A\beta42$ based on single reaction monitoring (SRM) mass spectrometry has recently been published (Leinenbach et al. 2014). This type of techniques will serve to harmonize different immunoassays with the aim to make uniform cutoff levels across different laboratories.

20.7 CSF Biomarkers in Clinical Research

The CSF biomarkers reviewed above play several important roles in clinical research on AD. They may be used as inclusion criteria in clinical trials of disease-modifying anti-AD drug candidates to verify that the included patients have the pathological changes against which the drug is targeted (Blennow et al. 2010). They may also be used as pharmacodynamic markers or markers of target engagement to test if the drug had the desired biochemical effect in patients on active treatment (Hampel et al. 2014). The markers may also be used in longitudinal studies of healthy volunteers and patients in different stages of AD to learn more about the time course of the different pathogenic processes in AD (Blennow et al. 2010). As an example, proteins secreted into the CSF from activated microglia could be used for determining the role of microglial activation in the AD process. If microglial activation is involved in the disease process and precedes neurodegeneration, a prediction would be that patients on route to AD first drop in CSF $A\beta42$ (as a sign of $A\beta$ buildup in the brain), then increase in markers of microglial activation, which ultimately is followed by cognitive symptoms and rise in CSF tau (as a sign of neurodegeneration). If microglial activation is a phenomenon downstream of neurodegeneration, such biomarker signals would appear after the rise in CSF tau. Finally, biomarkers for AD-related pathophysiological processes have also proven useful as quantitative traits for genetic analyses (Cruchaga et al. 2013; Andreasson et al. 2014).

20.8 CSF Biomarkers in Other Neurodegenerative Diseases

Pathologies relating to more than one neurodegenerative disorder are not an uncommon finding in postmortem brains. One autopsy study on brains of patients who had a clinical diagnosis of AD found that only 13.6 % of them had pure AD neuropathology, while the others displayed concomitant pathologies such as DLB and TDP (Toledo et al. 2013). This can have an impact in treatment studies targeting a certain pathology, since unknown pathologies may be affecting the outcome. Hence, it is important to find accurate biomarkers relating to pathologies from other diseases than AD.

In the brains of FTD patients, common findings are the neuronal inclusions of tau, TDP-43, or FUS protein (Seelaar et al. 2011). It is a heterogeneous disorder with around one third of the patients having an autosomal dominant variant with mutations in progranulin, microtubule-associated protein tau, or *C9orf72*. The search for CSF biomarkers for FTD has had limited success. TDP-43 has been measured in the CSF of FTD patients, but appears to originate mainly from blood and be of minor diagnostic importance (Feneberg et al. 2014). Patients with FTD typically have normal or mildly elevated levels of T-tau, but the use of T-tau to distinguish between AD and FTD only gives sensitivity and specificity figures around 80 % (Hampel and Teipel 2004). However, FTD patients have normal levels of P-tau, which can improve the diagnostic separation (Hampel et al. 2004). Further, FTD goes with increased CSF levels of NFL (de Jong et al. 2007).

Patients with DLB and PD belong to a group of diseases called *synucleinopathies*, based on the findings of α-synuclein in the Lewy bodies that constitute the pathologic hallmark of the diseases. Efforts have been made to quantify α-synuclein in CSF to find a diagnostic biomarker. Lower CSF levels of α-synuclein have been found in patients suffering from α-synucleinopathies (van Dijk et al. 2014; Hong et al. 2010; Mollenhauer et al. 2011; Shi et al. 2011; Hall et al. 2012b; Kasuga et al. 2010), although not in all studies (Spies et al. 2009; Reesink et al. 2010; Noguchi-Shinohara et al. 2009). Altogether, the levels of α-synuclein seem to be reduced in patients with α-synucleinopathies, but with overlap between diagnostic groups. The use of CSF α-synuclein as a biomarker for PD and DLB is also complicated by the finding that α-synuclein seems to reflect neuronal degeneration, with a very marked increase in disorders with marked neuronal loss, such as CJD (Mollenhauer et al. 2008). DLB patients have decreased levels of Aβ42 together with normal or only slightly elevated levels of T-tau in CSF (Parnetti et al. 2008; Zetterberg et al. 2010). Also here, P-tau may be utilized for increased discriminatory power against AD (Parnetti et al. 2008; Vanmechelen et al. 2001).

Due to the heterogenic nature of VaD and also the high degree of uncertainty in the clinical diagnosis of VaD, especially to exclude that a patient fulfilling the clinical criteria for VaD does not have concomitant AD pathology, it is difficult to make definite statements about CSF biomarker changes in patients suffering from this disorder (Roh and Lee 2014). However, findings of an increase in the CSF/serum albumin ratio and an increased CSF NFL level in a patient with a clinical picture suggestive of VaD add support to this diagnosis, while concomitant findings of low CSF Aβ42 and P-tau support a diagnosis of mixed AD/VaD (Blennow et al. 1990; Wallin et al. 1999; Skillback et al. 2013; Sjogren et al. 2001).

As mentioned above, patients with CJD have very high CSF levels of T-tau. As they tend to have normal or slightly elevated CSF levels of P-tau, the ratio of P-tau and T-tau may be used to differentiate CJD from AD (Riemenschneider et al. 2003; Skillback et al. 2014). Indeed, the CJD biomarker profile (T-tau >1,400 ng/L and T-tau/P-tau ratio >25) shows a very high positive likelihood ratio (LR+) for CJD, both in the differential diagnosis against AD (LR + 197) and against other dementias (LR + 109) (Skillback et al. 2014).

20.9 Summary

Three CSF biomarkers reflect the core pathological features of AD: T-tau (neurode-generation), P-tau (tau hyperphosphorylation and tangle formation), and $A\beta42$ (plaque pathology). According to revised clinical criteria, these markers may help diagnosing AD also in pre-dementia stages of the disease. At present, their most obvious utility is in clinical trials of novel disease-modifying treatments against AD. In the future, they may help in selecting the right treatment for individual patients by making it possible to assess what molecular pathology that is most likely to cause the patient's symptoms. Research is currently identifying and validating biomarkers for additional pathophysiological processes, including microglial activation and synapse loss.

References

Agren-Wilsson A, Lekman A, Sjoberg W et al (2007) CSF biomarkers in the evaluation of idiopathic normal pressure hydrocephalus. Acta Neurol Scand 116(5):333–339

Ahn HJ, Seo SW, Chin J et al (2011) The cortical neuroanatomy of neuropsychological deficits in mild cognitive impairment and Alzheimer's disease: a surface-based morphometric analysis. Neuropsychologia 49(14):3931–3945

Albert MS, DeKosky ST, Dickson D et al (2011) The diagnosis of mild cognitive impairment due to Alzheimer's disease: recommendations from the National Institute on Aging-Alzheimer's Association workgroups on diagnostic guidelines for Alzheimer's disease. Alzheimers Dement 7(3):270–279

Alzheimer A (1987) About a peculiar disease of the cerebral cortex. By Alois Alzheimer, 1907 (Translated by L. Jarvik and H. Greenson). Alzheimer Dis Assoc Disord 1(1):3–8

Andreasen N, Minthon L, Davidsson P et al (2001) Evaluation of CSF-tau and CSF-Abeta42 as diagnostic markers for Alzheimer disease in clinical practice. Arch Neurol 58(3):373–379

Andreasson U, Lautner R, Schott JM et al (2014) CSF biomarkers for Alzheimer's pathology and the effect size of APOE varepsilon4. Mol Psychiatry 19(2):148–149

Bateman RJ, Xiong C, Benzinger TL et al (2012) Clinical and biomarker changes in dominantly inherited Alzheimer's disease. N Engl J Med 367(9):795–804

Bennett DA, Wilson RS, Schneider JA et al (2002) Natural history of mild cognitive impairment in older persons. Neurology 59(2):198–205

Bian H, Van Swieten JC, Leight S et al (2008) CSF biomarkers in frontotemporal lobar degeneration with known pathology. Neurology 70(19 Pt 2):1827–1835

Blennow K (2004) Cerebrospinal fluid protein biomarkers for Alzheimer's disease. NeuroRx 1(2):213–225

Blennow K, Hampel H (2003) CSF markers for incipient Alzheimer's disease. Lancet Neurol 2(10):605–613

Blennow K, Wallin A, Fredman P, Karlsson I, Gottfries CG, Svennerholm L (1990) Blood-brain barrier disturbance in patients with Alzheimer's disease is related to vascular factors. Acta Neurol Scand 81(4):323–326

Blennow K, Wallin A, Agren H, Spenger C, Siegfried J, Vanmechelen E (1995) Tau protein in cerebrospinal fluid: a biochemical marker for axonal degeneration in Alzheimer disease? Mol Chem Neuropathol 26(3):231–245

Blennow K, Zetterberg H, Minthon L et al (2007) Longitudinal stability of CSF biomarkers in Alzheimer's disease. Neurosci Lett 419(1):18–22

Blennow K, Hampel H, Weiner M, Zetterberg H (2010) Cerebrospinal fluid and plasma biomarkers in Alzheimer disease. Nat Rev Neurol 6(3):131–144

Bruggink KA, Jongbloed W, Biemans EA et al (2012) Amyloid-beta oligomer detection by enzyme-linked immunosorbent assay in cerebrospinal fluid and brain tissue. Anal Biochem 433(2):112–120

Bruggink KA, Jongbloed W, Biemans EA et al (2013) Amyloid-beta oligomer detection by ELISA in cerebrospinal fluid and brain tissue. Anal Biochem 433(2):112–120

Brys M, Pirraglia E, Rich K et al (2009) Prediction and longitudinal study of CSF biomarkers in mild cognitive impairment. Neurobiol Aging 30(5):682–690

Buchhave P, Blennow K, Zetterberg H et al (2009) Longitudinal study of CSF biomarkers in patients with Alzheimer's disease. PLoS One 4(7):e6294

Buchhave P, Minthon L, Zetterberg H, Wallin AK, Blennow K, Hansson O (2012) Cerebrospinal fluid levels of beta-amyloid 1-42, but not of tau, are fully changed already 5 to 10 years before the onset of Alzheimer dementia. Arch Gen Psychiatry 69(1):98–106

Buerger K, Ewers M, Pirttila T et al (2006) CSF phosphorylated tau protein correlates with neocortical neurofibrillary pathology in Alzheimer's disease. Brain 129(Pt 11):3035–3041

Carrillo MC, Blennow K, Soares H et al (2013) Global standardization measurement of cerebral spinal fluid for Alzheimer's disease: an update from the Alzheimer's Association Global Biomarkers Consortium. Alzheimers Dement 9(2):137–140

Chalbot S, Zetterberg H, Blennow K, Fladby T, Grundke-Iqbal I, Iqbal K (2010) Cerebrospinal fluid secretory Ca2+-dependent phospholipase A2 activity: a biomarker of blood-cerebrospinal fluid barrier permeability. Neurosci Lett 478(3):179–183

Chartier-Harlin MC, Crawford F, Houlden H et al (1991) Early-onset alzheimer's disease caused by mutations at codon 717 of the beta-amyloid precursor protein gene. Nature 353(6347):844–846

Clark CM, Xie S, Chittams J et al (2003) Cerebrospinal fluid tau and beta-amyloid: how well do these biomarkers reflect autopsy-confirmed dementia diagnoses? Arch Neurol 60(12):1696–1702

Craig-Schapiro R, Fagan AM, Holtzman DM (2009) Biomarkers of Alzheimer's disease. Neurobiol Dis 35(2):128–140

Craig-Schapiro R, Perrin RJ, Roe CM et al (2010) YKL-40: a novel prognostic fluid biomarker for preclinical Alzheimer's disease. Biol Psychiatry 68(10):903–912

Cruchaga C, Kauwe JS, Harari O et al (2013) GWAS of cerebrospinal fluid tau levels identifies risk variants for Alzheimer's disease. Neuron 78(2):256–268

Das P, Murphy MP, Younkin LH, Younkin SG, Golde TE (2001) Reduced effectiveness of Abeta1-42 immunization in APP transgenic mice with significant amyloid deposition. Neurobiol Aging 22(5):721–727

Davidsson P, Puchades M, Blennow K (1999) Identification of synaptic vesicle, pre- and postsynaptic proteins in human cerebrospinal fluid using liquid-phase isoelectric focusing. Electrophoresis 20(3):431–437

De Felice FG, Wu D, Lambert MP et al (2008) Alzheimer's disease-type neuronal tau hyperphosphorylation induced by A beta oligomers. Neurobiol Aging 29(9):1334–1347

de Jong D, Jansen RW, Pijnenburg YA et al (2007) CSF neurofilament proteins in the differential diagnosis of dementia. J Neurol Neurosurg Psychiatry 78(9):936–938

Fagan AM, Mintun MA, Mach RH et al (2006) Inverse relation between in vivo amyloid imaging load and cerebrospinal fluid Abeta42 in humans. Ann Neurol 59(3):512–519

Fagan AM, Roe CM, Xiong C, Mintun MA, Morris JC, Holtzman DM (2007) Cerebrospinal fluid tau/beta-amyloid(42) ratio as a prediction of cognitive decline in nondemented older adults. Arch Neurol 64(3):343–349

Fagan AM, Head D, Shah AR et al (2009) Decreased cerebrospinal fluid Abeta(42) correlates with brain atrophy in cognitively normal elderly. Ann Neurol 65(2):176–183

Feneberg E, Steinacker P, Lehnert S et al (2014) Limited role of free TDP-43 as a diagnostic tool in neurodegenerative diseases. Amyotroph Lateral Scler Frontotemporal Degener 15:351–356

Fjell AM, Walhovd KB, Fennema-Notestine C et al (2010) Brain atrophy in healthy aging Is related to CSF levels of A{beta}1-42. Cereb Cortex 20:2069–2079

Forsberg A, Engler H, Almkvist O et al (2008) PET imaging of amyloid deposition in patients with mild cognitive impairment. Neurobiol Aging 29(10):1456–1465

Fukumoto H, Tokuda T, Kasai T et al (2010) High-molecular-weight beta-amyloid oligomers are elevated in cerebrospinal fluid of Alzheimer patients. FASEB J 24(8):2716–2726

Gabelle A, Roche S, Geny C et al (2010) Correlations between soluble alpha/beta forms of amyloid precursor protein and Abeta38, 40, and 42 in human cerebrospinal fluid. Brain Res 1357:175–183

Gao CM, Yam AY, Wang X et al (2010) Abeta40 oligomers identified as a potential biomarker for the diagnosis of Alzheimer's disease. PLoS One 5(12):e15725

Garcia-Alloza M, Subramanian M, Thyssen D et al (2009) Existing plaques and neuritic abnormalities in APP:PS1 mice are not affected by administration of the gamma-secretase inhibitor LY-411575. Mol Neurodegener 4:19

Georganopoulou DG, Chang L, Nam JM et al (2005) Nanoparticle-based detection in cerebral spinal fluid of a soluble pathogenic biomarker for Alzheimer's disease. Proc Natl Acad Sci U S A 102(7):2273–2276

Gisslen M, Hagberg L, Brew BJ, Cinque P, Price RW, Rosengren L (2007) Elevated cerebrospinal fluid neurofilament light protein concentrations predict the development of AIDS dementia complex. J Infect Dis 195(12):1774–1778

Goedert M, Spillantini MG, Potier MC, Ulrich J, Crowther RA (1989) Cloning and sequencing of the cDNA encoding an isoform of microtubule-associated protein tau containing four tandem repeats: differential expression of tau protein mRNAs in human brain. Embo J 8(2):393–399

Gomez-Isla T, Hollister R, West H et al (1997) Neuronal loss correlates with but exceeds neurofibrillary tangles in Alzheimer's disease. Ann Neurol 41(1):17–24

Grimmer T, Riemenschneider M, Forstl H et al (2009) Beta amyloid in Alzheimer's disease: increased deposition in brain is reflected in reduced concentration in cerebrospinal fluid Biol Psychiatry 65(11):927–934

Grundke-Iqbal I, Iqbal K, Tung YC, Quinlan M, Wisniewski HM, Binder LI (1986) Abnormal phosphorylation of the microtubule-associated protein tau (tau) in Alzheimer cytoskeletal pathology. Proc Natl Acad Sci U S A 83(13):4913–4917

Gustafson DR, Skoog I, Rosengren L, Zetterberg H, Blennow K (2007) Cerebrospinal fluid beta-amyloid 1-42 concentration may predict cognitive decline in older women. J Neurol Neurosurg Psychiatry 78(5):461–464

Hakala BE, White C, Recklies AD (1993) Human cartilage gp-39, a major secretory product of articular chondrocytes and synovial cells, is a mammalian member of a chitinase protein family. J Biol Chem 268(34):25803–25810

Hall S, Ohrfelt A, Constantinescu R et al (2012a) Accuracy of a panel of 5 cerebrospinal fluid biomarkers in the differential diagnosis of patients with dementia and/or parkinsonian disorders. Arch Neurol 69(11):1445–1452

Hall S, Ohrfelt A, Constantinescu R et al (2012b) Accuracy of a panel of 5 cerebrospinal fluid biomarkers in the differential diagnosis of patients with dementia and/or parkinsonian disorders. Arch Neurol 69:1445–1452, 1–8

Hampel H, Teipel SJ (2004) Total and phosphorylated tau proteins: evaluation as core biomarker candidates in frontotemporal dementia. Dement Geriatr Cogn Disord 17(4):350–354

Hampel H, Buerger K, Zinkowski R et al (2004) Measurement of phosphorylated tau epitopes in the differential diagnosis of Alzheimer disease: a comparative cerebrospinal fluid study. Arch Gen Psychiatry 61(1):95–102

Hampel H, Blennow K, Shaw LM, Hoessler YC, Zetterberg H, Trojanowski JQ (2010) Total and phosphorylated tau protein as biological markers of Alzheimer's disease. Exp Gerontol 45(1):30–40

Hampel H, Lista S, Teipel SJ et al (2014) Perspective on future role of biological markers in clinical therapy trials of Alzheimer's disease: a long-range point of view beyond 2020. Biochem Pharmacol 88(4):426–449

Handoko M, Grant M, Kuskowski M et al (2013) Correlation of specific amyloid-beta oligomers with tau in cerebrospinal fluid from cognitively normal older adults. JAMA Neurol 1–6

Hansson O, Zetterberg H, Buchhave P, Londos E, Blennow K, Minthon L (2006) Association between CSF biomarkers and incipient Alzheimer's disease in patients with mild cognitive impairment: a follow-up study. Lancet Neurol 5(3):228–234

Hardy J (2009) The amyloid hypothesis for Alzheimer's disease: a critical reappraisal. J Neurochem 110(4):1129–1134

Hardy JA, Higgins GA (1992) Alzheimer's disease: the amyloid cascade hypothesis. Science 256(5054):184–185

Hertze J, Minthon L, Zetterberg H, Vanmechelen E, Blennow K, Hansson O (2010) Evaluation of CSF biomarkers as predictors of Alzheimer's disease: a clinical follow-up study of 4.7 years. J Alzheimers Dis 21(4):1119–1128

Hesse C, Rosengren L, Andreasen N et al (2001) Transient increase in total tau but not phospho-tau in human cerebrospinal fluid after acute stroke. Neurosci Lett 297(3):187–190

Hollak CE, van Weely S, van Oers MH, Aerts JM (1994) Marked elevation of plasma chitotriosi-dase activity. A novel hallmark of Gaucher disease. J clin invest 93(3):1288–1292

Holsinger RM, McLean CA, Collins SJ, Masters CL, Evin G (2004) Increased beta-secretase activity in cerebrospinal fluid of Alzheimer's disease subjects. Ann Neurol 55(6):898–899

Holsinger RM, Lee JS, Boyd A, Masters CL, Collins SJ (2006) CSF BACE1 activity is increased in CJD and Alzheimer disease versus [corrected] other dementias. Neurology 67(4):710–712

Hong Z, Shi M, Chung KA et al (2010) DJ-1 and alpha-synuclein in human cerebrospinal fluid as biomarkers of Parkinson's disease. Brain 133(Pt 3):713–726

Jack CR Jr, Knopman DS, Jagust WJ et al (2010) Hypothetical model of dynamic biomarkers of the Alzheimer's pathological cascade. Lancet Neurol 9(1):119–128

Jack CR Jr, Albert MS, Knopman DS et al (2011) Introduction to the recommendations from the National Institute on Aging-Alzheimer's Association workgroups on diagnostic guidelines for Alzheimer's disease. Alzheimers Dement 7(3):257–262

Jarrett JT, Berger EP, Lansbury PT Jr (1993) The carboxy terminus of the beta amyloid protein is critical for the seeding of amyloid formation: implications for the pathogenesis of Alzheimer's disease. Biochemistry 32(18):4693–4697

Jin M, Shepardson N, Yang T, Chen G, Walsh D, Selkoe DJ (2011) Soluble amyloid beta-protein dimers isolated from Alzheimer cortex directly induce Tau hyperphosphorylation and neuritic degeneration. Proc Natl Acad Sci U S A 108(14):5819–5824

Johansson P, Mattsson N, Hansson O et al (2011a) Cerebrospinal fluid biomarkers for Alzheimer's disease: diagnostic performance in a homogeneous mono-center population. J Alzheimers Dis 24(3):537–546

Johansson P, Johansson JO, Labrie F et al (2011b) Mild dementia is associated with increased adrenal secretion of cortisol and precursor sex steroids in women. Clin Endocrinol (Oxf) 75(3):301–308

Karran E, Mercken M, De Strooper B (2011) The amyloid cascade hypothesis for Alzheimer's disease: an appraisal for the development of therapeutics. Nat Rev Drug Discov 10(9):698–712

Kasuga K, Tokutake T, Ishikawa A et al (2010) Differential levels of alpha-synuclein, beta-amyloid42 and tau in CSF between patients with dementia with Lewy bodies and Alzheimer's disease. J Neurol Neurosurg Psychiatry 81(6):608–610

Kohnken R, Buerger K, Zinkowski R et al (2000) Detection of tau phosphorylated at threonine 231 in cerebrospinal fluid of Alzheimer's disease patients. Neurosci Lett 287(3):187–190

Koopman K, Le Bastard N, Martin JJ, Nagels G, De Deyn PP, Engelborghs S (2009) Improved discrimination of autopsy-confirmed Alzheimer's disease (AD) from non-AD dementias using CSF P-tau(181P). Neurochem Int 55(4):214–218

Landqvist Waldo M, Frizell Santillo A, Passant U et al (2013) Cerebrospinal fluid neurofilament light chain protein levels in subtypes of frontotemporal dementia. BMC Neurol 13:54

Le Bastard N, Aerts L, Sleegers K et al (2013) Longitudinal stability of cerebrospinal fluid bio-marker levels: fulfilled requirement for pharmacodynamic markers in Alzheimer's disease. J Alzheimers Dis 33(3):807–822

Leinenbach A, Pannee J, Dülffer T et al (2014) Mass spectrometry-based candidate reference mea-surement procedure for quantification of Aβ42 in cerebrospinal fluid. Clin Chem 60:987–994

Levites Y, Das P, Price RW et al (2006) Anti-Abeta42- and anti-Abeta40-specific mAbs attenuate amyloid deposition in an Alzheimer disease mouse model. J Clin Invest 116(1):193–201

Lewczuk P, Kamrowski-Kruck H, Peters O et al (2010) Soluble amyloid precursor proteins in the cerebrospinal fluid as novel potential biomarkers of Alzheimer's disease: a multicenter study. Mol Psychiatry 15(2):138–145

Lewczuk P, Popp J, Lelental N et al (2012) Cerebrospinal fluid soluble amyloid-beta protein precursor as a potential novel biomarkers of Alzheimer's disease. J Alzheimers Dis 28(1):119–125

Li G, Sokal I, Quinn JF et al (2007) CSF tau/Abeta42 ratio for increased risk of mild cognitive impairment: a follow-up study. Neurology 69(7):631–639

Masters CL, Simms G, Weinman NA, Multhaup G, McDonald BL, Beyreuther K (1985) Amyloid plaque core protein in Alzheimer disease and down syndrome. Proc Natl Acad Sci U S A 82(12):4245–4249

Mattsson N, Zetterberg H, Hansson O et al (2009) CSF biomarkers and incipient Alzheimer disease in patients with mild cognitive impairment. JAMA 302(4):385–393

Mattsson N, Tabatabaei S, Johansson P et al (2011a) Cerebrospinal fluid microglial markers in Alzheimer's disease: elevated chitotriosidase activity but lack of diagnostic utility. Neuromolecular Med 13(2):151–159

Mattsson N, Andreasson U, Persson S et al (2011b) The Alzheimer's Association external quality control program for cerebrospinal fluid biomarkers. Alzheimers Dement 7(4):386–95 e6

Mattsson N, Rosen E, Hansson O et al (2012a) Age and diagnostic performance of Alzheimer disease CSF biomarkers. Neurology 78(7):468–476

Mattsson N, Portelius E, Rolstad S et al (2012b) Longitudinal cerebrospinal fluid biomarkers over four years in mild cognitive impairment. J Alzheimers Dis 30(4):767–778

May PC, Dean RA, Lowe SL et al (2011) Robust central reduction of amyloid-beta in humans with an orally available, non-peptidic beta-secretase inhibitor. J neurosci 31(46):16507–16516

McKhann G, Drachman D, Folstein M, Katzman R, Price D, Stadlan EM (1984) Clinical diagnosis of Alzheimer's disease: report of the NINCDS-ADRDA Work Group under the auspices of Department of Health and Human Services Task Force on Alzheimer's Disease. Neurology 34(7):939–944

Mollenhauer B, Cullen V, Kahn I et al (2008) Direct quantification of CSF alpha-synuclein by ELISA and first cross-sectional study in patients with neurodegeneration. Exp Neurol 213(2):315–325

Mollenhauer B, Locascio JJ, Schulz-Schaeffer W, Sixel-Doring F, Trenkwalder C, Schlossmacher MG (2011) alpha-Synuclein and tau concentrations in cerebrospinal fluid of patients presenting with parkinsonism: a cohort study. Lancet Neurol 10(3):230–240

Montine TJ, Beal MF, Cudkowicz ME et al (1999) Increased CSF F2-isoprostane concentration in probable AD. Neurology 52(3):562–565

Montine TJ, Kaye JA, Montine KS, McFarland L, Morrow JD, Quinn JF (2001) Cerebrospinal fluid abeta42, tau, and f2-isoprostane concentrations in patients with Alzheimer disease, other dementias, and in age-matched controls. Arch Pathol Lab Med 125(4):510–512

Montine TJ, Quinn J, Kaye J, Morrow JD (2007) F(2)-isoprostanes as biomarkers of late-onset alzheimer's disease. J Mol Neurosci 33(1):114–119

Moonis M, Swearer JM, Dayaw MP et al (2005) Familial Alzheimer disease: decreases in CSF Abeta42 levels precede cognitive decline. Neurology 65(2):323–325

Morrow JD, Roberts LJ (1997) The isoprostanes: unique bioactive products of lipid peroxidation Prog Lipid Res 36(1):1–21

Mulder SD, van der Flier WM, Verheijen JH et al (2010) BACE1 activity in cerebrospinal fluid and its relation to markers of AD pathology. J Alzheimers Dis 20(1):253–260

Mullan M, Crawford F, Axelman K et al (1992) A pathogenic mutation for probable Alzheimer's disease in the APP gene at the N-terminus of beta-amyloid. Nat Genet 1(5):345–347

Noguchi-Shinohara M, Tokuda T, Yoshita M et al (2009) CSF alpha-synuclein levels in dementia with Lewy bodies and Alzheimer's disease. Brain Res 1251:1–6

Olsson A, Hoglund K, Sjogren M et al (2003) Measurement of alpha- and beta-secretase cleaved amyloid precursor protein in cerebrospinal fluid from Alzheimer patients. Exp Neurol 183(1):74–80

Olsson B, Hertze J, Lautner R et al (2013) Microglial markers are elevated in the prodromal phase of Alzheimer's disease and vascular dementia. J Alzheimers Dis 33(1):45–53

Ost M, Nylen K, Csajbok L et al (2006) Initial CSF total tau correlates with 1-year outcome in patients with traumatic brain injury. Neurology 67(9):1600–1604

Otto M, Wiltfang J, Tumani H et al (1997) Elevated levels of tau-protein in cerebrospinal fluid of patients with Creutzfeldt-Jakob disease. Neurosci Lett 225(3):210–212

Palmqvist S, Zetterberg H, Blennow K et al (2014) Accuracy of brain amyloid detection in clinical practice using cerebrospinal fluid Aβ42: a cross-validation study against amyloid PET in non-demented individuals. JAMA Neurol 71:1282–1289

Parnetti L, Tiraboschi P, Lanari A et al (2008) Cerebrospinal fluid biomarkers in Parkinson's disease with dementia and dementia with Lewy bodies. Biol Psychiatry 64(10):850–855

Perl DP (2010) Neuropathology of Alzheimer's disease. Mt Sinai J Med 77(1):32–42

Perneczky R, Tsolakidou A, Arnold A et al (2011) CSF soluble amyloid precursor proteins in the diagnosis of incipient Alzheimer disease. Neurology 77(1):35–38

Perneczky R, Alexopoulos P, Alzheimer's Disease Neuroimaging Initiative (2014) Cerebrospinal fluid BACE1 activity and markers of amyloid precursor protein metabolism and axonal degeneration in Alzheimer's disease. Alzheimers Dement 10:S425–S429

Perrin RJ, Craig-Schapiro R, Malone JP et al (2011) Identification and validation of novel cerebrospinal fluid biomarkers for staging early Alzheimer's disease. PLoS One 6(1):e16032

Petersen RC (2003) Mild cognitive impairment: aging to Alzheimer's disease. Oxford University Press, New York

Petersen RC (2004) Mild cognitive impairment as a diagnostic entity. J Intern Med 256(3):183–194

Pitschke M, Prior R, Haupt M, Riesner D (1998) Detection of single amyloid beta-protein aggregates in the cerebrospinal fluid of Alzheimer's patients by fluorescence correlation spectroscopy. Nat Med 4(7):832–834

Portelius E, Hansson SF, Tran AJ et al (2008) Characterization of tau in cerebrospinal fluid using mass spectrometry. J Proteome Res 7(5):2114–2120

Portelius E, Bogdanovic N, Gustavsson MK et al (2010) Mass spectrometric characterization of brain amyloid beta isoform signatures in familial and sporadic Alzheimer's disease. Acta Neuropathol 120(2):185–193

Pratico D, Clark CM, Lee VM, Trojanowski JQ, Rokach J, FitzGerald GA (2000) Increased 8,12-iso-iPF2alpha-VI in Alzheimer's disease: correlation of a noninvasive index of lipid peroxidation with disease severity. Ann Neurol 48(5):809–812

Raina P, Santaguida P, Ismaila A et al (2008) Effectiveness of cholinesterase inhibitors and memantine for treating dementia: evidence review for a clinical practice guideline. Ann Intern Med 148(5):379–397

Reesink FE, Lemstra AW, van Dijk KD et al (2010) CSF alpha-synuclein does not discriminate dementia with Lewy bodies from Alzheimer's disease. J Alzheimers Dis 22(1):87–95

Reiman EM, Quiroz YT, Fleisher AS et al (2012) Brain imaging and fluid biomarker analysis in young adults at genetic risk for autosomal dominant Alzheimer's disease in the presenilin 1 E280A kindred: a case-control study. Lancet Neurol 11(12):1048–1056

Renkema GH, Boot RG, Au FL et al (1998) Chitotriosidase, a chitinase, and the 39-kDa human cartilage glycoprotein, a chitin-binding lectin, are homologues of family 18 glycosyl hydrolases secreted by human macrophages. Eur J Biochem 251(1–2):504–509

Riemenschneider M, Wagenpfeil S, Vanderstichele H et al (2003) Phospho-tau/total tau ratio in cerebrospinal fluid discriminates Creutzfeldt-Jakob disease from other dementias. Mol Psychiatry 8(3):343–347

Ringman JM, Younkin SG, Pratico D et al (2008) Biochemical markers in persons with preclinical familial Alzheimer disease. Neurology 71(2):85–92

Ringman JM, Coppola G, Elashoff D et al (2012) Cerebrospinal fluid biomarkers and proximity to diagnosis in preclinical familial Alzheimer's disease. Dement Geriatr Cogn Disord 33(1):1–5

Roh JH, Lee JH (2014) Recent updates on subcortical ischemic vascular dementia. J stroke 16(1):18–26

Rosén C, Andreasson U, Mattsson N et al (2012) Cerebrospinal fluid profiles of amyloid β-related biomarkers in Alzheimer's disease. Neuromolecular Med 14(1):65–73

Rosen C, Andreasson U, Mattsson N et al (2012) Cerebrospinal fluid profiles of amyloid beta-related biomarkers in Alzheimer's disease. Neuromolecular Med 14(1):65–73

Rosen C, Rosen H, Andreasson U et al (2014) Cerebrospinal fluid biomarkers in cardiac arrest survivors. Resuscitation 85(2):227–232

Rosén C, Andersson C, Andreasson U et al (2014) Increased levels of chitotriosidase and YKL-40 in CSF from patients with Alzheimer's disease. Dement Geriatr Cogn Dis Extra 4:297–304

Rosengren LE, Karlsson JE, Sjogren M, Blennow K, Wallin A (1999) Neurofilament protein levels in CSF are increased in dementia. Neurology 52(5):1090–1093

Samgard K, Zetterberg H, Blennow K, Hansson O, Minthon L, Londos E (2010) Cerebrospinal fluid total tau as a marker of Alzheimer's disease intensity. Int J Geriatr Psychiatry 25(4):403–410

Santos AN, Ewers M, Minthon L et al (2012) Amyloid-beta oligomers in cerebrospinal fluid are associated with cognitive decline in patients with Alzheimer's disease. J Alzheimers Dis 29(1):171–176

Schoonenboom NS, Reesink FE, Verwey NA et al (2012) Cerebrospinal fluid markers for differential dementia diagnosis in a large memory clinic cohort. Neurology 78(1):47–54

Schott JM, Bartlett JW, Fox NC, Barnes J, Alzheimer's Disease Neuroimaging Initiative Initiative (2010) Increased brain atrophy rates in cognitively normal older adults with low cerebrospinal fluid Abeta1-42. Ann Neurol 68(6):825–834

Seelaar H, Rohrer JD, Pijnenburg YA, Fox NC, van Swieten JC (2011) Clinical, genetic and pathological heterogeneity of frontotemporal dementia: a review. J Neurol Neurosurg Psychiatry 82(5):476–486

Selkoe DJ (2001) Alzheimer's disease: genes, proteins, and therapy. Physiol Rev 81(2):741–766

Seppala TT, Nerg O, Koivisto AM et al (2012) CSF biomarkers for Alzheimer disease correlate with cortical brain biopsy findings. Neurology 78(20):1568–1575

Seubert P, Vigo-Pelfrey C, Esch F et al (1992) Isolation and quantification of soluble Alzheimer's beta-peptide from biological fluids. Nature 359(6393):325–327

Shankar GM, Li S, Mehta TH et al (2008) Amyloid-beta protein dimers isolated directly from Alzheimer's brains impair synaptic plasticity and memory. Nat Med 14(8):837–842

Shaw LM, Vanderstichele H, Knapik-Czajka M et al (2009) Cerebrospinal fluid biomarker signature in Alzheimer's disease neuroimaging initiative subjects. Ann Neurol 65(4):403–413

Shi M, Bradner J, Hancock AM et al (2011) Cerebrospinal fluid biomarkers for Parkinson disease diagnosis and progression. Ann Neurol 69(3):570–580

Siemers ER (2009) How can we recognize "disease modification" effects? J Nutr Health Aging 13(4):341–343

Sjogren M, Blomberg M, Jonsson M et al (2001) Neurofilament protein in cerebrospinal fluid: a marker of white matter changes. J Neurosci Res 66(3):510–516

Skillback T, Zetterberg H, Blennow K, Mattsson N (2013) Cerebrospinal fluid biomarkers for Alzheimer disease and subcortical axonal damage in 5,542 clinical samples. Alzheimers Res Ther 5(5):47

Skillback T, Rosen C, Asztely F, Mattsson N, Blennow K, Zetterberg H (2014) Diagnostic performance of cerebrospinal fluid total tau and phosphorylated tau in Creutzfeldt-Jakob disease: results from the Swedish Mortality Registry. JAMA Neuro 71(4):476–483

Skoog I, Davidsson P, Aevarsson O, Vanderstichele H, Vanmechelen E, Blennow K (2003) Cerebrospinal fluid beta-amyloid 42 is reduced before the onset of sporadic dementia: a population-based study in 85-year-olds. Dement Geriatr Cogn Disord 15(3):169–176

Sperling RA, Aisen PS, Beckett LA et al (2011a) Toward defining the preclinical stages of Alzheimer's disease: recommendations from the National Institute on Aging-Alzheimer's Association workgroups on diagnostic guidelines for Alzheimer's disease. Alzheimers Dement 7(3):280–292

Sperling RA, Jack CR Jr, Aisen PS (2011b) Testing the right target and right drug at the right stage. Sci transl med 3(111):111cm33

Spies PE, Melis RJ, Sjogren MJ, Rikkert MG, Verbeek MM (2009) Cerebrospinal fluid alpha-synuclein does not discriminate between dementia disorders. J Alzheimers Dis 16(2):363–369

Spires-Jones TL, Stoothoff WH, de Calignon A, Jones PB, Hyman BT (2009) Tau pathophysiology in neurodegeneration: a tangled issue. Trends Neurosci 32(3):150–159

Stomrud E, Hansson O, Blennow K, Minthon L, Londos E (2007) Cerebrospinal fluid biomarkers predict decline in subjective cognitive function over 3 years in healthy elderly. Dement Geriatr Cogn Disord 24(2):118–124

Strozyk D, Blennow K, White LR, Launer LJ (2003) CSF Abeta 42 levels correlate with amyloid-neuropathology in a population-based autopsy study. Neurology 60(4):652–656

Sunderland T, Linker G, Mirza N et al (2003) Decreased beta-amyloid1-42 and increased tau levels in cerebrospinal fluid of patients with Alzheimer disease. Jama 289(16):2094–2103

Swardfager W, Lanctot K, Rothenburg L, Wong A, Cappell J, Herrmann N (2010) A meta-analysis of cytokines in Alzheimer's disease. Biol Psychiatry 68(10):930–941

Tabaraud F, Leman JP, Milor AM et al (2012) Alzheimer CSF biomarkers in routine clinical setting. Acta Neurol Scand 125(6):416–423

Tapiola T, Alafuzoff I, Herukka SK et al (2009) Cerebrospinal fluid {beta}-amyloid 42 and tau proteins as biomarkers of Alzheimer-type pathologic changes in the brain. Arch Neurol 66(3):382–389

Terry RD, Masliah E, Salmon DP et al (1991) Physical basis of cognitive alterations in Alzheimer's disease: synapse loss is the major correlate of cognitive impairment. Ann Neurol 30(4):572–580

Thorsell A, Bjerke M, Gobom J et al (2010) Neurogranin in cerebrospinal fluid as a marker of synaptic degeneration in Alzheimer's disease. Brain Res 1362:13–22

Tolboom N, van der Flier WM, Yaqub M et al (2009) Relationship of cerebrospinal fluid markers to 11C-PiB and 18F-FDDNP binding. J nucl med 50(9):1464–1470

Toledo JB, Cairns NJ, Da X et al (2013) Clinical and multimodal biomarker correlates of ADNI neuropathological findings. Acta neuropathol Commun 1(1):65

Tumani H, Nolker G, Reiber H (1995) Relevance of cerebrospinal fluid variables for early diagnosis of neuroborreliosis. Neurology 45(9):1663–1670

van Dijk KD, Bidinosti M, Weiss A, Raijmakers P, Berendse HW, van de Berg WD (2014) Reduced alpha-synuclein levels in cerebrospinal fluid in Parkinson's disease are unrelated to clinical and imaging measures of disease severity. Eur J Neurol 21(3):388–394

van Duijn CM, Hendriks L, Cruts M, Hardy JA, Hofman A, Van Broeckhoven C (1991) Amyloid precursor protein gene mutation in early-onset alzheimer's disease. Lancet 337(8747):978

van Harten AC, Visser PJ, Pijnenburg YA et al (2013) Cerebrospinal fluid Abeta42 is the best predictor of clinical progression in patients with subjective complaints. Alzheimers Dement 9(5):481–487

van Rossum IA, Vos SJ, Burns L et al (2012) Injury markers predict time to dementia in subjects with MCI and amyloid pathology. Neurology 79(17):1809–1816

Vanmechelen E, Vanderstichele H, Davidsson P et al (2000) Quantification of tau phosphorylated at threonine 181 in human cerebrospinal fluid: a sandwich ELISA with a synthetic phospho-peptide for standardization. Neurosci Lett 285(1):49–52

Vanmechelen E, Van Kerschaver E, Blennow K, et al (2001) CSF-phospho-tau (181P) as a promising marker for discriminating Alzheimer's disease from dementia with Lewy bodies, in alzheimer's disease: advances in etiology, pathogenesis and therapeutics. John Wiley and Sons, England. pp 285–291

Verheijen JH, Huisman LG, van Lent N et al (2006) Detection of a soluble form of BACE-1 in human cerebrospinal fluid by a sensitive activity assay. Clin Chem 52(6):1168–1174

Visser PJ, Verhey F, Knol DL et al (2009) Prevalence and prognostic value of CSF markers of Alzheimer's disease pathology in patients with subjective cognitive impairment or mild cognitive impairment in the DESCRIPA study: a prospective cohort study. Lancet Neurol 8(7):619–627

Wallin A, Sjogren M (2001) Cerebrospinal fluid cytoskeleton proteins in patients with subcortical white-matter dementia. Mech Ageing Dev 122(16):1937–1949

Wallin A, Blennow K, Rosengren L (1999) Cerebrospinal fluid markers of pathogenetic processes in vascular dementia, with special reference to the subcortical subtype. Alzheimer Dis Assoc Disord 13(Suppl 3):S102–S105

Wallin AK, Blennow K, Zetterberg H, Londos E, Minthon L, Hansson O (2010) CSF biomarkers predict a more malignant outcome in Alzheimer disease. Neurology 74(19):1531–1537

Walsh DM, Klyubin I, Fadeeva JV et al (2002) Naturally secreted oligomers of amyloid beta protein potently inhibit hippocampal long-term potentiation in vivo. Nature 416(6880):535–539

Watabe-Rudolph M, Song Z, Lausser L et al (2012) Chitinase enzyme activity in CSF is a powerful biomarker of Alzheimer disease. Neurology 78(8):569–577

Yang T, Hong S, O'Malley T, Sperling RA, Walsh DM, Selkoe DJ (2013) New ELISAs with high specificity for soluble oligomers of amyloid beta-protein detect natural Abeta oligomers in human brain but not CSF. Alzheimers Dement 9(2):99–112

Zempel H, Thies E, Mandelkow E, Mandelkow EM (2010) Abeta oligomers cause localized Ca(2+) elevation, missorting of endogenous Tau into dendrites, Tau phosphorylation, and destruction of microtubules and spines. J neurosci 30(36):11938–11950

Zetterberg H, Andreasen N, Blennow K (2004) Increased cerebrospinal fluid levels of transforming growth factor-beta1 in Alzheimer's disease. Neurosci Lett 367(2):194–196

Zetterberg H, Hietala MA, Jonsson M et al (2006) Neurochemical aftermath of amateur boxing. Arch Neurol 63(9):1277–1280

Zetterberg H, Pedersen M, Lind K et al (2007) Intra-individual stability of CSF biomarkers for Alzheimer's disease over two years. J Alzheimers Dis 12(3):255–260

Zetterberg H, Andreasson U, Hansson O et al (2008) Elevated cerebrospinal fluid BACE1 activity in incipient Alzheimer disease. Arch Neurol 65(8):1102–1107

Zetterberg H, Andreasson U, Blennow K (2009) CSF antithrombin III and disruption of the blood-brain barrier. J Clin Oncol 27(13):2302–2303; author reply 3–4

Zetterberg H, Mattsson N, Blennow K (2010) Cerebrospinal fluid analysis should be considered in patients with cognitive problems. Int J Alzheimers Dis 2010:163065

Zhong Z, Ewers M, Teipel S et al (2007) Levels of beta-secretase (BACE1) in cerebrospinal fluid as a predictor of risk in mild cognitive impairment. Arch Gen Psychiatry 64(6):718–726

Paraneoplastic Neurological Syndromes

21

Jan Lewerenz and Frank Leypoldt

Contents

Abstract

In this chapter, we summarise the current knowledge about a group of clinically diverse neurological syndromes that are unified by a common pathophysiology, mostly immune-mediated neuronal dysfunction or degeneration triggered by a distant tumour and thus are coined paraneoplastic neurological syndromes (PNS). In

J. Lewerenz (✉)
Universitätsklinik für Neurologie, Universitäts- und Rehabilitationskliniken Ulm,
Oberer Eselsberg 45, Ulm 89081, Germany
e-mail: jan.lewerenz@googlemail.com

F. Leypoldt
Neuroimmunologie, Klinische Chemie und Neuroimmunologische Ambulanz,
NeurologieUniversitätsklinik Schleswig-Holstein Campus,
Kiel Arnold-Heller-Str. 3, Kiel 24105, Germany

© Springer International Publishing Switzerland 2015
F. Deisenhammer et al. (eds.), *Cerebrospinal Fluid in Clinical Neurology*,
DOI 10.1007/978-3-319-01225-4_21

the majority of cases, antibodies against onconeural, intracellular antigens expressed by the tumour and the nervous system can be detected in serum and cerebrospinal fluid. Some clinical pictures are suggestive of an underlying PNS. These syndromes include progressive cerebellar degeneration, encephalomyelitis, limbic encephalitis, opsoclonus-myoclonus syndrome, subacute sensory neuronopathy, chronic gastro-intestinal pseudo-obstruction and Lambert-Eaton myasthenic syndrome. These clinical manifestations are called classical paraneoplastic syndromes. Other neurological syndromes like brainstem encephalitides or neuropathies can have diverse aetiologies, amongst which a tumour-triggered immune response is one possibility amongst many others. The detection of onconeural antibodies in suspected PNS confirms the diagnosis and aids in diagnosis, tumour search and therapy. Here, we summarise the practical approach, typical findings and the most important syndromes including electrophysiological tests, imaging and cerebrospinal fluid analysis. Not obligatorily paraneoplastic autoimmune encephalitides associated with antibodies against neuronal surface proteins are covered by a separate chapter of this book.

21.1   Definition and Introduction

By definition, all neurological complications of a neoplastic disorder that are not caused by (1) direct compression or infiltration of neuronal structures by tumour cells, (2) metabolic derangements, (3) toxic treatment effects or (4) infections are called "paraneoplastic". However, the current use of the term "paraneoplastic neurological syndrome (PNS)" generally implies an immune-mediated aetiology of neurological dysfunction or neurodegeneration that is triggered by an underlying tumour. In 1985, Graus and colleagues discovered that some of these cases harbour a distinct antibody in their serum that labels neuronal nuclei (Graus et al. 1985). This antibody became known as anti-Hu (Graus et al. 1987) or antineuronal nuclear antibody 1 (ANNA1) (Kimmel et al. 1988). Subsequently, additional antibodies associated with this or other paraneoplastic neurological syndromes were discovered, the second of which was the anti-Yo antibody. The anti-Yo antibody recognises the CDR (cerebellar-degeneration-related) 34 and 62 proteins expressed in Purkinje cells (Cunningham et al. 1986). It occurs in patients with mostly gynaecological tumours and subacute cerebellar degeneration (Anderson et al. 1988a). Within the following decades, the number of different antineuronal antibodies associated with PNS grew. Whereas the antibodies characterised first are named by the first two initials of the index patients (Hu = Hull, Ri = Richards, Yo = Young (Luque et al. 1991)) or by the order of detection (antineuronal nuclei antibody (ANNA)-1, ANNA-2 and Purkinje cell antibody (PCA)-1) (Lennon 1994), respectively, later on the names indicate the name of the proteins recognised by the antibody (e.g. anti-CRMP5 (Yu et al. 2001)). As a general rule, the more recently the antibodies were characterised, the rarer they occur. Currently, these "classical paraneoplastic antibodies" are categorised into two different subgroups: (1) well-characterised onconeural antibodies with a high probability of an underlying malignancy and (2) partially characterised onconeural antibodies with an unknown specificity for a tumour because of small numbers of reported patients. This classification, which was introduced in 2004, does not encompass the novel "synaptic" encephalitis syndromes with antibodies against neuronal surface antigens which occur with and without underlying tumours. For systematic reasons, this latter group of autoimmune encephalitides is discussed in detail in Chap. 6 of this book.

21.2 Practical Approach and General Aspects

Paraneoplastic neurological syndromes are rare diseases. Thus, the a priori chance of a paraneoplastic aetiology is low. Nevertheless, clinical syndromes can be divided into those with a high likelihood of paraneoplastic aetiology and those only rarely associated with underlying cancer. These have been termed "classical syndromes" and "nonclassical syndromes", which are discussed in detail below (Graus et al. 2004). While classical syndromes, e.g. limbic encephalitis (LE) or progressive cerebellar degeneration (PCD), have a high likelihood of an underlying paraneoplastic aetiology, nonclassical syndromes, e.g. brainstem encephalitis or optic neuritis, are usually caused by other diseases. Red flags for a paraneoplastic aetiology are the presence of a subacute, relentlessly progressive syndrome, consecutive or simultaneous affection of different areas of the central and/or peripheral nervous system and a high individual tumour risk (e.g. smoking, weight loss). Other neurological syndromes have diverse aetiolologies, amongst which a tumour-triggered immune response is only one remote possibility. These include brainstem encephalitis, optic neuritis, retinal degeneration, stiff-person syndrome, myelitis and motor neuron disease. Regarding the peripheral nervous system, diverse types of neuropathies including Guillain-Barré syndrome lookalikes and also vasculitic neuropathies, brachial neuritis and autonomic neuropathies can potentially be caused by an underlying malignancy. In some cases, also myasthenia gravis when associated with a thymoma can be regarded as a PNS, as well as some tumour-associated cases of acquired neuromyotonia (Graus et al. 2004).

The first step in the diagnostic workup of a neurological syndrome suspected to be paraneoplastic in origin is to prove its immune-mediated nature and rule out obvious differential diagnoses like meningeal disease, metastasis, toxic or metabolic causes. Next, if clinical suspicion of paraneoplastic aetiology remains high, screening for relevant onconeural or neuronal cell-surface antibodies should be initiated. Their presence or absence helps to further predict the probability and location of underlying cancer. Imaging studies are important to exclude differential diagnoses and in a minority of cases show abnormalities compatible with a PNS. The last step would be a tumour screening guided by the clinical information and antibody status.

Detecting antibodies against onconeural antigens, e.g. Hu, CV2/CRMP5, Yo and amphiphysin, together with a compatible neurological syndrome has a very high specificity for a PNS. However, most syndromes can be associated with different antibodies (Table 21.1) and different syndromes can occur with the same antibody.

Table 21.1 Syndromes of the CNS and relevant well-characterised onconeural or neuronal cell-surface antibodies

	Syndrome	Relevant antibodies
CNS	Subacute cerebellar degeneration 25 %	Hu, Yo, CV2/CRMP5, Ri, Tr[a], amphiphysin, VGCC
	Encephalomyelitis 6 %	Hu, CV2/CRMP5, amphiphysin
	Limbic encephalitis 10 %	Hu, Ma2, CV2/CRMP5, Ri, amphiphysin
		NMDAR, Lgi1[b], CASPR2[b], GABA(b)-R, AMPA-R, mGluR5, glyR[b], GAD[b]
	Opsoclonus-myoclonus syndrome (adults) 2 %	Ri, Hu, Ma/Ta, NMDAR
	Retinopathy 1 %	Hu, CV2/CRMP5, recoverin
	Stiff-person syndrome 1 %	Amphiphysin, glyR[b], GAD[b]

[a]Tr antibodies, are not considered well-characterised but should raise a high suspicion of underlying cancer
[b]Lgi1, GAD' glycine-receptor antibody-associated syndromes are rarely paraneoplastic

In addition, patients with PNS can harbour more than one onconeural antibody in serum and CSF (Pittock et al. 2003). Moreover, specific onconeural antibodies are associated with different types of cancer. The rather complex association of onconeural antibodies, different PNS and underlying cancers is summarised in Table 21.2. Of note, onconeural antibodies like anti-Hu antibodies, although at lower titres than those associated with PNS, occur in patients with tumours but without neurological syndromes (Monstad et al. 2009).

The probability of a PNS depends on (1) the occurrence of a classical or nonclassical syndrome, (2) absence or presence of a detectable tumour and (3) detection of a well-characterised antibody, partially characterised antibody or absence of known antibodies (Fig. 21.1). Classical syndromes and detectable tumours or any syndrome and detectable well-characterised antibodies can be classified as definite PNS. A nonclassical syndrome associated with a malignancy is considered to represent a definite PNS if either a well-characterised or partially characterised antibody can be detected or the neurological sign and symptoms respond to treatment of the underlying malignancy. Other situations can be classified as possible PNS after exclusion of differential diagnoses.

In most patients with PNS, neurological symptoms precede tumour diagnosis, because tumours are too small to be detectable with available techniques. If any classical or nonclassical syndrome co-occurs with a well-characterised onconeural (e.g. Hu, Yo) antibody, initial tumour screening should be carried out according to recently published European guidelines and close oncological follow-up every 3–6 months for 4 years is warranted (Titulaer et al. 2011a). A similar tumour screening approach is advisable for classical syndromes without well-characterised or with partially characterised antibodies. If the syndrome is nonclassical and no antibodies are found, the method of tumour screening and surveillance depends on the level of clinical suspicion and no clear guidelines exist. It is good clinical practice to perform close clinical follow-up visits and possibly repeat tumour screening but alternative diagnoses have to be considered frequently.

Table 21.2 Onconeural antibodies found in paraneoplastic syndromes

Antibody	Antigen	Associated syndromes and symptoms	Most common tumours
Onconeural antibodies (well-characterised, paraneoplastic antibodies tumour in >90 %)			
Anti-Hu (ANNA-1)	HuD	Encephalomyelitis, limbic encephalitis, cerebellar degeneration, brainstem encephalitis, multi-segmental myelitis, sensory neuronopathy, sensory-motor neuropathy, autonomic neuropathy	Lung cancer (85 %), mostly SCLC, neuroblastoma, prostate carcinoma
Anti-Yo (PCA-1)	CDR2, CDR62	Paraneoplastic cerebellar degeneration	Ovarian, breast cancer
Anti-CV2/ CRMP5	CRMP5	Encephalomyelitis, polyneuropathy, optic neuritis, limbic encephalitis, choreatic syndromes, cerebellar degeneration	SCLC, thymoma
Anti-Ta/Ma2[a]	MA-proteins	Limbic encephalitis, rhombencephalitis, m>>f	Testicular cancer
Anti-Ri (ANNA-2)	NOVA-1	Opsoclonus-myoclonus syndrome, rhombencephalitis, cerebellar degeneration, myelitis, jaw dystonia, laryngospasm	Breast, ovarian carcinoma, SCLC
Anti-amphiphysin	AMPHIPHYSIN	Stiff-person syndrome, limbic encephalitis, rhombencephalitis, cerebellar degeneration, polyneuropathy	Breast cancer, SCLC
Anti-recoverin	RECOVERIN	Retinopathy	SCLC
Anti-SOX-1 (AGNA)	SOX-1	Non syndrome-specific	Sensitivity 67 %, specificity 95 % for SCLC in LEMS
Partially characterised onconeural antibodies (antigen not characterised or positive predictive value for tumour unknown)			
Anti-Tr (PCA-Tr)	DNER	Cerebellar degeneration	Hodgkin lymphoma, non-Hodgkin lymphoma
Anti-Zic4	ZIC1-4	Cerebellar degeneration	SCLC
PCA-2	280 kD	Encephalitis, Lambert-Eaton myasthenic syndrome, polyneuropathy	SCLC
ANNA-3	170 kD	Neuropathy, cerebellar degeneration, limbic encephalitis	SCLC

Alternative names are given in brackets

DNER delta/notch-like epidermal growth factor-related receptor

[a]In some patients coexisting Ma1 antibodies, in which case often brainstem syndromes and non-testicular tumours predominate

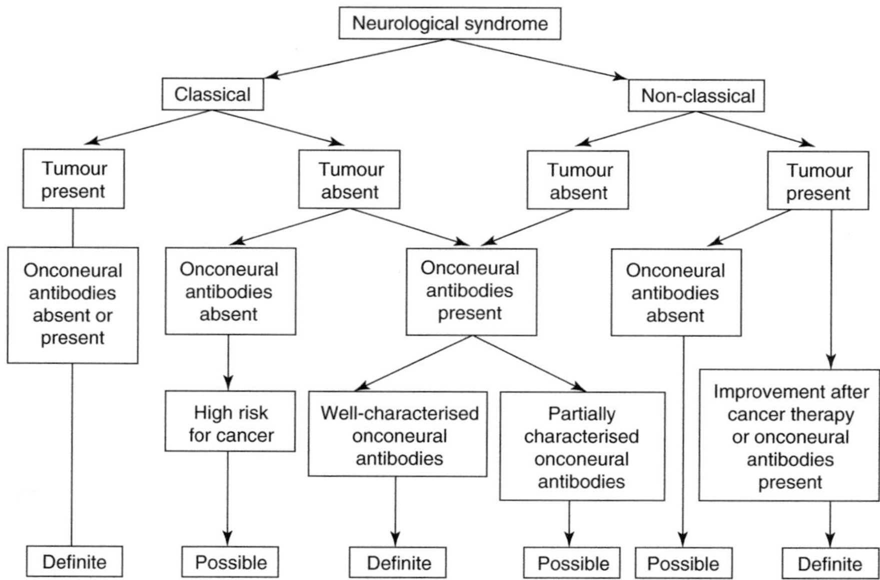

Fig. 21.1 Flow chart showing the level of diagnostic evidence of a paraneoplastic neurological syndrome depending on the neurological syndrome, the presence of absence of onconeural antibodies and a tumour. Of note, a definite and possible PNS without detection of a tumour requires regular tumour screenings for 4 years (Reprinted with permission from Graus et al. (2004))

21.3 Pathophysiology

In most paraneoplastic neurological syndromes described in this chapter, ectopic expression of neuronal antigens by systemic tumours drives an immune-mediated inflammatory response against central or peripheral nervous tissue. These *onconeural* antigens can be expressed by many tumours and most often by tumours of neuroectodermal lineage, e.g. small-cell lung cancer (SCLC). Antitumour immune responses are a common phenomenon, e.g. low titre anti-Hu antibodies are detectable in approximately 16 % of patients with SCLC without neurological symptoms (Dalmau et al. 1990; Graus et al. 1997). However, only a minority of these develop a paraneoplastic neurological syndrome. This might be due to intrinsic tumour factors (degree of inflammation, downregulation of HLA) (Maverakis et al. 2012), which causes breach of tolerance to self antigens. Furthermore, host factors like human leucocyte antigens (HLA) haplotypes likely contribute (Dalmau et al. 1995), but the main factors remain unclear.

Recent years have shown that the subcellular localisation of the detected antigen plays a major role for disease mechanisms. As already mentioned, onconeural antibodies are directed against intracellular antigens. These are not directly accessible to the antibodies. Most likely, the main pathogenic effect is carried out by cytotoxic T cells, resulting in neuronal cell death (Lancaster and Dalmau 2012). There are some exceptions to this rule. Amphiphysin antibodies might have a direct pathophysiological effect as suggested by in vivo models although the antigen is localised intracellularly (Sommer et al. 2005). Conversely, antibodies directed against neuronal surface proteins, δ/notch-like epidermal growth factor-related receptor (DNER), also known as anti-Tr (Greene et al. 2014; de Graaff et al. 2012), and antibodies against metabotropic glutamate receptor 5 (mGluR5) (Lancaster et al. 2011; Graus et al. 2014) can be found in PCD and LE in association with Hodgkin lymphomas (HL), respectively. However, beyond their atypical cellular localisation, the pathophysiology of anti-Tr and anti-mGluR5 antibody-associated PNS might differ with respect to cause of the autoimmune response as, in contrast to other onconeural antibodies, these antigens are not expressed in the underlying tumours (Graus et al. 2014). Nevertheless, this distinction helps to differentiate the paraneoplastic syndromes described in this chapter from the therapy-responsive encephalitis syndromes associated with neuronal surface and synaptic antibodies described in Chap. 6.

In Lambert-Eaton myasthenic syndrome (LEMS), antibodies directed against presynaptic P/Q-type voltage-gated calcium channels (VGCC) directly interfere with proper depolarisation-dependent acetylcholine release within the neuromuscular junction (Titulaer et al. 2011b). In paraneoplastic LEMS, the underlying SCLCs express VGCC (Roberts et al. 1985). However, as antibodies against VGCC also occur in non-paraneoplastic LEMS, which present about 50 % of the cases (Titulaer et al. 2011b), VGCC antibodies are not regarded as onconeural antibodies.

Not all paraneoplastic syndromes involving the nervous system are induced by an immune attack against structures of the nervous system. A notable exception is the POEMS syndrome. This acronym stands for polyneuropathy, organomegaly, edema, M-gradient and skin changes (Li and Zhou 2013). This subtype of monoclonal gammopathy-associated neuropathy normally shows an M-gradient representing IgA lambda. The assumed pathophysiology is a massively increased vascular endothelial growth factor (VEGF) contents in the patient's platelets somehow induced by the neoplastic plasma cells. VEGF is thought to induce a breakdown of the blood-nerve barrier with subsequent influx of serum proteins and demyelination. Highly increased serum VEGF levels are diagnostic.

21.4 Classical and Nonclassical Paraneoplastic Neurological Syndromes

21.4.1 Progressive Cerebellar Degeneration

PCD is one of the paraneoplastic syndromes with onconeural antibodies most frequently encountered in clinical practice (Giometto et al. 2010). Typical PCD clinically presents as a pancerebellar syndrome with both truncal and appendicular ataxia. Although initially, there can be asymmetrical involvement of the limbs, during the course of the disease the ataxia becomes symmetrical. Disability is usually severe so that most patients become unable to walk or even sit without support. Most patients have dysarthria, in part to an extend that speech becomes unintelligible, and nystagmus (Anderson et al. 1988a). Neurological symptoms progress over a few weeks or months and eventually stabilise, unfortunately most often with severe residual and permanent symptoms due to cerebellar dysfunction (Anderson et al. 1988a). Most patients have other signs of neuronal involvement beyond the cerebellum including extensor plantar responses, hyporeflexia or mild cognitive dysfunction. In some cases, progressive involvement of neuronal structures other than the cerebellum is observed leading to the diagnosis of progressive encephalomyelitis.

In an initial series, approximately 50 % of patients with PCD had detectable antineuronal antibodies upon screening using immunohistochemistry (Anderson et al. 1988a). In a later series of patients positive for antineuronal antibodies, five different antibody specificities were identified in PCD (Shams'ili et al. 2003): anti-Yo antibodies were most frequent, closely followed by anti-Hu antibodies. Anti-Tr (recently identified as directed against DNER) and anti-Ri occurred less often and anti-mGluR1 antibodies were rare. Another well-defined onconeural antibody detected in some cases of PCD is anti-CV2/CRMP5 (Honnorat et al. 1996). In addition, serum and CSF of patients with PCD and SCLC often harbours antibodies against VGCC (Graus et al. 2002) and in some cases against Zic4 (Bataller et al. 2004). Patients with PCD and VGCC antibodies should be examined for the presence of Lambert-Eaton myasthenic syndrome (Mason et al. 1997). One of four cases of anti-Ca/anti-ARHGAP26 antibodies and PCD has been reported to be paraneoplastic because of the coincidence with ovarian cancer (Jarius et al. 2013). In addition, two patients with antibodies against protein kinase Cγ, which is highly expressed in Purkinje cells, and cancer have been reported (Sabater et al. 2006; Hoftberger et al. 2013).

The severity of clinical impairment due to cerebellar dysfunction correlates with the antibodies detected. Compared to patients with anti-Yo, anti-Hu and anti-Tr, patients with anti-Ri antibodies retain their ability to walk far more often (Shams'ili et al. 2003). Anti-Ri antibodies were also associated with a lower incidence of dysarthria and nystagmus while anti-Hu positivity was associated with an increased incidence of additional neurological signs and symptoms. The median survival of patients with anti-Yo and anti- Hu antibodies and PCD was 13 and 7 months, respectively. This was much shorter than the survival in the group of patients with anti-Tr antibodies (>113 months). Also patients with anti-Ri-associated PCD tended to live longer. Interestingly, in a subset of patients with anti-Ri and anti-Tr antibodies, symptoms can improve considerably upon treatment (Shams'ili et al. 2003; Bernal et al. 2003), which only rarely occurs in anti-Yo-positive patients (Shams'ili et al. 2003).

Upon histopathological examination, PCD is characterised by a severe and diffuse loss of Purkinje cells throughout the cerebellum associated with CD8+ T-cell infiltrates and microglial activation throughout the brain (Giometto et al. 1997; Storstein et al. 2006).

Usually the neurological syndrome stabilises after several months but functionally on a very poor level with 90 % of patients being wheelchair bound (McKeon et al. 2011a). On magnetic resonance imaging (MRI) early during the disease, usually no abnormalities are found. Within months, atrophy may develop (McKeon et al. 2011a). In a few cases, fluor-deoxyglucose-positron-emission-tomography (FDG-PET) showed cerebellar hypermetabolism early during the disease (Choi et al. 2006).

The differential diagnosis of PCD is broad. Cerebellar ataxia can evolve as a predominant symptom in many neurological diseases, e.g. spinocerebellar ataxias, multiple system atrophy and non-paraneoplastic immune-mediated cerebellitis associated with antibodies against glutamic acid decarboxylase (GAD). However, paraneoplastic cerebellar degeneration is distinguished from these disorders by its relentless, subacute progression. In addition to its slower progression and indolent course, anti-GAD-positive cerebellar degeneration is also often associated with other autoimmune diseases including diabetes mellitus, thyroiditis and sometimes vitiligo (Honnorat et al. 2001). In some cases, Creutzfeldt-Jakob disease (CJD) can mimic PCD (Grau-Rivera et al. 2014). Cerebellitis of infectious origin, e.g. varicella zoster virus, can initially mimic PCD; however, it usually occurs in children (Bozzola et al. 2014). In rare occasions, HIV infection can induce progressive cerebellar ataxia (Tagliati et al. 1998) or it is a caused by infratentorial progressive multifocal leucoencephalopathy in the context of AIDS (Ali et al. 2013) or immunosuppression (Jones et al. 1982). The initial phase of Wernicke-Korsakoff syndrome due to thiamine deficiency can be dominated by subacute ataxia (Butterworth 1993).

21.4.2 Subacute Sensory Neuronopathy

Subacute sensory neuronopathy (SSN) is by far the most frequently encountered PNS affecting the peripheral nervous system (Giometto et al. 2010). This unique syndrome was initially described by Denny-Brown in two cases with neuropathy associated in bronchial carcinoma in 1948 (Denny-Brown 1948). Patients with SSN are characterised by subacutely spreading, frequently asymmetrical, non-length-dependent numbness and paraesthesias, including the face and trunk, which are associated with severe sensory ataxia. About half of the patients report neuropathic pains. Clinically, there is no motor involvement. Due to sensory ataxia, most patients become unable to walk without aid. In addition, frequently dysautonomia is observed. Just recently diagnostic criteria were published, which rely upon the characteristic clinical picture as well as on the typical result obtained in nerve conduction studies (Camdessanche et al. 2009). These reflect the pathophysiology with loss or reduced amplitude of sensory compound nerve action potentials. However, clinically inapparent involvement of motor axons with decreased amplitudes and nerve conductions velocity especially in the lower limb can be observed (Camdessanche et al. 2009). Sensory-evoked potentials are lost in most cases and abnormal when detectable (Camdessanche et al. 2009). Interestingly, upon electrophysiological examination, the masseter reflex in patients with SSN and facial hypaesthesia is unaffected while the blink reflex is abnormal (Valls-Sole et al. 1990). This observation was explained by the fact that perikaryons carrying the input from the masseter spindles are not localised in the trigeminal ganglion, which is affected by the disease. In contrast, they reside within mesencephalic nucleus of the trigeminal nerve. Thus, they are part of the central nervous system (Ongerboer de Visser 1983).

Approximately 80 % of patients with paraneoplastic SSN harbour anti-Hu antibodies. Other onconeural antibodies usually do not associate with SSN (Molinuevo et al. 1998). Small-cell carcinomas of the lung (SCLC) are by far the most common tumour found in anti-Hu-positive SSN. These are also frequently found in paraneoplastic SSN without known antibodies. In addition, a wide variety of cancers may be associated with SSN, including prostate, breast, pancreatic, neuroendocrine, bladder and ovarian cancer (Rudnicki and Dalmau 2005).

At autopsy, histological examination in SSN shows inflammatory infiltrates including CD8+ T cells in the spinal and autonomic ganglia (Panegyres et al. 1993; Wanschitz et al. 1997).

SSN is distinguished clinically from other forms of predominantly sensory neuropathy by the non-length-dependent development of sensory symptoms. Thus, sensory disturbances frequently involve the upper limb and may also include the face. In addition, sensory involvement is more often asymmetrical and presents predominantly as sensory ataxia. Finally, it is characterised by pronounced axonal loss upon sensory nerve conduction studies in the upper limbs while only minor changes can be found in motor nerve conduction studies (Camdessanche et al. 2009). Non-paraneoplastic SSN can evolve in the context of systemic autoimmune diseases, most often Sjögren's syndrome (Valls-Sole et al. 1990; Griffin et al. 1990). In addition, toxic SSN can occur upon chemotherapy including cisplatin (Gill and Windebank 1998) administered to cancer patients (Krarup-Hansen et al. 2007).

21.4.3 Limbic Encephalitis

The association of LE and cancer was initially described in 1968 by Corsellis et al. (1968). Diagnostic criteria, although not formally validated, include the following criteria: (a) a clinical picture with short-term memory loss, psychiatric symptoms or epileptic seizures suggesting the involvement of limbic structures; (b) an interval <4 years between onset of symptom and the diagnosis of cancer; (c) exclusion of other cancer-related explanations including metastasis, infections, nutritional or metabolic disturbances, cerebrovascular disease or side effect of cancer therapy; and (d) finally, either inflammatory cerebrospinal fluid (CSF) changes, unilateral or bilateral temporal hyperintensities in T2-/FLAIR-weighted MRI or temporal atrophy on T1-weighted images or EEG showing slow or sharp-wave activity in one or both temporal lobes need to underscore either the inflammatory origin or involvement of limbic structures (Gultekin et al. 2000).

In a recent European series, LE occurred in approximately 10 % of all PNS (Giometto et al. 2010). The neurological symptoms evolved in half of the patient before the diagnosis of cancer (Gultekin et al. 2000). Most cases present with short-term memory loss (84 %), seizures (50 %), acute confusional states (46 %) and/or and psychiatric symptoms (42 %) with affective symptoms, hallucinations and personality changes being most common. Symptoms usually evolve within days and weeks rather than months and years. A subset of patients also develops signs of hypothalamic dysfunction including hyperthermia, weight gain, endocrine dysfunction including diabetes insipidus and hypersomnia. In a few patients, cerebellar or brainstem involvement or neuropathy can occur (Gultekin et al. 2000). Especially in patients with anti-Hu antibodies, the syndrome can eventually evolve into an encephalomyelitis (Graus et al. 2001) (see below).

Anti-Hu antibodies most often associate with SCLC and the prognosis is generally unfavourable. In patients with anti-CV2/CRMP5 antibodies, optic neuritis and chorea can be associated features (Honnorat et al. 1996; Cross et al. 2003). Other onconeural antibodies are anti-Ma2 (also known as anti-Ta) and anti-amphiphysin. Most commonly associated tumours are lung cancers, especially SCLC. However, in women, breast and ovarian cancer are common, and in young male patients, one has to consider testicular cancer (anti-Ma2) (Voltz et al. 1999). Rarely, neuroectodermal skin cancer (Merkel-cell carcinoma) has been described (Greenlee et al. 2002). Furthermore, thymomas and lymphomas have to be considered in onconeural and neuronal cell-surface antibody-associated syndromes (Yu et al. 2001; Lancaster et al. 2011; Ingenito et al. 1990; Irani et al. 2012) (mGluR5, Chap. 6). Importantly, limbic encephalitis can be associated with onconeural (e.g. Hu) and neuronal cell-surface antibodies (e.g. against AMPA receptors, $GABA_B$ receptors, Chap. 6) or a combination of antibodies from both groups (e.g. Hu and $GABA_B$ receptors) (Lancaster and Dalmau 2012). Of the cases with paraneoplastic limbic encephalitis previously considered as seronegative, up to 40 % might harbour anti-$GABA_B$ receptor antibodies (Borcnat et al. 2011) (Chap. 6). In summary, in LE it is important to comprehensively test CSF and serum for known and unknown onconeural and neuronal surface antibodies. In cases with definite LE with well-characterised antibodies, about 50 % of the patients died during follow-up, and the minority showed improvement in response to therapy (Bataller et al. 2007). Patients with LE and neuronal surface or synaptic autoantibodies have a far better prognosis (Chap. 6).

In 70–80 % of cases with paraneoplastic LE, neuroimaging studies show medial temporal lobe hyperintensity on fluid-attenuated inversion recovery and T2-weighted images (Gultekin et al. 2000; Lawn et al. 2003). Upon neuropathological examination, brains of patients with classical paraneoplastic LE show neuronal loss, inflammatory infiltrates and microglial nodules in limbic structures including the hippocampus and amygdala (Alamowitch et al. 1997; Newman et al. 1990).

In oligosymptomatic cases of LE, schizophrenia or other psychiatric diseases might be considered as differential diagnosis. In addition, encephalopathy due to intoxication or metabolic disturbance might mimic some aspects of LE as does temporal lobe epilepsy or status epilepticus of complex-partial seizure due to other pathophysiologies. Infectious aetiologies, most importantly herpes simplex encephalitis have to be excluded (Granerod et al. 2010). Human herpes virus type 6 (HHV6) can induce LE-like encephalitis, including typical neuroimaging results, in patients after allogenic haematopoietic stem cell transplantation (Bhanushali et al. 2013). LE with antibodies against neuronal surface or synaptic proteins

(Chap. 6) are more common than the paraneoplastic LE variants described here (Granerod et al. 2010).

21.4.4 Encephalomyelitis

PCD, SSN as well as paraneoplastic LE can show signs and symptoms suggesting involvement of other parts of the nervous system. Thus, there is a spectrum from more localised syndromes (PCD, LE, SSN) to a widespread affection of the entire nervous system coined encephalomyelitis (EM) (Henson et al. 1965). The latter is characterised by a simultaneous or progressive involvement of different subsystems of the nervous system including the peripheral nervous system. This spectrum is best described in anti-Hu-associated syndromes with underlying SCLCs. Here, one quarter of patients show isolated involvement of the nervous system, while in three quarters of patients either two or three different areas of the nervous system are affected (Dalmau et al. 1992). SSN predominates in about 60 % of the cases, but motor neuron dysfunction, limbic involvement, cerebellar degeneration, brainstem encephalitis and autonomic dysfunction can also be dominating clinical features (10–20 %) (Dalmau et al. 1992). The distinction between encephalomyelitis and localised syndromes, e.g. PCD with minor brainstem involvement, remains somewhat arbitrary. According to the recommended diagnostic criteria, the diagnosis of EM should be avoided in cases with a clearly dominant localised syndrome (Graus et al. 2004) (Fig. 21.2). Nevertheless, the simultaneous or consecutive association of subacute dysfunction of different areas of the nervous system is highly suggestive of a paraneoplastic origin, and thus its recognition as (EM) is helpful for clinical practice.

Most patients suffering from (EM) have anti-Hu antibodies (Graus et al. 2001; Dalmau et al. 1992). However, (EM) was also reported in single cases with anti-CRMP5 antibodies (Honnorat et al. 1996). Although sharing parts of the name, the syndrome of progressive encephalomyelitis with rigidity and myoclonus, which is associated with a different subset of antibodies, is clinically more related with stiff-person syndrome and thus is discussed below.

21.4.5 Opsoclonus-Myoclonus Syndrome

The paraneoplastic opsoclonus-myoclonus syndrome (OMS), also named Kinsbourne syndrome after its first description in 1962 (Kinsbourne 1962), has a characteristic age distribution. Each age group has specific associated antibodies, underlying tumours and prognosis. In paediatric cases, the mean onset is 18–20 months with only 13 % of cases being older than 2 years (Boltshauser et al. 1979; Talon and Stoll 1985). Most of these patients suffer from neuroblastomas but onconeural antibodies are extremely rare. Young adults (median 22 years) have either idiopathic or teratoma-associated OMS and novel neuronal surface antibodies can be found in some of them (Armangue et al. 2014). Adult paraneoplastic cases

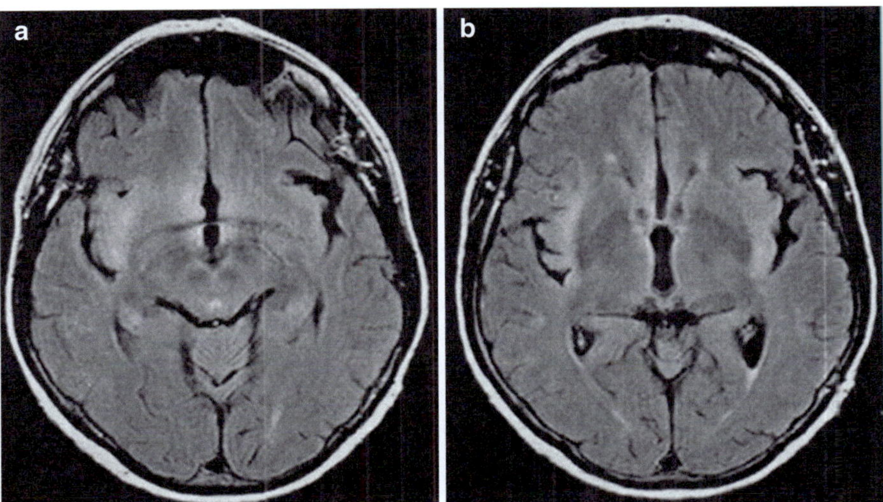

Fig. 21.2 Subclinical involvement of limbic structures in a patient with anti-Hu-associated subacute sensory neuropathy. The 69-year-old female with subacute sensory neuropathy (SSN) and high-titre anti-Hu antibodies presented with the typical clinical picture of SSN with paraesthesias of the limbs and severe sensory ataxia. In addition, mild neuropsychiatric abnormalities including apathy and mental slowness were noted Cranial MRI (FLAIR) showed hyperintensity of the temporal lobe (**a**), insular region (**a/b**) and the gyrus cinguli (**b**). Although these findings proved that the paraneoplastic syndrome affected areas of the nervous system beyond the spinal ganglia, the diagnosis of SSN not encephalomyelitis was made as the SSN was by far the predominant paraneoplastic syndrome. Although asbestosis was present, no lung tumour could be detected. After short-lived stabilisation in response to high-dose steroids, the patient's conditions deteriorated and she died 5 months after onset of symptoms

associated with other tumours were older than 40 years with a mean age of onset of 66 years reported (Anderson et al. 1988b; Bataller et al. 2001). Generally, paraneoplastic OMS is rare and occurs approximately tenfold less often than PCD or SSN (Giometto et al. 2010).

Opsoclonus is an ocular movement disorder defined by continuous, irregular and conjugated chaotic back-to-back saccades in all direction but preferentially horizontally without intersaccadic interval. Opsoclonus is normally increased by eye closure and fixation and persists during sleep (Bellur 1975). In OMS, opsoclonus is typically associated with action myoclonus of the extremities; also, asterixis may occur (Caviness et al. 1995). The neuronal generators of opsoclonus and myoclonus are distinct as there is no temporal association. In addition, opsoclonus and myoclonus are often associated with ataxia, which in comparison to PCD has been reported to be more truncal than appendicular (Anderson et al. 1988b). However, in many cases the presence of ataxia is difficult to ascertain due to severe myoclonus. Thus, its presence has even been questioned with the ataxic movement disorder interpreted rather as a result of the myoclonus (Pranzatelli 1992). The onset of OMS is usually subacute within days or weeks. Initially, patients frequently complain of vertigo. Both oscillopsias due to opsoclonus and stance and gait instability due to myoclonus (and ataxia) can become so severe that the patients lose their ability to walk unaided and prefer to lie supine with their eyes closed (Pranzatelli 1992). Encephalopathy has been reported repeatedly in OMS with altered mental status in the sense to apathy, lethargy or confusion occurring in approximately half of adult cases and progressing to stupor or coma in a minority of these. Dysphagia and dysarthria may be present (Pranzatelli 1992). Children that survive OMS frequently have neurological, neurocognitive and behavioural deficits, which can be severe in some cases (Hayward et al. 2001). If the tumour is not treated, patients with adult paraneoplastic OMS usually die from encephalopathy; antineoplastic treatment can improve symptoms considerably (Bataller et al. 2001).

Only a minority of both adult and paediatric patients with paraneoplastic OMS harbour antineuronal antibodies (Bataller et al. 2001; Antunes et al. 2000). The most common antibody found to be associated with adults paraneoplastic OMS is anti-Ri, which in a review of published cases occurred in 66 %. Much less often, anti-Hu and anti-amphiphysin as well as VGCC antibodies are found (Klaas et al. 2012). Neuronal surface antibodies of unknown specificity have been observed in young adult patients with teratomas or testis tumours (Armangue et al. 2014). In single cases, OMS might be part of the clinical presentation of NMDA receptor-antibody-associated encephalitis (Kurian et al. 2010; Smith et al. 2011); however, no tumour has been detected in these two cases, a patient with OMS and GABA$_B$ receptor antibodies (DeFelipe-Mimbrera et al. 2014) and OMS with GAD antibodies (Bhandari 2012). In addition, diverse autoantigens, including proteins of the post-synaptic density, have been found in paraneoplastic and non-paraneoplastic OMS but currently do not have diagnostic relevance (Bataller et al. 2003). In paediatric paraneoplastic OMS, cases with onconeural antibodies showed anti-Hu (Antunes et al. 2000; Fisher et al. 1994). In addition, antibodies against neurofilament (Connolly et al. 1997) and the cell surface of granule cells (Blaes et al. 2005) have been reported in paediatric OMS. However, the clinical or pathophysiological relevance of these findings remains to be explored.

Diverse tumours have been found associated with adult paraneoplastic OMS (Pranzatelli 1992). Lung cancer is the most frequent cancer followed by breast cancer (Klaas et al. 2012). Paediatric cases are associated with neuroblastoma, ganglioneuroblastoma or ganglioneuroma (Pranzatelli 1992). About 2 % of children with neuroblastomas develop OMS, and this is associated with a more favourable prognosis of the tumour (Altman and Baehner 1976).

Neuroimaging studies most frequently reveal pontine lesion in adult OMS (Kim et al. 2009; Hattori et al. 1988). Children with paraneoplastic OMS usually develop persisting cerebellar atrophy (Hayward et al. 2001) (Fig. 21.3).

Autopsy findings in paraneoplastic OMS did not reveal any specific abnormalities. Mostly, they report diffuse microglial proliferation and lymphocytic infiltrates in different brain areas including the cerebellum and brainstem (Anderson et al. 1988b; Young et al. 1993). However, mild Purkinje cell loss has been reported in some cases (Anderson et al. 1988b).

In adults, only a minority of cases with OMS are paraneoplastic (Klaas et al. 2012), whereas up to 40 % of children with OMS have neuroblastomas or related

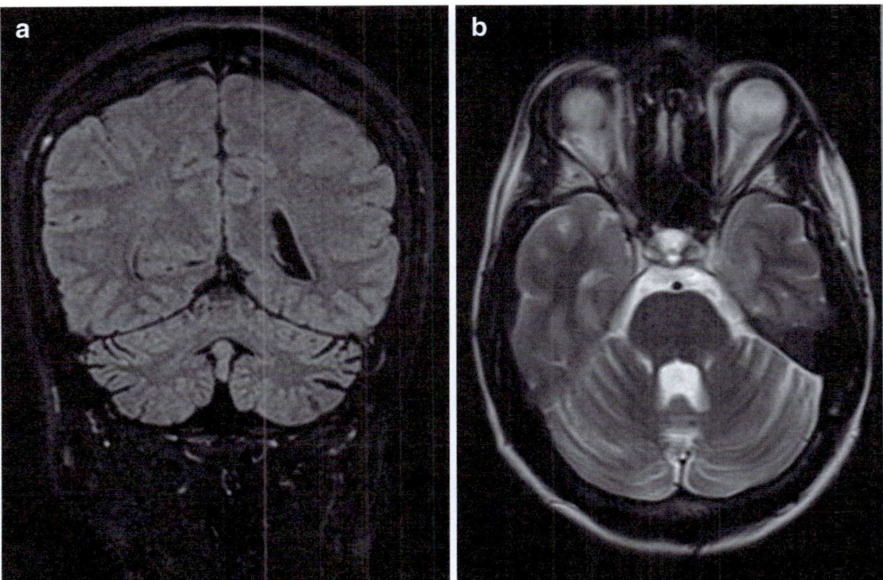

Fig. 21.3 Cerebellar atrophy as a residuum of childhood opsoclonus-myoclonus syndrome associated with neuroblastoma. Cranial MRI: (**a**) coronar FLAIR and (**b**) horizontal T2-weighted images. The 30-year-old female developed opsoclonus-myoclonus syndrome (OMS) at the age of 18 months. Several months later, a neuroblastoma of the left adrenal gland was diagnosed and surgically removed. After surgery and steroid therapy, the patient rapidly improved. However, cerebellar ataxia and behavioural-developmental deficits remained. Although the patient became ambulatory, frequent falls persistent. The patient is independent regarding activities of daily living; however, no school-leaving graduation could be obtained

tumours (Brunklaus et al. 2012). The rest remains idiopathic or infectious, parainfectious or toxic/metabolic (Pranzatelli 1992; Klaas et al. 2012). Infectious causes include HIV seroconversion, poliomyelitis, EBV, CMV, mumps, HHV6, West Nile virus and others (Pranzatelli 1992; Klaas et al. 2012; Belcastro et al. 2014; BirluTiu and BirluTiu 2014). A number of intoxications, including amitriptyline, lithium and carbamazepine, were found to induce OMS (for a more complete list, compare (Pranzatelli 1992)). The clinical course of non-paraneoplastic OMS is usually monophasic and, if the underlying infection is not life threatening, mostly benign.

21.4.6 Chronic Intestinal Pseudo-obstruction

Chronic intestinal pseudo-obstruction (CIPO) is subsumed under dysautonomia in epidemiological overviews about PNS (Giometto et al. 2010). Dysautonomia is a rather rare feature in PNS occurring approximately fivefold less often than SSN and as often as LEMS (Giometto et al. 2010). Thus, it can be concluded that paraneoplastic CIPO is even rarer. The first study indicating that CIPO can occur in the context of a PNS was reported in 1978 (Ahmed and Carpenter 1975). Soon, this was followed by larger case series of patients with SCLC or, in rare occasions, pulmonary carcinoids (Chinn and Schuffler 1988).

Per definition, CIPO is a clinical syndrome presenting with symptoms and signs of intestinal obstruction in the absence of mechanical blockade (Schuffler et al. 1981). Frequent complaints of patients with paraneoplastic CIPO are nausea and vomiting, abdominal pain and distension and severe obstipation. In some patients, additional neurological symptoms occur including other signs of dysautonomia including neurogenic bladder and orthostatic hypotension. Also peripheral neuropathy, cognitive disturbances or ataxia have been noted (Chinn and Schuffler 1988).

In a large series of 162 patients with PNS and anti-Hu antibodies, approximately 10 % presented with solely gastrointestinal symptoms (Lucchinetti et al. 1998). Some patients with medium to high titres of antibodies against α3 acetylcholine receptor antibodies develop limited dysautonomia with gastrointestinal dysmotility (McKeon et al. 2009).

The most frequent tumour associated with CIPO is SCLC (Lucchinetti et al. 1998; Lennon et al. 1991). CIPO has also been reported in a younger patients in association with neural crest tumours (Gohil et al. 2001), e.g. a ganglioneuroblastoma associated with high anti-Hu titres (Wildhaber et al. 2002). Dysautonomia with α3 acetylcholine receptor antibodies is frequently non-paraneoplastic but can occur in association with diverse tumours, most often adenocarcinomas (McKeon et al. 2009) but also thymomas (Rakocevic et al. 2003). CIPO in the context of a thymoma is sometimes associated with myasthenia gravis (Rakocevic et al. 2003; Kulling et al. 1997; Musthafa et al. 2006; Pande and Leis 1999).

Gastrointestinal hypo- or amotility in CIPO is demonstrated by oesophageal manometry, radiological investigations including barium meal examination and Gastrografin enemas (Chinn and Schuffler 1988). CT scan of the abdomen shows bowel distension without mechanical obstruction as does endoscopy of the gastrointestinal tract (Badari et al. 2012). Histopathological examination reveals inflammatory lymphocytic infiltrates in the myenteric plexus associated with Schwann cell proliferation and in most cases neuronal degeneration (Chinn and Schuffler 1988).

Paraneoplastic CIPO represents the minority of all cases with gastrointestinal dysmotility. A frequent cause is progressive systemic sclerosis followed by hollow visceral myopathy (Schuffler et al. 1981). Idiopathic cases of myenteric ganglionitis have been reported (Racalbuto et al. 2008). Familial cases with visceral myopathy associated with CIPO can occur (Sipponen et al. 2009). Amyloidosis may also present as CIPO (Wald et al. 1981). CIPO can develop as a late complication of radiotherapy (Conklin and Anuras 1981) and rarely in Chagas disease (Teixeira et al. 2006).

21.4.7 Lambert-Eaton Myasthenic Syndrome

Lambert-Eaton myasthenic syndrome (LEMS) is another classical PNS of the peripheral nervous systems. Paraneoplastic LEMS occurs approximately fivefold less frequent that SSN and PCD (Giometto et al. 2010). Clinically, it is characterised by predominantly proximal muscle weakness, loss of tendon reflexes, mild to moderate ptosis and autonomic dysfunction, especially dryness of the mouth (O'Neill et al. 1988). In about 10 % of patients with paraneoplastic LEMS, cerebellar ataxia can be found (Titulaer et al. 2011b).

In approximately 50 % of patients, an underlying cancer, almost exclusively SCLC, is detected (Titulaer et al. 2011b). Typically, if present, an initially occult SCLC is diagnosed within the first 2 years after onset by LEMS when thorough tumour screenings including thoracic CT, bronchoscopy and even FDG-PET are applied. In rare cases, prostate cancer, then differentiated in a neuroendocrine phenotype, has been reported associated with LEMS (Tetu et al. 1989; Agarawal et al. 1995). In addition, single patients with thymomas have been reported (Morimoto et al. 2010; Lauritzen et al. 1980).

Antibodies against VGCC are present in 90 % of LEMS (Roberts et al. 1985). However, this finding does not discriminate between paraneoplastic and non-paraneoplastic cases. In approximately 70 % of patients with paraneoplastic LEMS, high titre-antibodies against SOX proteins can be found (Titulaer et al. 2009). Upon immunofluorescence on cerebellar tissue, this antibody corresponds to the anti-glial nuclear antigen (AGNA) pattern (Sabater et al. 2008). Anti-Hu antibodies are found in 30 % of patients with paraneoplastic LEMS (Titulaer et al. 2009). About 10–15 % of patients with LEMS are negative for antibodies against VGCC (Nakao et al. 2002). However, these sera induce similar effects in functional assays. This indicates the presence of antibodies interfering with presynaptic acetylcholine release that are currently undetectable by the available diagnostic tests (Nakao et al. 2002).

Electrophysiological tests can prove the clinically suspected diagnosis of LEMS. Nerve conduction studies show an abnormally low compound muscle action potential (CMAP) in patients with LEMS, which further decreases with low-frequency stimulation (Anonymous 2001). Although this decrement is not specific for LEMS, there is a substantial increment of the CMAP either postexercise or upon high-frequency stimulation (50 Hz) (Hatanaka and Oh 2008).

Using autopsy material, Fukuda et al. could show that in patients with cerebellar ataxia associated with LEMS, there is a marked decrease in cerebellar P/Q-type calcium channel expression (Fukuda et al. 2003).

When the diagnosis of LEMS is established based on clinical and electrophysiological findings, the main differential diagnosis to paraneoplastic LEMS is non-paraneoplastic LEMS. The Dutch-English LEMS Tumor Association Prediction (DELTA-P) score has been reported to accurately predict SCLC in LEMS. This score gives one point each of the following item, if they occur within 3 months after onset of LEMS: age $\geq$50 years, smoking at diagnosis, weight loss $\geq$5 %, bulbar involvement, erectile dysfunction in male patients and Karnofsky performance status lower than 70. Whereas a score of 0 and 1 is associated with low risk of an SCLC, a score of 3 and higher is almost invariably associated with paraneoplastic LEMS (Titulaer et al. 2011c). The presence of anti-SOX antibodies has a sensitivity of 67 % and a specificity of 95 % for LEMS with SCLC (Titulaer et al. 2009).

21.4.8 Nonclassical Paraneoplastic Syndromes

Some frequent neurological syndromes can be paraneoplastic in rare occasions. These include brainstem encephalitides, optic neuritis, retinal degeneration, stiff-person syndrome, myelitis including necrotising myelopathy, motor neuron diseases, diverse forms of neuropathy as well as myasthenia gravis and acquired neuromyotonia (Graus et al. 2004) and are described in this section.

Brainstem encephalitis can be observed as part of a generalised paraneoplastic encephalomyelitis but isolated paraneoplastic brainstem encephalitis can also occur in rare cases. Anti-Hu antibodies are associated with a predominantly medullary brainstem dysfunction (Saiz et al. 2009). These patients present with dysarthria, dysphagia and central hypoventilation. Facial, abducens and oculomotor nerve palsies and nystagmus occur frequently, sometimes progressing to complete gaze palsy. In 50 % of the patients, the disease starts with pontine or mesencephalic dysfunction but rapidly descends to the medulla. In contrast, brainstem encephalitis associated with anti-Ma2 antibodies predominantly affects upper brainstem functions. Patients suffer from vertical gaze palsy, and most of these patients have a combination of brainstem, diencephalic and limbic symptoms, sometimes leading to Parkinsonism, excessive daytime sleepiness and chorea (Dalmau et al. 2004). In cases with anti-Ri antibodies and brainstem dysfunction, eye movement disorders, dysphagia and ptosis have been described. Most patients also show postural instability (Sutton et al. 2002). Laryngospasm and/or jaw dystonia has been reported (Pittock et al. 2010). Interestingly, whereas cranial MRI in anti-Hu-associated brainstem encephalitis invariably shows no abnormalities (Saiz et al. 2009), the localisation of clinical brainstem involvement corresponds to T2 or FLAIR hyperintensities in patients with anti-Ma2 antibodies (Dalmau et al. 2004).

Paraneoplastic optic neuritis occurs most frequently in association with anti-CRMP5 antibodies (Cross et al. 2003). These patients also frequently show basal ganglia involvement upon imaging studies and autopsy, which is clinically evident as chorea (Vernino et al. 2002).

Paraneoplastic stiff-person syndrome (SPS) was first described by Moersch and Woltman in 1956. Patients present with chronic fluctuating truncal and proximal muscle rigidity and spasms (Moersch and Woltman 1956). The syndrome is caused by hyperexcitability of spinal motor neurons due to dysregulation of inhibitory GABAergic and glycinergic neurotransmission (Levy et al. 1999; Khasani et al. 2004). The combination of SPS and limbic encephalitis together with prominent myoclonus, hyperekplexia and oculomotor involvement has been referred to as progressive encephalomyelitis with rigidity and myoclonus (PERM) (Meinck et al. 1994). About 80 % of patients with SPS have high titres of anti-GAD antibodies (McKeon et al. 2012). There is an overlap of patients with anti-GAD antibodies and antibodies against the glycine-receptor $\alpha 1$ subunit (McKeon et al. 2013). Only in about 5 % of patients with SPS, a paraneoplastic origin can be assumed due to the coexistence of cancer. SPS is definitely paraneoplastic when anti-amphiphysin antibodies are detected, a finding that is usually associated with breast cancer (McKeon et al. 2012; Murinson and Guarnaccia 2008). Seronegative paraneoplastic SPS have been reported in patients with Hodgkin lymphoma (McKeon et al. 2012). Less well-characterised antibodies associated with SPS include those against gephyrin (Butler et al. 2000) and antibodies against the potassium channel-associated protein DPPX, the latter in patients with a PERM-spectrum syndrome characterised by hyperekplexia and severe diarrhoea (Boronat et al. 2013).

Paraneoplastic myelitis is very rare. In a recent series of 31 cases of which 22 had onconeural antibodies, anti-amphiphysin and anti-CRMP5 antibodies (9 each) were the most common onconeural antibodies in isolated paraneoplastic myelitis (Flanagan et al. 2011). Aquaporin 4-antibodies can also occur in individual cases of paraneoplastic longitudinal extensive myelitis (LETM) (Pittock and Lennon 2008). Paraneoplastic necrotising myelopathy is a rare syndrome with rapidly progressive necrosis of the spinal cord, which clinically presents as ascending paraplegia followed by rapid deterioration and death (Ojeda 1984). This syndrome is usually not associated with onconeural antibodies (Graus et al. 2004).

Paraneoplastic retinal degeneration has also been recognised. The triad of photosensitivity, ring scotomas, visual field loss and attenuated retinal arteriole calibre has been reported as typical for this rare paraneoplastic disorder (Jacobson et al. 1990). Two different pathologies of the retina are distinguished: in melanoma-associated retinopathy, electrophysiological studies are consistent with a defect in intra-retinal transmission distal to the photoreceptors. Here, antibodies against bipolar retinal cells were reported, while the molecular mechanism remains unknown (Keltner et al. 2001; Weinstein et al. 1994). In contrast, in cancer-associated retinopathy, a degeneration of photoreceptor cells with limited signs of inflammation ensues (Buchanan et al. 1984). Here, antibodies against recoverin, a calcium-binding protein also expressed in underlying neoplasms, mostly SCLC (Polans et al. 1995), were identified (Polans et al. 1991). Retinitis can also occur in PNS associated with anti-CRMP5 antibodies but here visual loss is usually accompanied by additional neurological abnormalities (Cross et al. 2003).

There is no evidence for an increased frequency of motor neuron disease in cancer (Rosenfeld and Posner 1991). Generally, association of typical amyotrophic lateral sclerosis and cancer is most likely coincidental. However, a subset of patients with atypical MND suffer from paraneoplastic neurological syndromes. These include patients with subacutely progressive lower motor neuron disease, usually in association with anti-Hu antibodies and patients with isolated upper motor neuron disease, mostly associated with breast cancer (Forsyth et al. 1997). A recent survey supported the long acknowledged association of motor neuron disease with non-Hodgkin lymphomas; importantly none of the patients had inflammatory CSF changes, none showed improvement upon tumour treatment, and none had onconeural antibodies (Briani et al. 2011). Thus, a definite diagnosis of a PNS cannot be made in these cases.

Neuropathies are amongst the most frequent syndromes encountered by the clinical neurologist. The aetiologies encompass hereditary, metabolic, most frequently diabetic and inflammatory causes. Diverse forms of neuropathy including acute sensorimotor neuropathy mimicking Guillain-Barré syndrome (GBS), chronic inflammatory demyelinating polyradiculitis (CIDP), subacute to chronically progressive sensorimotor neuropathies, brachial plexusneuritis, vasculitic neuropathy

(Fig. 21.3) as well as dysautonomia can have a paraneoplastic origin (Koike et al. 2011). The detection of anti-Hu and anti-CRMP5 antibodies confirms the paraneoplastic origin in a subset of patients. Other subtypes that need to be mentioned specifically are neuropathies associated with monoclonal gammopathies of type IgM, mostly with antibodies against gangliosides or myelin-associated glycoprotein (Stork et al. 2014), which can also be considered as paraneoplastic. In POEMS syndrome, a monoclonal gammopathy, usually IgA lambda and a prominent increase in serum VEGF levels are confirmatory (Dispenzieri 2007).

Acquired neuromyotonia is a result of peripheral nerve hyperexcitability and leads to continuous involuntary muscle activity. Neuromyotonia and cramps-fasciculation syndrome represent a continuum (Hart et al. 2002). The likelihood that the acquired neuromyotonia is of paraneoplastic origin increases when the patient is older than 40 years and antibodies against voltage-gated potassium channels and acetylcholine receptors are found. The most common tumours are thymomas and SCLCs.

Myasthenia gravis, like LEMS, is a disorder with dysfunction of the neuromuscular junction. It is however initiated by antibodies against muscarinergic acetylcholine receptors. Myasthenia gravis is paraneoplastic in a minority of cases and then associated with thymoma (Skeie and Romi 2008). The presence of anti-titin antibodies in patients with myasthenia gravis is associated with an underlying thymoma (Yamamoto et al. 2001).

21.5　Cerebrospinal Fluid Studies

As already discussed in the section regarding the pathophysiology of PNS, the PNS sensu stricto is an inflammatory disease of the nervous system. Thus, it is common practice in clinical neurology to use CSF analysis to detect or exclude inflammatory changes, thereby implying that the absence of inflammatory CSF changes makes a PNS unlikely or even excludes a inflammatory disease of the nervous system and thereby a PNS.

CSF analysis is an invaluable diagnostic tool for comprehensive differential diagnosis in suspected PNS. As described in the previous sections on each clinical syndrome, these comprise infectious, other autoimmune, neoplastic, toxic and hereditary causes. For example, CSF analysis might help to identify LE due to HSV reactivation by CSF-PCR and serology with determination of antigen-specific intrathecal antibody synthesis and *Listeria* species by CSF culture in brainstem encephalitis. In addition, in some autoimmune encephalitides, determination of antibodies in CSF has a higher sensitivity and specificity than serum testing only. In anti-NMDA receptor antibody encephalitis, CSF testing revealed anti-NMDA receptor antibodies in 16 % of cases in which serum was tested as negative (Gresa-Arribas et al. 2014). Thus, some very experienced laboratories use CSF only to screen for these kinds of antibodies in cases with LE (Jerome Honnorat, Lyon, personal communication), and some use serum and CSF in parallel (Josep Dalmau, Barcelona, personal communication). Furthermore, neurological signs or symptoms in some cases of PNS, e.g. brainstem encephalitis or radiculitis, might be indistinguishable from those due to meningeosis carcinomatosa or leucemica or neurolymphomatosis. In these cases, even repeated CSF analysis including cytology or flow cytometry is advisable to exclude or confirm a direct effect of infiltrating neoplastic cells on the nervous system. In individual patients with PNS, the subacutely progressive course of the disease might lead to the differential diagnosis of CJD. Saiz et al. reported that the 14-3-3 protein in the CSF can be positive in 12.5 % of patients with PNS (Saiz et al. 1999). Thus, this marker is not reliable in distinguishing CJD from PNS. Taken together, CSF analysis is mandatory to clarify the differential diagnoses in cases with suspected PNS.

Whereas the specific findings to be expected upon CSF analysis in the diverse differential diagnoses of PNS will be covered in other chapters of this book, we will review here current knowledge about CSF findings in PNS. Even very early reports indicated that, in general, there are inflammatory CSF changes in PNS. However, since then there were only few systematic approaches to characterise the inflammatory CSF syndrome in PNS in detail. In these, methodological differences still leave room for ambiguity.

CSF results were reported in case series of PNS. An early series of patients with PCD with anti-Yo antibodies showed that 9 of 13 anti-Yo-positive cases had CSF abnormalities including mild lymphocytic pleocytosis and moderately elevated CSF protein, and-the numbers of patients tested were very low however-positive oligoclonal bands (OCB) in CSF or elevated IgG (Anderson et al. 1988a). In a series of eight cases with paraneoplastic LE each with and without anti-Hu antibodies, the majority of cases had increased protein and CSF white blood cell (WBC) counts. OCBs were positive in five of six patients with anti-Hu antibodies (Alamowitch et al. 1997). In a larger series of patients with paraneoplastic LE, CSF showed inflammatory changes in 40/49 patients (24/47 increased total protein, 24/47 CSF pleocytosis, 15/15 increased IgG synthesis, 10/13 oligoclonal IgG) (Gultekin et al. 2000). In series of 19 patients with anti-Ri-associated PNS, less than 50 % had increased WBC count in the CSF or increased total protein but the absence or presence of OCB was not reported (Pittock et al. 2003). Lymphocytic pleocytosis, increased protein and isolated OCB in CSF were noted in most patients with paraneoplastic optic neuritis associated with anti-CRMP5 antibodies (Cross et al. 2003). In adult paraneoplastic OMS, 10/19 patients showed increased total protein or pleocytosis; two of these patients had oligoclonal IgG in the CSF (Anderson et al. 1988b). In most of these studies, the number of patients who neither had positive OCB, increased cell count or protein was not reported. Thus, the important question of the negative predictive value of normal CSF studies remains unanswered by these studies. In anti-Tr-associated PNS (mostly PCD), routine CSF analysis was normal in 9/22 patients; the remaining 13 patients had mild CSF pleocytosis with a median WBC count/µl of 50 (range 14–150/µl) (Bernal et al. 2003). Although as a group, anti-Tr-associated PNS had pleocytosis or CSF protein increase not different from other PNS, none of three patients tested had OCBs in the CSF (Psimaras et al. 2010). In 5 of 11 cases with Hodgkin lymphoma and PNS, CSF was reportedly normal (Briani et al. 2011). Although larger confirmatory studies are missing, inflammatory CSF changes might be less frequent in PNS of the central nervous system associated with lymphomas than in PNS associated with other tumours. Correspondingly, in PNS of the peripheral nervous system, e.g. paraneoplastic demyelinating polyradiculoneuritis associated with lymphoma, CSF studies were normal except for increased total protein (Briani et al. 2011). However, in all these studies and many other reports about CSF abnormalities in patients with PNS, there are technical issues which limit comparability. It is often unknown which technique for the detection of OCB was used and whether serum and CSF were analysed in parallel. Thus, sensitivity between studies may vary considerably. Usually quantitative intrathecal IgG synthesis is reported as IgG index (e.g. (Cross et al. 2003)) or elevated CSF IgG (e.g.(Anderson et al. 1988a)) instead of the more accurate method developed by Reiber and Felgenhauer (1987).

The largest case series to date was published in 2010 by Psimaras et al. on behalf of the PNS Euronetwork (Psimaras et al. 2010). In this series, three basic values of CSF analysis were evaluated: WBC count, CSF protein levels and presence or absence of CSF OCB. Combining all these three values, abnormal CSF was found in 93 % of the patients; in 10 % of cases, the only abnormality was positive OCB. Pleocytosis, if present (39 %), was moderate, maximally 110 cells/µl, and CSF/blood-barrier dysfunction (>500 mg/l, present in 67 %) in some cases (13/281, 5 %) was substantial (>2,000 mg/l, maximally 4,000 mg/l). However, as it remained unclear whether the OCB detected in the CSF were actually isolated and not present in both serum and CSF, the value of this conclusion remains somewhat limited. Moreover, OCB were only analysed in 135/295 patients (46 %) and reported to be positive in 63 %. However, a small case series which definitely analysed OCB in serum and CSF in parallel led to similar results (10/18, 55 %: 3/5 patients with anti-Ri antibodies (Jarius et al. 2008), 3/3 anti-CV2 positive cases, 0/1 with anti-amphiphysin (Stich and Rauer 2007), 4/9 patients with anti-Yo-positive PCD (Stich et al. 2003)). In addition, the data published by Psimaras et al. indicated that lymphocytic pleocytosis as well as CSF/brain barrier dysfunction may subside during the course of the disease. Thus, normal results upon CSF analysis may be more often in the late stage of the disease (Psimaras et al. 2010). Counterintuitively, a higher cell count seems to be associated with a better prognosis regarding survival (Psimaras et al. 2010).

In the unpublished series of 13 patients with definite PNS, we cared for in the last years, using comprehensive CSF analysis, we observed similar results. In our patients, pleocytosis was present in 31 %. Upon routine cytology, lymphocytes dominated. Frequently, activated lymphocytes (up to 5 %) and plasma cells (up to 17 %) were observed. The CSF/serum albumin ratio (Q_{Alb}) was moderately increased in 69 %. The highest value was 27.9×10^{-3} in a case with SSN associated with uterus carcinoma. The majority of patients had isolated OCB in the CSF (69 %). Quantitative intrathecal IgG synthesis analysed by the formulas developed by Reiber occurred in 31 %; intrathecal IgA synthesis was not observed; only one patient had intrathecal IgM synthesis upon quantitative analysis (Reiber and Felgenhauer 1987). Three of 13 patients, a 63-year-old male with adenocarcinoma of the lung and motor neuron disease involving the upper and lower motor neuron, a 60-year-old female with HL and motor neuropathy involving the cranial nerves and a 58-year-old male with squamous cell lung carcinoma, PCD and neuropathy, all without onconeural antibodies, had entirely normal CSF results. However, an isolated mild CSF/blood-barrier dysfunction was found in another patient. Thus, in our series strong indicators of an inflammatory disease, e.g. pleocytosis or intrathecal Ig synthesis, occurred in 69 % of patients only. In three of our patients with intrathecal IgG synthesis, the so-called MRZ reaction, a polyclonal increase of IgG against measles, rubella and varicella zoster, was tested. As in previous reports (Jarius et al. 2009), the MRZ reaction was negative in all patients.

Another question is whether CSF analysis can complement clinical monitoring for the efficacy of immunosuppressive and antitumour therapy. As indicated above, during the course of the disease, both pleocytosis and CSF/blood-brain barrier dysfunction may normalise without association of a better prognosis (Psimaras et al. 2010). We have followed a case with anti-Ri-positive myelitis without tumour and surprisingly good response to immunosuppression. In this case, over a period of more than 2 years, increases in the CSF/serum albumin ratio and CSF pleocytosis closely indicated relapses and both markers of inflammatory activity responded well to enforced immune suppression (Fig. 21.4) (Leypoldt et al. 2006). Thus, in individual cases, serial CSF analysis might be beneficial to guide therapeutic decisions (Fig. 21.5).

Importantly, CSF cannot only be used to detect and monitor inflammatory changes but also to look for the antibodies against onconeural antibodies that confirm the diagnosis of PNS (Graus et al. 2004). Already very early reports indicated that there is, at least in some cases, an intrathecal synthesis of onconeural antibodies as shown by Graus et al. in two patients with PCD and anti-Yo antibodies (Graus et al. 1988). A similar observation was published using quantitative western blotting in all of six patients harbouring anti-Ri antibodies in serum and CSF (Luque et al. 1991). Four of five patients with anti-Ma2 antibodies showed intrathecal synthesis (Voltz et al. 1999). These observations were supported by the detection of oligoclonal IgG specific for onconeural proteins in anti-Ri- (Jarius et al. 2008), anti-amphiphysin-, anti-CV2- (Stich and Rauer 2007), anti-Yo- (Stich et al. 2003) and anti-Hu-associated (Rauer and Kaiser 2000) PNS. Using ELISA to quantify antibody titres against onconeural antibodies, quantitative intrathecal synthesis of anti-Hu-IgG defined as an CSF/serum antibody index >1.5 was detected in 60 % of the patients (Rauer and Kaiser 2001). Presence or absence of intrathecal synthesis of anti-Hu antibodies in anti-Hu-positive PNS seemed to correlate with the presence or absence of oligoclonal IgG in the CSF (Rauer and Kaiser 2001). In the majority of patients (88 %) with primarily CNS involvement of the PNS and diverse antibodies, quantitative intrathecal synthesis was observed, while none of three patients with a PNS involving the peripheral nervous system had specific intrathecal antibody synthesis (Stich et al. 2007).

The 25-year experience of the laboratory at the MAYO Clinic in Rochester revealed that most cases of PNS with classical onconeural antibodies upon screening using indirect immunofluorescence show titres that are readily detectable in both serum and CSF (McKeon et al. 2011b). However, in 2 % of patients with

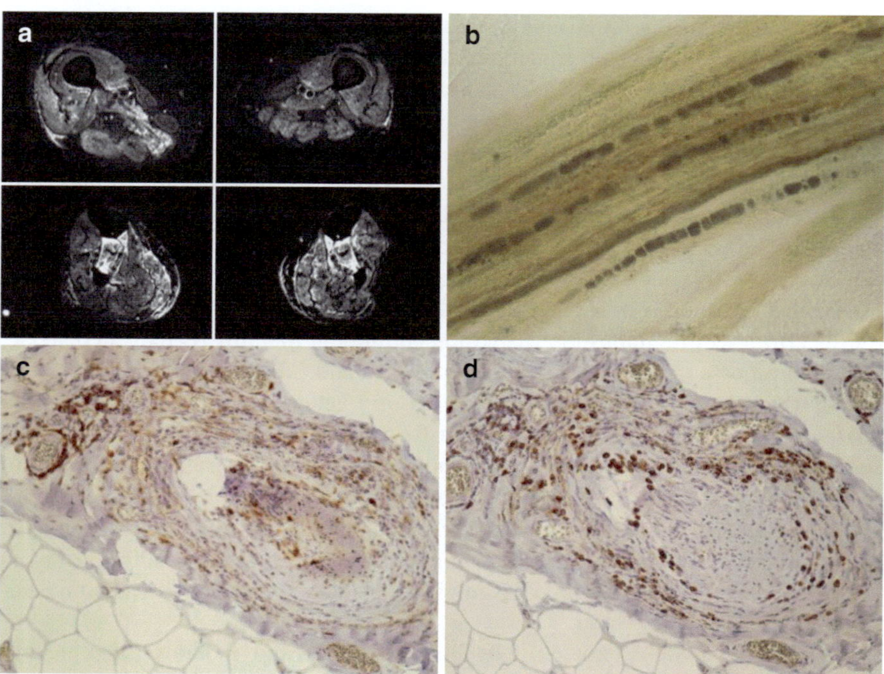

Fig. 21.4 Paraneoplastic vasculitic neuropathy associated with CRMP5- and amphiphysin antibodies and small- cell bladder carcinoma. The 74-year old patient with a present with chronically asymmetric painful sensorimotor neuropathy of the lower limbs. Four months before onset of symptoms a urothel carcinoma had been surgically removed. Cerebrospinal fluid (CSF) analysis showed lymphocytic pleocytosis (16 cells/µl), blood brain barrier dysfunction (Q_{Alb}15.7 x 10_{-3}) and prominent intrathecal IgG synthesis (Q_{IgG} 22.6 x 10_{-3}, isolated oligoclonal bands in the CSF upon isoelectric focussing). (**a**) Muscle MRI showed scattered edema of legs muscles. (**b**) Nerve fiber teasing showed secondary myelin sheath degeneration. (**c/d**) Sural nerve biopsy showed vasculitis of the endoneurial vessels with lymphocytic infiltrates containing B cells (**c**, anti-CD20) and T cells (**d**, anti-CD3). Antibody testing of the patients serum revealed high-titre anti-CRMP5 (1 : 245,760) and antiamphiphysin antibodies (1 : 61.400) (Antibody testing was kindly performed by the Professor Vanda Lennon, Department of Laboratory Medicine and Pathology, Mayo Clinic, Rochester, MN, US; micrographs were provided by the courtesy of Professor Christian Hagel, Institute for Neuropathology, University Medical Center Hamburg-Eppendorf)

anti-Hu syndrome, antibodies were positive in either serum or CSF only. Seventeen per cent of patients with anti-Ri syndrome were positive in CSF only, while anti-Ri antibodies were detectable in serum only in 8 %. Six per cent of anti-Yo-positive patients were found to harbour anti-Yo antibodies in CSF only, while only 1 % were positive in serum. Three per cent of patients showed isolated anti-CRMP5 antibodies in either serum or CSF. Twenty per cent of patients with paired CSF and serum evaluated with positive results for anti-amphiphysin antibodies had detectable levels in CSF only, while 5 % were positive in serum only. Finally, two of 28 patients with anti-Tr-positive PNS showed anti-Tr antibodies in CSF but not in serum. Thus, in patients with classical well-characterised antibodies (including anti-Tr), detection

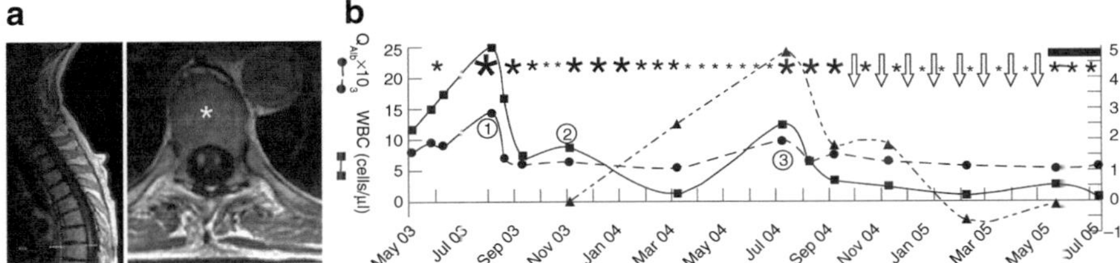

Fig. 21.5 Serial CSF analysis in a patient with anti-Ri-positive myelitis without tumour detected. The 65-year-old female presented with subacutely progressive spastic paraparesis due to myelitis demonstrated by MRI (**a**). Coronal and sagittal sections of gadolinium-enhanced T1-weighted spinal magnetic resonance image showing symmetrical contrast enhancement of the lateral aspects of the spinal cord. *Asterisk* indicates TH12. *Dashed line* indicates the level of axial section. (**b**) Clinical course including serial CSF analysis. *Continuous line* with *closed boxes*, white blood cells (WBCs (cells/µl), left y-axis, normal <5/µl); *dashed line* with *filled circles*, Q_{Alb} (CSF/ serum albumin ratio × 10^3, left y-axis, normal <8.4); *dashed line* with *filled triangles*, differences of left peroneal somatosensory-evoked potential (*SEP*) latencies compared with those from November 2003 (ms, right y-axis). *Encircled numbers*, numbered clinical relapses; *open arrows*, cyclophosphamide pulses; *line of asterisks*, steroid treatment, roughly corresponding in size of dose; *filled line* above *asterisks*, azathioprine treatment (Reprinted with permission from Leypoldt et al. (2006))

of antibodies in CSF only occurred twice as often as serum only positives (5 % vs. 2.5 %) (McKeon et al. 2011b).

In summary, in cases of suspected PNS, CSF analysis is (1) helpful in detecting CSF inflammation and (2) can complement serum testing for paraneoplastic antibodies. Unfortunately, commercially available tissues for immunofluorescence screening are mostly validated with serum only. Nevertheless, CSF testing for paraneoplastic antibodies should be performed in cases where the diagnosis of PNS is clinically suspected and serum antibody testing for onconeural antibodies remains negative.

21.6 Treatment

Treatment of paraneoplastic syndromes consists of tumour and/or immunosuppressive therapy. Prompt initiation of therapy is important. Unfortunately, most of the syndromes described in this chapter respond poorly to immunotherapy.

In large case series, elimination of tumour tissue in has been shown to be beneficial (Shams'ili et al. 2003; Graus et al. 2001; Candler et al. 2004). For example, in patients with a paraneoplastic encephalomyelitis associated with anti-Hu antibodies, tumour treatment was associated with recovery or stabilisation with an odds ratio of 4.56 (95 % confidence interval 1.62–12.86) (Graus et al. 2001). Patients with a paraneoplastic cerebellar degeneration with onconeural antibodies lived significantly longer if their tumour was treated (Shams'ili et al. 2003). Tumour therapy should be instituted according to current oncological guidelines; there is no evidence suggesting a different tumour treatment in paraneoplastic neurological syndromes. However, in clinical oncology, the administration of aggressive chemotherapies is guided by the Karnofsky performance status. This measure can be quite low in patients with PNS due to neurological disturbances but not due to the cancer itself. This difference has to be thoroughly communicated by the treating neurologist. Efficacy of immunosuppression in paraneoplastic neurologic syndromes with onconeural antibodies is not supported by higher level evidence (Mason et al. 1997; Giometto et al. 2012; Greenlee 2013). However, expert opinion recommends immunosuppression in the absence of a detectable tumour or in combination with a tumour therapy in cases not improving or stabilising. No systematic studies exist concerning the type of immunosuppression. Mostly steroids, plasmapheresis, intravenous immunoglobulins (ivIG) or immunoadsorption in combination with cyclophosphamide-based immunosuppression are used. Biological therapies, e.g. rituximab, alemtuzumab and tocilizumab, can be considered but systematic evidence is lacking. Rituximab has been utilised with encouraging results in childhood opsoclonus-myoclonus syndrome (Battaglia et al. 2012). Immunosuppressants (azathioprine, methotrexate, cyclosporin A, tacrolimus, mycophenolate mofetil) are commonly used as steroid-sparing agents. In LEMS, treatment with steroids and azathioprine and in some cases immunoglobulins can be considered (Titulaer et al. 2011b; Keogh et al. 2011).

References

Agarawal SK, Birch BR, Abercrombie GF (1995) Adenocarcinoma of the prostate and Eaton-Lambert syndrome. A previously unreported association. Scand J Urol Nephrol 29:351–353

Ahmed MN, Carpenter S (1975) Autonomic neuropathy and carcinoma of the lung. Can Med Assoc J 113:410–412

Alamowitch S, Graus F, Uchuya M et al (1997) Limbic encephalitis and small cell lung cancer. Clinical and immunological features. Brain 120(Pt 6):923–928

Ali K, Amin R, Yoganathan KG et al (2013) Rapidly progressive cerebellar ataxia in West Wales. BMJ Case Rep 2013

Altman AJ, Baehner RL (1976) Favorable prognosis for survival in children with coincident opso-myoclonus and neuroblastoma. Cancer 37:846–852

Anderson NE, Rosenblum MK, Posner JB (1988a) Paraneoplastic cerebellar degeneration: clinical-immunological correlations. Ann Neurol 24:559–567

Anderson NE, Budde-Steffen C, Rosenblum MK et al (1988b) Opsoclonus, myoclonus, ataxia, and encephalopathy in adults with cancer: a distinct paraneoplastic syndrome. Medicine (Baltimore) 67:100–109

Anonymous (2001) Practice parameter for repetitive nerve stimulation and single fiber EMG evaluation of adults with suspected myasthenia gravis or Lambert-Eaton myasthenic syndrome: summary statement. Muscle Nerve 24:1236–1238

Antunes NL, Khakoo Y, Matthay KK et al (2000) Antineuronal antibodies in patients with neuroblastoma and paraneoplastic opsoclonus-myoclonus. J Pediatr Hematol Oncol 22:315–320

Armangue T, Titulaer MJ, Sabater L et al (2014) A novel treatment-responsive encephalitis with frequent opsoclonus and teratoma. Ann Neurol 75:435–441

Badari A, Farolino D, Nasser E et al (2012) A novel approach to paraneoplastic intestinal pseudo-obstruction. Support Care Cancer 20:425–428

Bataller L, Graus F, Saiz A et al (2001) Clinical outcome in adult onset idiopathic or paraneoplastic opsoclonus-myoclonus. Brain 124:437–443

Bataller L, Rosenfeld MR, Graus F et al (2003) Autoantigen diversity in the opsoclonus-myoclonus syndrome. Ann Neurol 53:347–353

Bataller L, Wade DF, Graus F et al (2004) Antibodies to Zic4 in paraneoplastic neurologic disorders and small-cell lung cancer. Neurology 62:778–782

Bataller L, Kleopa KA, Wu GF et al (2007) Autoimmune limbic encephalitis in 39 patients: immunophenotypes and outcomes. J Neurol Neurosurg Psychiatry 78:381–385

Battaglia T, De Grandis E, Mirabelli-Badenier M et al (2012) Response to rituximab in 3 children with opsoclonus-myoclonus syndrome resistant to conventional treatments. Eur J Paediatr Neurol 16:192–195

Belcastro V, Piola M, Binda S et al (2014) Opsoclonus-myoclonus syndrome associated with human herpes virus-6 rhomboencephalitis. J Neurol Sci 341:165–166

Bellur SN (1975) Opsoclonus: its clinical value. Neurology 25:502–507

Bernal F, Shams'ili S, Rojas I et al (2003) Anti-Tr antibodies as markers of paraneoplastic cerebellar degeneration and Hodgkin's disease. Neurology 60:230–234

Bhandari HS (2012) Presentation of opsoclonus myoclonus ataxia syndrome with glutamic acid decarboxylase antibodies. BMJ Case Rep 2012

Bhanushali MJ, Kranick SM, Freeman AF et al (2013) Human herpes 6 virus encephalitis complicating allogeneic hematopoietic stem cell transplantation. Neurology 80:1494–1500

BirluTiu V, BirluTiu RM (2014) Opsoclonus-myoclonus syndrome attributable to West Nile encephalitis: a case report. J Med Case Rep 8:232

Blaes F, Fuhlhuber V, Korfei M et al (2005) Surface-binding autoantibodies to cerebellar neurons in opsoclonus syndrome. Ann Neurol 58:313–317

Boltshauser E, Deonna T, Hirt HR (1979) Myoclonic encephalopathy of infants or "dancing eyes syndrome". Report of 7 cases with long-term follow-up and review of the literature (cases with and without neuroblastoma). Helv Paediatr Acta 34:119–133

Boronat A, Sabater L, Saiz A et al (2011) GABA(B) receptor antibodies in limbic encephalitis and anti-GAD-associated neurologic disorders. Neurology 76:795–800

Boronat A, Gelfand JM, Gresa-Arribas N et al (2013) Encephalitis and antibodies to dipeptidyl-peptidase-like protein-6, a subunit of Kv4.2 potassium channels. Ann Neurol 73:120–128

Bozzola E, Bozzola M, Tozzi AE et al (2014) Acute cerebellitis in varicella: a ten year case series and systematic review of the literature. Ital J Pediatr 40:57

Briani C, Vitaliani R, Grisold W et al (2011) Spectrum of paraneoplastic disease associated with lymphoma. Neurology 76:705–710

Brunklaus A, Pohl K, Zuberi SM et al (2012) Investigating neuroblastoma in childhood opsoclonus-myoclonus syndrome. Arch Dis Child 97:461–463

Buchanan TA, Gardiner TA, Archer DE (1984) An ultrastructural study of retinal photoreceptor degeneration associated with bronchial carcinoma. Am J Ophthalmol 97:277–287

Butler MH, Hayashi A, Ohkoshi N et al (2000) Autoimmunity to gephyrin in Stiff-Man syndrome. Neuron 26:307–312

Butterworth RF (1993) Pathophysiology of cerebellar dysfunction in the Wernicke-Korsakoff syndrome. Can J Neurol Sci 20(Suppl 3):S123–S126

Camdessanche JP, Jousserand G, Ferraud K et al (2009) The pattern and diagnostic criteria of sensory neuronopathy: a case–control study. Brain 132:1723–1733

Candler PM, Hart PE, Barnett M et al (2004) A follow up study of patients with paraneoplastic neurological disease in the United Kingdom. J Neurol Neurosurg Psychiatry 75:1411–1415

Caviness JN, Forsyth PA, Layton DD et al (1995) The movement disorder of adult opsoclonus. Mov Disord 10:22–27

Chinn JS, Schuffler MD (1988) Paraneoplastic visceral neuropathy as a cause of severe gastrointestinal motor dysfunction. Gastroenterology 95:1279–1286

Choi KD, Kim JS, Park SH et al (2006) Cerebellar hypermetabolism in paraneoplastic cerebellar degeneration. J Neurol Neurosurg Psychiatry 77:525–528

Conklin JL, Anuras S (1981) Radiation-induced recurrent intestinal pseudo-obstruction. Am J Gastroenterol 75:440–444

Connolly AM, Pestronk A, Mehta S et al (1997) Serum autoantibodies in childhood opsoclonus-myoclonus syndrome: an analysis of antigenic targets in neural tissues. J Pediatr 130:878–884

Corsellis JA, Goldberg GJ, Norton AR (1968) "Limbic encephalitis" and its association with carcinoma. Brain 91:481–496

Cross SA, Salomao DR, Parisi JE et al (2003) Paraneoplastic autoimmune optic neuritis with retinitis defined by CRMP-5-IgG. Ann Neurol 54:38–50

Cunningham J, Graus F, Anderson N et al (1986) Partial characterization of the Purkinje cell antigens in paraneoplastic cerebellar degeneration. Neurology 36:1163–1168

Dalmau J, Furneaux HM, Gralla RJ et al (1990) Detection of the anti-Hu antibody in the serum of patients with small cell lung cancer–a quantitative western blot analysis. Ann Neurol 27:544–552

Dalmau J, Graus F, Rosenblum MK et al (1992) Anti-Hu–associated paraneoplastic encephalomyelitis/sensory neuronopathy. A clinical study of 71 patients. Medicine (Baltimore) 71:59–72

Dalmau J, Graus F, Cheung NK et al (1995) Major histocompatibility proteins, anti-Hu antibodies, and paraneoplastic encephalomyelitis in neuroblastoma and small cell lung cancer. Cancer 75:99–109

Dalmau J, Graus F, Villarejo A et al (2004) Clinical analysis of anti-Ma2-associated encephalitis. Brain 127:1831–1844

de Graaff E, Maat P, Hulsenboom E et al (2012) Identification of delta/notch-like epidermal growth factor-related receptor as the Tr antigen in paraneoplastic cerebellar degeneration. Ann Neurol 71:815–824

DeFelipe-Mimbrera A, Masjuan J, Corral I et al (2014) Opsoclonus-myoclonus syndrome and limbic encephalitis associated with GABAB receptor antibodies in CSF. J Neuroimmunol 272:91–93

Denny-Brown D (1948) Primary sensory neuropathy with muscular changes associated with carcinoma. J Neurol Neurosurg Psychiatry 11:73–87

Dispenzieri A (2007) POEMS syndrome. Blood Rev 21:285–299

Fisher PG, Wechsler DS, Singer HS (1994) Anti-Hu antibody in a neuroblastoma-associated paraneoplastic syndrome. Pediatr Neurol 10:309–312

Flanagan EP, McKeon A, Lennon VA et al (2011) Paraneoplastic isolated myelopathy: clinical course and neuroimaging clues. Neurology 76:2089–2095

Forsyth PA, Dalmau J, Graus F et al (1997) Motor neuron syndromes in cancer patients. Ann Neurol 41:722–730

Fukuda T, Motomura M, Nakao Y et al (2003) Reduction of P/Q-type calcium channels in the postmortem cerebellum of paraneoplastic cerebellar degeneration with Lambert-Eaton myasthenic syndrome. Ann Neurol 53:21–28

Gill JS, Windebank AJ (1998) Cisplatin-induced apoptosis in rat dorsal root ganglion neurons is associated with attempted entry into the cell cycle. J Clin Invest 101:2842–2850

Giometto B, Marchiori GC, Nicolao P et al (1997) Sub-acute cerebellar degeneration with anti-Yo autoantibodies: immunohistochemical analysis of the immune reaction in the central nervous system. Neuropathol Appl Neurobiol 23:468–474

Giometto B, Grisold W, Vitaliani R et al (2010) Paraneoplastic neurologic syndrome in the PNS Euronetwork database: a European study from 20 centers. Arch Neurol 67:330–335

Giometto B, Vitaliani R, Lindeck-Pozza E et al (2012) Treatment for paraneoplastic neuropathies. Cochrane Database Syst Rev 12, CD007625

Gohil A, Croffie JM, Fitzgerald JF et al (2001) Reversible intestinal pseudoobstruction associated with neural crest tumors. J Pediatr Gastroenterol Nutr 33:86–88

Granerod J, Ambrose HE, Davies NW et al (2010) Causes of encephalitis and differences in their clinical presentations in England: a multicentre, population-based prospective study. Lancet Infect Dis 10:835–844

Grau-Rivera O, Sanchez-Valle R, Saiz A et al (2014) Determination of neuronal antibodies in suspected and definite Creutzfeldt-Jakob disease. JAMA Neurol 71:74–78

Graus F, Cordon-Cardo C, Posner JB (1985) Neuronal antinuclear antibody in sensory neuronopathy from lung cancer. Neurology 35:538–543

Graus F, Elkon KB, Lloberes P et al (1987) Neuronal antinuclear antibody (anti-Hu) in paraneoplastic encephalomyelitis simulating acute polyneuritis. Acta Neurol Scand 75:249–252

Graus F, Segurado OG, Tolosa E (1988) Selective concentration of anti-Purkinje cell antibody in the CSF of two patients with paraneoplastic cerebellar degeneration. Acta Neurol Scand 78:210–213

Graus F, Dalmou J, Rene R et al (1997) Anti-Hu antibodies in patients with small-cell lung cancer: association with complete response to therapy and improved survival. J Clin Oncol 15:2866–2872

Graus F, Keime-Guibert F, Rene R et al (2001) Anti-Hu-associated paraneoplastic encephalomyelitis: analysis of 200 patients. Brain 124:1138–1148

Graus F, Lang B, Pozo-Rosich P et al (2002) P/Q type calcium-channel antibodies in paraneoplastic cerebellar degeneration with lung cancer. Neurology 59:764–766

Graus F, Delattre JY, Antoine JC et al (2004) Recommended diagnostic criteria for paraneoplastic neurological syndromes. J Neurol Neurosurg Psychiatry 75:1135–1140

Graus F, Arino H, Dalmau J (2014) Paraneoplastic neurological syndromes in Hodgkin and non-Hodgkin lymphomas. Blood 123:3230–3238

Greene M, Lai Y, Baella N et al (2014) Antibodies to Delta/notch-like epidermal growth factor-related receptor in patients with anti-Tr, paraneoplastic cerebellar degeneration, and Hodgkin lymphoma. JAMA Neurol 71:1003–1008

Greenlee JE (2013) Treatment of paraneoplastic cerebellar degeneration. Curr Treat Options Neurol 15:185–200

Greenlee JE, Steffens JD, Clawson SA et al (2002) Anti-Hu antibodies in Merkel cell carcinoma. Ann Neurol 52:111–115

Gresa-Arribas N, Titulaer MJ, Torrents A et al (2014) Antibody titres at diagnosis and during follow-up of anti-NMDA receptor encephalitis: a retrospective study. Lancet Neurol 13:167–177

Griffin JW, Cornblath DR, Alexander E et al (1990) Ataxic sensory neuropathy and dorsal root ganglionitis associated with Sjogren's syndrome. Ann Neurol 27:304–315

Gultekin SH, Rosenfeld MR, Voltz R et al (2000) Paraneoplastic limbic encephalitis: neurological symptoms, immunological findings and tumour association in 50 patients. Brain 123(Pt 7):1481–1494

Hart IK, Maddison P, Newsom-Davis J et al (2002) Phenotypic variants of autoimmune peripheral nerve hyperexcitability. Brain 125:1887–1895

Hatanaka Y, Oh SJ (2008) Ten-second exercise is superior to 30-second exercise for post-exercise facilitation in diagnosing Lambert-Eaton myasthenic syndrome. Muscle Nerve 37:572–575

Hattori T, Hirayama K, Imai T et al (1988) Pontine lesion in opsoclonus-myoclonus syndrome shown by MRI. J Neurol Neurosurg Psychiatry 51:1572–1575

Hayward K, Jeremy RJ, Jenkins S et al (2001) Long-term neurobehavioral outcomes in children with neuroblastoma and opsoclonus-myoclonus-ataxia syndrome: relationship to MRI findings and anti-neuronal antibodies. J Pediatr 139:552–559

Henson RA, Hoffman HL, Urich H (1965) Encephalomyelitis with carcinoma. Brain 88:449–464

Hoftberger R, Kovacs GG, Sabater L et al (2013) Protein kinase C gamma antibodies and paraneoplastic cerebellar degeneration. J Neuroimmunol 256:91–93

Honnorat J, Antoine JC, Derrington E et al (1996) Antibodies to a subpopulation of glial cells and a 66 kDa developmental protein in patients with paraneoplastic neurological syndromes. J Neurol Neurosurg Psychiatry 61:270–278

Honnorat J, Saiz A, Giometto B et al (2001) Cerebellar ataxia with anti-glutamic acid decarboxylase antibodies: study of 14 patients. Arch Neurol 58:225–230

Ingenito GG, Berger JR, David NJ et al (1990) Limbic encephalitis associated with thymoma. Neurology 40:382

Irani SR, Pettingill P, Kleopa KA et al (2012) Morvan syndrome: clinical and serological observations in 29 cases. Ann Neurol 72:241–255

Jacobson DM, Thirkill CE, Tipping SJ (1990) A clinical triad to diagnose paraneoplastic retinopathy. Ann Neurol 28:162–167

Jarius S, Stich O, Rasiah C et al (2008) Qualitative evidence of Ri specific IgG-synthesis in the cerebrospinal fluid from patients with paraneoplastic neurological syndromes. J Neurol Sci 268:65–68

Jarius S, Eichhorn P, Jacobi C et al (2009) The intrathecal, polyspecific antiviral immune response: specific for MS or a general marker of CNS autoimmunity? J Neurol Sci 280:98–100

Jarius S, Martinez-Garcia P, Hernandez AL et al (2013) Two new cases of anti-Ca (anti-ARHGAP26/GRAF) autoantibody-associated cerebellar ataxia. J Neuroinflammation 10:7

Jones HR Jr, Hedley-Whyte ET, Freidberg SR et al (1982) Primary cerebellopontine progressive multifocal leukoencephalopathy diagnosed premortem by cerebellar biopsy. Ann Neurol 11:199–202

Keltner JL, Thirkill CE, Yip PT (2001) Clinical and immunologic characteristics of melanoma-associated retinopathy syndrome: eleven new cases and a review of 51 previously published cases. J Neuroophthalmol 21:173–187

Keogh M, Sedehizadeh S, Maddison P (2011) Treatment for Lambert-Eaton myasthenic syndrome. Cochrane Database Syst Rev (2):CD003279

Khasani S, Becker K, Meinck HM (2004) Hyperekplexia and stiff-man syndrome: abnormal brainstem reflexes suggest a physiological relationship. J Neurol Neurosurg Psychiatry 75:1265–1269

Kim H, Lim Y, Kim KK (2009) Anti-ri-antibody-associated paraneoplastic syndrome in a man with breast cancer showing a reversible pontine lesion on MRI. J Clin Neurol 5:151–152

Kimmel DW, O'Neill BP, Lennon VA (1988) Subacute sensory neuronopathy associated with small cell lung carcinoma: diagnosis aided by autoimmune serology. Mayo Clin Proc 63:29–32

Kinsbourne M (1962) Myoclonic encephalopathy of infants. J Neurol Neurosurg Psychiatry 25:271–276

Klaas JP, Ahlskog JE, Pittock SJ et al (2012) Adult-onset opsoclonus-myoclonus syndrome. Arch Neurol 69:1598–1607

Koike H, Tanaka F, Sobue G (2011) Paraneoplastic neuropathy: wide-ranging clinicopathological manifestations. Curr Opin Neurol 24:504–510

Krarup-Hansen A, Helweg-Larsen S, Schmalbruch H et al (2007) Neuronal involvement in cisplatin neuropathy: prospective clinical and neurophysiological studies. Brain 130:1076–1088

Kulling D, Reed CE, Verne GN et al (1997) Intestinal pseudo-obstruction as a paraneoplastic manifestation of malignant thymoma. Am J Gastroenterol 92:1564–1566

Kurian M, Lalive PH, Dalmau JO et al (2010) Opsoclonus-myoclonus syndrome in anti-N-methyl-D-aspartate receptor encephalitis. Arch Neurol 67:118–121

Lancaster E, Dalmau J (2012) Neuronal autoantigens–pathogenesis, associated disorders and antibody testing. Nat Rev Neurol 8:380–390

Lancaster E, Martinez-Hernandez E, Titulaer MJ et al (2011) Antibodies to metabotropic glutamate receptor 5 in the Ophelia syndrome. Neurology 77:1698–1701

Lauritzen M, Smith T, Fischer-Hansen B et al (1980) Eaton-Lambert syndrome and malignant thymoma. Neurology 30:634–638

Lawn ND, Westmoreland BF, Kiely MJ et al (2003) Clinical, magnetic resonance imaging, and electroencephalographic findings in paraneoplastic limbic encephalitis. Mayo Clin Proc 78:1363–1368

Lennon VA (1994) The case for a descriptive generic nomenclature: clarification of immunostaining criteria for PCA-1, ANNA-1, and ANNA-2 autoantibodies. Neurology 44:2412–2415

Lennon VA, Sas DF, Busk MF et al (1991) Enteric neuronal autoantibodies in pseudoobstruction with small-cell lung carcinoma. Gastroenterology 100:137–142

Levy LM, Dalakas MC, Floeter MK (1999) The stiff-person syndrome: an autoimmune disorder affecting neurotransmission of gamma-aminobutyric acid. Ann Intern Med 131:522–530

Leypoldt F, Eichhorn P, Saager C et al (2006) Successful immunosuppressive treatment and long-term follow-up of anti-Ri-associated paraneoplastic myelitis. J Neurol Neurosurg Psychiatry 77:1199–1200

Li J, Zhou DB (2013) New advances in the diagnosis and treatment of POEMS syndrome. Br J Haematol 161:303–315

Lucchinetti CF, Kimmel DW, Lennon VA (1998) Paraneoplastic and oncologic profiles of patients seropositive for type 1 antineuronal nuclear autoantibodies. Neurology 50:652–657

Luque FA, Furneaux HM, Ferziger R et al (1991) Anti-Ri: an antibody associated with paraneoplastic opsoclonus and breast cancer. Ann Neurol 29:241–251

Mason WP, Graus F, Lang B et al (1997) Small-cell lung cancer, paraneoplastic cerebellar degeneration and the Lambert-Eaton myasthenic syndrome. Brain 120(Pt 8):1279–1300

Maverakis E, Goodarzi H, Wehrli LN et al (2012) The etiology of paraneoplastic autoimmunity. Clin Rev Allergy Immunol 42:135–144

McKeon A, Lennon VA, Lachance DH et al (2009) Ganglionic acetylcholine receptor autoantibody: oncological, neurological, and serological accompaniments. Arch Neurol 66: 735–741

McKeon A, Tracy JA, Pittock SJ et al (2011a) Purkinje cell cytoplasmic autoantibody type 1 accompaniments: the cerebellum and beyond. Arch Neurol 68:1282–1289

McKeon A, Pittock SJ, Lennon VA (2011b) CSF complements serum for evaluating paraneoplastic antibodies and NMO-IgG. Neurology 76:1108–1110

McKeon A, Robinson MT, McEvoy KM et al (2012) Stiff-man syndrome and variants: clinical course, treatments, and outcomes. Arch Neurol 69:230–238

McKeon A, Martinez-Hernandez E, Lancaster E et al (2013) Glycine receptor autoimmune spectrum with stiff-man syndrome phenotype. JAMA Neurol 70:44–50

Meinck HM, Ricker K, Hulser PJ et al (1994) Stiff man syndrome: clinical and laboratory findings in eight patients. J Neurol 241:157–166

Moersch FP, Woltman HW (1956) Progressive fluctuating muscular rigidity and spasm ('stiff-man" syndrome); report of a case and some observations in 13 other cases. Proc Staff Meet Mayo Clin 31:421–427

Molinuevo JL, Graus F, Serrano C et al (1998) Utility of anti-Hu antibodies in the diagnosis of paraneoplastic sensory neuropathy. Ann Neurol 44:976–980

Monstad SE, Knudsen A, Salvesen HB et al (2009) Onconeural antibodies in sera from patients with various types of tumours. Cancer Immunol Immunother 58:1795–1800

Morimoto M, Osaki T, Nagara Y et al (2010) Thymoma with Lambert-Eaton myasthenic syndrome. Ann Thorac Surg 89:2001–2003

Murinson BB, Guarnaccia JB (2008) Stiff-person syndrome with amphiphysin antibodies: distinctive features of a rare disease. Neurology 71:1955–1958

Musthafa CP, Moosa A, Chandrashekharan PA et al (2006) Intestinal pseudo-obstruction as initial presentation of thymoma. Indian J Gastroenterol 25:264–265

Nakao YK, Motomura M, Fukudome T et al (2002) Seronegative Lambert-Eaton myasthenic syndrome: study of 110 Japanese patients. Neurology 59:1773–1775

Newman NJ, Bell IR, McKee AC (1990) Paraneoplastic limbic encephalitis: neuropsychiatric presentation. Biol Psychiatry 27:529–542

O'Neill JH, Murray NM, Newsom-Davis J (1988) The Lambert-Eaton myasthenic syndrome. A review of 50 cases. Brain 111(Pt 3):577–596

Ojeda VJ (1984) Necrotizing myelopathy associated with malignancy. A clinicopathologic study of two cases and literature review. Cancer 53:1115–1123

Ongerboer de Visser BW (1983) Anatomical and functional organization of reflexes involving the trigeminal system in man: jaw reflex, blink-reflex, corneal reflex and exteroceptive suppression. In: Desmedt JE (ed) Motor control mechanisms in health and disease. Raven Press, New York, pp 727–738

Pande R, Leis AA (1999) Myasthenia gravis, thymoma, intestinal pseudo-obstruction, and neuronal nicotinic acetylcholine receptor antibody. Muscle Nerve 22:1600–1602

Panegyres PK, Reading MC, Esiri MM (1993) The inflammatory reaction of paraneoplastic ganglionitis and encephalitis: an immunohistochemical study. J Neurol 240:93–97

Pittock SJ, Lennon VA (2008) Aquaporin-4 autoantibodies in a paraneoplastic context. Arch Neurol 65:629–632

Pittock SJ, Lucchinetti CF, Lennon VA (2003) Anti-neuronal nuclear autoantibody type 2: paraneoplastic accompaniments. Ann Neurol 53:580–587

Pittock SJ, Parisi JE, McKeon A et al (2010) Paraneoplastic jaw dystonia and laryngospasm with antineuronal nuclear autoantibody type 2 (anti-Ri). Arch Neurol 67:1109–1115

Polans AS, Buczylko J, Crabb J et al (1991) A photoreceptor calcium binding protein is recognized by autoantibodies obtained from patients with cancer-associated retinopathy. J Cell Biol 112:981–989

Polans AS, Witkowska D, Haley TL et al (1995) Recoverin, a photoreceptor-specific calcium-binding protein, is expressed by the tumor of a patient with cancer-associated retinopathy. Proc Natl Acad Sci U S A 92:9176–9180

Pranzatelli MR (1992) The neurobiology of the opsoclonus-myoclonus syndrome. Clin Neuropharmacol 15:186–228

Psimaras D, Carpentier AF, Rossi C (2010) Cerebrospinal fluid study in paraneoplastic syndromes. J Neurol Neurosurg Psychiatry 81:42–45

Racalbuto A, Magro G, Lanteri R et al (2008) Idiopathic myenteric ganglionitis underlying acute 'dramatic' intestinal pseudoobstruction: report of an exceptional case. Case Rep Gastroenterol 2:461–468

Rakocevic G, Barohn R, McVey AL et al (2003) Myasthenia gravis, thymoma, and intestinal pseudo-obstruction: a case report and review. J Clin Neuromuscul Dis 5:93–95

Rauer S, Kaiser R (2000) Demonstration of anti-HuD specific oligoclonal bands in the cerebrospinal fluid from patients with paraneoplastic neurological syndromes. Qualitative evidence of anti-HuD specific IgG-synthesis in the central nervous system. J Neuroimmunol 111:241–244

Rauer S, Kaiser R (2001) Enzyme linked immunosorbent assay using recombinant HuD-autoantigen for serodiagnosis of paraneoplastic neurological syndromes. Acta Neurol Scand 103:248–254

Reiber H, Felgenhauer K (1987) Protein transfer at the blood cerebrospinal fluid barrier and the quantitation of the humoral immune response within the central nervous system. Clin Chim Acta 163:319–328

Roberts A, Perera S, Lang B et al (1985) Paraneoplastic myasthenic syndrome IgG inhibits 45Ca2+ flux in a human small cell carcinoma line. Nature 317:737–739

Rosenfeld MR, Posner JB (1991) Paraneoplastic motor neuron disease. In: Rowland LP (ed) Advances in neurology: amyotrophic lateral sclerosis and other motor neuron diseases. Raven Press, New York, pp 445–459

Rudnicki SA, Dalmau J (2005) Paraneoplastic syndromes of the peripheral nerves. Curr Opin Neurol 18:598–603

Sabater L, Bataller L, Carpentier AF et al (2006) Protein kinase C gamma autoimmunity in paraneoplastic cerebellar degeneration and non-small-cell lung cancer. J Neurol Neurosurg Psychiatry 77:1359–1362

Sabater L, Titulaer M, Saiz A et al (2008) SOX1 antibodies are markers of paraneoplastic Lambert-Eaton myasthenic syndrome. Neurology 70:924–928

Saiz A, Graus F, Dalmau J et al (1999) Detection of 14-3-3 brain protein in the cerebrospinal fluid of patients with paraneoplastic neurological disorders. Ann Neurol 46:774–777

Saiz A, Bruna J, Stourac P et al (2009) Anti-Hu-associated brainstem encephalitis. J Neurol Neurosurg Psychiatry 80:404–407

Schuffler MD, Rohrmann CA, Chaffee RG et al (1981) Chronic intestinal pseudo-obstruction. A report of 27 cases and review of the literature. Medicine (Baltimore) 60:173–196

Shams'ili S, Grefkens J, de Leeuw B et al (2003) Paraneoplastic cerebellar degeneration associated with antineuronal antibodies: analysis of 50 patients. Brain 126:1409–1418

Sipponen T, Karikoski R, Nuutinen H et al (2009) Three-generation familial visceral myopathy with alpha-actin-positive inclusion bodies in intestinal smooth muscle. J Clin Gastroenterol 43:437–443

Skeie GO, Romi F (2008) Paraneoplastic myasthenia gravis: immunological and clinical aspects. Eur J Neurol 15:1029–1033

Smith JH, Dhamija R, Moseley BD et al (2011) N-methyl-D-aspartate receptor autoimmune encephalitis presenting with opsoclonus-myoclonus: treatment response to plasmapheresis. Arch Neurol 68:1069–1072

Sommer C, Weishaupt A, Brinkhoff J et al (2005) Paraneoplastic stiff-person syndrome: passive transfer to rats by means of IgG antibodies to amphiphysin. Lancet 365:1406–1411

Stich O, Rauer S (2007) Antigen-specific oligoclonal bands in cerebrospinal fluid and serum from patients with anti-amphiphysin- and anti-CV2/CRMP5 associated paraneoplastic neurological syndromes. Eur J Neurol 14:650–653

Stich O, Graus F, Rasiah C et al (2003) Qualitative evidence of anti-Yo-specific intrathecal antibody synthesis in patients with paraneoplastic cerebellar degeneration. J Neuroimmunol 141:165–169

Stich O, Jarius S, Kleer B et al (2007) Specific antibody index in cerebrospinal fluid from patients with central and peripheral paraneoplastic neurological syndromes. J Neuroimmunol 183:220–224

Stork AC, van der Pol WL, Franssen H et al (2014) Clinical phenotype of patients with neuropathy associated with monoclonal gammopathy: a comparative study and a review of the literature. J Neurol 261:1398–1404

Storstein A, Krossnes B, Vedeler CA (2006) Autopsy findings in the nervous system and ovarian tumour of two patients with paraneoplastic cerebellar degeneration. Acta Neurol Scand Suppl 183:69–70

Sutton IJ, Barnett MH, Watson JD et al (2002) Paraneoplastic brainstem encephalitis and anti-Ri antibodies. J Neurol 249:1597–1598

Tagliati M, Simpson D, Morgello S et al (1998) Cerebellar degeneration associated with human immunodeficiency virus infection. Neurology 50:244–251

Talon P, Stoll C (1985) Opsomyoclonus syndrome in children. A new case. Review of the literature (110 cases). Pediatrie 40:441–449

Teixeira AR, Nitz N, Guimaro MC et al (2006) Chagas disease. Postgrad Med J 82:788–798

Tetu B, Ro JY, Ayala AG et al (1989) Small cell carcinoma of prostate associated with myasthenic (Eaton-Lambert) syndrome. Urology 33:148–152

Titulaer MJ, Klooster R, Potman M et al (2009) SOX antibodies in small-cell lung cancer and Lambert-Eaton myasthenic syndrome: frequency and relation with survival. J Clin Oncol 27:4260–4267

Titulaer MJ, Soffietti R, Dalmau J et al (2011a) Screening for tumours in paraneoplastic syndromes: report of an EFNS task force. Eur J Neurol 18:19–e13

Titulaer MJ, Lang B, Verschuuren JJ (2011b) Lambert-Eaton myasthenic syndrome: from clinical characteristics to therapeutic strategies. Lancet Neurol 10:1098–1107

Titulaer MJ, Maddison P, Sont JK et al (2011c) Clinical Dutch-English Lambert-Eaton Myasthenic syndrome (LEMS) tumor association prediction score accurately predicts small-cell lung cancer in the LEMS. J Clin Oncol 29:902–908

Valls-Sole J, Graus F, Font J et al (1990) Normal proprioceptive trigeminal afferents in patients with Sjogren's syndrome and sensory neuronopathy. Ann Neurol 28:786–790

Vernino S, Tuite P, Adler CH et al (2002) Paraneoplastic chorea associated with CRMP-5 neuronal antibody and lung carcinoma. Ann Neurol 51:625–630

Voltz R, Gultekin SH, Rosenfeld MR et al (1999) A serologic marker of paraneoplastic limbic and brain-stem encephalitis in patients with testicular cancer. N Engl J Med 340:1788–1795

Wald A, Kichler J, Mendelow H (1981) Amyloidosis and chronic intestinal pseudoobstruction. Dig Dis Sci 26:462–465

Wanschitz J, Hainfellner JA, Kristoferitsch W et al (1997) Ganglionitis in paraneoplastic subacute sensory neuronopathy: a morphologic study. Neurology 49:1156–1159

Weinstein JM, Kelman SE, Bresnick GH et al (1994) Paraneoplastic retinopathy associated with anti-retinal bipolar cell antibodies in cutaneous malignant melanoma. Ophthalmology 101:1236–1243

Wildhaber B, Niggli F, Stallmach T et al (2002) Intestinal pseudoobstruction as a paraneoplastic syndrome in ganglioneuroblastoma. Eur J Pediatr Surg 12:429–431

Yamamoto AM, Gajdos P, Eymard B et al (2001) Anti-titin antibodies in myasthenia gravis: tight association with thymoma and heterogeneity of nonthymoma patients. Arch Neurol 58:885–890

Young CA, MacKenzie JM, Chadwick DW et al (1993) Opsoclonus-myoclonus syndrome: an autopsy study of three cases. Eur J Med 2:239–241

Yu Z, Kryzer TJ, Griesmann GE et al (2001) CRMP-5 neuronal autoantibody: marker of lung cancer and thymoma-related autoimmunity. Ann Neurol 49:146–154

Laboratory Diagnosis of Subarachnoid Haemorrhage

22

Markus Otto, Karin Nagy, and Niklas Mattson

Contents

Abstract

The diagnosis of CT-negative subarachnoid haemorrhage (SAH) is an important clinical challenge in clinical neurology. Cerebrospinal fluid (CSF) analysis via lumbar puncture is the method of first choice. The diagnosis of SAH in CSF is based on a bloody or xanthochromic discoloration of the CSF as well as on findings in nonautomated CSF cytology including the detection of erythrophages and siderophages. The automated determination of CSF ferritin concentrations or spectrophotometric detection of xanthochromia may contribute to the diagnosis but are only useful with regard to the overall clinical picture. Generally, the

M. Otto (✉)
Department of Neurology, University of Ulm, Oberer Eselsberg 45, 89081 Ulm, Germany
e-mail: markus.otto@uni-ulm.de

K. Nagy • N. Mattson
Department of Psychiatry and Neurochemistry, Institute of Neuroscience and Physiology,
Sahlgrenska Academy, University of Gothenburg, Gothenburg, Sweden
e-mail: niklas.mattsson@neuro.gu.se

© Springer International Publishing Switzerland 2015
F. Deisenhammer et al. (eds.), *Cerebrospinal Fluid in Clinical Neurology*,
DOI 10.1007/978-3-319-01225-4_22

knowledge of the time flow of the CSF changes associated with SAH (8–12 h after onset of headache) is essential for a correct interpretation of CSF findings.

22.1 Introduction

Subarachnoid haemorrhage (SAH) accounts for approximately 5 % of all strokes and has a yearly incidence of approximately 1 in 10,000 persons (Feigin et al. 2003). Importantly, SAH both has a high fatality (30–70 %) (Hop et al. 1997) and may occur at an early age compared with other causes of stroke (Johnston et al. 1998). In the majority of cases, SAH is caused by a spontaneous rupture of an aneurysm in the arterial circulation of the brain. Typical initial symptoms are severe headache with a sudden onset ("thunderclap headache"), neck stiffness, vomiting, confusion, or loss of consciousness. However sometimes SAH presents only with a mild headache which makes the differential diagnosis difficult (Marton and Gean 1986; Linn et al. 1996).

Early diagnosis is of utmost importance: A delayed diagnosis and therapy increases the risk of mortality. The risk for a rebleeding increases from 5 % within the first day to 15–20 % within 2 weeks up to 50 % within 6 months (Morgenstern et al. 1998).

The most commonly used first line of investigation is noncontrast computed tomography (CT) of the brain. CT has an excellent sensitivity for SAH in the acute stage, especially using modern scanners, with sensitivities up to 98–100 % within the first hours from symptom onset (Perry et al. 2011).

However, because subarachnoid blood is rapidly cleared from the brain, the sensitivity drops quickly. Six hours after onset, the sensitivity of a CT scan for finding

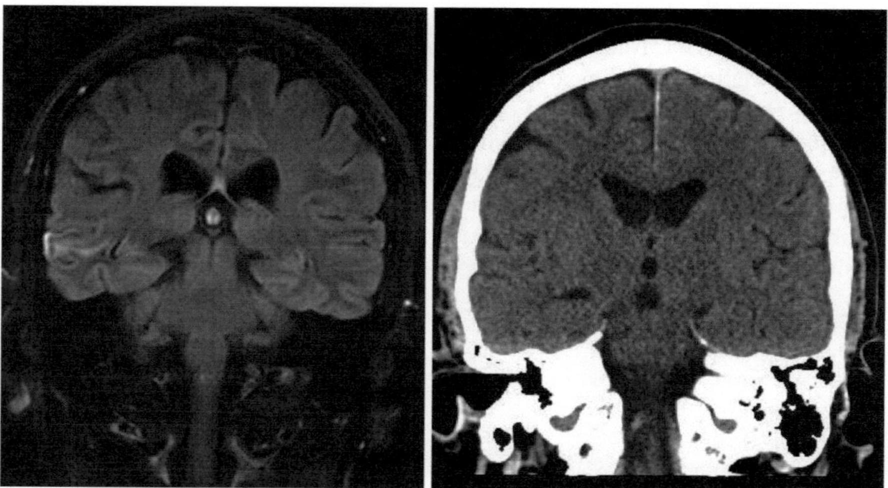

Fig. 22.1 CT-negative SAH. *Left side* MRI (FLAIR): hyperintense signal clearly visible; *right side* CT scan: no sign for SAH

an SAH is approximately 86–93 %, and it decreases to approximately 50 % after 1 week (Perry et al. 2011).

MRI investigation with FLAIR sequence and gradient spin echo do have a similar sensitivity in the early phase of the bleeding, but in contrast to CT investigations, older bleedings can be seen with a higher sensitivity (Noguchi et al. 1997). But MRI is not always available and then the exact timing of the bleeding is not always possible (Fig. 22.1).

22.2 Laboratory Diagnostic Methods

There are several widely used CSF analyses for SAH with different diagnostic performance, availability, and technical requirements. The laboratory diagnostic methods were reviewed recently (Tumani et al. 2010; Nagy et al. 2013).

22.2.1 Visual Inspection

The most basic CSF method for SAH is the visual evaluation of discoloration. For this, the sample is usually centrifuged and the supernatant compared with a tube of water, held against a well-illuminated white background. Normal CSF is uncolored and transparent. After an SAH, a yellowish or reddish tint is seen due to bilirubin (called xanthochromia) or oxyhaemoglobin. However, the sensitivity of the human colour vision is not sufficient to detect a very small amount of bilirubin, which may appear as transparent as water (Petzold et al. 2005; Sidman et al. 2005).

A traumatic tap may occur when the needle punctuates a blood vessel. This might be differentiated by the three-tube method – visual inspection or cell count in serial tubes, to detect declining red blood cell counts, indicating a traumatic tap – but especially in the very early phase of a bleeding, this might not always be helpful for the differentiation (Fig. 22.2 and Table 22.1).

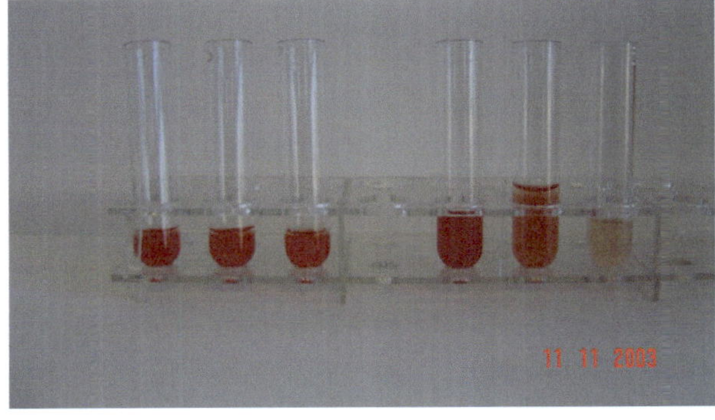

Fig. 22.2 Three-tube method

Table 22.1 Differentiation artificial versus SAH

	SAH	Artificial
3 tubes	All reddish	Clear in the last tube
Cytology	Macrophages	No macrophages
Cell-free CSF	Xanthochromia	Clear
Ferritin	>15 ng/ml	<15 ng/ml
Spectrophotometer	Pos.	Neg.

Table 22.2 Time series of different CSF finding after subarachnoid haemorrhage

	<12 h	12 h to 3 days	>3 days
Pleocytosis	+++	++	+
Erythrocytes	+++	++	+
Oxy-Hb	+	+++	+
Erythrophages	+	++	
Bilirubin	(+)	++	+++
Siderophages		+	++
Ferritin	+	++	+++
Haematoidin crystals		(+)	++

22.2.2 Spectrophotometry

More reliable than visual inspection is the spectrophotometry. By this the absorption of bilirubin can be quantified and documented, so that an objective rating of xanthochromia is possible (Petzold et al. 2004, 2006).

It is a rapid (<1 min) technique that requires a small sample amount (50–500 μL). Because sensitivity and specificity vary for different markers that may be elevated depending on the duration since symptom onset, the laboratory technician must know the time point of symptom debut, sampling, and centrifugation to perform a sound interpretation (Table 22.2).

22.2.3 Oxyhaemoglobin

After an SAH, the erythrocytes in the CSF will gradually lyse and release their intracellular haemoglobin. This process starts shortly (2–4 h) after the bleeding, and oxyhaemoglobin can be detected in CSF from approximately 2–12 h after ictus (Cruickshank 2001). Oxyhaemoglobin, the oxygenated form of haemoglobin, has an absorbance maximum around 415 nm, in the violet region of the optical spectrum.

22.2.4 Bilirubin

Oxyhaemoglobin is metabolized to bilirubin through enzymatic reactions by macrophages in vivo. This does not occur in vitro in tapped CSF (except in samples with very high white blood cell count), which strongly reduces the risk for false-positive results caused by a traumatic tapping. Bilirubin has a broad maximum absorption peak in the blue region of the optical spectrum at 450–460 nm (Petzold et al. 2006). As an alternative to using a spectrophotometer, CSF (Shah and Edlow 2002) bilirubin may also be measured by the modification of the direct diazo methods used for bilirubin measurements in serum or plasma. But difficulties regarding technical analyses and method standardization may hinder a broad implementation of this tentative approach (Beetham et al 2006).

22.2.5 Methaemoglobin

Methaemoglobin is haemoglobin with ferric (Fe 3+) instead of ferrous iron (Fe 2+) in the haem group, with a broad absorbance maximum peak at 403–410 nm. Normally, methaemoglobin is present in very small amounts, but it has been reported in CSF of patients with subdural haematoma or an enclosed bleeding, giving the CSF a brownish colour (Barrows et al. 1955). A spontaneous oxidation of the haem group occurs around 10 days after a bleed, irrespective of cause (Wahlgren and Lindquist 1987), which may be useful to distinguish between a traumatic tap and a cerebral haemorrhage (Trbojevic-Cepe et al. 1992).

22.2.6 Ferritin

Ferritin is an iron-storage protein complex that removes toxic iron released from the metabolized haemoglobin. The production of this large protein takes some time, and therefore, CSF ferritin has a lower sensitivity in the first hours after SAH and is not advocated for diagnostic use at an early stage (Watson et al. 2008; Petzold et al. 2009). A first increase is possibly due to the activation of macrophages. It takes approximately 3 days for the CSF ferritin levels to consistently increase and 7–10 days to reach over 1,000 ng/mL (Petzold et al. 2011).

One conservative reference limit that has been proposed is 12 ng/mL, and in a prospective study, a cut-off of 15 ng/mL achieved 95 % sensitivity and specificity for SAH (Wick and Pfister 1999). Importantly, CSF ferritin levels remain high long after CSF bilirubin decreases or becomes undetectable (Tumani et al. 2010; Petzold et al. 2011).

In the German-speaking countries (Germany, Austria, and Switzerland), the use of CSF ferritin measurement is the method of choice at most centres because it is easily available on the routine laboratory instruments that already measure CSF total protein, glucose, and lactate.

22.2.7 Cytology

Within 1–2 h after an SAH, large quantities of erythrocytes can be found and CSF on visual inspection is bloody (see above). But there is no cut-off established from

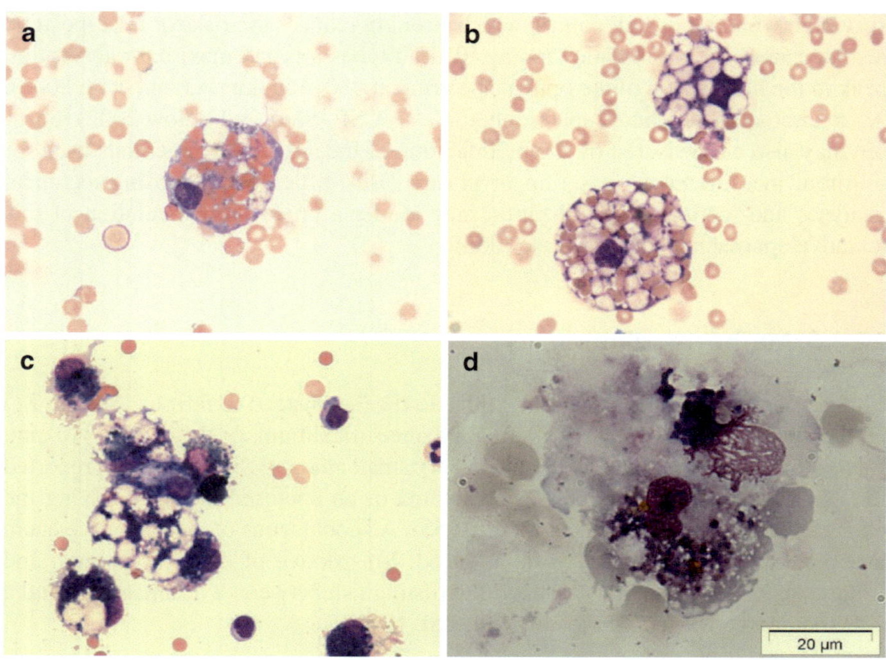

Fig. 22.3 Cytology of SAH at different time points: (**a**) bleeding (2–10 h) with erythrophages, (**b**) 1–2-day-old bleeding with erythro- or siderophages, (**c**) transition fresh to old bleeding with no erythrophages, and (**d**) old bleeding with haematoidin crystals >10 days

which an SAH can be excluded (Shah and Edlow 2002), until a cell count of 400 erythrocytes per microL CSF can still look clear under visual inspection.

SAH induces an inflammatory response that includes macrophage activation. Macrophages that have consumed erythrocytes develop haemosiderin storage and are called siderophages. Detection of CSF siderophages have a low sensitivity within the first 3 days after an intracranial bleeding, making them unsuitable for early diagnosis, but later in the process, they have high sensitivity and specificity, and they may even be detected for several months after an insult (Veuger et al. 1977). In combination with erythrophages (macrophages that do not have haemosiderin inside), they can give important clues about the age and dynamics of the bleeding (Tumani et al. 2010) (Fig. 22.3).

22.3   Summary and Practical Approach

Early CSF diagnostics is the method of choice for CT-negative SAH. The exact knowledge of the time course of different biochemical changes is necessary to come to a conclusive laboratory diagnosis. With the increasing use of MRI and incidental finding of bleedings especially in the T2-star sequence, CSF diagnostics might help in the judgement of how acute these findings are.

References

Barrows LJ, Hunter FT, Banker BQ (1955) The nature and clinical significance of pigments in the cerebrospinal fluid. Brain 78(1):59–80

Beetham R, Monk C, Keating L, Benger JR, Kendall J (2006) Effects of storage at -20 degrees C on ischaemia-modified albumin results. Ann Clin Biochem 43(Pt 6):500–502

Cruickshank AM (2001) ACP Best Practice No 166: CSF spectrophotometry in the diagnosis of subarachnoid haemorrhage. J Clin Pathol 54(11):827–830

Feigin VL, Lawes CM, Bennett DA, Anderson CS (2003) Stroke epidemiology: a review of population-based studies of incidence, prevalence, and case-fatality in the late 20th century. Lancet Neurol 2(1):43–53

Hop JW, Rinkel GJ, Algra A, van Gijn J (1997) Case-fatality rates and functional outcome after subarachnoid hemorrhage: a systematic review. Stroke 28(3):660–664

Johnston SC, Selvin S, Gress DR (1998) The burden, trends, and demographics of mortality from subarachnoid hemorrhage. Neurology 50(5):1413–1418

Linn FH, Rinkel GJ, Algra A, van Gijn J (1996) Incidence of subarachnoid hemorrhage: role of region, year, and rate of computed tomography: a meta-analysis. Stroke 27(4):625–629

Marton KI, Gean AD (1986) The spinal tap: a new look at an old test. Ann Intern Med 104(6):840–848

Morgenstern LB, Luna-Gonzales H, Huber JC Jr, Wong SS, Uthman MO, Gurian JH, Castillo PR, Shaw SG, Frankowski RF, Grotta JC (1998) Worst headache and subarachnoid hemorrhage: prospective, modern computed tomography and spinal fluid analysis. Ann Emerg Med 32(3 Pt 1):297–304

Nagy K, Skagervik I, Tumani H, Petzold A, Wick M, Kuhn HJ, Uhr M, Regeniter A, Brettschneider J, Otto M, Kraus J, Deisenhammer F, Lautner R, Blennow K, Shaw L, Zetterberg H, Mattsson N (2013) Cerebrospinal fluid analyses for the diagnosis of subarachnoid haemorrhage and experience from a Swedish study. What method is preferable when diagnosing a subarachnoid haemorrhage? Clin Chem Lab Med 1–14

Noguchi K, Ogawa T, Inugami A, Fujita H, Hatazawa J, Shimosegawa E, Okudera T, Uemura K, Seto H (1997) MRI of acute cerebral infarction: a comparison of FLAIR and T2-weighted fast spin-echo imaging. Neuroradiology 39(6):406–410

Perry JJ, Stiell IG, Sivilotti ML, Bullard MJ, Emond M, Symington C, Sutherland J, Worster A, Hohl C, Lee JS, Eisenhauer MA, Mortensen M, Mackey D, Pauls M, Lesiuk H, Wells GA (2011) Sensitivity of computed tomography performed within six hours of onset of headache for diagnosis of subarachnoid haemorrhage: prospective cohort study. BMJ 343:d4277

Petzold A, Keir G, Sharpe LT (2004) Spectrophotometry for xanthochromia. N Engl J Med 351(16):1695–1696

Petzold A, Keir G, Sharpe TL (2005) Why human color vision cannot reliably detect cerebrospinal fluid xanthochromia. Stroke 36(6):1295–1297

Petzold A, Sharpe LT, Keir G (2006) Spectrophotometry for cerebrospinal fluid pigment analysis. Neurocrit Care 4(2):153–162

Petzold A, Worthington V, Pritchard C, Appleby I, Kitchen N, Smith M (2009) The longitudinal profile of bilirubin and ferritin in the cerebrospinal fluid following a subarachnoid hemorrhage: diagnostic implications. Neurocrit Care 11(3):398–402

Petzold A, Worthington V, Appleby I, Kerr ME, Kitchen N, Smith M (2011) Cerebrospinal fluid ferritin level, a sensitive diagnostic test in late-presenting subarachnoid hemorrhage. J Stroke Cerebrovasc Dis 20(6):489–493

Shah KH, Edlow JA (2002) Distinguishing traumatic lumbar puncture from true subarachnoid hemorrhage. J Emerg Med 23(1):67–74

Sidman R, Spitalnic S, Demelis M, Durfey N, Jay G (2005) Xanthrochromia? By what method? A comparison of visual and spectrophotometric xanthrochromia. Ann Emerg Med 46(1):51–55

Trbojevic-Cepe M, Vogrinc Z, Brinar V (1992) Diagnostic significance of methemoglobin determination in colorless cerebrospinal fluid. Clin Chem 38(8 Pt 1):1404–1408

Tumani H, Petzold A, Wick M, Kuhn HJ, Uhr M, Otto M, Regeniter A, Brettschneider J (2010) Cerebrospinal fluid-based diagnostics of CT-negative subarachnoid haemorrhage. Nervenarzt 81(8):973–979

Veuger AJ, Kortbeek LH, Booij AC (1977) Siderophages in differentiation of blood in cerebrospinal fluid. Clin Neurol Neurosurg 80(1):46–56

Wahlgren NG, Lindquist C (1987) Haem derivatives in the cerebrospinal fluid after intracranial haemorrhage. Eur Neurol 26(4):216–221

Watson ID, Beetham R, Fahie-Wilson MN, Holbrook IB, O'Connell DM (2008) What is the role of cerebrospinal fluid ferritin in the diagnosis of subarachnoid haemorrhage in computed tomography-negative patients? Ann Clin Biochem 45(Pt 2):189–192

Wick M, Pfister HW (1999) Ferritin and iron metabolism in cerebrospinal fluid (CSF) subarachnoid hemorrhage (SAH). IFCC– WorldLab 77

CSF-orrhoea

23

Geoffrey Keir and Ligy Thomas

Contents

Abstract

CSF-orrhoea is defined as the leakage or transfer of CSF from any of its normal compartments. Head trauma or surgical interventions probably account for 80–90 % of all cases of CSF rhinorrhoea, whilst spontaneous CSF leaks account for 3–4 % of cases. Most spontaneous CSF leaks will self-repair in 7–10 days, although persistent leaks will usually require surgical management typically involving an endoscopic trans-nasal procedure. Transsphenoidal pituitary sur-

G. Keir (✉)
Neuroimmunology and CSF Laboratory,
Walton Centre for Neurology and Neurosurgery,
Liverpool, UK
e-mail: Geoffrey.Keir@thewaltoncentre.nhs.uk

L. Thomas
Department of Otorhinolaryngology,
Lancashire Teaching Hospital,
Preston, UK

© Springer International Publishing Switzerland 2015
F. Deisenhammer et al. (eds.), *Cerebrospinal Fluid in Clinical Neurology*,
DOI 10.1007/978-3-319-01225-4_23

gery and transmastoid schwannoma surgery can lead to CSF leaks manifesting as rhinorrhoea or otorrhoea. CSF leaks are also relatively common following spinal surgery and can prove problematic to differentiate from seromas and focal infections. The management algorithm in a suspected CSF leak is first to identify the discharge fluid as being or containing CSF. Currently, the best laboratory approach is to test for asialotransferrin and beta-trace protein. Glucose and chloride measurements are now considered inadequately specific, and their use is discouraged. Magnetic resonance imaging, including the use of intrathecal gadolinium, and computerised tomography are applied to localising the site of leakage.

Non-standard Definitions Throughout

CSF-orrhoea	The leakage or transfer of CSF from any of its normal compartments.
CSF rhinorrhoea	The leakage of CSF into the sinonasal tract.
CSF otorrhoea	The leakage of CSF into the ear/Eustachian canals.
Liquorrhoea	An alternative term for CSF-orrhoea.
CSF shunt	A tubular surgical implant intended for the bulk movement of CSF. Used most often in a treatment of hydrocephalus, shunts will divert CSF either into the peritoneal cavity (ventriculoperitoneal shunt, VPS), directly into the blood (ventriculoatrial shunt; VAS), into the pleural cavity (VPS) or simply from the lateral ventricles into the cisterna magna (VCS).
CSF drain	This, by contrast, is intended to remove CSF from the body. It is most commonly inserted into the lumbar sac (lumbar drain). CSF is drained *ex corpus* into a collection bottle.

23.1   Introduction

CSF-orrhoea is most commonly encountered as the leakage of CSF from the skull, although CSF fistulae can also occur anywhere along the spine, particularly following surgery or trauma. CSF fistulae are often under-diagnosed, difficult to localise and clinically silent. CSF leakage can lead to the accumulation in (and discharge from) the nasal sinuses (CSF rhinorrhoea) and/or the ear canals/ Eustachian tube (CSF otorrhoea). Leakage elsewhere can result in the formation of an abscess.

The primary causes of CSF-orrhoea include the following:

- Traumatic head injury
- Surgery
- Erosive bone disease, e.g. secondary to infections or tumours

- Increased intracranial pressure, which can rupture the membranes covering the cranial foramina through which nerves, blood vessels and other structures pass

23.2 CSF-orrhoea

23.2.1 CSF Rhinorrhoea

Patients with CSF rhinorrhoea typically present with a clear rhinorrhoea (unilateral or bilateral). CSF leaking to the middle ear space can drain through Eustachian tube (when eardrum is intact) into postnasal space and manifest as CSF rhinorrhoea. Patients can also present with symptoms of orthostatic headache, pneumocephalus, recurrent meningitis, brain abscess or unilateral intranasal masses. Whilst not significantly hazardous in itself (assuming that the cause is benign) CSF-orrhoea does carry a cumulative risk of CNS infections, with an overall risk of ~20 % and an individual incidence of 0.3 episodes/year (Daudia et al. 2007). Differential diagnosis includes perennial allergic rhinitis, vasomotor rhinitis, chronic rhinosinusitis and sinonasal polyps. CSF rhinorrhoea commonly occurs following surgical trauma (endoscopic sinus surgery and/or tumour resection) or head trauma (frontobasal skull fractures), which probably accounts for 80–90 % of all causes. Other conditions include osteomyelitis and congenital abnormalities, such as meningoceles or meningoencephaloceles and skull base tumours. Idiopathic intracranial hypertension (IIH, also termed benign intracranial hypertension and pseudotumour cerebri) is a disorder of elevated intracranial pressure of unknown cause with an annual incidence of around 0.9/100,000. It is thought that outflow resistance to CSF resorption is increased, leading to the rise in intracranial pressure. Less benign cause of raised intracranial pressure (ICP) should always be considered, including hydrocephalus, tumours and brain cysts. A raised ICP may explain the observation of empty enlarged sella turcica in some patients with non-traumatic CSF rhinorrhoea (Bjerre 1990; Naing and Frohman 2007). It is thought that an empty sella develops when CSF under pressure enters the sella through a tear in the sellar diaphragm causing compression of the pituitary tissue (Lenz and Root 2012). If this is so, then empty sella syndrome could be considered a form of 'internal CSF-orrhoea' – in which the CSF is entering an area from which it is normally excluded.

23.2.2 Management Algorithm

The management of CSF-orrhoea is as follows:

- To confirm that the discharge fluid is CSF and not simply rhinitis fluid.

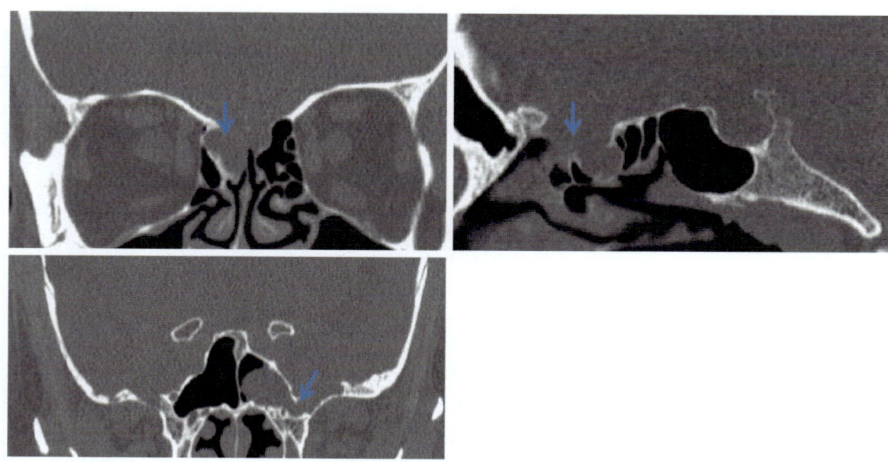

Fig. 23.1 CT scans showing defects in anterior skull base with encephalocoeles, *arrows* pointing towards the bony defects (Courtesy Dr. S. Mathur, Royal Preston Hospital)

- To determine the site and size of the CSF leak; generally this will involve either high-resolution CT scan using coronal and axial planes in bone window setting (Fig. 23.1), CT cisternography, MR cisternography following intrathecal Gd-DTPA, endoscopy or the use of peri-operative intrathecal fluorescent tracer.
- To rule out high intracranial pressure or malignant lesions as a causative factor. If there is tumour or raised intracranial pressure, then these have to be appropriately managed before considering any surgical repair.
- To undertake necessary corrective measures. The choice will usually be between surgical intervention and a conservative approach, insofar as some leaks will repair themselves. Some post-traumatic CSF leaks may spontaneously settle. The decision concerning which approach to adopt needs to be made on a case-by-case basis.

Spontaneous CSF leaks can be challenging to manage owing to frequent recurrences. Furthermore, individuals with this disorder seem also to rise from a distinct demographic group. Spontaneous CSF leaks account for 3–4 % of cases of CSF rhinorrhoea, and recurrences of spontaneous CSF leaks are seen mainly in patients who have raised intracranial pressure. In one study, patients with a spontaneous CSF leak and raised ICP had a 46 % recurrence rate (Mirza et al. 2005). Paradoxically, the presence of a CSF leak may keep patients with raised ICP symptom-free; classic signs may only develop after the leak is repaired (Pérez et al. 2013). Most spontaneous CSF leaks will self-repair within 7–10 days, and this may be helped by oral acetazolamide, an inhibitor of carbonic anhydrase, which is now the standard treatment for benign intracranial hypertension (Chaaban et al. 2013).

In tracing the source of a leak, the intrathecal contrast-enhanced MR cisternography (CEMRC), which can identify 90 % of surgically proven cases, is more sensitive than T2-weighted MR cisternography (T2MRC), identifying 65 % of cases

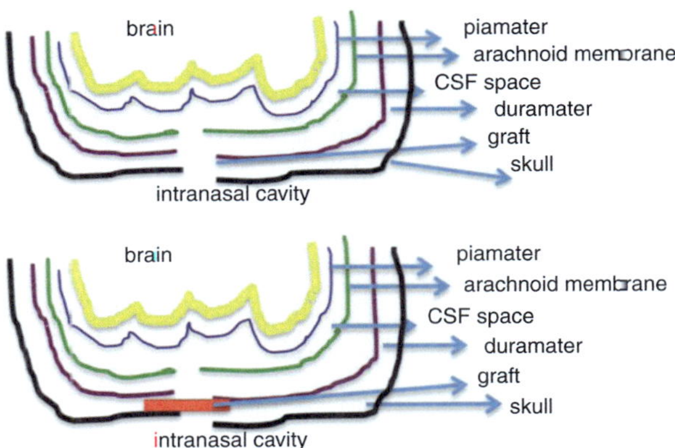

Fig. 23.2 Schematic diagram for CSF leak and placement of graft for repair of defect

(Ecin et al. 2013). The overall, detection sensitivity, specificity, positive predictive values and negative predictive values are typically 92, 80, 76 and 93 % for CEMRC and 56, 77, 64 and 71 % for T2MRC, respectively (Aydin et al. 2008; Reiche et al. 2012). High-resolution CT was accurate in 93 % of patients, whilst MR cisternography was accurate in 89 % (Shetty et al. 1998).

Although relatively safe, the use of intrathecal fluorescein injection is not without risk (Keerl et al. 2004; Jacob et al. 2008). As an alternative to this invasive approach, endoscopic endonasal topical application of fluorescein has been suggested (Saafan et al. 2006). This relies on either detecting a colour change in the fluorescence triggered by the pH of CSF or simply observing the washing away of the fluorescein solution by flowing CSF. Such an approach was reported to accurately identifying the presence of CSF fistulae, though not always possible to identify the accurate site of the leak. It has the advantage that it is a quick and simple outpatient clinic test, although further studies are required.

When CSF rhinorrhoea is identified postoperatively, there is a role for conservative management with lumbar drain, bed rest with head elevation and stool softeners up to 4–6 weeks. Persistent rhinorrhoea, however, will need surgical management due to the risk of ascending meningitis and consequent catastrophic sequelae. Generally, all cases of spontaneous CSF leak, intermittent CSF leak, delayed post-traumatic leak, CSF leak with history of meningitis and CSF otorrhoea presenting as rhinorrhoea require surgical closure. Open craniotomy surgery was prevalent prior to the advent of endoscopic surgery, but endoscopic intranasal management of CSF leaks is now preferred, as this approach is generally associated with high success rates and less morbidity. The key is to place a graft between the skull base bone and dura mater across the CSF leak site (Fig. 23.2). The graft material can be free tissue: fascia lata, abdominal fat, septal or turbinate mucosa or composite grafts with perichondrium or periosteum and mucosa. Multiple techniques have been described and include endonasal repair using septal flap or osteomucoperiosteal flaps through an external ethmoidectomy approach or endoscopic intranasal approach. After the graft is placed, the graft is supported with use of fibrin glue. Gelfoam pieces/Surgicel or other absorbable nasal packs first. The rest of nasal cavity can be packed with rapid Rhino pack/Merocel/BIPP according to surgeon preference. Patient should be advised bed rest with head end elevation of 45° and stool softeners for at least 48 h. Although endoscopic closure is now the treatment of choice (Martin and Loehrl 2007), there remains a recurrence rate of ~10 %.

Whilst trauma-related CSF fistulas can also resolve without intervention, these cases carry a greater risk of an ascending infection, and surgical closure of leaks and defects should be considered. Although the value of prophylactic antibiotics in CSF leaks is debatable (Brodie 1997), this precaution likely justified until the remaining questions are answered. Contemporary surgical innovations towards repair include the use of fibrin glue (Yang et al. 2013).

23.2.3 Transsphenoidal Pituitary Surgery and Transmastoid Schwannoma Surgery

CSF leak can occur after pituitary surgery through the sphenoid sinus. Transsphenoidal surgery has been the gold standard for intra- and suprasellar lesions for nearly half a century. Following this approach, CSF fistulas occur in ~2 % of cases (Malik et al. 2012). Intra-operative CSF leakage can occur in ~20 % of cases (Nishioka et al. 2005). In such cases after covering the defect with graft, the sphenoid sinus is obliterated with abdominal fat (Zie and Jimenez 2013). Similarly following vestibular schwannoma surgery, it is important to have watertight dural closure, typically involving the use of fascia lata over the dural closure, obliteration of the mastoid cavity with abdominal fat, occlusion of all air cell tracts with bone wax and use of palva periosteal flap to reduce the risk of CSF leak.

23.2.4 Spinal Surgery

CSF leaks are relatively common following spinal surgery, and surgeons can be confronted with a draining operative wound with or without deep lying fluid accumulation. Most frequently, the differential diagnoses include seroma, infection and CSF leakage. Imaging can show fluid accumulation but does not necessarily differentiate between diagnoses. Duro-pleural fistula will result in a chronic transudative pleural effusion with a watery fluid having a low total protein (Huggins and Sahn 2003) that can prove problematic to distinguish from a true CSF leak. Testing for asialotransferrin can be an effective means of identifying CSF leakage in such cases (Nyunoya et al. 2003; Haft et al. 2004).

Whilst postspinal surgery midline dural tears are easy to repair, ventral tears are more problematic. As with transsphenoidal surgery, spinal surgery approaches to sealing a leak involve using a sheet of fat from a patient's subcutaneous tissue to cover the dural suture site, exposed dura, followed by application of fibrin glue and surgical/Gelfoam (Black 2002).

Post-lumbar puncture (LP) headache is probably the most common consequence of spinal intervention and is caused by a persistent CSF leak. One common approach to minimising the risk of this is to use the patient's own blood to form a clot over the puncture site extradurally (epidural blood patch).

23.2.5 Shunt CSF-orrhoea

Extreme examples of CSF-orrhoea are seen in abdominal CSF pseudocysts, infrequent but well recognised complications of ventriculoperitoneal shunts (VPS). In CSF pseudocysts, litres of fluid can accumulate, and presenting symptoms and signs are mainly related to abdominal complaints (Ersahin et al. 1996). The mechanisms by which CSF pseudocysts form are not clear. They may take years to develop, and it is often the case that the patient has not undergone any prior abdominal surgery (other than shunt placement). Manifest shunt malfunction is not a prominent feature. Whilst antecedent shunt infections associate only rarely, CSF obtained at the time of surgery is infected in about one third of cases (Hahn et al. 1985–1986). Suggested surgical management consists of either a contralateral VPS or placement of a ventriculoatrial shunt (Hahn et al. vide supra). Diagnosis is usually by abdominal ultrasound and/or CT scan. An intra-abdominal inflammatory process is widely accepted as a hypothesis for the formation of a pseudocyst. In a meta-review the rate of mechanical malfunction ranged from 8 to 64 %, whilst the rate of infection ranged from 3 to 12 % of shunt operations (Wong et al. 2012). Non-cystic variations include CSF ascites (Dean and Keller 1972)

23.3   Confirmation of CSF

The identification of an unknown fluid as being, or containing, CSF clearly depends upon identifying a components or components that characterise CSF. In times past this involved measuring chloride (Cl-), glucose and total protein. It is now widely realised that these tests do not offer the necessary discriminatory efficiency (Chan et al. 2004) and this analytical approach is no longer tenable (Mantur et al. 2011), even though there have been brave efforts to maintain their use (Baker et al. 2005).

Contemporary methods approach the problem by measuring molecular biomarkers, typically CSF-enriched proteins (Tabaouti et al. 2009).

23.3.1 Biomarkers of CSF

23.3.1.1 Asialotransferrin

Transferrin is protein used to transport iron throughout the body. All body fluids contain transferrin. Transferrin is also a glycoprotein, which means that it has oligosaccharide carbohydrate (glycan) chains incorporated into its structure. These glycan chains terminate in sialic acid (N-acetylneuraminic acid) moieties. One significant feature of sialic acid is that it carries a negative charge. This means that sialic acid contributes to the overall charge on the transferrin molecule. Electrophoresis is a method that is used to separate protein molecules on the basis

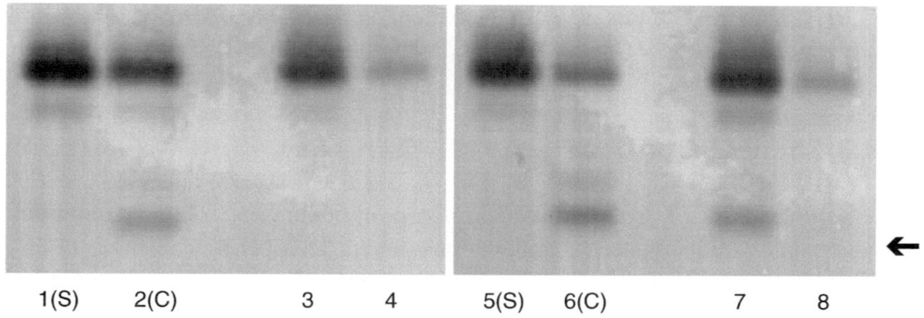

Fig. 23.3 Immunoblotting for transferrin glycoforms in rhinorrhoea fluids. *Lanes 1, 2, 5 and 6* are control serum (S) and CSF (C). *Lanes 3, 4 and 8* are rhinorrhoea fluids negative for CSF. *Lane 7* is a sample of CSF rhinorrhoea. The asialotransferrin band in indicated by the *arrow*

of their charge. The most common form of transferrin in blood serum has 4 sialic acid residues. Asialotransferrin is a rare form of transferrin that has no sialic acid residues. Asialotransferrin, however, is present in significant amounts in perilymph, aqueous humour and CSF. Significantly, it is not present in either tears or rhinitis fluid. Using a combination of electrophoresis and immunoblotting, it is possible to separate and identify glycoforms of transferrin that can be used to distinguish CSF from other serum-based fluids (Fig. 23.3). CSF is characterised by the presence of a significant proportion of asialotransferrin. Approximately 30 % of CSF transferrin is in the form of asialotransferrin. Asialotransferrin is also referred to as *tau-transferrin* and *β₂-transferrin*, although the use of *asialotransferrin* is preferred, as this is less ambiguous.

Identifying an unknown fluid as containing CSF simply requires performing electrophoresis and immunoblotting for transferrin (Keir et al. 1992). The presence of the asialotransferrin band signifies the presence of CSF. The immunoblotting method is sufficiently sensitive to identify CSF even when contaminated with either tears or nasal secretion. Indeed, CSF can be detected when it comprises 10 % or more of an admixture with other non-CSF fluids. Although technically straightforward, the main limitation to the asialotransferrin test is the time taken to perform the electrophoresis and immunoblotting.

In cases of CSF rhinorrhoea and skull base fistulas, asialotransferrin has a detection sensitivity of 94–100 % and specificity of 98–100 % (Marshall et al. 1999). Of course, asialotransferrin testing can also be useful to exclude rhinorrhoea feigning as CSF leak (Bateman and Jones 2000). The test has also been successful in identifying cases of CSF pleural effusion following placement of a ventriculoperitoneal shunt (Smith and Cohen 2009).

Asialotransferrin is found in perilymphatic fluid produced by the cochlea. A perilymph fistula is defined as a leak of perilymph at the oval or round window and is most commonly caused by either barometric trauma associated with either flying or diving, ear surgery or, rarely, head trauma. The very existence and definition of perilymph fistulas remains a contentious area that is fraught with difficulties (Hornibrook 2012). Not least of the problems is that the volume of perilymph is only some 75 µl in toto, so collecting and analysing the fluid is difficult; a typical clinical sample is typically less than 10 µl and is often contaminated with other fluids. This makes the laboratory analysis challenging. Furthermore, the concentration of asialotransferrin in perilymph is only half that of CSF (Thalmann et al. 1994). Irrespective of these technical barriers, asialotransferrin has been successfully applied to the detection of perilymphatic fluid leaks (Skedros et al. 1993). Future developments, such as detection of cochlin-tomoprotein (CTP) may yet prove to be a more specific marker for this fluid (Ikezeno et al. 2010).

23.3.1.2 Beta-Trace Protein

β-Trace protein is one of the dominant proteins within CSF and has been shown to have prostaglandin D2 synthase activity. It is produced by the leptomeninges, which probably explains its rostrocaudal concentration gradient, which increases from 1.5 mg/L in ventricular CSF to 16.6 ± 5.8 mg/L for lumbar CSF. The first study applying β-trace protein to identify CSF liquorrhoea was that of Felgenhauer et al. (1987). Like asialotransferrin the β-trace protein test has the benefit that the level of β-trace in nasal secretions is very low (median 0.016; range <0.003–0.12 mg/L) (Reiber et al. 2003) and is undetectable in tears.

Although β-trace has been detected using 2D electrophoresis (Lescuyer et al. 2012), nephelometry is a rapid and more convenient method (Petereit et al. 2001), and values greater than 0.35–0.5 mg/L have been recommended as levels above which CSF rhinorrhoea is plausible (Reiber et al. 2003; Sampaio et al. 2009). β-Trace is present in normal serum at a concentration of 0.59 ± 0.13 mg/L. Renal disease can raise this to 1.2–6.6 mg/L. Conversely meningitis, which increases CSF total protein, reduces the proportion that is β-trace. Both of these limit the value of the test in such circumstances (Meco et al. 2003). An alternative approach is to measure the ratio of β-trace in fluid to that of paired serum. A value >2.0 indicates that CSF comprises ≥5 % of the unknown fluid volume (Kleine et al. 2000).

Unfortunately β-trace cannot be used for the detecting CSF in ascites or pleural effusions, as these fluids contain β-trace in their own right (Dietzel et al. 2012).

The quantitative measurement of β-trace is non-invasive, quick, sensitive and inexpensive. Where doubt remains, then reflex testing should include asialotransferrin or sodium fluorescein test.

23.3.1.3 Prealbumin

Prealbumin (transthyretin) is another protein that is selectively enriched in CSF. Prealbumin is locally synthesised by the choroid plexus and supports transport of thyroid hormones into the brain (Kassem et al. 2006).

Although the serum concentration of prealbumin is higher than that of CSF, the protein comprises a greater proportion of the CSF total protein. Prealbumin is the third most common protein in CSF. The ratio of prealbumin to albumin in CSF is

0.07; whereas in serum and other fluids, this value is tenfold less (0.007). Measuring the prealbumin/albumin ratio in rhinorrhoea fluid has therefore been advocated to identify CSF (Reisinger et al. 1987). The analysis has been thoroughly modernised using a rapid immunosubtraction microfluidic approach, with results available within 15 min, and reported to have a high clinical specificity (Apori et al. 2013). Unfortunately, the use of prealbumin as a biomarker for CSF rhinorrhoea in general is prone to false negative results, so its use alone cannot be recommended for routine clinical purposes.

23.4 Summary

CSF-orrhoea remains an important clinical entity that requires input from several specialities, including ENT, surgery, chemical pathology and imaging. Currently, the best biomarkers of CSF are asialotransferrin and beta-trace protein. Asialotransferrin is arguably the more specific, but beta-trace protein has the advantage of allowing more rapid testing. Identifying more specific biomarkers is the challenge for the laboratory, whilst improving resolution of minimally invasive imaging techniques is that for radiology.

References

Apori AA, Brozynski MN, El-Sayed IH, Herr AE (2013) Microfluidic validation of diagnostic protein markers for spontaneous cerebrospinal fluid rhinorrhea. J Proteome Res 12:1254–1265

Aydin K, Terzibasioglu E, Senser S, Senser A, Suoglu Y, Karasu A, Kiris T, Turantan MI (2008) Localisation of cerebrospinal fluid leaks by gadolinium-enhanced magnetic resonance cisternography: a 5-year single-centre experience. Neurosurgery 62:584–589

Baker EH, Wood DM, Brennan A, Baines DL, Philips BJ (2005) New insights into the glucose oxidase stick test for cerebrospinal fluid rhinorrhoea. Emerg Med J 22:556–557

Bateman N, Jones NS (2000) Rhinorrhoea feigning cerebrospinal fluid leak: nine illustrative cases. J Laryngol Otol 114:462–464

Bjerre P (1990) The empty sella. A reappraisal of etiology and pathogenesis. Acta Neurol Scand Suppl 130:1–25

Black P (2002) Cerebrospinal fluid leaks following spinal surgery: use of fat grafts for prevention and repair. Technical note. J Neurosurg 96(Suppl 2):250–252

Brodie HA (1997) Prophylactic antibiotics in posttraumatic cerebrospinal fistulae. A meta-analysis. Arch Otolaryngol Head Neck Surg 123:749–752

Chaaban MR, Illing E, Riley KO, Woodworth BA (2013) Acetazolamide for high intracranial pressure cerebrospinal fluid leaks. Int Forum Allergy Rhinol 3:718–721

Chan DT, Poon WS, IP CP, Chiu PW, Goh KY (2004) How useful is glucose detection in diagnosing cerebrospinal fluid leak? The rational use of CT and Beta-2 transferrin assay in detection of cerebrospinal fluid fistula. Asian J Surg 27:39–42

Daudia A, Biswas D, Jones NS (2007) Risk of meningitis with cerebrospinal fluid rhinorrhea. Ann Otol Rhinol Laryngol 116:902–905

Dean DF, Keller IB (1972) Cerebrospinal fluid ascites: a complication of a vetriculoperitoneal shunt. J Neurol Neurosurg Psychiatry 35:474–476

Dietzel J, Krebs A, Böttcher D, Sieb M, Glocker MO, Lüdemann J, Roser M, Dressel A (2012) Beta-trace protein in ascites and pleural effusions: limits of CSF leakage detection. J Neurotrauma 29:1817–1820

Ecin G, Oner AY, Tokgoz N, Ucan M, Aykol S, Tali T (2013) T2-weighted vs intrathecal contrast-enhanced MR cisternography in the evaluation of CSF rhinorrhea. Acta Radiol 54:698–701

Ersahin Y, Mutluer S, Tekeli G (1996) Abdominal cerebrospinal fluid pseudocysts. Childs Nerv System 12:755–758

Felgenhauer K, Schädlich HJ, Nekic M (1987) β-trace protein as marker for cerebrospinal fluid fistula. Klin Wochenschr 65:764–768

Haft GF, Mendoza SA, Weinstein SL, Nyunoya T, Smoker W (2004) Use of beta-2-transferrin to diagnose CSF leakage following spinal surgery a case report. Iowa Orthop J 24:115–118

Hahn YS, Engelhard H, McLone DG (1985–1986) Abdominal CSF pseudocyst. Clinical features and surgical management. Paediatr Neurosci 12:75–79

Hornibrook J (2012) Perilymph fistula: fifty years of controversy. ISRN Otolaryngol 2012:Article ID 281248, 9 p. doi:10.5402/2012/281248

Huggins JT, Sahn SA (2003) Duro-pleural fistula diagnosed by β2-transferrin case report. Respiration 70:423–425

Ikezeno T, Shindo S, Sekiguchi S, Morizane T, Pawankar R, Watanabe A, Miura M, Yagi T (2010) The performance of Cochlin-tomoprotein detection test in the diagnosis of perilymphatic fistula. Audiol Neurootol 15:168–174

Jacob AK, Dilger JA, Hebl JR (2008) Status epilepticus and intrathecal fluorescein: anesthesia providers beware. Anesth Analg 107:229–231

Kassem NA, Deane R, Segal MB, Preston JE (2006) Role of transthyretin in thyroxine transfer from cerebrospinal fluid to brain and choroid plexus. Am J Physiol Regul Integr Comp Physiol 291:R1310–R1315

Keerl R, Weber RK, Draf W, Wienke A, Shaefer SD (2004) Use of sodium fluorescein solution for detection of cerebrospinal fluid fistulas: an analysis of 420 administrations and reported complications in Europe and the United States. Laryngoscope 114:266–272

Keir G, Zeman A, Brookes G, Porter M, Thompson EJ (1992) Immunoblotting of transferrin in the identification of cerebrospinal fluid ctorrhoea and rhinorrhoea. Ann Clin Biochem 29:210–213

Kleine TO, Damm T, Althaus H (2000) Quantification of beta-trace protein and detection of transferrin isoforms in mixtures of cerebrospinal fluid and blood serum as models of rhinorrhea and otorrhea diagnosis. Fresenius J Anal Chem 366:382–386

Lenz AM, Root AW (2012) Empty sella syndrome. Paediatr Endocrinol Rev 9:710–715

Lescuyer P, Auer L, Converset V, Hochstrasser DF, Landis BN, Burkhard PR (2012) Comparison of gel-based methods for the detection of cerebrospinal fluid rhinorrhea. Clin Chim Acta 413:1145–1450

Malik MU, Aberle JC, Flitsch J (2012) CSF fistulas after transsphenoidal pituitary surgery – a solved problem? J Neurol Surg A Cent Eur Neurosurg 73:275–280

Mantur M, Łukaszewicz-Zajac M, Mroczko B, Kułakowska A, Ganslandt O, Kemona H, Szmitkowski M, Drozdowski W, Zimmermann R, Kornhuber J, Lewczuk P (2011) Cerebrospinal fluid leakage – reliable diagnostic methods. Clin Chim Acta 412:837–840

Marshall AH, Jones NS, Robertson JJ (1999) An algorithm for the management of CSF rhinorrhea illustrated by 36 cases. Rhinology 37:181–185

Martin TJ, Loehrl TA (2007) Endoscopic CSF leak repair. Curr Opin Otolaryngol Head Neck Surg 15:35–39

Meco C, Oberascher G, Arrer E, Moser G, Albegger K (2003) Beta-trace protein test: new guidelines for the reliable diagnosis of cerebrospinal fluid fistula. Otolaryngol Head Neck Surg 129:508–517

Mirza S, Thaper A, McClelland L, Jones NS (2005) Sinonasal cerebrospinal fluid leaks: management of 97 patients over 10 years. Laryngoscope 115:1774–1777

Naing S, Frohman LA (2007) The empty sella. Paediatr Endocinol Rev 4:335–342

Nishioka H, Haraoke J, Ikeda Y (2005) Risk factors of cerebrospinal fluid rhinorrhoea following transsphenoidal surgery. Acta Neurochir (Wien) 147:1163–1166

Nyunoya T, Gross T, Rooney C, Mendoza S, Kline J (2003) Massive pleural transudate following a vertebral fusion in a 49-year-old woman. Chest 123:1280–1283

Pérez MA, Bialer OY, Bruce BB, Newman NJ, Biousse V (2013) Primary spontaneous cerebrospinal fluid leaks and idiopathic intracranial hypertension. J Neuroophthalmol 33:330–337

Petereit HF, Bachmann G, Nekic M, Althaus H, Pukrop R (2001) A new nephelometric assay for b-trace protein (prostaglandin D synthase) as an indicator of liquorrhoea. J Neurol Neurosurg Psychiatry 71:347–351

Reiber H, Walther K, Althaus H (2003) Beta-trace protein as sensitive marker for CSF rhinorhea and CSF otorhea. Acta Neurol Scand 108:359–362

Reiche W, Komenda Y, Schick B, Grunwald I, Steudel WI, Reith W (2012) MR cisternography after intrathecal Gd-DTPA application. Eur J Radiol 12:2943–2949

Reisinger PW, Lempart K, Hochstrasser K (1987) New methods of diagnosing cerebrospinal fluid fistulas using beta 2-transferrin or prealbumin-principles and methodology. Laryngol Rhinol Otol (Stuttg) 66:255–259

Saafan ME, Ragab SM, Albirmawy OA (2006) Topical intranasal fluorescein: the missing partner in algorithms of cerebrospinal fluid fistula detection. Laryngoscope 116:1158–1161

Sampaio MH, de Barros-Mazon S, Sakano E, Chone CT (2009) Predictability of quantification of beta-trace protein for diagnosis of cerebrospinal fluid leak: cutoff determination in nasal fluids with two control groups. Am J Rhinol Allergy 23:585–590

Shetty PG, Shroff MM, Sahani DV, Kirtane MV (1998) Evaluation of high-resolution CR and MR cisternography in the diagnosis of cerebrospinal fluid fistula. AJNR Am J Neuroradiol 19:633–639

Skedros DG, Cass SP, Hirsch BE, Kelly RH (1993) Beta-2 transferrin assay in clinical management of cerebrospinal and perilymphatic leaks. J Otolaryngol 22:341–344

Smith JC, Cohen E (2009) Beta-2 transferrin to detect cerebrospinal fluid pleural effusion: a case report. J Med Case Rep 3:6495

Tabaouti K, Kraoul L, Alyousef L, Abi Lahoud G, Brivedani Rousset S, Lancelin F, Mouchet E, Piketty M-L (2009) The role of biology in the diagnosis of cerebrospinal fluid leaks. Ann Biol Clin 67:141–145

Thalmann I, Kohut RI, Ryu J, Comegys TH, Serarita M, Thalmann R (1994) Protein profile of human perilymph: in search of markers for the diagnosis of perilymph fistula and other inner ear disease. Otolaryngol Head Neck Surgery 111:273–280

Wong JD, Ziewacz JE, Allen LH, Panchmatia JR, Bader AM, Garton HJ, Laws ER, Gawande AA (2012) Patterns in neurosurgical adverse events: cerebrospinal fluid shunt surgery. Neurosurg Focus 33:E13

Yang L, Wu J, Zhang G, Zhao Z, Fan Z, Wang B (2013) A novel technology: percutaneous injection of fibrin glue as a treatment for frontal sinus cerebrospinal fluid rhinorrhea. J Craniofac Surg 24:1646–1649

Zie M, Jimenez DF (2013) The history of autologous fat graft use for prevention of cerebrospinal fluid rhinorrhoea after transsphenoidal approaches. World Neurosurg 80:554–562

Guidelines on Cerebrospinal Fluid Analysis

24

Harald Hegen, Charlotte E. Teunissen, Finn Sellebjerg, Hayrettin Tumani, and Florian Deisenhammer

Contents

H. Hegen (✉)
Department of Neurology,
Innsbruck Medical University,
Anichstrasse 35, Innsbruck 6020, Austria
e-mail: harald.hegen@i-med.ac.at

C.E. Teunissen
Neurochemistry Laboratory and Biobank,
Department of Clinical Chemistry, VU University Medical Center Amsterdam,
Amsterdam, The Netherlands

F. Sellebjerg
Danish Multiple Sclerosis Center,
Department of Neurology Rigshospitalet, University of Copenhagen,
Copenhagen, Denmark

H. Tumani
Department of Neurology,
University of Ulm,
Ulm, Germany

F. Deisenhammer
Department of Neurology,
Innsbruck Medical University,
Innsbruck, Austria

© Springer International Publishing Switzerland 2015
F. Deisenhammer et al. (eds.), *Cerebrospinal Fluid in Clinical Neurology*,
DOI 10.1007/978-3-319-01225-4_24

Abstract

The examination of cerebrospinal fluid (CSF) is invaluable for the diagnosis of various neurological diseases. Whereas routine parameters such as white blood cell count, CSF/serum albumin quotient, CSF/serum glucose ratio, intrathecal fraction of immunoglobulins or cytological examination are used to obtain an integrative CSF report, there are also single disease-specific CSF biomarkers contributing to clinical diagnosis making. Furthermore, infectious agents can be detected in CSF either directly by microscopy and culture or indirectly by detection of antigens via polymerase chain reaction or of specific antibodies via serology. In this chapter, we discuss the diagnostic value of CSF referring to existing guidelines.

24.1   Introduction

A considerable number of neurological diseases require examination of cerebrospinal fluid (CSF) to confirm diagnosis or to exclude relevant differential diagnoses. To facilitate clinical diagnosis making, expert panels have provided guidelines on routine CSF analysis as well as on disease-specific CSF biomarkers, e.g. defining cut-off values for single parameters or presenting typical constellations of results in different diseases. All recommendations refer to CSF collected by lumbar puncture. Furthermore, several position papers have given instructions for assay implementation in order to increase the reliability of tests and addressed pre-analytic aspects, which can be a significant source of variation in CSF results. In this chapter, we review existing guidelines and address issues that have not been covered in the preceding chapters. Besides the few published guidelines (see Table 24.1), there exist also recommendations of different national societies, e.g. the German Society for Cerebrospinal Fluid Diagnostics and Neurochemistry, which, however, are not discussed here if they have not been published in peer-reviewed journals.

24.2   Recommendations on Routine CSF Analysis

Basic CSF analysis is invaluable for the evaluation of inflammatory infectious and non-infectious conditions of the central nervous system (CNS), in cases of computed tomography (CT)-negative subarachnoid haemorrhage (SAH) or leptomeningeal metastases. It includes visual inspection of the sample, cytological

Table 24.1 Guidelines on CSF diagnostics

Main topic of guideline	Reference
Routine CSF analysis	Deisenhammer et al. (2006)
Examination of infectious CSF	
Qualitative IgG assessment in CSF	Freedman et al. (2005)
CSF collection and biobanking	Teunissen et al. (2009)
Control groups in CSF biomarker studies	Teunissen et al. (2013)
Disease-specific CSF investigation (including CSF amyloid-β_{1-42}, tau, 14-3-3, hypocretin-1, β-trace, β2-transferrin)	Deisenhammer et al. (2009)
CSF analysis for diagnosis of Creutzfeldt-Jakob disease	Muayqil et al. (2012)
	Sorbi et al. (2012)
CSF analysis for diagnosis of multiple sclerosis	Polman et al. (2011)
	Freedman et al. (2005)
CSF analysis for diagnosis of Lyme neuroborreliosis	Mygland et al. (2010)
CSF amyloid-β_{1-42} and tau protein in Alzheimer's disease	Albert et al. (2011)
	McKhann et al. (2011)
	Sperling et al. (2011)
	Dubois et al. (2007)
	Hort et al. (2010)

A literature search in PubMed using the search terms "cerebrospinal fluid" and "guidelines" limited to July 1, 2014, returned 516 references. Abstracts that primarily did not deal with guidelines on CSF diagnostics were excluded. Only original articles written in English were considered

Table 24.2 Recommended normal limits for routine CSF parameters

CSF parameter	Normal limit
RBC count	$\leq 0/\mu L$
WBC count	$< 5/\mu L$
CSF total protein	< 0.45 g/L
Glucose ratio	>0.4–0.5
CSF lactate	<2.8–3.5 mmol/L
Q_{alb}	NA
Intrathecal IgG synthesis	Detection of OCB only in CSF but not in serum *and/or* calculation by non-linear function, e.g. Reiber hyperbolic formula
Intrathecal IgA and IgM synthesis	Calculation by non-linear function, e.g. Reiber hyperbolic formula
Cytological examination	Lymphocytes and monocytes (at resting phase), occasionally ependymal cells

RBC red blood cell, *WBC* white blood cell, *CSF* cerebrospinal fluid, Q_{alb} CSF albumin/serum albumin ratio, *OCB* oligoclonal bands, *NA* not available, *Ig* immunoglobulin

examination, determination of red blood cell (RBC) and white blood cell (WBC) count, CSF total protein, CSF/serum glucose (CSF/S_{Glu}) ratio and/or CSF lactate as well as measurement of albumin and immunoglobulins (Ig) in CSF and serum for assessment of blood-CSF barrier (BCB) function and intrathecal Ig synthesis. Recommended reference values for all routine CSF parameters are displayed in Table 24.2 (Deisenhammer et al. 2006).

24.2.1 White Blood Cell Count and Cytological Examination

WBC count is typically increased in inflammatory CNS diseases but also in leptomeningeal metastases. Cytological examination allows identification of the underlying cell type in the case of inflammation (e.g. mononuclear versus polymorphonuclear) as well as of tumour cells (Deisenhammer et al. 2006). Currently available guidelines established by a task force of the European Federation of Neurological Societies (EFNS) define a WBC count $<5/\mu L$ as normal, indicating noninflammatory CSF. Cytological examination usually yields lymphocytes and monocytes at resting phase and occasionally ependymal cells (Deisenhammer et al. 2006).

In recent years, there was an increasing interest in automated cell counting and cell sorting for CSF. Therefore, recommendations on at least advantages and disadvantages compared to the conventional methods of cell counting in a chamber under microscopy as well as performing cytology would be desirable. So far, studies comparing WBC count determined automatically and visually remain contradictory showing good overall correlation of results but still weak concordance rates at low WBC counts (Sandhaus et al. 2010; Zimmermann et al. 2011). The reliability of cell sorting is still equivocal at low WBC counts, and pathological cell types such as tumour cells are most likely only detected by microscopic cytological examination (Sandhaus et al. 2010; Zimmermann et al. 2011; Danise et al. 2013).

24.2.2 Red Blood Cell Count

RBC count is essential for the diagnosis of SAH especially in patients with normal CT scan (refer to chapter 24.4.1) as well as to estimate whether blood contamination of CSF (by traumatic puncture) could affect the results of other CSF parameters. In general, the extent of interference with the analyte depends on its serum concentration, e.g. blood contamination can lead more easily to a false positive result of a CSF parameter in the case of high serum concentration. There are no recommendations at which RBC count a particular CSF parameter should not be determined or whether and how calculative corrections should be performed. Research recommendations consider CSF samples as blood contaminated if RBC count exceeds $500/\mu L$; however, this cut-off value was based on proteomic data (Teunissen et al. 2009) and, thus, does not necessarily apply to routine CSF analysis.

Since the ratio of WBC to RBC in blood is roughly 1:750, some authors suggested to subtract 1–2 WBC per 1,000 counted RBC in CSF (Delank 1972; Olischer and von Suchodoletz 1972). Reske et al. recommended to correct 1 WBC per 666 RBC (Reske et al. 1981) and others even calculated a formula involving leukocytes and erythrocytes both in blood and CSF ($WBC_{CSF}/RBC_{CSF} \times RBC_{blood}/WBC_{blood}$) in order to obtain the "true" WBC count in CSF (Pfausler et al. 2004). Concerning CSF total protein concentration, Reske et al. suggested the formula $Protein_{CSF}$ (mg/L) $- RBC_{CSF}$ (/μL)/333×5.25 (Reske et al. 1981), but the method used for the determination of CSF total protein has to be considered in this context (see below) (Boer et al. 2007). Although blood contamination in CSF also influences CSF Ig concentrations and calculated intrathecal Ig synthesis, there are so far no suggestions for a corrective approach.

24.2.3 CSF Total Protein and CSF/Serum Albumin Quotient

Both measures, CSF total protein and CSF/serum albumin quotient (Q_{alb}), are increased in case of blood-CSF barrier (BCB) dysfunction, which is evident in different conditions such as meningitis, leptomeningeal metastases or inflammatory polyneuropathy (Reiber and Peter 2001). Q_{alb} should be preferred to CSF total protein concentration in order to assess BCB function (Deisenhammer et al. 2006). The superiority of Q_{alb} is based on the fact that it is not influenced by intrathecal Ig synthesis, is corrected for serum concentrations of albumin and is a technology-independent value (Deisenhammer et al. 2006). Although it is known that the protein concentration in CSF increases with age (Tibbling et al. 1977; Garton et al. 1991; Blennow et al. 1993; Eeg-Olofsson et al. 1981), no specific age-dependent upper normal limit for Q_{alb} has been recommended. Reiber et al. suggested the approximate formula "Age/15 + 4 ' (Reiber et al. 2001), but this still returns false positive/elevated results in roughly 15 % of patients without evidence of neurological disorders (ruled out by clinical, laboratory and imaging diagnostics) (Brettschneider et al. 2005).

Regarding CSF total protein, concentrations less than 0.45 g/L are considered as normal (Deisenhammer et al. 2005). However, there is no recommendation for age correction, and existing literature even provides evidence that the upper normal limit has to be corrected to levels ranging between 0.5 and 0.6 g/L (Tibbling et al. 1977; Garton et al. 1991; Ahonen et al. 1979; Gilland 1967; Dufour-Rainfray et al. 2013; Mertin et al. 1971; Breebaart et al. 1978). Comments on the methodology for CSF total protein measurement are lacking too (not relevant for Q_{alb}, as a ratio is dimensionless and method independent given that the same method is used for CSF and serum measurements).

In a subgroup of patients such as in SAH patients developing hydrocephalus and requiring ventricular drain, CSF samples are collected from the ventricular lumen (via the drain). The site of CSF collection (due to a rostrocaudal protein concentration gradient) has a significant impact on levels of CSF total protein concentration and CSF albumin (therefore also on Q_{alb}) with levels in lumbar CSF roughly 2.2 times higher than in ventricular CSF (Weisner and Bernhardt 1978). Cut-off values for CSF total protein or Q_{alb} in ventricular CSF have not been formally investigated; nevertheless, it is common practice to use cut-off values of lumbar CSF divided by 2.2.

24.2.4 CSF/Serum Glucose Ratio

CSF glucose and, thus, the CSF/S_{Glu} ratio are typically decreased in bacterial or fungal infectious CNS disease as well as in leptomeningeal metastases. According to EFNS guidelines, a CSF/S_{Glu} ratio between 0.5 and 0.6 is considered as normal and values below 0.4–0.5 are pathologic (albeit, e.g. the German Society of Neurology recommends to consider a CSF/S_{Glu} <0.3 for an accurate diagnosis of bacterial meningitis (Diener 2012)). It has to be stated that despite the long-term and widespread use of glucose measurement in routine CSF diagnostics, the level of evidence for the recommended cut-off is low (Deisenhammer et al. 2006). Although it is well known that CSF/S_{Glu} ratio decreases with increasing serum glucose level in a non-linear manner (Leen et al. 2012), proposed normal and cut-off values are not serum glucose adapted. A recent study linked CSF/S_{Glu} ratio to specific serum glucose concentrations and suggested CSF/S_{Glu} ratio >0.5 as normal for patients with serum glucose concentrations <1 g/L, >0.4 for those with a serum glucose level of 1 g/L up to 1.49 g/L and >0.3 for values exceeding 1.5 g/L (Hegen et al. 2014). Other factors which might influence CSF/S_{Glu} ratio such as age, WBC count and CSF total protein (i.e. lower CSF/S_{Glu} ratio with increase of these parameters) could be ruled out in this study by regression analysis revealing only serum glucose concentration as a significant covariant for CSF/S_{Glu} ratio (Hegen et al. 2014).

24.2.5 Intrathecal Immunoglobulin Synthesis

Intrathecal Ig production can be found in various, mainly inflammatory, conditions of the CNS (Deisenhammer et al. 2006), and specific Ig patterns are indicative for certain diseases, e.g. IgM dominance for neuroborreliosis or IgA dominance for neurotuberculosis and brain abscess (Reiber and Peter 2001). Evidence on the frequency of intrathecal IgG, IgA and IgM synthesis in different neurological diseases is summarised in Table 24.3. Nevertheless, existing guidelines conclude that there is no evidence to support the routine use of quantitative assessment of intrathecal Ig synthesis (Deisenhammer et al. 2006; Freedman et al. 2005). This might be due to several reasons: Calculation of intrathecal IgG synthesis, e.g. by non-linear formula such as Reiber hyperbolic function (Reiber 1994), has lower diagnostic accuracy in terms of sensitivity and specificity compared to oligoclonal band (OCB) evaluation for diseases such as multiple sclerosis (MS) (Reiber et al. 1998; Rudick et al. 1989). Regarding intrathecal IgM synthesis, there are reports of falsely positive results in patients with noninflammatory diseases without IgM oligoclonal bands in CSF (Sharief et al. 1990), and the same applies for IgA. Further ambiguities arise from recommendations such as those of the German Society for Cerebrospinal Fluid Diagnostics and Neurochemistry to consider intrathecal fractions of IgA and IgM, indicated by the percentage of intrathecally synthesised Ig, of less than 10 % as non-pathological (DGLN DGfLuKN 2004).

It is known that besides intact immunoglobulins, plasma cells secrete an excess of free light chains (FLC) (Nakano et al. 2011), which accumulate in the CSF in the case of intrathecal B-cell activity. Several studies have already indicated the potential diagnostic value of κFLC in MS (Rudick et al. 1989; Krakauer et al. 1998; Desplat-Jego et al. 2005; Senel et al. 2014; Duranti et al. 2013); however, there have been no recommendations on FLC as a measure for intrathecal B-cell activity.

Table 24.3 Percentage of patients with quantitative intrathecal immunoglobulin synthesis in different diseases

	IgG (%)	IgA (%)	IgM (%)
No inflammatory and no CNS disease	<5	<5	<5
Noninflammatory CNS disease[d]	<25[a]	<5	<5
Infections of the nervous system	25–50	25	25
Bacterial infections	25–50	25–50	<25
Viral infections	25–50	<25	<25
Lyme neuroborreliosis	25–50	<25	75
Multiple sclerosis	70–80	<25	<25
Clinically isolated syndrome	40–60	<10	<25
Inflammatory neuropathies	25–50[a]	25–50[a]	25–50[a]
Neoplastic disorders (in general)	<25[a]	ND	ND
Paraneoplastic syndromes	<25	ND	ND
Meningeal carcinomatosis	25–50	ND	ND
Other neuroinflammatory diseases	25–50[b]	ND[c]	ND

Adapted from Deisenhammer et al. (2006). Intrathecal Ig synthesis was determined by elevated IgA, IgG, IgM index or by non-linear formula values

[a]Usually not associated with oligoclonal bands (artefact in presence of barrier impairment)

[b]Rare in biopsy-proven neurosarcoidosis

[c]Prominent IgA synthesis in adrenoleukodystrophy

[d]Including degenerative and vascular diseases

CNS central nervous system, *ND* not determined

24.2.6 Oligoclonal Bands

Detection of OCB by isoelectric focusing (IEF) on agarose gels followed by immunoblotting is the gold standard method for the determination of an intrathecal IgG synthesis (Freedman et al. 2005). As mentioned above, intrathecal IgG synthesis is found primarily in inflammatory CNS diseases indicating a long-lasting B-cell activity (Deisenhammer et al. 2006), and its detection by OCB shows significantly higher sensitivity and specificity than IgG quantitation in CSF and serum followed by calculation of any formulae (e.g. Reiber IgG synthesis) (Reiber et al. 1998; Rudick et al. 1989). The incidence of OCB in different neurological diseases is shown in Table 24.4.

OCB are of high importance especially in the diagnosis of MS. A recent large meta-analysis showed that OCB (detected by IEF followed by immunofixation) were positive in roughly 90 % of more than 12,000 MS patients and 70 % of more than 2,600 patients with clinically isolated syndrome, the first manifestation of the disease (Dobson et al. 2013). In cases of primary progressive MS, the detection of intrathecal IgG synthesis (e.g. by OCB) is still included in the diagnostic criteria, as one of three criteria supporting evidence for dissemination in space (Polman et al. 2011). Although no longer required for diagnosis of relapsing MS (Polman et al. 2011), CSF analysis is still required for exclusion of differential diagnoses (Freedman et al. 2005; Polman et al. 2011; Miller et al. 2008; Tumani et al. 2011). Findings of mild lymphocytic pleocytosis and intrathecal IgG

Table 24.4 Incidence of OCB in different inflammatory CNS diseases

Disease	OCB positive (%)
Autoimmune	
Multiple sclerosis	95
Neuro-SLE	50
Neuro-Behcet's	20
Neuro-sarcoid	40
Harada's meningitis-uveitis	60
Infectious	
Acute viral encephalitis (<7 days)	<5
Acute bacterial meningitis (<7 days)	<5
Subacute sclerosing panencephalitis	100
Progressive rubella panencephalitis	100
Neurosyphilis	95
Neuro-AIDS	80
Neuroborreliosis	80
Tumour	<5
Hereditary	
Ataxia-telangiectasia	60
Adrenoleukodystrophy (encephalitic)	100

Adapted from Deisenhammer et al. (2006)

OCB oligoclonal band, *CNS* central nervous system, *SLE* systemic lupus erythematosus, *AIDS* acquired immunodeficiency syndrome

synthesis prove the inflammatory nature of the underlying condition in MS (the only test besides brain biopsy) (Freedman et al. 2005; Polman et al. 2011; Miller et al. 2008; Tumani et al. 2011).

As detection of OCB is a technically demanding method, clear recommendations exist on how to perform it. Freedman et al. provide a list of 12 red flags, which should be considered in order to achieve and guarantee high diagnostic accuracy of this method (Table 24.5) (Freedman et al. 2005). Furthermore, it is clearly defined how to interpret test results, classified into five different patterns (see chapter 10) (Freedman et al. 2005). In general, a positive result is found if two or more OCB are present in CSF but not in serum. The cut-off of two bands ensures the high specificity of the test for MS. In cases of a single detected band (most likely reflecting incomplete OCB in CSF but not in serum), if other (clinical or MRI) criteria clearly point to MS, CSF analysis might be repeated (after several months) for re-evaluation (Freedman et al. 2005; Davies et al. 2003).

24.2.7 Disease-Related Patterns of Routine CSF Parameters

Not a single CSF parameter but the integrative report allows reliable diagnosis making in a variety of neurological disorders. Here, we would like to highlight this

Table 24.5 Recommendations for qualitative assessment of IgG in CSF

1.	IEF followed by immunodetection (blotting or fixation)
2.	Unconcentrated CSF
3.	Parallel run of CSF and serum samples at similar IgG concentrations
4.	Positive and negative controls on each gel
5.	Standardised reporting: staining patterns I–V
6.	Interpretation by an individual experienced in the technique
7.	Full CSF reports most helpful
8.	Detection of light chains in certain cases
9.	Repeat CSF analysis if clinical suspicion is high but test result is negative (or shows only a single band in CSF)
10.	Quantitative IgG analysis is complementary but not a substitute for OCB detection
11.	Non-linear formulas should be used to calculate intrathecal IgG synthesis considering BCB integrity (by Q_{alb})
12.	Quality controls, both internal and external

CSF cerebrospinal fluid, *IEF* isoelectric focusing, *OCB* oligoclonal bands, Q_{alb} CSF albumin/serum albumin ratio, *BCB* blood-CSF barrier

Table 24.6 Typical constellation of CSF parameters in various neurological disorders

	WBC count	CSF total protein	CSF/S_{Glu} ratio	CSF lactate	Typical cytology
Acute bacterial meningitis	> 1,000	↑	↓	↑	PNC
Viral neuro-infections	10–1,000	=/↑	=/↓	=	PNC/MNC
Autoimmune polyneuropathy	=	↑	=	=	
Infectious polyneuropathy	↑	↑	=	=	MNC
Subarachnoidal haemorrhage	↑	↑	=	=/↑	RBC, MAC, SID, MNC
Multiple sclerosis	=/↑	=	=	=	MNC
Leptomeningeal metastases	=/↑	↑	↓	n.a.	Malignant cells, MNC

Adapted from Deisenhammer et al. (2006)

CSF cerebrospinal fluid, *MNC* mononuclear cells, *PNC* polymorphonuclear cells, *n.a.* no evidence, *SID* siderophages, *MAC* macrophages, *CSF/S_{Glu} ratio* CSF/serum glucose ratio, *WBC* white blood cells (per µL), *RBC* red blood cells

special feature in CSF analysis by the following example: Whereas WBC count alone could not reliably distinguish between viral and bacterial meningitis (in a cohort of patients published by Spanos et al.), the combination of different parameters, i.e. of CSF glucose concentration <0.34 g/L, a CSF/S_{Glu} ratio <0.23, a CSF total protein concentration >2.2 g/L and a CSF WBC count of >2,000/µL, enables the correct assignment of patients with bacterial meningitis with ≥99 % certainty (Spanos et al. 1989). Table 24.6 summarises typical constellations of CSF results in different neurological conditions (Deisenhammer et al. 2006).

24.3 Recommendations on Diagnostic Workup of CSF for Infectious CNS Diseases

In the case of infectious CNS disease, the detection of the pathogen is necessary for a target-specific antimicrobial treatment. There are many small- to medium-sized studies investigating diagnostic sensitivity and specificity of tests for various infectious agents but no controlled study evaluating a workup of infectious CSF in general, i.e. how to proceed with CSF in obvious CNS infections. Existing proposals for the general workup of infectious CSF are based on clinical practice and theoretically plausible procedures. Available guidelines recommend different detection methods for different infectious agents: directly by microscopy and culture or indirectly by detection of antigens via polymerase chain reaction or by detection of specific antibodies via serology (Table 24.7) (Deisenhammer et al. 2006).

In several infectious CNS diseases, evidence of an intrathecal synthesis of specific antibodies (Ab) significantly contributes to diagnosis. For example, an increased *Borrelia burgdorferi* sensu lato-specific antibody index is necessary for a definitive diagnosis of neuroborreliosis (besides appropriate clinical signs and CSF pleocytosis) (Mygland et al. 2010). The antibody-specific index (ASI) discriminates between blood-derived (in the case of solely systemic infection) and brain-derived specific antibody fraction (in the case of CNS infection) taking into account individual BCB function (Reiber and Lange 1991). The relative intrathecal synthesis of specific antibodies is calculated by the following formula:

$$\text{ASI} = \frac{\dfrac{\text{Ab}_{\text{CSF}}}{\text{Ab}_{\text{Serum}}}}{\dfrac{\text{IgG}_{\text{CSF}}}{\text{IgG}_{\text{Serum}}}}$$

In the case of a polyclonal intrathecal IgG synthesis, it has been proposed to use Q_{Lim}, a parameter representing the IgG fraction in CSF at a specific Q_{alb} originating only from the blood, instead of the CSF/serum IgG ratio (Reiber and Lange 1991). However, this adaptation (although used in clinical routine for many years) has never been included in CSF guidelines:

$$\text{ASI} = \frac{\dfrac{\text{Ab}_{\text{CSF}}}{\text{Ab}_{\text{Serum}}}}{Q_{\text{Lim}}}$$

In general, an antibody index ≥ 1.5 is considered as pathologic (Deisenhammer et al. 2006). Calculation of ASI is used for different pathogens such as herpes simplex, varicella zoster, human immunodeficiency virus, cytomegalovirus, Toxoplasma gondii and *Borrelia* burgdorferi sensu lato (Reiber and Lange 1991); nevertheless, there are so far no recommendations on the clinical utility of these pathogen-specific antibodies except for anti-*Borrelia* antibodies.

Table 24.7 List of infectious agents responsible for the vast majority of infectious CNS diseases

Pathogen	Recommended diagnostic method[a]
Bacteria	
Should be considered in first line	
Neisseria meningitides	Microscopy, culture
Streptococcus pneumoniae	Microscopy, culture
Haemophilus influenzae	Microscopy, culture
Staphylococcus aureus	Microscopy, culture
Escherichia coli	Microscopy, culture
Borrelia burgdorferi sensu lato	Serology
Treponema pallidum	Serology
Mycobacterium tuberculosis	PCR[a], culture, positive tuberculin test
Should be considered especially in immunosuppressed patients	
Actinobacteria species	Culture
Bacteroides fragilis	Culture
JC virus	PCR
Listeria monocytogenes	Microscopy, culture
Nocardia asteroides	Microscopy (modified Ziehl-Neelsen stain and culture from brain biopsy)
Pasteurella multocida	Culture
Streptococcus mitis	Culture
Should be considered in special situations	
Brucella spp.	Culture
Campylobacter fetus	Microscopy, culture
Coxiella burnetii	Serology
Leptospira interrogans	Culture, serology
Mycoplasma pneumoniae	Serology
Rickettsia	Serology
Coagulase-negative staphylococci	Culture
Group B streptococci	Microscopy, culture
Tropheryma whipplei	PCR
Viruses	
Should be considered in first line	
Herpes simplex virus (HSV) types 1 and 2	PCR, serology
Varicella zoster virus (VZV)	PCR, serology
Enteroviruses (echovirus, coxsackievirus A and B)	PCR, serology
Human immunodeficiency virus (HIV) type 1 or 2	PCR, serology
Epstein–Barr virus (EBV)	PCR

(continued)

Table 24.7 (continued)

Pathogen	Recommended diagnostic method[a]
Cytomegalovirus (CMV)	PCR
Should be considered in special situations	
Adenovirus	PCR, culture, antigen detection
Human T-cell leukaemia virus type I (HTLV-I)	Serology
Influenza and parainfluenza virus	Serology
Lymphocytic choriomeningitis (LCM) virus	Serology
Mumps virus	Serology
Poliovirus	PCR
Rabies virus	PCR from CSF, root of hair, cornea
Rotavirus	Antigen detection in stool specimens
Rubella virus	Serology
Sandfly fever	Serology
Fungi	
Aspergillus fumigatus	Antigen detection in CSF, where required culture from brain biopsy
Cryptococcus neoformans	Antigen detection in CSF, India ink stain, less sensitive than antigen detection, culture
Parasites	
Toxoplasma gondii	CSF, PCR and serology; brain biopsy, PCR
Strongyloides stercoralis	Pathogen detection in stool

24.4 Recommendations on Disease-Specific CSF Biomarkers

The analysis of routine CSF parameters (as outlined above) and interpretation of their specific constellation often lead to a clear diagnosis, such as purulent meningitis (e.g. in case of massive granular pleocytosis, decreased CSF/S_{Glu} ratio and detection of coccus in cytological examination), or contribute to diagnosis making such as in MS (in case of lymphocytic pleocytosis with intrathecal IgG synthesis); however, there are also cases where routine CSF diagnostics is inconclusive or even normal. That is why there has been a long history in CSF research to fill this gap, and a multitude of molecules in CSF have been investigated in various neurological disorders in order to receive in the best case one disease-specific either diagnostic or prognostic biomarker. However, only a few of them achieved implementation in clinical setting. A summary of markers that are recommended for use in clinical routine is shown in Table 24.8 (making no claim to be complete).

24.4.1 Subarachnoid Haemorrhage

SAH is a serious potentially life-threatening disease characterised by arterial bleeding into the subarachnoid space. In patients with normal cerebral CT scan, it is

Table 24.8 Recommendations on disease-specific biomarkers in clinical routine

CSF biomarker	Disease	Description
Tau	Alzheimer's disease	Increased
		Tau can also be increased in CSF from patients with diseases other than AD
P-Tau		Increased
		P-Tau can also be increased in CSF from patients with dementias other than AD, such as dementia with Lewy bodies
Amyloid-β_{1-42}		Decreased
		Amyloid-β_{1-42} can also be decreased in CSF from patients with dementias other than AD
14-3-3 protein	Creutzfeldt-Jakob disease	Sensitivity >90 %, specificity >80 % for sCJD
		14-3-3 can also be detected in CSF from patients with more common diseases
Hypocretin-1	Narcolepsy	Hypocretin-1 (orexin-1) levels of <110 pg/mL are diagnostic for narcolepsy with cataplexy. The value of measuring hypocretin-1 (orexin-1) in CSF of other sleep disorders is controversial
β-Trace protein	Oto- and rhinorrhoea	>90 % sensitivity and 100 % specificity in combination with CT investigation
Bilirubin, net oxyhaemoglobin, ferritin	Subarachnoid haemorrhage	Increased
		At least 12 h after symptom onset

CSF cerebrospinal fluid, *CT* computed tomography, *AD* Alzheimer's disease, *CJD* Creutzfeldt-Jakob disease

important to detect bleeding by CSF analysis (Cruickshank et al. 2008). One difficulty is to distinguish blood of intrathecal origin from blood contamination in a CSF sample due to traumatic lumbar puncture, which is estimated to happen in roughly 20 % of all punctures (Marton and Gean 1986). Several studies reported different parameters to distinguish between these two scenarios. Approximately 60 % of patients with SAH were reported (in Walton's series published in the pre-CT era) to have elevated CSF pressure (>20 cm of H_2O) (Walton 1956). A positive "3-tube test" argues for traumatic lumbar puncture, i.e. blood is gradually clearing with further CSF collection, whereas in SAH the bloody appearance persists (Buruma et al. 1981). Reliability of this method is limited and is considered only really helpful when RBC count is zero in the last collected tube (Shah and Edlow 2002). RBC count per se is not a reliable parameter, as SAH has also been reported with only low RBC counts (Walton 1956) and, to our knowledge, no cut-off for RBC count exists specifying at least a certain probability for traumatic tab and risk for SAH, respectively. Visual inspection (and perception of yellow-orange colour) might give further information but has repeatedly been shown to lack the required sensitivity for reliably detecting the presence of bilirubin (Cruickshank et al. 2005; Petzold et al. 2005). Guidelines suggest measuring the absorbance of bilirubin and net oxyhaemoglobin in CSF, feasible at least 12 hours after symptom onset (corresponding to the time bilirubin needs to occur in CSF in case of SAH) (Cruickshank et al. 2008). Erythrophages, siderophages or haematoidin (crystallised bilirubin) are signs of a previous subarachnoid bleeding but found inconsistently in CSF of SAH patients (Page et al. 1994) (therefore lacking diagnostic sensitivity). The use of D-dimer levels in CSF has proved inconsistent, too (Page et al. 1994; Lang et al. 1990). CSF ferritin, a well-established parameter in routine analysis, is increased in patients with intracranial bleedings with temporal dynamics similar to siderophages and bilirubin and has been suggested to stay elevated longer than bilirubin but might have a lower specificity (Watson et al. 2008). Where spectrophotometry is not available (to measure bilirubin), the combination of CSF cytology for erythrophages or siderophages and measurement of ferritin in CSF is an alternative. However, the implementation of these parameters varies in different countries (Nagy et al. 2013), and the contribution of the parameters mentioned above for correct assignment of artificial and intrathecal blood has not been sufficiently addressed in currently available guidelines.

24.4.2 Creutzfeldt-Jakob Disease

Creutzfeldt-Jakob disease (CJD) is a rapidly progressive neurodegenerative disorder characterised by dementia and multifocal neurological findings such as myoclonus or cerebellar signs. Diagnosis making is challenging due to various differential diagnoses and the wide spectrum of clinical manifestations of sporadic CJD (Meissner et al. 2005; Appleby et al. 2009). Current diagnostic criteria as defined by the World Health Organization (2003) require, besides progressive dementia and at least two typical clinical features, a supportive paraclinical finding demonstrated either by EEG or positive 14-3-3 assay in CSF (Muayqil et al. 2012). According to the Guideline Development Subcommittee of the American Academy of Neurology (AAN), CSF 14-3-3 assays should be performed in patients who have rapidly progressive dementia and are strongly suspected of having sporadic CJD (Muayqil et al. 2012). A meta-analysis including more than 1,800 patients with suspected CJD showed that CSF 14-3-3 assay reaches a sensitivity of 92 % and specificity of 80 % (Muayqil et al. 2012). In terms of specificity, it has been clearly stated that 14-3-3 protein is an unspecific biomarker, which is also found in other forms of dementia. Due to the very low incidence of CJD (1:1.000.000 (Ladogana et al. 2005)), it is important to increase pretest probability in clinical context, i.e. to perform testing only in a selected patient group, when CJD is suspected due to other clinical findings than dementia (Muayqil et al. 2012). Variations in the sensitivity of 14-3-3 assay have been reported on the basis of the duration of illness (lower in early and late disease course) and CJD subtype (e.g. lower in MV2 or MM2 molecular subtype) (Collins et al. 2006). Limitations of 14-3-3 also arise from variations due to different laboratory techniques. Whereas Western blot technique implies subjective evaluation of a protein-antibody band, ELISA techniques need a cut-off value (to decide whether the test result is positive or negative), having a considerable impact on sensitivity and specificity of the test (Aksamit 2003).

Furthermore, different isoforms (β or γ) of 14-3-3 protein have been used so far (Muayqil et al. 2012). Concluding, there is a need for an international standardisation of the 14-3-3 assays.

Other proteins such as tau or S100B have also been proposed as diagnostic CSF biomarker in CJD showing at least equal diagnostic performance compared to 14-3-3 protein (Coulthart et al. 2011; Sorbi et al. 2012). EFNS guidelines on dementia, in contrast to the recommendations of the AAN, recommend determining CSF tau protein besides 14-3-3 protein in rapidly progressive dementia when CJD is suspected; however, they also clearly state that CSF tau is an unspecific marker as well and that there are overlaps to other forms of dementia, e.g. Alzheimer's disease (see chapter 24.4.3) (Sorbi et al. 2012). A new development known as a real-time quaking-induced conversion (RT-QUIC) assay seems to be promising. This assay classified CSF samples from two different CJD cohorts as compared to patients with other neurodegenerative diseases correctly in more than 80 % of cases; and there were no false positive results (meaning a specificity of 100 %) (Atarashi et al. 2011). Future revision of the guidelines on CSF diagnostics in CJD might include comments on these new developments.

24.4.3 Alzheimer's Disease

Alzheimer's disease (AD) is the most common cause of dementia in elderly people. Clinical diagnosis making is still demanding, as the ability to distinguish between Alzheimer's disease and other dementias shows still quite low accuracy (Ballard et al. 2011). Two major sets of criteria for the diagnosis of AD have been published. Both criteria aim to support a clinical diagnosis with in vivo evidence of AD pathology, using brain imaging techniques as well as CSF biomarker analysis (Dubois et al. 2007; Sperling et al. 2011; Albert et al. 2011; McKhann et al. 2011).

Apart from the clinical core feature of episodic memory impairment, an International Working Group suggested to include several supportive features, one of which is abnormal CSF biomarkers, i.e. low amyloid-β_{1-42} concentrations, increased total tau concentrations or increased phospho-tau concentrations or combinations of the three (Dubois et al. 2007). Experts convened by the National Institute on Aging and the Alzheimer's Association in the United States have applied a more pathophysiologically driven approach (Sperling et al. 2011; Albert et al. 2011; McKhann et al. 2011). Both amyloid-β_{1-42} (Aβ_{1-42}) and tau protein should be used in the preclinical phase to establish the presence of AD pathophysiological process in subjects with no (or very subtle) symptoms (see Table 24.9) (Sperling et al. 2011). In the minimal cognitive impairment (MCI) phase, these markers are used to establish the underlying aetiology responsible for the clinical deficit and indicate the likelihood of progression to AD dementia. Decreased Aβ_{1-42} and elevated tau levels indicate high likelihood to convert from MCI to AD (Albert et al. 2011). In the AD phase, the markers are used to increase the level of certainty that AD pathology underlies the dementia in an individual (McKhann et al. 2011).

Table 24.9 Staging categories for preclinical Alzheimer's disease

Stage	Description	Amyloid-β_{1-42}	Tau	Cognitive change
I	Asymptomatic cerebral amyloidosis	Positive	Negative	Negative
II	Asymptomatic amyloidosis and "downstream" neurodegeneration	Positive	Positive	Negative
III	Amyloidosis and neuronal injury and subtle cognitive behavioural decline	Positive	Positive	Positive

However, these guidelines also highlight several limitations of CSF biomarker in AD stating that more research needs to be done to ensure that criteria including the use of biomarkers are appropriately designed. Biomarker assays need more standardisation; and no uniform cut-off levels have been established (probably leading to higher between-centre variability and, thus, lower test accuracy) (McKhann et al. 2011; Morris et al. 2014).

24.4.4 Narcolepsy

Narcolepsy is a rare sleep disorder, which is characterised by hypersomnia, cataplexy, sleep paralysis and hypnagogic hallucinations and is probably caused by dysfunction of the hypocretin-1 (alias orexin-1) neurotransmitter system of the hypothalamus (Leschziner 2014). There exists a clear recommendation that hypocretin-1 levels of <110 pg/mL in CSF measured by radioimmunoassay is diagnostic for narcolepsy with cataplexy (Deisenhammer et al. 2009).

24.4.5 Cerebrospinal Fluid Rhinorrhoea

CSF rhinorrhoea occurs in case of fistula between the intrathecal compartment and nasal cavity, mostly following traumatic frontobasal skull fractures, surgery or destructive, neoplastic processes. To clearly identify CSF, measurement of either ß2-transferrin or ß-trace protein is eligible; due to procedural advantages, ß-trace protein should be used as first line. In combination with cerebral CT scan (and clinical investigation), determination of these biomarkers allows the detection of CSF fistulas with high sensitivity and specificity (Deisenhammer et al. 2009).

24.5 Recommendations on Pre-analytic Aspects

Pre-analytical variability and errors are an important source of variation in CSF biomarker analysis. In general, pre-analytic issues account for roughly 60 % of total laboratory errors and include patient-related factors as well as variations in laboratory processing or assay performance (Plebani 2006). In recent years, these aspects

Table 24.10 Control groups in CSF biomarker studies in multiple sclerosis

Control group	Definition and examples
Inflammatory neurological disease control (INDC)	Infectious CNS diseases, e.g. neuroborreliosis Autoimmune CNS diseases, e.g. MS Paraneoplastic CNS syndromes
Peripheral inflammatory neurological disease control (PINDC)	Inflammatory demyelinating neuropathies, e.g. GBS Inflammatory neuritis, e.g. radiculitis
Noninflammatory neurological disease control (NINDC)	Neurodegenerative diseases, e.g. ALS, Parkinson syndromes, dementia disorders Vascular diseases, e.g. stroke CNS expansions, e.g. glioblastoma Metabolic encephalopathies, e.g. CADASIL Noninflammatory PNS involvement, e.g. polyneuropathy CSF flow abnormalities, e.g. normotensive hydrocephalus
Symptomatic control (SC)	Sensory disturbances (if brain/spinal MRI and CSF normal) Dizziness (if brain MRI and CSF normal) Headache, e.g. tension headache Vertebrogenic syndromes, e.g. disc herniation
Healthy controls (HC)	Volunteers without specific medical complaints and normal CSF
Spinal anaesthesia subjects (SAS)	No history of any neurological deficit and normal CSF

CNS central nervous system, *MS* multiple sclerosis, *GBS* Guillain-Barré syndrome, *ALS* amyotrophic lateral sclerosis, *CADASIL* cerebral autosomal dominant arteriopathy with subcortical infarcts and leukoencephalopathy, *PNS* peripheral nervous system, *CSF* cerebrospinal fluid, *MRI* magnetic resonance imaging

have become of more broad international interest and several recommendations have been published.

Addressing patient-related factors, an international CSF biomarker consortium defined different categories of control groups in MS research, as their choice inevitably influences study outcome (Teunissen et al. 2013), e.g. CSF CXCL13 levels are higher in MS patients compared to several control groups, including inflammatory controls, though not higher than in patients with a viral or bacterial infection (Khademi et al. 2011). Table 24.10 displays the suggested control groups (for MS CSF biomarker studies).

To minimise variations due to different laboratory processing, international consensus guidelines have recently been published, which have been detailed in chapter 5 (Teunissen et al. 2009).

Whereas some analytes are probably stable for a certain time, others such as CSF WBC count (Steele et al. 1986) or serum glucose concentration (Dujmovic and Deisenhammer 2010) decrease with increasing time delay to sample processing. There is only scarce evidence dealing with this pre-analytic aspect, explaining why it has not been addressed in existing CSF guidelines. An example to adapt for time delay is a correction formula for the CSF/S_{Glu} ratio that has been recently published (Dujmovic and Deisenhammer 2010).

Regarding disease-specific CSF biomarkers, there are several consensus papers on standardisation of pre-analytic aspects in AD (del Campo et al. 2012; Vanderstichele et al. 2012), Parkinson disease (Vanderstichele et al. 2012) and amyotrophic lateral sclerosis (Otto et al. 2012), which are all based on the original BioMS guidelines (Teunissen et al. 2009).

References

Ahonen A, Myllyla VV, Hokkanen E (1979) Cerebrospinal fluid protein findings in various lower back pain syndromes. Acta Neurol Scand 60(2):93–99. PubMed PMID: 158934

Aksamit AJ (2003) Cerebrospinal fluid 14-3-3 protein: variability of sporadic Creutzfeldt-Jakob disease, laboratory standards, and quantitation. Arch Neurol 60(6):803–804. PubMed PMID: 12810481

Albert MS, DeKosky ST, Dickson D, Dubois B, Feldman HH, Fox NC et al (2011) The diagnosis of mild cognitive impairment due to Alzheimer's disease: recommendations from the National Institute on Aging-Alzheimer's Association workgroups on diagnostic guidelines for Alzheimer's disease. Alzheimers Dement 7(3):270–279. PubMed PMID: 21514249. Pubmed Central PMCID: 3312027

Appleby BS, Appleby KK, Crain BJ, Onyike CU, Wallin MT, Rabins PV (2009) Characteristics of established and proposed sporadic Creutzfeldt-Jakob disease variants. Arch Neurol 66(2):208–215. PubMed PMID: 19204157

Atarashi R, Satoh K, Sano K, Fuse T, Yamaguchi N, Ishibashi D et al (2011) Ultrasensitive human prion detection in cerebrospinal fluid by real-time quaking-induced conversion. Nat Med 17(2):175–178. PubMed PMID: 21278748

Ballard C, Gauthier S, Corbett A, Brayne C, Aarsland D, Jones E (2011) Alzheimer's disease. Lancet 377(9770):1019–1031. PubMed PMID: 21371747

Blennow K, Fredman P, Wallin A, Gottfries CG, Karlsson I, Langstrom G et al (1993) Protein analysis in cerebrospinal fluid. II. Reference values derived from healthy individuals 18–88 years of age. Eur Neurol 33(2):129–133. PubMed PMID: 8467819

Boer K, Isenmann S, Deufel T (2007) Strong interference of hemoglobin concentration on CSF total protein measurement using the trichloroacetic acid precipitation method. Clin Chem Lab Med 45(1):112–113. PubMed PMID: 17243927

Breebaart K, Becker H, Jongebloed FA (1978) Investigation of reference values of components of cerebrospinal fluid. J Clin Chem Clin Biochem 16(10):561–565. PubMed PMID: 712336

Brettschneider J, Claus A, Kassubek J, Tumani H (2005) Isolated blood-cerebrospinal fluid barrier dysfunction: prevalence and associated diseases. J Neurol 252(9):1067–1073. PubMed PMID: 15789126

Buruma OJ, Janson HL, Den Bergh FA, Bots GT (1981) Blood-stained cerebrospinal fluid: traumatic puncture or haemorrhage? J Neurol Neurosurg Psychiatry 44(2):144–147. PubMed PMID: 7217970. Pubmed Central PMCID: 490846

Collins SJ, Sanchez-Juan P, Masters CL, Klug GM, van Duijn C, Poleggi A et al (2006) Determinants of diagnostic investigation sensitivities across the clinical spectrum of sporadic Creutzfeldt-Jakob disease. Brain 129(Pt 9):2278–2287. PubMed PMID: 16816392

Coulthart MB, Jansen GH, Olsen E, Godal DL, Connolly T, Choi BC et al (2011) Diagnostic accuracy of cerebrospinal fluid protein markers for sporadic Creutzfeldt-Jakob disease in Canada: a 6-year prospective study. BMC Neurol 11:133. PubMed PMID: 22032272. Pubmed Central PMCID: 3216246

Cruickshank A, Beetham R, Holbrook I, Watson I, Wenham P, Keir G et al (2005) Spectrophotometry of cerebrospinal fluid in suspected subarachnoid haemorrhage. BMJ 330(7483):138. PubMed PMID: 15649929. Pubmed Central PMCID: 544435

Cruickshank A, Auld P, Beetham R, Burrows G, Egner W, Holbrook I et al (2008) Revised national guidelines for analysis of cerebrospinal fluid for bilirubin in suspected subarachnoid haemorrhage. Ann Clin Biochem 45(Pt 3):238–244. PubMed PMID: 18482910

Danise P, Maconi M, Rovetti A, Avino D, Di Palma A, Gerardo Pirofalo M et al (2013) Cell counting of body fluids: comparison between three automated haematology analysers and the manual microscope method. Int J Lab Hematol 35(6):608–613. PubMed PMID: 23647736

Davies G, Keir G, Thompson EJ, Giovannoni G (2003) The clinical significance of an intrathecal monoclonal immunoglobulin band: a follow-up study. Neurology 60(7):1163–1166. PubMed PMID: 12682325

Deisenhammer F, Bartos A, Egg R, Gilhus NE, Giovannoni G, Rauer S et al (2006) Guidelines on routine cerebrospinal fluid analysis. Report from an EFNS task force. Eur J Neurol 13(9):913–922. PubMed PMID: 16930354

Deisenhammer F, Egg R, Giovannoni G, Hemmer B, Petzold A, Sellebjerg F et al (2009) EFNS guidelines on disease-specific CSF investigations. Eur J Neurol 16(6):760–770. PubMed PMID: 19475759

del Campo M, Mollenhauer B, Bertolotto A, Engelborghs S, Hampel H, Simonsen AH et al (2012) Recommendations to standardize preanalytical confounding factors in Alzheimer's and Parkinson's disease cerebrospinal fluid biomarkers: an update. Biomark Med 6(4):419–430. PubMed PMID: 22917144

Delank HW (1972) Clinical cerebrospinal fluid diagnostics. Nervenarzt 43(2):57–68. PubMed PMID: 4622639. Klinische Liquordiagnostik

Desplat-Jego S, Feuillet L, Pelletier J, Bernard D, Cherif AA, Boucraut J (2005) Quantification of immunoglobulin free light chains in cerebrospinal fluid by nephelometry. J Clin Immunol 25(4):338–345. PubMed PMID: 16133990

DGLN DGfLuKN (2004) Ausgewählte Methoden der Liquordiagnostik und Klinischen Neurochemie. http://www.uke.de/extern/dgln/pdf/Methodenkatalog.pdf

Diener H, Weimar C, Berlit P, Deuschl G, Elger C, Gold R, et al. Leitlinen für Diagnostik und Therapie in der Neurologie. 2012;5. Available from: http://www.dgn.org/images/stories/dgn/leitlinien/LL_2012/pdf/ll_34_ambulant_erworbene_bakterielle_eitrige_meningoenzephalitis.pdf

Dobson R, Ramagopalan S, Davis A, Giovannoni G (2013) Cerebrospinal fluid oligoclonal bands in multiple sclerosis and clinically isolated syndromes: a meta-analysis of prevalence, prognosis and effect of latitude. J Neurol Neurosurg Psychiatry 84(8):909–914. PubMed PMID: 23431079

Dubois B, Feldman HH, Jacova C, Dekosky ST, Barberger-Gateau P, Cummings J et al (2007) Research criteria for the diagnosis of Alzheimer's disease: revising the NINCDS-ADRDA criteria. Lancet Neurol 6(8):734–746. PubMed PMID: 17616482

Dufour-Rainfray D, Beaufils E, Vourc'h P, Vierron E, Mereghetti L, Gendrot C et al (2013) Total protein level in cerebrospinal fluid is stable in elderly adults. J Am Geriatr Soc 61(10):1819–1821. PubMed PMID: 24117297

Dujmovic I, Deisenhammer F (2010) Stability of cerebrospinal fluid/serum glucose ratio and cerebrospinal fluid lactate concentrations over 24 h: analysis of repeated measurements. Clin Chem Lab Med 48(2):209–212. PubMed PMID: 19958211

Duranti F, Pieri M, Centonze D, Buttari F, Bernardini S, Dessi M (2013) Determination of kappaFLC and kappa Index in cerebrospinal fluid: a valid alternative to assess intrathecal immunoglobulin synthesis. J Neuroimmunol 263(1–2):116–120. PubMed PMID: 23916392

Eeg-Olofsson O, Link H, Wigertz A (1981) Concentrations of CSF proteins as a measure of blood brain barrier function and synthesis of IgG within the CNS in 'normal' subjects from the age of 6 months to 30 years. Acta Paediatr Scand 70(2):167–170. PubMed PMID: 7234400

Freedman MS, Thompson EJ, Deisenhammer F, Giovannoni G, Grimsley G, Keir G et al (2005) Recommended standard of cerebrospinal fluid analysis in the diagnosis of multiple sclerosis: a consensus statement. Arch Neurol 62(6):865–870. PubMed PMID: 15956157

Garton MJ, Keir G, Lakshmi MV, Thompson EJ (1991) Age-related changes in cerebrospinal fluid protein concentrations. J Neurol Sci 104(1):74–80. PubMed PMID: 1717663

Gilland O (1967) Lumbar cerebrospinal fluid total protein in healthy subjects. Acta Neurol Scand 43(4):526–529. PubMed PMID: 6081215

Hegen H, Auer M, Deisenhammer F (2014) Serum glucose adjusted cut-off values for normal cerebrospinal fluid/serum glucose ratio: implications for clinical practice. Clin Chem Lab Med 52(9):1335–1340. PubMed PMID: 24731954

Hort J et al (2010) EFNS guidelines for the diagnosis and management of Alzheimer's disease. Eur J Neurol 17:1236–1248

Khademi M, Kockum I, Andersson ML, Iacobaeus E, Brundin L, Sellebjerg F et al (2011) Cerebrospinal fluid CXCL13 in multiple sclerosis: a suggestive prognostic marker for the disease course. Mult Scler 17(3):335–343. PubMed PMID: 21135023

Krakauer M, Schaldemose Nielsen H, Jensen J, Sellebjerg F (1998) Intrathecal synthesis of free immunoglobulin light chains in multiple sclerosis. Acta Neurol Scand 98(3):161–165. PubMed PMID: 9786611

Ladogana A, Puopolo M, Croes EA, Budka H, Jarius C, Collins S et al (2005) Mortality from Creutzfeldt-Jakob disease and related disorders in Europe, Australia, and Canada. Neurology 64(9):1586–1591. PubMed PMID: 15883321

Lang DT, Berberian LB, Lee S, Ault M (1990) Rapid differentiation of subarachnoid hemorrhage from traumatic lumbar puncture using the D-dimer assay. Am J Clin Pathol 93(3):403–405. PubMed PMID: 2309662

Leen WG, Willemsen MA, Wevers RA, Verbeek MM (2012) Cerebrospinal fluid glucose and lactate: age-specific reference values and implications for clinical practice. PLoS One 7(8):e42745. PubMed PMID: 22880096. Pubmed Central PMCID: 3412827

Leschziner G (2014) Narcolepsy: a clinical review. Pract Neurol 15. PubMed PMID: 24830461

Marton KI, Gean AD (1986) The spinal tap: a new look at an old test. Ann Intern Med 104(6):840–848. PMID: 3518565

McKhann GM, Knopman DS, Chertkow H, Hyman BT, Jack CR Jr, Kawas CH et al (2011) The diagnosis of dementia due to Alzheimer's disease: recommendations from the National Institute on Aging-Alzheimer's Association workgroups on diagnostic guidelines for Alzheimer's disease. Alzheimers Dement 7(3):263–269. PubMed PMID: 21514250. Pubmed Central PMCID: 3312024

Meissner B, Westner IM, Kallenberg K, Krasnianski A, Bartl M, Varges D et al (2005) Sporadic Creutzfeldt-Jakob disease: clinical and diagnostic characteristics of the rare VV1 type. Neurology 65(10):1544–1550. PubMed PMID: 16221949

Mertin J, Wisser H, Doerr P (1971) [Studies on the normal concentration range of total protein and the total protein fractions of the cerebrospinal fluid by electrophoresis on cellulose acetate (author's transl)]. Z Klin Chem Klin Biochem 9(4):337–340. PubMed PMID: 4142825. Untersuchung uber den Normalbereich des Gesamteiweisses und der Eiweissfraktionen des Liquor cerebrospinalis nach elektrophoretischer Trennung auf Celluloseacetatfolie

Miller DH, Weinshenker BG, Filippi M, Banwell BL, Cohen JA, Freedman MS et al (2008) Differential diagnosis of suspected multiple sclerosis: a consensus approach. Mult Scler 14(9):1157–1174. PubMed PMID: 18805839. Pubmed Central PMCID: 2850590

Morris JC, Blennow K, Froelich L, Nordberg A, Soininen H, Waldemar G et al (2014) Harmonized diagnostic criteria for Alzheimer's disease: recommendations. J Intern Med 275(3):204–213. PubMed PMID: 24605805

Muayqil T, Gronseth G, Camicioli R (2012) Evidence-based guideline: diagnostic accuracy of CSF 14-3-3 protein in sporadic Creutzfeldt-Jakob disease: report of the guideline development subcommittee of the American Academy of Neurology. Neurology 79(14):1499–1506. PubMed PMID: 22993290. Pubmed Central PMCID: 3525296

Mygland A, Ljostad U, Fingerle V, Rupprecht T, Schmutzhard E, Steiner I et al (2010) EFNS guidelines on the diagnosis and management of European Lyme neuroborreliosis. Eur J Neurol 17(1):8–16, e1–4. PubMed PMID: 19930447

Nagy K, Skagervik I, Tumani H, Petzold A, Wick M, Kuhn HJ et al (2013) Cerebrospinal fluid analyses for the diagnosis of subarachnoid haemorrhage and experience from a Swedish study.

What method is preferable when diagnosing a subarachnoid haemorrhage? Clin Chem Lab Med 51(11):2073–2086. PubMed PMID: 23729569

Nakano T, Matsui M, Inoue I, Awata T, Katayama S, Murakoshi T (2011) Free immunoglobulin light chain: its biology and implications in diseases. Clin Chim Aacta 412(11–12):843–849. PubMed PMID: 21396928

Olischer RM, von Suchodoletz W (1972) [Evaluation of quantitative cell findings in cerebrospinal fluid containing blood]. Z Arztl Fortbild 66(4):213–218. PubMed PMID: 5036811. Zur Bewertung quantitativer Zellbefunde im bluthaltigen Liquor cerebrospinalis

Otto M, Bowser R, Turner M, Berry J, Brettschneider J, Connor J et al (2012) Roadmap and standard operating procedures for biobanking and discovery of neurochemical markers in ALS. Amyotroph Lateral Scler 13(1):1–10. PubMed PMID: 22214350

Page KB, Howell SJ, Smith CM, Dabbs DJ, Malia RG, Porter NR et al (1994) Bilirubin, ferritin, D-dimers and erythrophages in the cerebrospinal fluid of patients with suspected subarachnoid haemorrhage but negative computed tomography scans. J Clin Pathol 47(11):986–989. PubMed PMID: 7829694. Pubmed Central PMCID: 503057

Petzold A, Keir G, Sharpe TL (2005) Why human color vision cannot reliably detect cerebrospinal fluid xanthochromia. Stroke 36(6):1295–1297. PubMed PMID: 15879320

Pfausler B, Beer R, Engelhardt K, Kemmler G, Mohsenipour I, Schmutzhard E (2004) Cell index– a new parameter for the early diagnosis of ventriculostomy (external ventricular drainage)-related ventriculitis in patients with intraventricular hemorrhage? Acta Neurochir 146(5):477–481. PubMed PMID: 15118885

Plebani M (2006) Errors in clinical laboratories or errors in laboratory medicine? Clin Chem Lab Med 44(6):750–759. PubMed PMID: 16729864

Polman CH, Reingold SC, Banwell B, Clanet M, Cohen JA, Filippi M et al (2011) Diagnostic criteria for multiple sclerosis: 2010 revisions to the McDonald criteria. Ann Neurol 69(2):292–302. PubMed PMID: 21387374. Pubmed Central PMCID: 3084507

Reiber H (1994) Flow rate of cerebrospinal fluid (CSF)–a concept common to normal blood-CSF barrier function and to dysfunction in neurological diseases. J Neurol Sci 122(2):189–203. PubMed PMID: 8021703

Reiber H, Lange P (1991) Quantification of virus-specific antibodies in cerebrospinal fluid and serum: sensitive and specific detection of antibody synthesis in brain. Clin Chem 37(7):1153–1160. PubMed PMID: 1855284

Reiber H, Peter JB (2001) Cerebrospinal fluid analysis: disease-related data patterns and evaluation programs. J Neurol Sci 184(2):101–122. PubMed PMID: 11239944

Reiber H, Ungefehr S, Jacobi C (1998) The intrathecal, polyspecific and oligoclonal immune response in multiple sclerosis. Mult Scler 4(3):111–117. PubMed PMID: 9762657

Reiber H, Otto M, Trendelenburg C, Wormek A (2001) Reporting cerebrospinal fluid data: knowledge base and interpretation software. Clin Chem Lab Med 39(4):324–332. PubMed PMID: 11383657

Reske A, Haferkamp G, Hopf HC (1981) Influence of artificial blood contamination of the analysis of cerebrospinal fluid. J Neurol 226(3):187–193. PubMed PMID: 6172566

Rudick RA, French CA, Breton D, Williams GW (1989) Relative diagnostic value of cerebrospinal fluid kappa chains in MS: comparison with other immunoglobulin tests. Neurology 39(7):964–968. PubMed PMID: 2500621

Sandhaus LM, Ciarlini P, Kidric D, Dillman C, O'Riordan M (2010) Automated cerebrospinal fluid cell counts using the Sysmex XE-5000: is it time for new reference ranges? Am J Clin Pathol 134(5):734–738. PubMed PMID: 20959656

Senel M, Tumani H, Lauda F, Presslauer S, Mojib-Yezdani R, Otto M et al (2014) Cerebrospinal fluid immunoglobulin kappa light chain in clinically isolated syndrome and multiple sclerosis. PLoS One 9(4):e88680. PubMed PMID: 24695382. Pubmed Central PMCID: 3973621

Shah KH, Edlow JA (2002) Distinguishing traumatic lumbar puncture from true subarachnoid hemorrhage. J Emerg Med 23(1):67–74. PubMed PMID: 12217474

Sharief MK, Keir G, Thompson EJ (1990) Intrathecal synthesis of IgM in neurological diseases: a comparison between detection of oligoclonal bands and quantitative estimation. J Neurol Sci 96(2–3):131–142. PubMed PMID: 2115907

Sorbi S, Hort J, Erkinjuntti T, Fladby T, Gainotti G, Gurvit H et al (2012) EFNS-ENS Guidelines on the diagnosis and management of disorders associated with dementia. Eur J Neurol 19(9):1159–1179. PubMed PMID: 22891773

Spanos A, Harrell FE Jr, Durack DT (1989) Differential diagnosis of acute meningitis. An analysis of the predictive value of initial observations. JAMA 262(19):2700–2707. PubMed PMID: 2810603

Sperling RA, Aisen PS, Beckett LA, Bennett DA, Craft S, Fagan AM et al (2011) Toward defining the preclinical stages of Alzheimer's disease: recommendations from the National Institute on Aging-Alzheimer's Association workgroups on diagnostic guidelines for Alzheimer's disease. Alzheimers Dement 7(3):280–292. PubMed PMID: 21514248. Pubmed Central PMCID: 3220946

Steele RW, Marmer DJ, O'Brien MD, Tyson ST, Steele CR (1986) Leukocyte survival in cerebrospinal fluid. J Clin Microbiol 23(5):965–966. PubMed PMID: 3711287. Pubmed Central PMCID: 268763

Teunissen CE, Petzold A, Bennett JL, Berven FS, Brundin L, Comabella M et al (2009) A consensus protocol for the standardization of cerebrospinal fluid collection and biobanking. Neurology 73(22):1914–1922. PubMed PMID: 19949037. Pubmed Central PMCID: 2839806

Teunissen C, Menge T, Altintas A, Alvarez-Cermeno JC, Bertolotto A, Berven FS et al (2013) Consensus definitions and application guidelines for control groups in cerebrospinal fluid biomarker studies in multiple sclerosis. Mult Scler 19(13):1802–1809. PubMed PMID: 23695446

Tibbling G, Link H, Ohman S (1977) Principles of albumin and IgG analyses in neurological disorders. I. Establishment of reference values. Scand J Clin Lab Invest 37(5):385–390. PubMed PMID: 337459

Tumani H, Deisenhammer F, Giovannoni G, Gold R, Hartung HP, Hemmer B et al (2011) Revised McDonald criteria: the persisting importance of cerebrospinal fluid analysis. Ann Neurol 70(3):520; author reply 1. PubMed PMID: 21710627

Vanderstichele H, Bibl M, Engelborghs S, Le Bastard N, Lewczuk P, Molinuevo JL et al (2012) Standardization of preanalytical aspects of cerebrospinal fluid biomarker testing for Alzheimer's disease diagnosis: a consensus paper from the Alzheimer's Biomarkers Standardization Initiative. Alzheimers Dement 8(1):65–73. PubMed PMID: 22047631

Walton J (1956) Subarachnoid hemorrhage. E & S Livingstone Ltd., Edinburgh

Watson ID, Beetham R, Fahie-Wilson MN, Holbrook IB, O'Connell DM (2008) What is the role of cerebrospinal fluid ferritin in the diagnosis of subarachnoid haemorrhage in computed tomography-negative patients? Ann Clin Biochem 45(Pt 2):189–192. PubMed PMID: 18325184

Weisner B, Bernhardt W (1978) Protein fractions of lumbar, cisternal, and ventricular cerebrospinal fluid. Separate areas of reference. J Neurol Sci 37(3):205–214. PubMed PMID: 681976

Zimmermann M, Ruprecht K, Kainzinger F, Heppner FL, Weimann A (2011) Automated vs. manual cerebrospinal fluid cell counts: a work and cost analysis comparing the Sysmex XE-5000 and the Fuchs-Rosenthal manual counting chamber. Int J Lab Hematol 33(6):629–637. PubMed PMID: 21668655

Index